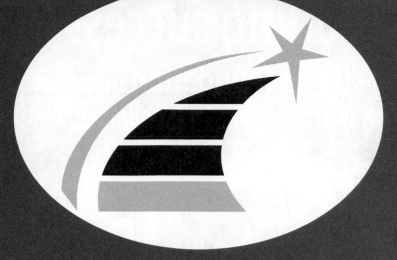

Step 1: Learn

"A journey of a thousand miles begins with a single step."

— Lao-tzu

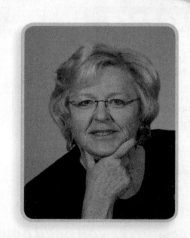

Congratulations! You are embarking on an exciting and rewarding career, and you have taken a great first step. Coding is a career that gives you a chance to pursue excellence at a variety of levels, and I am happy that you have chosen to start with my *Step* line of products. As a lifelong coder and educator, I am dedicated to giving you the tools you need to succeed. ***So, get out there and code!***

— Carol J. Buck, MS, CPC-I, CPC, CPC-H, CCS-P

Track your progress!

See the checklist in the back of this book to learn more about your next step toward coding success!

The tools for your
total coding success are here!

Build a **strong foundation** for career success with the proven leader in coding education.

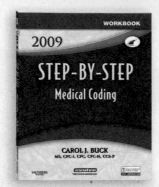

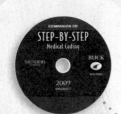

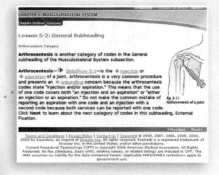

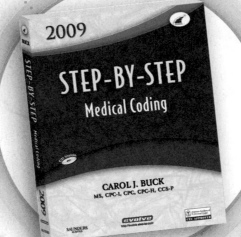

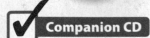

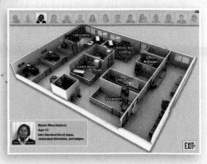

SL80266

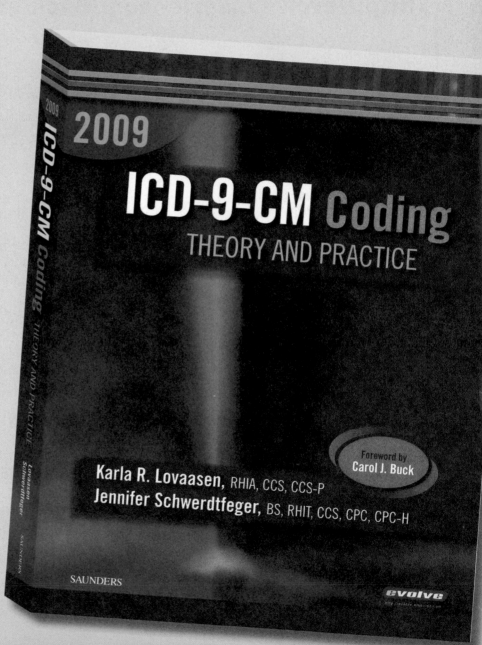

ELSEVIER

evolve

STEP-BY-STEP
Medical Coding

2009

STEP-BY-STEP
Medical Coding

CAROL J. BUCK
MS, CPC-I, CPC, CPC-H, CCS-P

Program Director, Retired
Medical Secretary Programs
Northwest Technical College
East Grand Forks, Minnesota

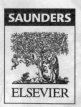

SAUNDERS

ELSEVIER

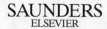

11830 Westline Industrial Drive
St. Louis, Missouri 63146

STEP-BY-STEP MEDICAL CODING, 2009 EDITION   ISBN: 978-1-4160-4566-3

Library of Congress Cataloging-in-Publication Data

Buck, Carol J.
  Step-by-step medical coding / Carol J. Buck. -- 2009 ed.
      p. ; cm.
  Includes bibliographical references and indexes.
  ISBN 978-1-4160-4566-3 (pbk. : alk. paper) 1. Nosology--Code numbers. I. Title. II. Title: Medical coding. III. Title: 2009 step-by-step medical coding.
  [DNLM: 1. Disease--classification. 2. Terminology as Topic. 3. Forms and Records Control--methods. 4. Insurance, Health, Reimbursement. WB 15 B922s 2009]
  RB115.B83 2009
  616.001'48--dc22

                                                                     2008035112

Publisher: Michael S. Ledbetter
Developmental Editor: Joshua S. Rapplean
Publishing Services Manager: Pat Joiner-Myers
Senior Designer: Amy Buxton

Working together to grow
libraries in developing countries

www.elsevier.com | www.bookaid.org | www.sabre.org

ELSEVIER   BOOK AID International   Sabre Foundation

Printed in the United States of America

Last digit is the print number: 9 8 7 6 5 4 3 2 1

*To the students, whose drive and determination to learn serve as
my endless source of inspiration and enrichment.*

*To teachers, whose contributions are immense and workloads daunting.
May this work make your preparation for class a little easier.*

*To Mary and Richard Garden, whose friendship and
enthusiasm have been so greatly appreciated
and a bright spot in many days.*

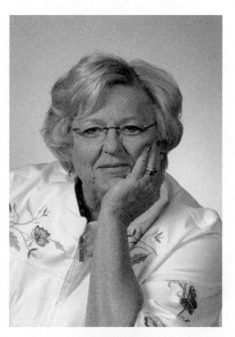

Carol J. Buck

ACKNOWLEDGMENTS

This book was developed in collaboration with educators and employers in an attempt to meet the needs of students preparing for careers in the medical coding allied health profession. Obtaining employers' input about the knowledge, skills, and abilities desired of entry-level coding employees benefits educators tremendously. This text is an endeavor to use this information to better prepare our students.

There are several other people who deserve special thanks for their efforts in making this text possible.

Joan E. Wolfgang, who joined the effort and has lent her expertise and unending patience to this project and many others. She is a highly regarded member of our team.

Jacqueline Grass, Research Assistant, for her technical knowledge, interest in student learning, and long hours of dedicated service to developing education materials. Her gentle and quiet demeanor is a gift beyond measure.

Jody Klitz, Research Assistant, for her meticulous approach to myriad complex assignments. Her professionalism is beyond compare.

Nancy Maguire, for her dedication to superior education and a lifetime of devotion to the coding career.

Lindsay-Anne Jenkins, who has spent hours carefully reviewing and improving this work. Her attention to detail is outstanding.

Michael Ledbetter, Publisher, who managed to maintain an excellent sense of humor while jumping into the fray and who is a valued member of the team. **Josh Rapplean,** Developmental Editor, who manages the developmental duties of this text with calm, confidence, and tremendous efficiency. **Laura Slown Sullivan** and **Rhoda Bontrager,** Production Editors, Graphic World, who assumed responsibility for many projects while maintaining a high degree of professionalism.

Victoria Tsitlik and her students, whose careful attention to detail we are so thankful for.

Linda Krecklau, Provider Education and Communications Specialist, BCBS, Eagan, Minnesota, for translating the *Federal Register* into "ordinary words."

The publisher would also like to acknowledge and thank the following people:

Judy Breuker, Patricia Champion, Beverly Comsa, Maria Coslett, Ellen Dooley, Chris Galeziewski, Patricia Cordy Henricksen, Stephanie A. Lewis, Nancy Maguire, John R. Neumann III, Barbara Oviatt, Christine A. Patterson, Letitia Patterson, Keith Russell, Patricia Sommerfeld, Cynthia Stahl, Jane A. Tuttle, and Joan E. Wolfgang for their enthusiasm and dedication to the coding profession.

UnicorMed (http://www.unicormed.com) for providing the valued use of the Alpha II *i*Coder resource.

Dennis Bishop of Bishop & Associates, Inc., for his talent, enthusiasm, and quality photographs.

Skip Stowers of Photography by Skip Stowers, for his talent, patience, and photographs.

Thank you for purchasing *Step-by-Step Medical Coding*, the leading textbook for medical coding education. This 2009 edition has been carefully reviewed and updated with the latest content, making it the most current textbook for your class. The author and publisher have made every effort to equip you with skills and tools you will need to succeed on the job. To this end, *Step-by-Step Medical Coding* presents essential information for all health care coding systems and covers the skills needed to be a successful medical coder. No other text on the market brings together such thorough coverage of all coding systems in one source.

ORGANIZATION OF THIS TEXTBOOK

Developed in collaboration with employers and educators, *Step-by-Step Medical Coding, 2009 Edition* takes a practical approach to training for a successful career in medical coding. The text is divided into three units— Current Procedural Terminology (CPT); International Classification of Diseases, 9th Revision, Clinical Modification (ICD-9-CM); and An Overview of Reimbursement.

Unit I, Current Procedural Terminology (CPT), begins with an introduction to the CPT manual, followed by in-depth explanation of the sections found in the code set. Organized by body systems to follow the CPT codes, the chapters include important information about anatomy, terminology, and various procedures, as well as demonstration and examples of how to code each service.

Unit II, International Classification of Diseases, 9th Revision, Clinical Modification (ICD-9-CM), provides an overview of the ICD-9-CM codes and their use in medical coding. A highlight of this unit is the inclusion of the *ICD-9-CM Official Guidelines for Coding and Reporting* within the chapter text, as they apply to the content.

Unit III, An Overview of Reimbursement, is a chapter that ties everything in the book together with the reimbursement process, making the connections between coding and reimbursement.

DISTINCTIVE FEATURES OF OUR APPROACH

This book was designed to be the first step in your coding career, and it has many unique features to help you along the way.

- The repetition of skills in each chapter reinforces the material and creates a logical progression for learning and applying each skill—a truly "step-by-step" approach!

- In-text exercises further reinforce important concepts and allow you to check your comprehension as you read.

- The format for exercise and review answers guides you in the development of your coding ability by including three response variations:

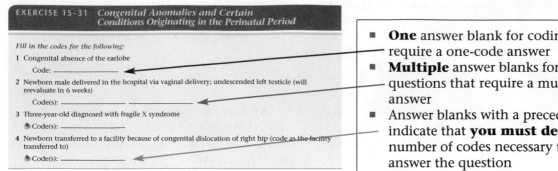

EXERCISE 15-31 *Congenital Anomalies and Certain Conditions Originating in the Perinatal Period*

Fill in the codes for the following:

1 Congenital absence of the earlobe
   Code: _____

2 Newborn male delivered in the hospital via vaginal delivery; undescended left testicle (will reevaluate in 6 weeks)
   Code(s): _____ _____ _____

3 Three-year-old diagnosed with fragile X syndrome
   🌐 Code(s): _____

4 Newborn transferred to a facility because of congenital dislocation of right hip (code as the facility transferred to)
   🌐 Code(s): _____

- **One** answer blank for coding questions that require a one-code answer
- **Multiple** answer blanks for coding questions that require a multiple-code answer
- Answer blanks with a preceding symbol (🌐) indicate that **you must decide** the number of codes necessary to correctly answer the question

- *Quick Checks* are located throughout the chapters, providing short follow-up questions after a key concept has been covered to immediately assess learning. Answers to the *Quick Checks* are located at the end of each chapter.

QUICK CHECK 6-1

Rhinoplasty can be performed either _____, through external skin incisions, or closed, through _____ incisions.

- A full-color design brings a fresh look to the material, enhancing illustrations and visually reinforcing new concepts and examples.

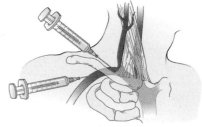

FIGURE 7-20 Percutaneous method of catheterization (Seldinger technique).

APPENDIX E

Alpha II *iCoder* Exercises

Note: It is recommended that you wait to access this feature until you've finished working through the main text.
   As an additional bonus feature, we have included 30-day access to Alpha II *iCoder* online code editor from UnicorMed.

CASES 1 THROUGH 15
Your supervisor has asked you to use the *iCoder* to check the accuracy of several cases that were coded by another coder.

CASES 16 THROUGH 20
For Cases 16 through 20, you are to assign the correct CPT and ICD-9-CM codes. Be sure to check the codes you assign with the *iCoder*. Once you have finished, your instructor will provide you with answers for Cases 16-20 so you can check your work.

USING ALPHA II ICODER ONLINE CODE EDITOR
Note: The User Name and Password will only be valid during the current coding year.
   Also, if you are logged in to *iCoder* and leave without clicking on Sign Out, you will not be able to re-enter for 15 minutes. If you are logged in to *iCoder* and the system doesn't detect any input from you for 15 minutes, you will be automatically logged out, and you will not be able to re-enter for 15 minutes.
   Here are some easy steps to start using your free trial of the Alpha II *iCoder*.
1. Start at the Evolve Learning Resources at
   http://evolve.elsevier.com/ Buck/step
2. Click on the *iCoder* section, and click on the link to be taken to the *iCoder login page.*
3. Enter your **User Name** and **Password** from the card you received with your textbook. (You may want to check the **Remember My User Name** box for faster access in subsequent logins.)
4. The first page that opens in *iCoder* is the main page. Click on **My Settings.** This will take you to a settings page.

- Medical procedures or conditions are illustrated and discussed in the text to help you understand the services being coded.

- Using the login information on the bind-in card, access to UnicorMed's Alpha II *iCoder* online code editor is available with this edition. The *iCoder* can be used with the exercises in Appendix E as a capstone experience after completing work with the textbook.

- Chapter learning objectives and end of chapter review questions help readers focus on essential chapter content.

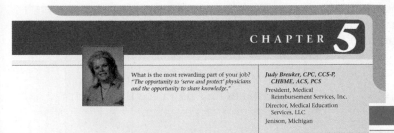

CHAPTER 5

What is the most rewarding part of your job? *"The opportunity to 'serve and protect' physicians and the opportunity to share knowledge."*

Judy Breuker, CPC, CCS-P, CHBME, ACS, PCS
President, Medical
Reimbursement Services, Inc.
Director, Medical Education
Services, LLC
Jenison, Michigan

Musculoskeletal System

Chapter Topics

Format

Coding Highlights

General

Application of Casts and Strapping

Endoscopy/Arthroscopy

Chapter Review

Quick Check Answers

Learning Objectives

After completing this chapter, you should be able to

1 Differentiate among fracture treatment types.
2 Understand types of traction.
3 Identify services/procedures included in the General subheading.
4 Understand elements of arthroscopic procedures.
5 Analyze cast application and strapping procedures.
6 Demonstrate the ability to code musculoskeletal services and procedures.

CHAPTER REVIEW

CHAPTER 5, PART I, THEORY

Without the use of reference material, complete the following:

1 The Musculoskeletal System subsection is formatted according to what type of sites?

2 Which physician subspecialty can use the codes from the Musculoskeletal System subsection?

3 List the three types of fracture treatments and briefly describe each:

4 It is the _____ of the fracture that determines the type of treatment.

5 _____ is the application of pulling force to hold a bone in place.

6 What is the term that describes the physician's actions of bending, rotating, pulling, or guiding the bone back into place?

7 What term is used to mean "put the bone back in place"?

8 What term describes a bone that is not in its normal location?

9 What term describes the cleaning of a wound?

10 This is a hollow needle that is often used to withdraw samples of fluid from a joint:

11 Would a biopsy code usually include the administration of any necessary local anesthesia?

- Concrete "real-life" examples illustrate the application of important coding principles and practices.

Example
During a cardiac catheterization procedure, contrast medium is injected into a bypass graft and into the coronary arteries. CPT codes would be used to identify each of the areas of injection as follows:
93540 injection into the bypass graft
93545 injection into selective coronary arteries

OFFICIAL GUIDELINES FOR CODING AND REPORTING

INTRODUCTION (Paragraph 3)

These guidelines are based on the coding and sequencing instructions in Volumes I, II and III of ICD-9-CM, but provide additional instruction. Adherence to these guidelines when assigning ICD-9-CM diagnosis and procedure codes is required under the Health Insurance Portability and Accountability Act (HIPAA). The diagnosis codes (Volumes 1-2) have been adopted under HIPAA for all healthcare settings. Volume 3 procedure codes have been adopted for inpatient procedures reported by hospitals.

Symptoms, Signs, and Ill-Defined Conditions

OFFICIAL GUIDELINES FOR CODING AND REPORTING

SECTION II. A. Codes for symptoms, signs, and ill-defined conditions

Codes for symptoms, signs, and ill-defined conditions from Chapter 16 are not to be used as a principal diagnosis when a related definitive diagnosis has been established.

OFFICIAL GUIDELINES FOR CODING AND REPORTING

SECTION IV. E. Codes that describe symptoms and signs

Codes that describe symptoms and signs, as opposed to diagnoses, are acceptable for reporting purposes when a diagnosis has not been established (confirmed) by the provider. Chapter 16 of ICD-9-CM, Symptoms, Signs, and Ill-defined conditions (codes 780.0-799.9), contains many, but not all codes for symptoms.

- *ICD-9-CM Official Guidelines for Coding and Reporting* boxes in Chapter 15 contain excerpts of the actual guidelines, presenting the official wording alongside in-text discussions, and visually indicate Inpatient vs. Outpatient use.

- *From the Trenches* boxes highlight a different real-life medical coding practitioner in each chapter, with photographs throughout the chapter alongside quotes that offer practical advice or motivational comments.

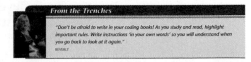

From the Trenches

"Don't be afraid to write in your coding books! As you study and read, highlight important rules. Write instructions 'in your own words' so you will understand when you go back to look at it again."
BEVERLY

- *Coding Shots* contain tips for the new coder.

CODING SHOT Included in the Biopsy codes are codes that are to be used for biopsies of mucous membranes. A mucous membrane is tissue that covers a variety of body parts, such as the tongue and the nasal cavities.

● **STOP** *You were just presented with some very important information about the use of certain codes in the CPT manual. The plus (+) symbol next to any CPT code—not just next to Qualifying Circumstances codes—indicates that that code cannot be used alone. Throughout the remaining sections of the CPT manual, the plus symbol will appear to caution you to use the code only as an adjunct code (with other codes).*

- *Stop!* notes halt you for a reality check, offering a brief summary of material that was just covered and providing a transition into the next topic.

CAUTION *Some CPT codes are for bilateral procedures and do not require a bilateral modifier. For example, 27395 is for a bilateral lengthening of the hamstring tendon, and it would be incorrect to place a bilateral modifier on the code.*

- *Caution!* notes warn you about common coding mistakes and reinforce the concept of coding as an exact science.

CHECK THIS OUT The American Medical Association (AMA) has a Website located at http://www.ama-assn.org

- *Check This Out!* boxes offer notes about accessing reference information related to coding, primarily via the Internet.

ICD-9-CM AND ICD-10 CODES

21.1: 472
24.04: 466
27.54: 472, 491
39.21: 485
39.51: 488
39.61: 485
40.9: 491
42.40-42.42: 484
42.6: 484, 485
42: 634
43.1: 484
43.19: 486
45.51: 489
57.87: 489
68.49: 483
75.36: 557
78.4: 490
80.00: 489
80.10: 489
80.12: 489
80.17: 489
81.92: 489
82.69: 491
83.86: 491
86.22: 573
86.28: 573
87-99: 482
90: 490
91: 490
99: 97
99.25: 519
C50.4: 479

- A *Coder's Index* can be found in the back of the book, providing easy reference when looking for specific codes.

EXTENSIVE SUPPLEMENTAL RESOURCES

Considering the broad range of students, programs, and institutions in which this textbook is used, we have developed an extensive package of supplements designed to complement *Step-by-Step Medical Coding*. Each of these comprehensive supplements has been developed with the needs of both students and instructors in mind.

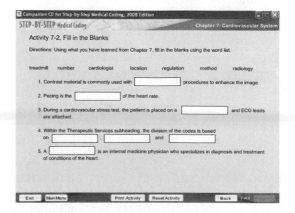

Student Companion CD

The companion CD supplements the text with 35 chapter activities and 29 coding cases. The variety of activity styles include multiple choice, fill in the blank, matching, and coding exercises. These activities will reinforce material learned in the text and offer students another study tool. Answers can be found in the TEACH Instructor Resources.

Student Workbook

The fully updated workbook supplements the text with more than 1000 questions and terminology exercises, as well as over 80 original source documents to familiarize the user with documents he or she will encounter in practice. Reports are included in a variety of areas, including arthroscopy, muscle repair, thoracentesis, tubal ligation, and endoarterectomy. The workbook questions also follow the same answer format of the main text, improving coding skills and promoting critical thinking.

CHAPTER 10 • General Surgery II

PRACTICAL

Using the CPT manual, code the following:

78. Injection procedure for identification of the sentinel node.

Code: _____

79. Radical cervical lymphadenectomy, unilateral.

Code: _____

80. Drainage of an extensive lymph node abscess.

Code: _____

81. Autologous bone marrow transplant.

Code: _____

82. Incision and drainage of an infected thyroglossal duct cyst.

Code(s): _____

83. Removal of a complete cerebrospinal fluid shunt system; without replacement.

Code(s): _____

84. Suture of the posterior tibial nerve.

Code(s): _____

85. Incision and drainage of conjunctival cysts of left and right eyes.

Code(s): _____

86. Optic nerve decompression of the right eye.

Code(s): _____

87. Removal of a embedded foreign body of the eyelid.

Code(s): _____

88. Myringoplasty of the left ear.

Code(s): _____

89. Single stage reconstruction of the external auditory canal for congenital atresia.

Code(s): _____

User to decide number of codes necessary to correctly answer the question.

76

TEACH Instructor Resources with CD-ROM

No matter what your level of teaching experience, this total-teaching solution will help you plan your lessons with ease, and the author has developed all the curriculum materials necessary to use *Step-by-Step Medical Coding* in the classroom. Included in the printed material are all answers to the textbook, companion CD, and workbook exercises; extra coding cases with answers; a course calendar and syllabus; curriculum with lesson plans; alternative TEACH Lesson Plans and Lecture Outlines; and ready-made tests for easy assessment. The CD-ROM, bound free with this item, includes all printed content, a comprehensive PowerPoint collection of the entire text, interactive PowerPoint slides, and a test bank in ExamView. The slides can be easily customized to support your lectures or formatted with PowerPoint as overhead transparencies or handouts for student note-taking. The ExamView test generator will help you quickly and easily prepare quizzes and exams, and the test banks can be customized to your specific teaching methods.

STEP-BY-STEP
Medical Coding
2009
CAROL J. BUCK
MS, CPC-I, CPC, CPC-H, CCS-P

SAUNDERS

CHAPTER 1

INTRODUCTION TO THE CPT

MEDICAL CODING

- Transforms services/procedures/supplies/drugs into CPT/HCPCS codes
- Transforms diagnosis and procedures into ICD-9-CM codes

2

Evolve Learning Resources

The Evolve Learning Resources offer helpful material that will extend your studies beyond the classroom. Chapter WebLinks offer you the opportunity to expand your knowledge base and stay current with this ever-changing field, while extra Coding Cases and Coding Tips are available online to check your understanding. Instructors can also download all materials available from the Instructor's Resource Manual, as well as content updates and industry news.

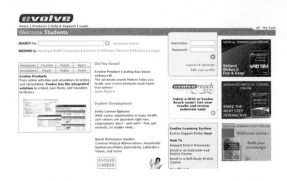

A Course Management System (CMS) is also available free to instructors who adopt this textbook. This web-based platform gives instructors yet another resource to facilitate learning and to make medical coding content accessible to students. In addition to the Evolve Learning Resources available to both faculty and students, there is an entire suite of tools available that allows for communication between instructors and students. Students can log on through the Evolve portal to take online quizzes, participate in threaded discussions, post assignments to instructors, or chat with other classmates, while instructors can use the online grade book to follow class progress.

To access this comprehensive online resource, simply go to the Evolve home page at http://evolve.elsevier.com and enter the user name and password provided by your instructor. If your instructor has not set up a Course Management System, you can still access the free Evolve Learning Resources at http://evolve.elsevier.com/Buck/step/.

Step-by-Step Medical Coding Online

Designed to accommodate diverse learning styles and environments, *Step-by-Step Medical Coding Online* is an online course supplement that works in conjunction with the textbook to provide you with a wide range of visual, auditory, and interactive learning materials. The course amplifies course content, synthesizes concepts, reinforces learning, and demonstrates practical applications in a dynamic and exciting way. As you move through the course, interactive exercises, quizzes, and activities allow you to check your comprehension and learn from immediate feedback, while still allowing you to use your textbook as a resource. Because of its design, this course offers students a unique and innovative learning experience.

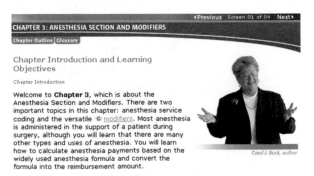

DEVELOPMENT OF THIS EDITION

This book would not have been possible without a team of educators and professionals, including practicing coders and technical consultants. The combined efforts of the team members have made this text an incredible learning tool.

SENIOR ICD-9-CM CODING REVIEWER

Karla R. Lovaasen, RHIA, CCS, CCS-P
Coding and Consulting Services
Abingdon, Maryland

—Co-author of *ICD-9-CM Coding: Theory and Practice, 2009 Edition,* St. Louis, 2009, Saunders.

CODING SPECIALISTS

Joan E. Wolfgang, BA, CPC, CPC-H
Consultant, Educator, PMCC Certified Instructor
Milwaukee, Wisconsin

Jacqueline Klitz Grass, MA, CPC
Coding Specialist
Grand Forks, North Dakota

Lindsay-Anne Jenkins, CRNA, CPC, CPC-H, CPC-I
Coding and Auditing Specialist
Healthcare Strategic Initiatives
St. Louis, Missouri

Nancy Maguire, ACS, CRT, PCS, FCS, CPC, CPC-H, HCS-D, APC, AFC
Physician Consultant for Auditing and Education
Universal City, Texas

To ensure the accuracy of the material presented in this textbook, many reviewers have provided feedback over several editions of this text. We are deeply grateful to the numerous people who have shared their suggestions and comments. Reviewing a book or supplement takes an incredible amount of energy and attention, and we are glad so many colleagues were able to take the time to give us their feedback on the material.

EDITORIAL REVIEW BOARD

Karen Drummond, CPC, CPC-H, CMC, ACS-OB/GYN, ACS-RA, PCS, FCS, CMBS-I
Instructor and Consultant
Stark State College
Portage Lakes Career Center
Uniontown, Ohio

Teena Gregory-Gooding, MS, CMRS, CPC
Medical Education Consultant
New Horizons Computer Learning Centers
Rapid City, South Dakota

Debra Kroll, RHIT
Altru Health System
Grand Forks, North Dakota

Patricia Harrison Skibbe
Welcoming Officer
AAPC Richardson, Texas, Chapter
Richardson, Texas

Victoria Tsitlik, MS, CCS-P
Advanced Coding Program Instructor
Computer Career Institute at Johns Hopkins University
Columbia, Maryland

The number of people seeking health care services has increased as a result of an aging population, technologic advances, and better access to health care. At the same time, there is an increase in the use of outpatient facilities. This increase is due in part to the government's introduction of tighter controls over inpatient services. The government continues to increase its involvement in and control over health care through reimbursement of services for Medicare patients. Other insurance companies are following the government's lead and adopting reimbursement systems that have proved effective in reducing third-party payer costs.

Health care in America has undergone tremendous change in the recent past, and more changes are promised for the future. These changes have resulted in an ever-increasing demand for qualified medical coders. The Bureau of Labor Statistics states that medical records and health information technicians job growth will be "much faster than average" with three out of five of these jobs being in the physician/outpatient setting.[1] The national shortage has increased the salary for the coding occupation, and salaries in general show a solid upward trend.

There is also a greater demand for coders due to the increase in the number of medical tests, treatments, and procedures and the increase in the claims review by third-party payers. Certified coders are on average paid more than the noncertified coder. According to the 2007 Medical Coding Salary Survey,* the certified coder earns an average of 17% higher salary than a noncertified coder![2] Figure 1 illustrates the earnings by state; Figure 2 shows the average salary by experience; and Figure 3 lists the certification and salary. Note that the CPC-H®, the hospital outpatient certification, pays significantly more than the CPC®, the physician outpatient certification. Dual certification as a CPC and CPC-H is also gaining popularity. Further information can be obtained about the AAPC and the certifications offered by the organization at http://www.aapc.com.

---

*Check your Evolve resources for the latest AAPC Salary Survey information.

From the Trenches

"Coding can really open doors to a variety of things. You're not tied into one job— there are many roads you can take and many things you can do with a coding background."

MARIA

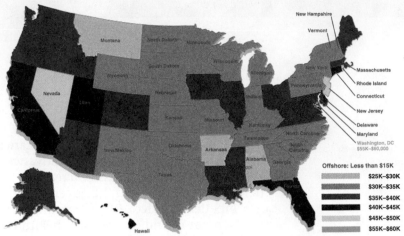

FIGURE 1 Earnings by State. (From American Academy of Professional Coders: *2007 Medical Coding Salary Survey* [website] http://www.aapc.com/documents/Salary_Survey2007.pdf. Accessed February 19, 2008.)

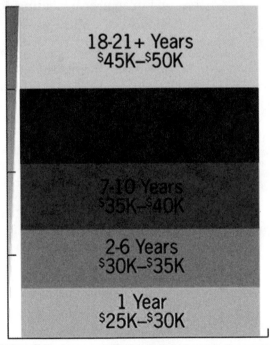

FIGURE 2 Average Salary by Experience. (From American Academy of Professional Coders: *2007 Medical Coding Salary Survey* [website] http://www.aapc.com/documents/Salary_Survey2007.pdf. Accessed February 19, 2008.)

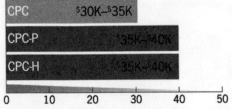

FIGURE 3 Average Salary by Certification. (From American Academy of Professional Coders: *2007 Medical Coding Salary Survey* [website] http://www.aapc.com/documents/Salary_Survey2007.pdf. Accessed February 19, 2008.)

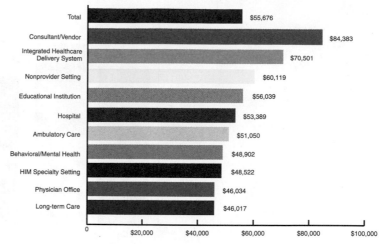

FIGURE 4   Average Salaries by Work Setting. (From American Health Information Management Association: *The Results Are In: 2006 Salary Study* [website]: http://www.ahima.org/membership/member_profile_data.asp. Accessed January 16, 2008.)

Average Salary by Setting Category	Director	Manager	Coder
Ambulatory Care	$68,164	$56,949	$43,262
Behavioral/Mental Health	$58,257	$51,002	$33,777
Consultant/Vendor	$101,067	$80,877	$58,488
Educational Institution	$65,514	$51,348*	$40,522
HIM Specialty Setting	$62,563*	$56,520*	$46,007
Hospital	$72,698	$58,401	$44,064
Integrated Healthcare Delivery System	$92,818	$69,444	$45,297
Long-term Care	$47,495	$49,062	$39,084
Nonprovider Setting	$93,553	$67,784	$44,610
Physician Office	$79,074	$50,150	$39,608
Total	$72,140	$58,942	$43,995
			*fewer than 30 cases in the sample

FIGURE 5   Average Salary by Setting Category. (From American Health Information Management Association: *The Results Are In: 2006 Salary Study* [website]: http://www.ahima.org/membership/member_profile_data.asp. Accessed January 16, 2008.)

The American Health Information Management Association (AHIMA) is a health care organization that offers the Certified Coding Specialist—Physician-based (CCS-P) certification. The AHIMA 2006 Salary Study indicated, ". . . the average annual full-time HIM salary across all work settings is $55,676."[3] Figure 4 illustrates the average salary by the work setting. For coding professionals, while each region shows that the majority is earning in the $30,000 to $49,999 range, variances are most apparent at the ends of the salary spectrum. Figure 5 illustrates the average salary by job setting. Figure 6 illustrates the average salary for coders by credential. Further information about AHIMA and the certifications offered can be accessed at the organization's website, http://www.ahima.org.

Medical coding is far more than assigning numbers to services and diagnoses. Coders abstract information from the patient record and combine it with their knowledge of reimbursement and coding guidelines to optimize physician payment. Coders have been called the "fraud squad" because they optimize but never maximize and code only for services provided to the patient that are documented in the patient record.

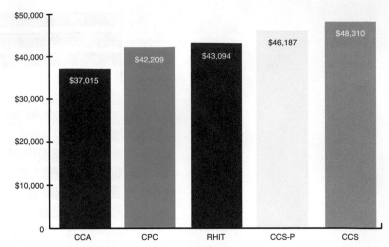

FIGURE 6 Average Coder Salaries by Credential. (From American Health Information Management Association: *The Results Are In: 2006 Salary Study* [website]: http://www.ahima.org/membership/member_profile_data.asp. Accessed January 16, 2008.)

From the Trenches

"You need to be committed . . . Be prepared to spend some time and effort to study and work hard. Do whatever you have to do to get your foot in the door."

BARBARA

There is a demand for skilled coders, and you can be one of those in demand. Put your best efforts into building the foundation of your career, and you will be rewarded for a lifetime.

References

1. U.S. Department of Labor, Bureau of Labor Statistics, Employment Projections, 2000-2010. http://www.bls.gov/oco/ocos103.htm#emply
2. 2007 Salary Survey, *AAPC Coding Edge,* Salt Lake City, UT. http://www.aapc.com/documents/Salary_Survey2007.pdf
3. American Health Information Management Association. http://www.ahima.org/membership/member_profile_data.asp

CONTENTS

Contents

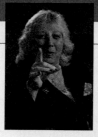

"Educate yourself—you are always learning in this field. Let supervisors know what your goals are! Find out what it takes to move into that position—then make sure you become empowered with whatever it takes to move up!"

Beverly Comsa, CPC
HealthCare Training Manager
New Horizons Learning Center
Anaheim, California

Introduction to the CPT

Chapter Topics

The Purpose
of the CPT Manual

Updating the CPT Manual

The CPT Manual Format

Starting with the Index

Chapter Review

Quick Check Answers

Learning Objectives

After completing this chapter, you should be able to

1 Identify the uses of the CPT manual.

2 Name the developers of the CPT manual.

3 Know the importance of using the current-year CPT manual.

4 Identify placement of CPT codes on the CMS-1500 insurance form.

5 Recognize the symbols used in the CPT manual.

6 List the major sections found in the CPT manual.

7 Interpret the information contained in the section Guidelines and notes.

8 Describe the CPT code format.

9 Append modifiers.

10 Describe what is meant by unlisted procedures/services.

11 State the purposes of a special report.

12 Review Category II and III CPT codes.

13 Locate the terms in the CPT index.

14 Identify the content of the CPT appendices.

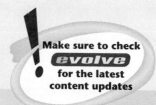

Make sure to check
evolve
for the latest
content updates

THE PURPOSE OF THE CPT MANUAL

Current Procedural Terminology (CPT), also known as CPT-4, is a coding system developed by the American Medical Association (AMA) to convert widely accepted, uniform descriptions of medical, surgical, and diagnostic services rendered by health care providers into five-digit numeric codes. The use of the CPT codes enables health care providers to communicate both effectively and efficiently with third-party payers (i.e., commercial insurance companies, Medicare, Medicaid) about the procedures and services provided to the patient. For example, on an insurance form you can report a service by entering 21182 rather than "Reconstruction of orbital walls, rims, forehead, nasoethmoid complex following intra- and extracranial excision of benign tumor of the cranial bone (e.g., fibrous dysplasia) with multiple autografts (includes obtaining grafts); total area of bone grafting less than 40 sq cm." By using 21182, you are able to communicate not only quickly but also exactly about a very detailed service.

The majority of CPT codes are Category I codes and have been approved by the Editorial Panel of the AMA. Category II codes are optional performance measures. Category III codes are temporary codes that are used to help identify emerging technologies, services, and procedures.

Health care providers are reimbursed based on the codes submitted on a claim form for the procedures and services rendered. For an example of placement of the CPT codes on a claim form, refer to Fig. 1–1.

Reporting the correct code is essential because incorrect coding can result in a provider's being reimbursed incorrectly or in some cases being penalized by the government for submitting inappropriate claims. The CPT coding system is used by clinics, outpatient hospital departments, ambulatory surgery centers, and third-party payers to describe health care services. Although there are differences in the rules governing coding in various health care settings, CPT codes offer increased compatibility and comparability of data among users and providers, allowing for comparative analysis, research, and reimbursement.

The CPT coding system was first developed and published by the AMA in 1966 as a method of reporting medical and surgical procedures and services using standard terminology. Three editions of *Current Procedural Terminology* were published in the 1970s, and updates and revisions reflected changes in the technology and practices of health care. Use of the CPT manual was increased in 1983 when the Centers for Medicare and Medicaid Services (CMS), formerly the Health Care Financing Administration (HCFA), incorporated CPT codes into the Healthcare Common Procedural Coding System (HCPCS) to provide a uniform system of reporting services, procedures, and supplies. CPT codes are Level I codes and, for the most part, define professional services. Level II national codes (HCPCS) are alphanumeric codes that are used by providers to report services, supplies, and equipment provided to Medicare and Medicaid patients for which no CPT codes exist.

UPDATING THE CPT MANUAL

Because the practice of medicine is ever changing, the CPT manual is ever changing. It is updated annually to reflect technologic advances and editorial revisions. It is very important to use the most current CPT manual available so as to provide quality data and ensure appropriate reimbursement. The AMA is anticipating the publication of the next generation of CPT updates, CPT-5. The major changes in the CPT-5 will be the use of terminology that more clearly describes services and procedures. Currently, definitions include many vague terms such as "with or without," "and/or," and "by use of any method." This unclear terminology is being replaced with more precise definitions, making code selection a much easier process. The clarification of

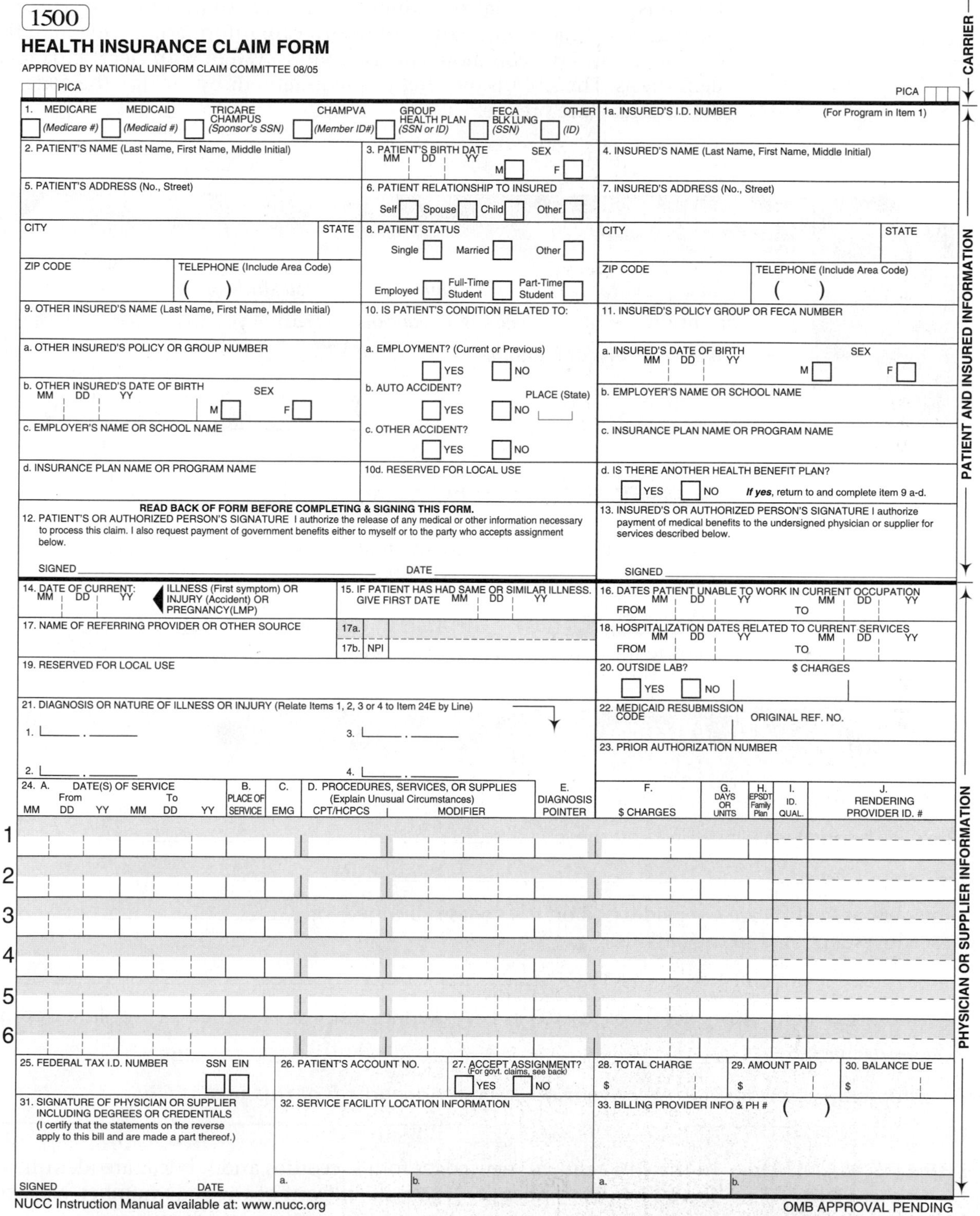
1500

HEALTH INSURANCE CLAIM FORM

APPROVED BY NATIONAL UNIFORM CLAIM COMMITTEE 08/05

PICA | PICA

CARRIER

1. MEDICARE (Medicare #) | MEDICAID (Medicaid #) | TRICARE CHAMPUS (Sponsor's SSN) | CHAMPVA (Member ID#) | GROUP HEALTH PLAN (SSN or ID) | FECA BLK LUNG (SSN) | OTHER (ID)

1a. INSURED'S I.D. NUMBER (For Program in Item 1)

2. PATIENT'S NAME (Last Name, First Name, Middle Initial)

3. PATIENT'S BIRTH DATE MM DD YY | SEX M F

4. INSURED'S NAME (Last Name, First Name, Middle Initial)

5. PATIENT'S ADDRESS (No., Street)

6. PATIENT RELATIONSHIP TO INSURED Self Spouse Child Other

7. INSURED'S ADDRESS (No., Street)

CITY | STATE

8. PATIENT STATUS Single Married Other

CITY | STATE

ZIP CODE | TELEPHONE (Include Area Code) ( )

Employed | Full-Time Student | Part-Time Student

ZIP CODE | TELEPHONE (Include Area Code) ( )

9. OTHER INSURED'S NAME (Last Name, First Name, Middle Initial)

10. IS PATIENT'S CONDITION RELATED TO:

11. INSURED'S POLICY GROUP OR FECA NUMBER

a. OTHER INSURED'S POLICY OR GROUP NUMBER

a. EMPLOYMENT? (Current or Previous) YES NO

a. INSURED'S DATE OF BIRTH MM DD YY | SEX M F

b. OTHER INSURED'S DATE OF BIRTH MM DD YY | SEX M F

b. AUTO ACCIDENT? YES NO | PLACE (State)

b. EMPLOYER'S NAME OR SCHOOL NAME

c. EMPLOYER'S NAME OR SCHOOL NAME

c. OTHER ACCIDENT? YES NO

c. INSURANCE PLAN NAME OR PROGRAM NAME

d. INSURANCE PLAN NAME OR PROGRAM NAME

10d. RESERVED FOR LOCAL USE

d. IS THERE ANOTHER HEALTH BENEFIT PLAN? YES NO *If yes,* return to and complete item 9 a-d.

READ BACK OF FORM BEFORE COMPLETING & SIGNING THIS FORM.

12. PATIENT'S OR AUTHORIZED PERSON'S SIGNATURE I authorize the release of any medical or other information necessary to process this claim. I also request payment of government benefits either to myself or to the party who accepts assignment below.

SIGNED ____ DATE ____

13. INSURED'S OR AUTHORIZED PERSON'S SIGNATURE I authorize payment of medical benefits to the undersigned physician or supplier for services described below.

SIGNED ____

PATIENT AND INSURED INFORMATION

14. DATE OF CURRENT: MM DD YY | ILLNESS (First symptom) OR INJURY (Accident) OR PREGNANCY(LMP)

15. IF PATIENT HAS HAD SAME OR SIMILAR ILLNESS. GIVE FIRST DATE MM DD YY

16. DATES PATIENT UNABLE TO WORK IN CURRENT OCCUPATION FROM MM DD YY TO MM DD YY

17. NAME OF REFERRING PROVIDER OR OTHER SOURCE | 17a. | 17b. NPI

18. HOSPITALIZATION DATES RELATED TO CURRENT SERVICES FROM MM DD YY TO MM DD YY

19. RESERVED FOR LOCAL USE

20. OUTSIDE LAB? YES NO | $ CHARGES

21. DIAGNOSIS OR NATURE OF ILLNESS OR INJURY (Relate Items 1, 2, 3 or 4 to Item 24E by Line)

1. ___ . ___ 3. ___ . ___

2. ___ . ___ 4. ___ . ___

22. MEDICAID RESUBMISSION CODE | ORIGINAL REF. NO.

23. PRIOR AUTHORIZATION NUMBER

24. A. DATE(S) OF SERVICE From MM DD YY	To MM DD YY	B. PLACE OF SERVICE	C. EMG	D. PROCEDURES, SERVICES, OR SUPPLIES (Explain Unusual Circumstances) CPT/HCPCS MODIFIER	E. DIAGNOSIS POINTER	F. $ CHARGES	G. DAYS OR UNITS	H. EPSDT Family Plan	I. ID. QUAL.	J. RENDERING PROVIDER ID. #
1										
2										
3										
4										
5										
6										

25. FEDERAL TAX I.D. NUMBER SSN EIN

26. PATIENT'S ACCOUNT NO.

27. ACCEPT ASSIGNMENT? (For govt. claims, see back) YES NO

28. TOTAL CHARGE $

29. AMOUNT PAID $

30. BALANCE DUE $

31. SIGNATURE OF PHYSICIAN OR SUPPLIER INCLUDING DEGREES OR CREDENTIALS (I certify that the statements on the reverse apply to this bill and are made a part thereof.)

SIGNED ____ DATE ____

32. SERVICE FACILITY LOCATION INFORMATION a. b.

33. BILLING PROVIDER INFO & PH # ( ) a. b.

PHYSICIAN OR SUPPLIER INFORMATION

NUCC Instruction Manual available at: www.nucc.org

OMB APPROVAL PENDING

FIGURE 1–1 The CMS-1500 Health Insurance Claim Form was revised to accommodate reporting of the National Provider Identifier (NPI) number mandated for April 2007. (Courtesy U.S. Department of Health and Human Services, Centers for Medicare and Medicaid Services.)

terminology is not the only change in the CPT-5 project. The revisions were necessary to address requirements of the Health Insurance Portability and Accountability Act of 1996 (HIPAA). HIPAA requires the Secretary of Health and Human Services to adopt national uniform standards for the electronic transmission of financial and administrative health information. These standards include a wide variety of health care information. One item that HIPAA requires is a common, concise coding system with clear, expandable definitions. The AMA is meeting this requirement by making the code definitions more precise.

From the Trenches

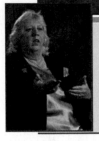

"Don't be afraid to write in your coding books! As you study and read, highlight important rules. Write instructions 'in your own words' so you will understand when you go back to look at it again."

BEVERLY

CHECK THIS OUT ☞ HIPAA legislation at http://www.cms.hhs.gov/

Updated editions of the CPT manual are available for purchase in November for use beginning the following January 1.

CHECK THIS OUT ☞ The American Medical Association (AMA) has a website located at http://www.ama-assn.org

EXERCISE 1–1 *The Purpose of the CPT Manual*

Complete the following:

1 The CPT manual was developed by the _____.

2 CPT stands for _____ _____ _____.

3 Providers of health care are paid based on the codes submitted for _____ or procedures provided to the patient.

4 The first CPT was published in this year: _____.

5 In which year were CPT codes incorporated as Level I codes into the Healthcare Procedure Coding System (HCPCS)? _____.

After completing Exercise 1–1, check your answers in Appendix B of this text.

THE CPT MANUAL FORMAT

In the CPT manual, new codes for procedures and services are identified by the bullet (●) symbol that is placed in front of the code number. Note the location of this symbol in Fig. 1–2.

Important Symbols and Appendices

A triangle (▲) placed in front of a code indicates that the description for the code has been **changed** or modified since the previous edition. Changes may be additions, deletions, or revisions in code descriptions (Fig. 1–3).

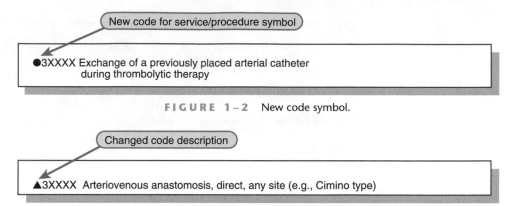

FIGURE 1–2 New code symbol.

FIGURE 1–3 Changed code symbol.

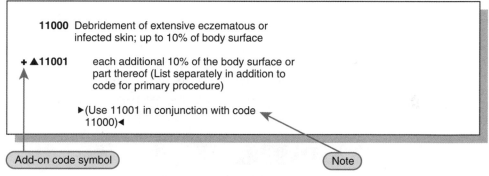

FIGURE 1–4 Changed text symbols.

```
    11000  Debridement of extensive eczematous or
           infected skin; up to 10% of body surface

+ ▲11001        each additional 10% of the body surface or
                part thereof (List separately in addition to
                code for primary procedure)

                ►(Use 11001 in conjunction with code
                  11000)◄
```

Add-on code symbol   Note

FIGURE 1–5 Add-on code symbol.

When the text has changed, a right and a left triangle (► ◄) indicate the beginning and end of the text changes, as illustrated in Fig. 1–4.

The plus symbol (+) placed in front of a code indicates an **add-on code** (Fig. 1–5).

Add-on codes are never used alone; rather, they are used with another primary procedure or service code. For example, code 11000 describes a debridement (removal of contaminated tissue) of up to 10% of the body surface. Add-on code 11001 is used for each additional 10% of the body surface debrided or part thereof. Code 11001 cannot be used unless code 11000 is used first. Also notice in Fig. 1–5 that there is a note in parentheses that indicates that code 11001 can be used only in conjunction with code 11000. **Appendix D** in the CPT manual lists all add-on codes.

The circle with a line through it (⊘) identifies a **modifier -51 exempt code** (Fig. 1–6).

Modifier -51 indicates that more than one (multiple) procedure was performed. **Appendix E** in the CPT manual contains the complete list of modifier -51 exempt codes.

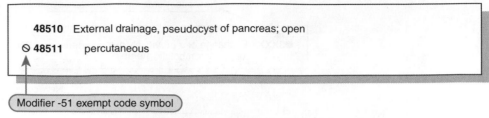

FIGURE 1–6   Modifier -51 exempt code symbol.

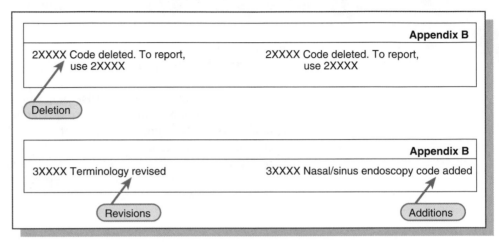

FIGURE 1–7   CPT manual Appendix B, showing types of changes.

Modifier -51 is discussed later in greater detail in Chapter 3.

Appendix A lists all modifiers used to alter or modify codes. Modifiers will be discussed in detail later in the chapter.

Appendix B of the CPT manual contains a complete list of the additions to, deletions from, and revisions of the CPT manual. When a code is listed in Appendix B, the type of change is also listed (Fig. 1–7).

Appendix C of the CPT manual contains clinical examples of many of the Evaluation and Management (E/M) service codes (Fig. 1–8).

The examples are meant to offer a broad idea of the type of presenting problem that each code could represent. But a word of caution: only the patient's record and the particular services rendered by the physician to a particular patient can determine the level of service provided. Appendix C is not meant to be an exhaustive list of E/M services.

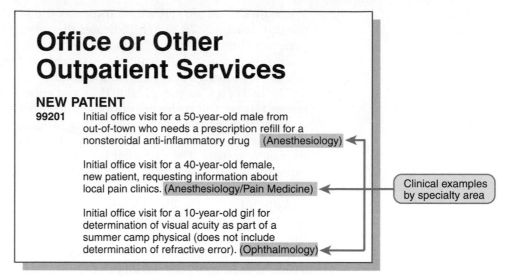

FIGURE 1-8 Appendix C of the CPT manual contains clinical examples in the use of E/M codes.

Appendix F of the CPT manual contains the summary of CPT codes that are Modifier -63 exempt. Modifier -63 identifies procedures that are performed on infants who weigh less than 4 kg or 8.8 pounds.

Appendix G is a summary of Moderate (Conscious) Sedation Codes identified by a bullseye (⊙) that denotes a procedure that includes moderate (conscious) sedation. For example, 32201, Pneumonostomy, with percutaneous drainage of abscess or cyst, has a bullseye before the code indicating that bundled into the code is both the insertion of the catheter and any conscious sedation provided. Moderate or conscious sedation is the type that leaves the patient alert enough to follow directions but still sedated enough to alleviate pain.

Appendix H is the Alphabetic Index of Performance Measures by Clinical Condition or Topic and lists the Category II codes. Category II codes are optional tracking codes that are used to identify performance measures of clinical components that may be typically included in evaluation and management services. The codes make it easier to collect data about certain services or test results that contribute to the health and quality of care of the patient. Another advantage of these measures is that their use will decrease the need for record abstraction and chart review. The codes are updated twice a year (January 1 and July 1) on the American Medical Association's website, http://www.ama-assn.org. The codes are four digits with "F" in the last position of each code (i.e., 0000F). The categories are arranged in the SOAP (subjective, objective, assessment, plan) format, which is a standard clinical documentation format. The categories and codes are:

- Composite Measures
- Patient Management
- Patient History
- Physical Examination
- Diagnostic/Screening Processes or Results
- Therapeutic, Preventive, or Other Interventions
- Follow-up, Patient Safety, and Other Outcomes

Appendix H provides further information about the code categories and the four modifiers (1P, 2P, 3P, and 8P) that are used with Category II codes.

These modifiers are -1P, which indicates the service was not provided due to medical reasons, -2P, which indicates the service was not provided due to the patient's choice, -3P, which reports service not provided due to a system reason (equipment not available, insurance coverage limitations, etc.), and -8P, for situations not otherwise specified.

The use of a Category II code does not substitute for a Category I code, rather Category II codes are optional and provide supplemental data.

Appendix I lists the Genetic Testing Modifiers. The modifiers in this appendix are reported with molecular laboratory procedures that are related to genetic testing. The first digit is a number that indicates the disease category and the second digit is a letter that denotes the gene type. For example, 0M is the modifier that indicates retinoblastoma (Rb).

Appendix J is the Electrodiagnostic Medicine Listing of Sensory, Motor and Mixed Nerves that identifies the sensory, motor, and mixed nerves with the corresponding conduction study code (95900, 95903, and 95904). Codes 95900 and 95903 are used to report motor nerve conduction studies, and 95904 is used to report sensory nerve conduction studies. Appendix J identifies the nerves in each of the nerve groups. Sensory and motor nerves are part of the peripheral nervous system (PNS) and run from the stimulus receptors to the central nervous system (CNS). A table in Appendix J lists the "reasonable maximum number of studies performed per diagnostic category necessary for a physician to arrive at a diagnosis in 90% of the patients with that final diagnosis." The recommended number of studies for each indication (condition) is identified. For example, if the indication was myopathy, it is recommended that the physician perform two needle electromyographies (EMGs), two motor nerve conduction studies (NCS), two sensory NCS, and two neuromuscular junction testings.

Appendix K, Products Pending FDA Approval, contains the lightning bolt symbol (⚡) that identifies codes that are being tracked by the AMA to monitor Food and Drug Administration (FDA) status for approval of a drug. In the 2009 CPT, six codes are listed in Appendix K. The internet site http://www.ama-assn.org/ama/pub/category/10902.html provides updates to the list of FDA pending approval codes.

Appendix L, Vascular Families, is a helpful listing of the orders of the vascular families. Listed are the first order, second order branch, third order branch, and beyond third order branches. The assumption is made that the starting point is the aorta. If the vessel is accessed at some other location, the branches, of course, would not be correct. You will find this appendix very helpful when you are coding catheterizations in the later chapters.

Appendix M, Crosswalk to Deleted CPT Codes, lists the current-year code to replace a deleted code.

EXERCISE 1-2 *Symbols*

Match the following code symbols with the correct definition:

1 ▲ _____ a. beginning and end of text changes

2 ►◄ _____ b. modifier -51 exempt

3 ● _____ c. revised description

4 ⊘ _____ d. add-on

5 + _____ e. moderate (conscious) sedation

6 ⊙ _____ f. pending FDA approval status

7 ✗ _____ g. new

8 Where is a complete list of additions, deletions, and revisions located in the CPT manual?

_____

9 Which CPT manual appendix contains a complete list of all modifier -51 exempt codes?

_____

10 Which CPT manual appendix contains a complete list of add-on codes? _____

_____

The CPT Sections

The CPT manual is composed of six chapters into which all codes and descriptions are categorized. These chapters are called **sections.**

THE SECTIONS OF THE CPT MANUAL

- Evaluation and Management   99201-99499
- Anesthesia   00100-01999, 99100-99140
- Surgery   10021-69990
- Radiology   70010-79999
- Pathology and Laboratory   80047-89356
- Medicine   90281-99199, 99500-99607

The sections are further divided into subsections, subheadings, categories, and subcategories. A section is a chapter that covers one of the six topics included in the CPT manual: Evaluation/Management (E/M), Anesthesia, Surgery, Radiology, Pathology/Laboratory, and Medicine codes. The CPT codes are arranged in numerical order in each section. Let's review these six sections.

Sections are divided into subsections. For example, the Surgery section includes subsections of Integumentary, Musculoskeletal, Respiratory, Cardiovascular, and so forth.

Subsections, subheadings, categories, and subcategories are divisions of sections that are based on anatomy, procedure, condition, description, or approach.

Examples

Section:	Surgery
Subsection:	Cardiovascular System
Subheading:	Arteries and Veins
Category:	Embolectomy/Thrombectomy
Subcategory:	Arterial, With or Without Catheter

Section:	Surgery
Subsection:	Nervous System
Subheading:	Skull, Meninges, and Brain
Category:	Approach Procedures
Subcategory:	Anterior Cranial Fossa

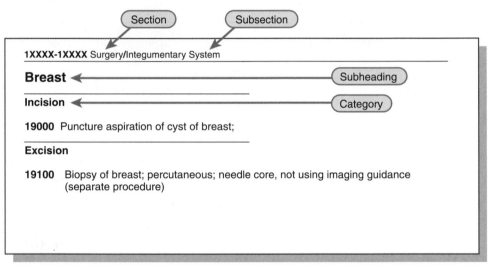

FIGURE 1–9 Section, subsection, subheading, and category.

EXERCISE 1-3 *Section, Subsection, Subheading, and Category*

To see an example of section, subsection, subheading, and category, locate the code 19000 Puncture aspiration of cyst of breast in the CPT in the Surgery section.

With a CPT beside you, open to the page where CPT code 19000 is located, or referring to Fig. 1–9 find the information on the top of the CPT manual page:

Section. At the top of the page, the word "Surgery" indicates the section. Note that this word is followed by a range of numbers, which is a list of all the code numbers located on that page.

Subsection. Also at the top of the page, the phrase "Integumentary System" indicates the subsection.

Subheading. The word "Breast" indicates the subheading.

Category. The word "Incision" indicates the category.

In summary, the divisions for the previous example are

Section: Surgery

Subsection: Integumentary System

Subheading: Breast

Category: Incision

Now you try one.

With a CPT manual open to the page that contains code 30100, locate the following information for the 30100 code:

1 Section: _____

2 Subsection: _____

3 Subheading: _____

4 Category: _____

Using the section, subsection, subheading, and category information makes it much faster and easier to get around in the CPT manual.

The Guidelines   Each section in the CPT manual includes Guidelines. The Guidelines provide specific information about coding in that section and contain valuable information for the coder. Guidelines that are applicable to all codes in the section are found at the beginning of each section (Fig. 1–10).

Notes pertaining to specific codes or groups of codes are listed before or after the codes (Fig. 1–11).

The Guidelines and notes may contain definitions of terms, applicable modifiers, subsection information, unlisted services, special reports information, or clinical examples. Always read the Guidelines and notes before coding to help ensure accurate assignment of the CPT codes.

Section Guidelines applicable to all Surgery codes

Surgery Guidelines

Items used by all physicians in reporting their services are presented in the **Introduction**. Some of the commonalities are repeated here for the convenience of those physicians referring to this section on **Surgery**. Other definitions and items unique to Surgery are also listed.

FIGURE 1–10 Section guidelines.

Specific notes applicable to a group of codes

SURGERY OF SKULL BASE
The surgical management of lesions involving the skull base (base of anterior, middle, and posterior cranial fossae) often requires the skills of several surgeons of different surgical specialties working together or in tandem during the operative session. These operations are usually…

FIGURE 1–11 Specific notes.

EXERCISE 1–4 *Guidelines*

Using the Guidelines for each of the sections, answer the following questions:

1 Write the definition of a chief complaint using the E/M Guidelines. _____

_____

_____

_____

2 According to the Surgery Guidelines, surgical destruction is a part of a surgical procedure and _____ methods of destruction are not usually listed separately.

3 According to the Radiology Guidelines, who must sign a written report to have the report considered part of the radiologic procedure? _____

4 Under whose supervision are Pathology and Laboratory services provided? _____

5 What is the code listed in the Medicine Guidelines that is to be used to identify materials supplied by the physician that are beyond those ordinarily included in the service provided? _____

Code Format   Procedure and service descriptions are located after the code (Fig. 1–12). They are commonly accepted descriptions of procedures or services that are provided to patients.

There are two types of codes: **stand-alone codes** and **indented codes** (Fig. 1–13).

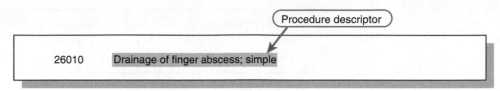

FIGURE 1–12 Code and description format.

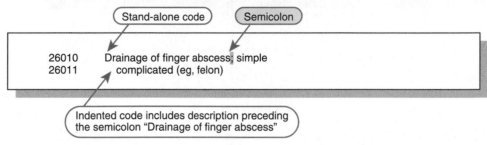

FIGURE 1–13 Stand-alone codes and indented codes.

Only the stand-alone codes have the full description; indented codes are listed under associated stand-alone codes. It is understood that descriptions for indented codes include the portion of the stand-alone code description that precedes the semicolon. The purpose of the semicolon is to save space.

 CAUTION *You may not have realized it, but you've just been given a critical clue to coding—the semicolon. The following information will help you understand why the semicolon is so important.*

In Fig. 1–13, the code 26011 is an indented code—the indentation serves to represent the words "Drainage of finger abscess," which appear before the semicolon in CPT code 26010. The semicolon is a powerful tool in the CPT manual; when you see it, be sure to read the words before it carefully.

The words following the semicolon can indicate alternative anatomic sites, alternative procedures, or a description of the extent of the service.

Example

ALTERNATIVE ANATOMIC SITE:

27705	Osteotomy; tibia
27707	fibula
27709	tibia and fibula

ALTERNATIVE PROCEDURE:

31505	Laryngoscopy, indirect; diagnostic (separate procedure)
31510	with biopsy
31511	with removal of foreign body
31512	with removal of lesion
31513	with vocal cord injection

DESCRIPTION OF EXTENT OF THE SERVICE:

20520	Removal of foreign body in muscle or tendon sheath; simple
20525	deep or complicated

CAUTION *Before assigning an indented code, make sure you refer to the preceding stand-alone code and read the words that precede the semicolon. That is the only way to ensure a full description and select a correct code.*

EXERCISE 1–5 *Code Format*

Complete the following:

1 Describe a stand-alone code. _____

_____

_____

2 Describe an indented code. _____

_____

_____

3 Words following the semicolon in stand-alone codes can indicate the following three things:

a. _____

b. _____

c. _____

Modifiers

Modifiers provide additional information to the third-party payer about services provided to a patient. At times, the five-digit CPT code may not reflect completely the service or procedure provided. Because numeric codes, not written procedure descriptions, are required by third-party payers, additional numbers or letters may be added to the basic five-digit code to modify the CPT code and thereby provide further specificity. These additional modifiers may be two numbers, two letters, or a letter and a number and are appended, or "tacked on," to the basic five-digit CPT code. In the HCPCS, two-place modifiers such as -RC and -F1 are used.

In the CPT system, a modifier is an appended two-digit number, such as:

Example

-62

or

-51

Modifier

-62 **Two Surgeons:** When two surgeons work together as primary surgeons performing distinct part(s) of a procedure, each surgeon should report his/her distinct operative work by adding the modifier '-62' to the procedure code and any associated add-on code(s) for that procedure as long as both surgeons continue to work together as primary surgeons. Each surgeon should report the co-surgery once using the same procedure code. If additional procedure(s) (including add-on procedure(s)) are performed during the same surgical session, separate codes(s) may be reported without the modifier '-62' added. Note: If a co-surgeon acts as an assistant in the performance of additional procedure(s) during the same surgicial session, those services may be reported using separate procedure code(s) with the modifier '-80' or modifier '-82' added, as appropriate.

FIGURE 1–14 Two-digit modifier.

Appendix A lists all modifiers with complete directions for use

Appendix A
Modifiers

Deleted in 2009

-21 **Prolonged Evaluation and Management Services:** When the face-to-face or floor/unit service(s) provided is prolonged or otherwise greater than that usually required for the highest level of evaluation and management services within a given category, it may be identified by adding modifier '-21' to the evaluation and management code number. A report may also be appropriate.

FIGURE 1–15 Modifiers in Appendix A.

The two-digit modifier is added to the five-digit CPT code.

Example

Code 43820 is the CPT procedure code for a gastrojejunostomy, without vagotomy. If two surgeons with different surgical skills participated as primary surgeons, each performing a specific part of the procedure, the procedure code 43820 could be altered by the addition of the modifier -62 to indicate co-surgeons (Fig. 1–14).

The code would be 43820-62 for a gastrojejunostomy, without vagotomy, in which two surgeons participated as primary surgeons. Each physician would submit his or her own bill, indicating code 43820-62.

For a complete listing of all modifiers, see Appendix A in the CPT manual. Refer to Fig. 1–15 for an example of the information found in Appendix A. Further information regarding modifiers is presented throughout the following chapters of this text.

CPT modifiers are listed first in descending numeric order (e.g., -62-50), and CPT modifiers are listed before HCPCS modifiers (e.g., -62-RT).

EXERCISE 1–6 *Modifiers*

Using Appendix A of the CPT manual and the information you just learned, fill in the blank with the correct number:

1 What is the two-digit modifier that indicates two primary surgeons? _____

2 If the CPT code is 43820 (gastrojejunostomy without vagotomy) and two primary surgeons

   performed the service, the service could be stated this way:_____ ,
   by each surgeon.

Use Appendix A of the CPT manual to list the correct two-digit modifier in the following examples.

3 Bilateral inguinal herniorrhaphy:_____

4 A postoperative ureterotomy patient has to be returned to the operating room for a related

   procedure during the postoperative period:_____

5 A decision to perform surgery is made during an evaluation, and management service on the day

   before or the day of surgery:_____

6 There is a need for multiple procedures to be performed during the same surgical

   session:_____

7 A surgical team is required:_____

8 Physician A assists physician B:_____

Unlisted Procedures

When developing the CPT manual, the AMA realized that not every surgical and diagnostic procedure could be listed. There may not be a code for many procedures that are considered experimental, newly approved, or seldom used. In addition, medical advancements often create a variation of procedures currently performed. A procedure or service not found in the CPT manual can be coded as an unlisted procedure if no Category I or III code exists to describe the procedure/service provided. For example, when the first heart transplant was performed, there was no code to use to report the new surgical procedure. Until a code was available, the unlisted code for cardiac surgery was used to report this procedure (Fig. 1–16).

The Surgery Guidelines have unlisted procedure codes listed by body site or type of procedure. Individually unlisted procedure codes are also at the end of the subsection or subheading to which they refer. For example, at the end of the Cardiovascular System subsection, Heart and Pericardium subheading, is the unlisted cardiac procedure code 33999, and at the end of the Respiratory System subsection, Lungs and Pleura subheading is the unlisted lungs/pleura code 32999.

EXERCISE 1–7 *Unlisted Procedures*

Assuming there is no Category III code available for the procedure you are reporting, using the Guidelines in the front of the sections indicated below, locate the five-digit unlisted procedure code for each of the following:

1 Surgery

Unlisted procedure; middle ear: Code(s): _____

    arthroscopy: Code(s): _____

    esophagus: Code(s): _____

2 Pathology and Laboratory

Unlisted procedure; cytogenetic study: Code(s): _____

    urinalysis procedure: Code(s): _____

    chemistry procedure: Code(s): _____

3 Medicine

Unlisted procedure; special service, procedure, or report: Code(s): _____

4 Radiology

Unlisted procedure; clinical brachytherapy: Code(s): _____

Unlisted miscellaneous procedures;
diagnostic nuclear medicine: Code(s): _____

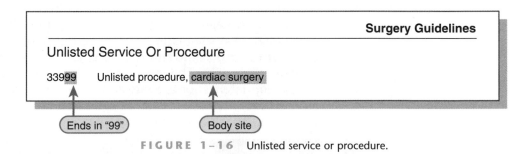

FIGURE 1–16 Unlisted service or procedure.

Category III Codes   Category III contains codes for emerging technology; they are temporary codes used for up to 5 years. If there is a Category III code for the service or procedure you are reporting, you must use the Category III code, not the Category I unlisted code.

Category I codes are those that are widely used to describe services and procedures that have been approved by the Food and Drug Administration (FDA), if appropriate. Category I codes also relate to services and procedures that have been proven to have clinical effectiveness. Category III codes describe services and procedures that may not have been approved by the FDA, may not be widely offered, and may not have been proven to be clinically effective. The use of the Category III codes allows physicians, other health care professionals, third-party payers, researchers, and health policy experts to identify emerging trends in health care.

Format of Category III Codes

The codes have five digits—four numbers and a letter: for example, 0030T (antiprothrombin). Prior to the existence of Category III codes, you would have reported this procedure using an unlisted code, because there was no specific code that described the procedure. But because there now is a Category III code available that describes the procedure, you must report the procedure using the Category III code, not the unlisted code from Category I.

Category III codes may or may not eventually receive Category I code status and be placed in the main part of the CPT.

QUICK CHECK 1-2

A Category III code would be reported rather than a Category I _____ code.

Publication of Category III Codes

New Category III codes are released twice a year (January and July) via the AMA website. The full set of temporary codes is then published in the next edition of the CPT in a section following the Medicine section.

Special Reports

Special reports must accompany claims when an unusual, new, seldom used, unlisted, or Category III procedure is performed. The special report should include an adequate definition or description of the **nature, extent,** and **need** for the procedure and the **time, effort,** and **equipment** necessary to provide the service. The special report helps the third-party payer determine the appropriateness of the care and the medical necessity of the service provided.

QUICK CHECK 1-3

Special reports must be submitted with claims for procedures that are unusual, new, seldom used, or use Category I _____ codes or Category _____ codes.

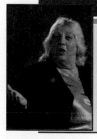

From the Trenches

"You will probably feel a bit 'lost' in the beginning, but don't let that slow you down! You are learning to identify the little pieces to a big puzzle. Wait until the puzzle is completed before deciding if you like the 'big picture;' you will be greatly rewarded."
BEVERLY

STARTING WITH THE INDEX

Locating the Terms

The CPT index is located at the back of the CPT manual and is arranged alphabetically. Index headings located at the top right and left corners of the index pages direct the coder to the entries that are included on that page, much like a dictionary. Use of index headings speeds location of the term (Fig. 1–17).

Code numbers are displayed in the CPT index in one of the ways shown in the following example.

Example

single code:	38115
multiple codes:	26645, 26650
range:	22305-22325

See Fig. 1–18 for an example of the display in the index using the single, multiple, and range formats.

Single Code

When only one code number is stated, you should verify the code in the main (tabular) portion of the CPT manual to ensure its accuracy.

Multiple Codes

The use of a **comma** between code numbers indicates the presence of only those numbers displayed. If more than one code number is listed, then all codes must be reviewed in the tabular to make an accurate choice.

Range of Codes

A range is indicated by a **hyphen.** When a range is given in the index, you must look up each code within the range in the tabular of the CPT manual to select the appropriate code from the range. There may even be multiple ranges listed.

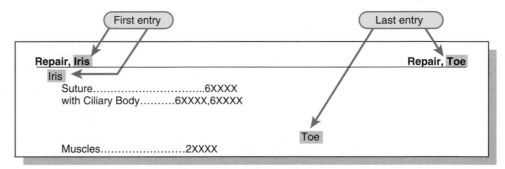

FIGURE 1–17 CPT manual index headings.

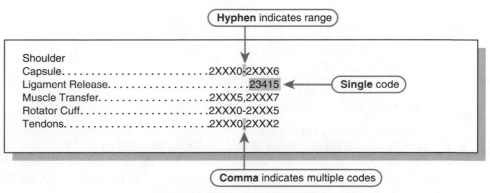

FIGURE 1–18 Code display.

> **CAUTION** *Never code directly from the index. You can't be sure you have the right code until you have located the code in the main portion of the CPT manual and read the information presented there regarding the specifics of the code.*

The index is in alphabetic order by main terms and is further divided by subterms. Fig. 1–19 illustrates the main term and subterm as used in the index. Having identified the main term of the service or procedure, you can locate the term in the index. When you are just beginning to use the CPT manual, it may be difficult to locate the main term. Not being able to locate a term in the index can be very frustrating, but don't be discouraged if you don't identify the main term on the first try. This is a skill that is learned by practice, and part of the practice is making mistakes. Soon you'll be locating those main terms quickly. Just keep thinking about the service or procedure and looking up the words in the index.

Some basic location methods will help you to locate these main terms.

LOCATION METHODS

- Service or Procedure
- Anatomic Site
- Condition or Disease
- Synonym
- Eponym
- Abbreviation

Let's take these location methods and apply each one to locating "repair of a fracture of a femur."

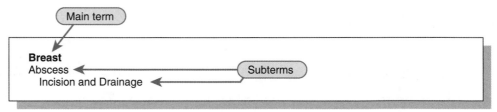

FIGURE 1–19 CPT manual index indicating main terms and subterms.

EXERCISE 1–8 *Term Practice*

SERVICE OR PROCEDURE

1 When using the service or procedure location method, "repair" would be the main term in "*repair of a fracture of a femur.*"

  a. Locate "Repair" in the index of the CPT manual. Using this location method, "Repair" is the main term and the subterms are "Fracture" and "Femur."

  b. Under the main term "Repair," locate the subterm "Femur." If you were to look under "Repair" and then look for the term "Fracture," you wouldn't find "Fracture," because listed under "Repair" are the anatomic divisions that can be repaired. "Fracture" isn't an anatomic division, so it isn't located under "Repair." It can be just as difficult to locate the correct subterm as it is to find the main term.

Right now, don't be concerned with looking up the codes in the main part of the CPT manual; we will come to that in Chapter 2. For now, concentrate on learning how to locate the main term and subterms in the index of the CPT manual.

ANATOMIC SITE

2 The second method of locating an anatomic site uses the word "femur" as the main term, and the subterms are "fracture" and "repair."

a. Locate "Femur" in the index of the CPT manual.

b. Under the main term "Femur," locate the subterm "Fracture."

c. Notice that the entry "Fracture" is further divided based on repair type (e.g., closed treatment) or anatomic location (e.g., distal).

CONDITION OR DISEASE

3 The third location method focuses on the condition or disease. In this instance you would use the main term "fracture" as a condition.

a. Locate the main term "Fracture" in the index.

b. Locate the subterm "Femur."

The use of the first three location methods will usually get you to the applicable codes in the index. If you try each of the first three methods and still can't locate the codes in the index, don't despair; try one of the other location methods: synonym, eponym, or abbreviation.

SYNONYM

4 The fourth location method involves synonyms. Synonyms are words with similar meanings.

a. Toe joint is a synonym for interphalangeal joint or metatarsophalangeal joint. Suppose, then, you couldn't think of the correct medical term, but you could think of the word "toe." In that case, you could look up "Toe" in the CPT manual index, and that entry would direct you to:

See Interphalangeal Joint, Toe; Metatarsophalangeal Joint, Phalanx

EPONYM

5 The fifth location method uses eponyms. Eponyms are things that are named after people. For example, the Barr Procedure—a tendon-transfer procedure—was named after the person who developed it.

a. Locate "Barr Procedure" in the CPT manual index. You are directed to:

See Tendon, Transfer, Leg, Lower.

ABBREVIATION

6 The sixth location method uses abbreviations. Abbreviations are common in medicine for names of drugs, diseases, and procedures.

a. Locate the abbreviation "INH" in the index of the CPT manual. You are directed to:

See Drug Assay.

Medicine uses many synonyms, eponyms, and abbreviations. A good medical dictionary that contains the most common synonyms, eponyms, and abbreviations will be a necessity for you.

Locate each of the following main terms in the CPT manual index, and then locate the subterms and secondary subterms and fill in the code(s) you find there:

MAIN TERM	SUBTERM	SECONDARY SUBTERM	
1 Repair	Abdomen	Suture	Code(s): _____
2 Femur	Abscess	Incision	Code(s): _____
3 Fracture	Ankle	Lateral	Code(s): _____

CAUTION *Never code directly from the index. The index does not include the information necessary for appropriate code selection. Locate the code in the index and then verify the code in the main part of the CPT manual to ensure that the code is the correct one to apply to the given procedure. Don't rely on memory. Always follow the steps outlined for coding.*

You are now ready to put your term location skills to work by doing the next exercise.

EXERCISE 1–9 *Main Term Location*

Identify the main terms in the following examples and write the main term on the line provided. Then locate the main terms and any subterms in the CPT manual index. Write the code listed in the index for that service or procedure on the line provided.

1 Description: Emergency Department Services, Physician Direction of Advanced Life Support

   a. Main term: _____

   b. Locate the code available in the index of the CPT manual for Emergency Department Services, Physician Direction of Advanced Life Support.

      Code: _____

2 Condition/Disease: intertrochanteric femoral fracture (closed treatment)

   a. Main term: _____

   b. Locate the code available in the index of the CPT manual for intertrochanteric femoral fracture (closed treatment).

      Code: _____

3 Procedure: removal of gallbladder calculi

   a. Main term: _____

   b. Locate the code available in the index of the CPT manual for removal of gallbladder calculi.

      Code: _____

4 Anatomic site: lung, bullae excision

   a. Main term: _____

   b. Locate the code available in the index of the CPT manual for excision of bullae of lung.

      Code: _____

As you can probably see from this exercise, there are often many ways to locate an item in the index. The same word can serve as a main term or a subterm, depending on the location method you are using. In addition, the annual updating of the CPT results in numerous changes within the index.

You will be locating terms in the CPT manual index throughout your study of this text. For your ready reference, there is a guideline at the beginning of the index in the CPT manual that contains directions for the use of the CPT manual index. Beginning with Chapter 2 of this text, Appendix B will list not only the correct code answer, but also one index location for that code. For example, if the correct answer is 99203, the following appears after the code: (Office and/or Other Outpatient Services, New Patient). It is difficult to locate items in the CPT index when you begin coding, so if you get stuck and just cannot locate the index entry, you will be able to find one location in Appendix B of this text.

QUICK CHECK 1-4

In the CPT manual there are instructions for using the CPT index. The headings on this page are _____ Terms, _____ Terms, Code Ranges and Conventions.

See   "See" is a **cross-reference** term found in the index of the CPT manual. The term directs you to another term or other terms.

"See" indicates that the correct code will be found elsewhere.

Example

Anticoagulant   *See* Clotting Inhibitors

 CAUTION *Never code directly from the index. To ensure correct coding, the code number must be located in the main portion of the CPT manual.*

EXERCISE 1–10 *See*

Complete the following:

1 Locate the term "Renal Disease Services" in the CPT index. You are directed to

_____.

2 Locate the abbreviation "ANA" in the CPT index. The entry you find is _____.

3 Locate the term "Arm" in the CPT index. You are directed to _____.

CHAPTER REVIEW

CHAPTER 1, PART I, THEORY

Do not use your CPT manual for this part of the review.

1 CPT stands for _____.

2 The CPT manual often reflects the technologic advances made in medicine with

_____.

3 The CPT manual is ever changing and is updated annually to reflect technologic advances

and editorial _____.

4 What type of code ends with 99?

_____

5 Coding information that pertains to an entire

section is located in the _____.

6 These codes provide supplemental information and do not substitute for a Category I code.

_____

7 What is the name of the two-digit number that is located after the CPT code number and provides more detail about the code?

_____

8 Where is a list of all the modifiers

located? _____

9 When using an unlisted or Category III code, third-party payers usually require the submission

of what? _____

10 Additions, deletions, and revisions are listed in which Appendix? _____

11 A listing of all add-on codes is located in which Appendix? _____

12 The symbol used between two code numbers to indicate that a range is available is a

_____.

Using Fig. 1–20, identify the category, section, subheading, and subsection.

13 _____.

14 _____.

15 _____.

16 _____.

17 The symbol that indicates a product is pending FDA approval is the

_____.

18 A complete list of the codes designated with the symbol that indicates a product is pending FDA approval is listed in this appendix of the CPT manual.

_____

19 The Genetic Testing Code Modifiers are listed in this appendix of the CPT manual.

_____

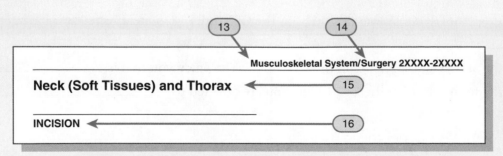

FIGURE 1–20 Identify the section, subsection, subheading, and category.

CHAPTER 1, PART II, PRACTICAL

Use your CPT manual for this part of the review. Using Appendix A of the CPT manual, list the correct two-digit modifiers for the following services:

20 Repeat procedure by the same physician:

_____

21 Surgical care only: _____

22 Anesthesia by the surgeon:

_____

23 Bilateral procedure: _____

Assuming there is no Category III code for the unlisted procedure you are reporting, locate the following unlisted procedure codes using the Surgery Guidelines:

24 Orbit: Code: _____

25 Rectum: Code: _____

26 Lips: Code: _____

27 General musculoskeletal:

Code: _____

Using the index of the CPT manual, locate an example of each of the following types of code display:

28 Single code _____

29 Multiple code _____

30 Range _____

Using the index of the CPT manual, locate the following terms and write what the index note directs you to do:

31 T4 Total _____

32 SHBG _____

33 Radius _____

34 Physical Therapy _____

Using the index of the CPT manual, locate the code(s) for the following:

35 Repair, Abdomen _____

36 Bypass Graft, Excision, Abdomen

_____

37 Catheterization, Arteriovenous Shunt

_____

38 Cystotomy, with Drainage

_____

39 Fracture, Femur, Intertrochanteric, Closed

Treatment _____

40 Alveoloplasty _____

41 Duodenotomy _____

QUICK CHECK ANSWERS

QUICK CHECK 1-1
True

QUICK CHECK 1-2
unlisted

QUICK CHECK 1-3
unlisted, III

QUICK CHECK 1-4
Main, Modifying

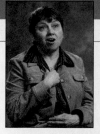

"I think having a goal of being a lifelong learner is important. One also has to have a great degree of integrity. It takes knowledge and character to adhere to the correct way to do things, and not be swayed by other factors, such as how to 'get it paid.'"

Joan E. Wolfgang, BA, CPC, CPC-H
Consultant, Educator, PMCC Certified Instructor
Milwaukee, Wisconsin

Evaluation and Management (E/M) Section

Chapter Topics

Contents of the E/M Section

Three Factors of E/M Codes

Various Levels of E/M Service

An E/M Code Example

Using the E/M Codes

Documentation Guidelines

Chapter Review

Quick Check Answers

Learning Objectives

After completing this chapter, you should be able to

1   Identify and explain the three factors of E/M code assignment.
2   Differentiate between a new and an established patient.
3   Differentiate between an inpatient and an outpatient.
4   Explain the levels of E/M service.
5   Review the key components.
6   Analyze the key component history.
7   Analyze the key component examination.
8   Analyze the key component medical decision making.
9   List contributory factors.
10 Analyze code information.
11 Analyze the types of E/M codes.
12 Identify CMS Documentation Guidelines.
13 Demonstrate the ability to code E/M services.

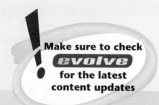

Make sure to check **evolve** for the latest content updates

CONTENTS OF THE E/M SECTION

The information in Chapter 1 described the basic format of the CPT manual. The information and exercises in this chapter will familiarize you with the first section of the CPT manual, Evaluation and Management (E/M). Locate Table 1, Categories and Subcategories of Service, in the E/M Guidelines of the CPT manual, which indicates all the E/M categories/subcategories.

Office or Other Outpatient Services	
New Patient	99201-99205
Established Patient	99211-99215
Hospital Observation Services	
Hospital Observation Discharge Services	99217
Initial Hospital Observation Services	99218-99220
Hospital Observation or Inpatient Care Services (Including Admission and Discharge Services)	99234-99236
Hospital Inpatient Services	
Initial Hospital Care	99221-99223
Subsequent Hospital Care	99231-99233
Hospital Discharge Services	99238-99239
Consultations	
Office Consultations	99241-99245
Inpatient Consultations	99251-99255
Emergency Department Services	99281-99288
Critical Care Services	
Adult (over 24 months of age)	99291-99292
Nursing Facility Services	
Initial Nursing Facility Care	99304-99306
Subsequent Nursing Facility Care	99307-99310
Nursing Facility Discharge Services	99315-99316
Other Nursing Facility Services	99318
Domiciliary, Rest Home (e.g., Boarding Home), or Custodial Care Services	
New Patient	99324-99328
Established Patient	99334-99337

Domiciliary, Rest Home (e.g., Assisted Living Facility), or Home Care Plan Oversight Services	99339-99340
Home Services	
New Patient	99341-99345
Established Patient	99347-99350
Prolonged Services	
With Direct Patient Contact	99354-99357
Without Direct Patient Contact	99358-99359
Physician Standby Services	99360
Case Management Services	
Anticoagulation Management	99363, 99364
Medical Team Conferences	99366-99368
Care Plan Oversight Services	99374-99380
Preventive Medicine Services	
New Patient	99381-99387
Established Patient	99391-99397
Counseling Risk Factor Reduction and Behavior Change Intervention	99401-99429
Non-Face-to-Face Physician Services	99441-99444
Special E/M Services	99450-99456
Newborn Care	99460-99465
Neonatal and Pediatric Critical Care Services	99466-99480
Other E/M Services	99499

THREE FACTORS OF E/M CODES

Code assignment in the E/M section varies according to three factors:

1. Place of service   2. Type of service   3. Patient status

Place of Service

The first factor you must consider in code assignment is the place of service (Fig. 2–1).

Place of service explains the setting in which the services were provided to the patient. Codes vary depending on the place of the service. Places of service can be a physician's office, hospital, emergency department, nursing home, and so on.

Type of Service

The second factor in code assignment is the type of service (Fig. 2–2).

Type of service is the reason the service is requested or performed. Examples of types of service are consultation, admission, newborn care, and office visit.

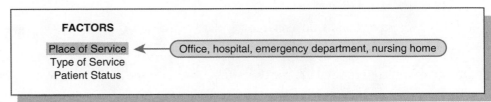

FACTORS

Place of Service ◄— Office, hospital, emergency department, nursing home
Type of Service
Patient Status

FIGURE 2-1   Place of service.

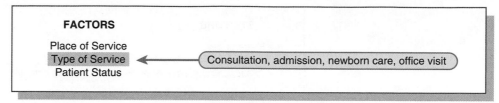

FIGURE 2–2   Type of service.

- Consultation is requested to obtain an opinion or advice about a diagnosis or management option from another physician.
- Admission is attention to an acute illness or injury that results in admission to a hospital.
- Newborn care is the evaluation and determination of care management of a newly born infant.
- Office visit is a face-to-face encounter between a physician and a patient to allow for primary management of the patient's health care status.

Patient Status   The third factor in code assignment is patient status (Fig. 2–3).

The four types of patient status are new patient, established patient, outpatient, and inpatient. Codes are often grouped in the CPT manual according to the type of patient involved.

- New patient is one who has not received professional face-to-face services from the physician or another physician of the same specialty in the same group within the past 3 years.
- Established patient is one who has received professional face-to-face services from the physician or another physician of the same specialty in the same group within the past 3 years.
- Outpatient is one who has not been formally admitted to a health care facility or a patient admitted for observation.
- Inpatient is one who has been formally admitted to a health care facility.

EXERCISE 2–1   *Three Factors of E/M Codes*

Using a CPT manual, locate the subsection Office and Other Outpatient Services and then the category New Patient in the E/M section to answer the following questions:

1 Where is the place of service? _____

2 What is the type of service? _____

3 What is the patient status? _____

4 What is the first code number listed under the subheading New Patient?

   Code: _____

5 Each code represents a different level of service. How many codes are listed under Office or Other

   Outpatient Services for a new patient? _____

6 How many codes are listed for the established patient in the Office or Other Outpatient Services

   category? _____

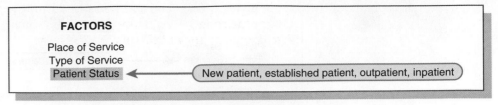

FIGURE 2-3   Patient status.

Medical Records Documentation

Patient information is located in the medical record. This information is referred to as the documentation. The documentation in the medical record has many uses, such as evaluation of the patient's treatment, communications regarding the patient's health care, reimbursement claims, review of the use of the health care facility, research/education, and legal documentation. Seven organizations (American Health Information Management Association, American Hospital Association, Managed Care and Review Association, American Medical Association, American Medical Peer Review Association, Blue Cross and Blue Shield Association, and the Health Insurance Association of America) developed minimum documentation guidelines, as follows:

1. The medical record should be complete and legible.

2. Documentation of each encounter should include the date, reason for encounter, appropriate history and physical examination, review of ancillary services, assessment, and plan of care.

3. Past and present diagnoses should be accessible to the treating and/or consulting physician.

4. The reasons for and results of x-rays, lab tests, and other ancillary services should be clear.

5. Relevant risk factors should be identified.

6. The patient's progress and response to treatment, any change in treatment or change in diagnosis, and any patient noncompliance should be documented.

7. A written plan of treatment should include, when appropriate, treatments and medications, specifying frequency and dosage, any referrals or consultations, patient or family education, and any specific instructions for follow-up care.

8. Documentation should report the intensity of the patient evaluation and/or the treatment, including thought processes and the complexity of the medical decision making.

9. All entries should be dated and authenticated.

10. The CPT/ICD-9-CM codes reported on the insurance claim or billing statement should reflect the documentation in the medical record.

VARIOUS LEVELS OF E/M SERVICE

The levels of E/M service are based on documentation located in the patient's medical record supporting various amounts of skill, effort, time, responsibility, and medical knowledge used by the physician to provide the service to the patient. The levels of service are based on **key components** (history, examination, and medical decision making complexity) and **contributory factors** (counseling, coordination of care, nature of presenting problem, and time). The components contain a great deal of information that you need to know before you learn about factors. Let's look at each of these components and factors individually.

Key Components

- History
- Examination
- Medical decision making

The key components of history, examination, and medical decision making reflect the clinical information that is recorded by the physician in the patient's medical record. Key components are present in every patient case except counseling encounters, which are discussed later in the chapter. Key components enable you to choose the appropriate level of service. New patient encounters, consultations, emergency-department visits, and admissions require documentation of all three of the key components. Subsequent visits such as daily hospital visits or outpatient visits for an established patient require that only two of the three key components be present for assignment to a given code. For example, to assign code 99214—established patient, office visit—at least two of the three key components must be documented in the patient's medical record.

Example

99214   Office or other outpatient visit for the evaluation and management of an established patient, which requires **at least two of these three key components:**

- **a detailed history;**
- **a detailed examination;**
- **medical decision making of moderate complexity.**

QUICK CHECK 2-1

The following categories/subcategories must meet or _exceed_ ~~three~~ of three key components.

According to the E/M Guidelines, the following categories/subcategories must meet or exceed the stated level of the key components:

- Office, New Patient
- Hospital Observation Services
- Initial Hospital Care
- Office Consultation
- Inpatient Consultation
- Emergency Department Services
- Initial Nursing Facility Care
- Domiciliary Care, New Patient
- Home, New Patient

Of the following categories/subcategories, **two** of the **three** key components must be met or exceeded before the code may be assigned:

- Office, Established Patient
- Subsequent Hospital Care
- Subsequent Nursing Facility Care
- Domiciliary Care, Established Patient
- Home, Established Patient

History. The history is the *subjective* information the patient tells the physician based on the four elements of a history—chief complaint (CC); history of present illness (HPI); review of systems (ROS); and past, family, and/or social history (PFSH). The history contains the information the physician needs to appropriately assess the patient's condition. Not all histories have all elements. The inclusion of each of the elements and the extent to which each of the elements is contained in a history are determined by the physician, based on the need for more or less subjective information, and will determine the extent of the history level. The documentation of the history is found in the patient's medical record and is recorded by the physician.

Ancillary staff (nurses, physician assistants, and so forth) are allowed to document some of the history, such as chief complaint and past, family, and social histories, but the physician must authenticate the entries. Also, a physician can have the patient complete a form composed of questions concerning the review of systems; however, the physician must evaluate the form and indicate in the medical record that the form has been reviewed (authenticated).

QUICK CHECK 2-2

Some history elements may be documented by ancillary staff or the patient. True or False?

THE FOUR ELEMENTS OF A HISTORY

- Chief Complaint (CC)
- History of Present Illness (HPI)
- Review of Systems (ROS)
- Past, Family, and/or Social History (PFSH)

History Elements. You need to be able to identify the various elements and levels of a history by reading the notes entered into the medical record by the physician.

1. **Chief Complaint (CC)** is a concise statement describing the symptom, problem, condition, diagnosis, physician-recommended return, or other factor that is the reason for the encounter, usually stated in the patient's words.
2. **History of Present Illness (HPI)** is a chronological description of the development of the patient's present illness from the first sign and/or symptom or from the previous encounter to the present. The HPI may include the following elements.

Example

Location: thoracic spine (site on body)

Quality: burning, throbbing (characteristics)

Severity: on a scale of 1 to 10, an 8 (intensity)

Duration: 3 days (how long is an episode or how long has the problem existed)

Timing: throughout the day: continuously, at night, in the morning, etc., indicates the frequency (when does it occur)

Context: when bending over (under what circumstances does it occur)

Modifying factors: better when lying down (what circumstances make it better or worse)

Associated signs and symptoms: weakness (what else is happening when it occurs)

The HPI must be documented in the medical record by the physician.

3. **Review of Systems (ROS)** is an inventory of body systems obtained through a series of questions seeking to identify signs and/or symptoms that the patient may be experiencing or has experienced. According to Huffman's *Health Information Management,** the "ROS is an inventory of systems to reveal subjective symptoms that the patient either forgot to describe or which at the time seemed relatively unimportant. In general, an analysis of the subjective findings will indicate the nature and extent of examination required." The inventory of systems may be made by means of a questionnaire filled out by the patient or ancillary staff; but the physician must evaluate the questionnaire and document in the medical record that the questionnaire has been reviewed in order for it to qualify as an ROS. For the purposes of an ROS, the following systems are recognized*:

- Constitutional symptoms

  Usual weight, recent weight changes, fever, weakness, fatigue

- Eyes (Ophthalmologic)

  Glasses or contact lenses, last eye examination, visual glaucoma, cataracts, eyestrain, pain, diplopia, redness, lacrimation, inflammation, blurring

- Ears, Nose, Mouth, Throat (Otolaryngologic)

  Ears: hearing, discharge, tinnitus, dizziness, pain

  Nose: head colds, epistaxis, discharges, obstruction, postnasal drip, sinus pain

  Mouth and Throat: condition of teeth and gums, last dental examination, soreness, redness, hoarseness, difficulty in swallowing

- Cardiovascular

  Chest pain, rheumatic fever, tachycardia, palpitation, high blood pressure, edema, vertigo, faintness, varicose veins, thrombophlebitis

- Respiratory

  Chest pain, wheezing, cough, dyspnea, sputum (color and quantity), hemoptysis, asthma, bronchitis, emphysema, pneumonia, tuberculosis, pleurisy, last chest radiograph (Note: also shortness of breath)

---

*Definitions from Huffman E: Health Information Management, 10th ed. Revised by the American Medical Record Association. Berwyn, IL, Physician's Record Company, 1994, pp 57–62.

■ Gastrointestinal

Appetite, thirst, nausea, vomiting, hematemesis, rectal bleeding, change in bowel habits, diarrhea, constipation, indigestion, food intolerance, flatus, hemorrhoids, jaundice

■ Genitourinary

Urinary: frequent or painful urination, nocturia, pyuria, hematuria, incontinence, urinary infection

Genito-reproductive: male—venereal disease, sores, discharge from penis, hernias, testicular pain or masses; female—age at menarche and menstruation (frequency, type, duration, dysmenorrhea, menorrhagia; symptoms of menopause), contraception, pregnancies, deliveries, abortions, last Papanicolaou smear

■ Musculoskeletal

Joint pain or stiffness, arthritis, gout, backache, muscle pain, cramps, swelling, redness, limitation in motor activity

■ Integumentary (skin and/or breast)

Skin: rashes, eruptions, dryness, cyanosis, jaundice, changes in skin, hair, or nails*

Breast: lumps, dimpling, nipple discharge*

■ Neurologic *(neurological)*

Faintness, blackouts, seizures, paralysis, tingling, tremors, memory loss

■ Psychiatric

Personality type, nervousness, mood, insomnia, headache, nightmares, depression

■ Endocrine

Thyroid trouble, heat or cold intolerance, excessive sweating, thirst, hunger, or urination, blood sugar levels

■ Hematologic/Lymphatic

Anemia, easy bruising or bleeding, past transfusions

■ Allergic/Immunologic

Sneezing, itching eyes, rhinorrhea, nasal obstruction, or recurrent infections

4. **Past, Family, and/or Social History (PFSH)****

■ Past history is the patient's past experience with illnesses, operations, injuries, and treatments; that includes significant information about:

Prior major illnesses and injuries

Prior operations

Prior hospitalizations

Current medications

Allergies (e.g., drug, food)

Age-appropriate immunization status

Age-appropriate feeding/dietary status

---

*Modified from Huffman E: Health Information Management, 10th ed. Revised by the American Medical Record Association. Berwyn, IL, Physician's Record Company, 1994, pp 57–62.

**Definitions from 2009 CPT, Evaluation and Management Guidelines, p 4. CPT codes, descriptions, and materials only are © 2008 American Medical Association.

- ▪ Social history is an age-appropriate review of past and current activities that includes significant information about:

  Marital status and/or living arrangements

  Current employment

  Occupational history

  Use of drugs, alcohol, and tobacco

  Level of education

  Sexual history

  Other relevant social factors

- ▪ Family history is a review of medical events in the patient's family that includes significant information about:

  The health status or cause of death of parents, siblings, and children

  Specific diseases related to problems identified in the Chief Complaint or History of the Present Illness, and/or System Review

  Diseases of family members that may be hereditary or place the patient at risk

Three of the elements of a history (HPI, ROS, and PFSH) are included to varying degrees in all patient encounters. The degree or level of HPI, ROS, and PFSH is determined by the chief complaint or presenting problem of the patient.

History Levels. Now that you have reviewed the elements of a history you are prepared to choose a history level. There are four history levels; the level is based on the extent of the history during the history-taking portion of the physician-patient encounter.

HISTORY LEVELS

- ▪ Problem focused
- ▪ Expanded problem focused
- ▪ Detailed
- ▪ Comprehensive

1. **Problem focused:** The physician focuses on the chief complaint and a brief history of the present problem of a patient.

   A brief history would include a review of the history regarding pertinent information about the present problem or chief complaint. Brief history information would center around the severity, duration, and/or symptoms of the problem or complaint. The brief history does not have to include the past, family, or social history or a review of systems.

2. **Expanded problem focused:** The physician focuses on a chief complaint, obtains a brief history of the present problem, and also performs a problem pertinent review of systems. The expanded problem focused history does not have to include the past, family, or social history.

   This history would center around specific questions regarding the system involved in the presenting problem or chief complaint. The review of systems for this history would cover the organ system most closely related to the chief complaint or presenting problem and any related or associated organ system. For example, if the presenting problem or chief complaint is a red, swollen knee, the system reviewed would be the musculoskeletal system.

3. **Detailed:** The physician focuses on a chief complaint, obtains an extended history of the present problem, an extended review of systems, and a pertinent PFSH.

  The system review in this history is extended, which means that positive responses and pertinent negative responses relating to multiple organ systems should be documented.

4. **Comprehensive:** This is the most complex of the history types: the physician documents the chief complaint, obtains an extended history of the present problem, does a complete review of systems, and obtains a complete PFSH.

For a summary of the elements required for each level of history (according to the 1995 Documentation Guidelines), see Fig. 2–4.

Some third-party payers have established standards for the number of elements that must be documented in the medical record to qualify for a given level of service. For example, a third-party payer may state that to qualify as a comprehensive history the medical record must document that an extended HPI was conducted and that it included four of the eight elements (e.g., location, quality, severity, duration), a complete ROS, including a review of at least 10 of the 14 organ systems, and a complete review of all three areas of the PFSH.

CODING SHOT

When selecting a history level, the choice goes to the lowest level. For example, if the HPI is a level 2, the ROS is a level 2, but the PFSH is a level 1, the history level is a 1. Another example is if the HPI is a level 3, the ROS is a level 2, and the PFSH is a level 2, the history is a level 2.

QUICK CHECK 2-3

Which levels of history require the documentation of the Chief Complaint (CC)?

a. Problem focused
b. Expanded problem focused
c. Detailed
d. Comprehensive
e. All of the above

History Elements

Chief Complaint (CC)
Reason for the encounter in the patient's words

History of Present Illness (HPI)
Location
Quality
Severity
Duration*
Timing
Context
Modifying factors
Associated signs and symptoms

Review of Systems (ROS)
Constitutional symptoms (fever, weight loss, etc.)
Ophthalmologic (eyes)
Otolaryngologic (ears, nose, mouth, throat)
Cardiovascular
Respiratory
Gastrointestinal
Genitourinary
Musculoskeletal
Integumentary (skin and/or breast)
Neurological
Psychiatric
Endocrine
Hematologic/Lymphatic
Allergic/Immunologic

Past, Family, and/or Social History (PFSH)
Past major illnesses, operations, injuries, and treatments
Family medical history for heredity and risk
Social activities, both past and current

Elements Required for Each Level of History

History		Problem Focused	Expanded Problem Focused	Detailed	Comprehensive
	HPI	Brief 1-3	Brief 1-3	Extended 4+	Extended 4+
	ROS	None	Problem-pertinent 1	Extended 2-9	Complete 10+
	PFSH	None	None	Pertinent 1	Complete 2-3

* Not listed in the CPT E/M Guidelines, but listed in the 1995 Documentation Guidelines.

FIGURE 2-4 History elements required for each level of history.

Copyright © 2009, 2008, 2007, 2006, 2005, 2004, 2002, 2000, 1998, 1996 by Saunders, an imprint of Elsevier Inc. All rights reserved.

EXERCISE 2-2 *History Levels*

Using the CPT manual, locate the Office or Other Outpatient Services subsection, New Patient category, to identify the history level on each of the following codes:

CODE	HISTORY LEVEL
1 99201	_____
2 99202	_____
3 99203	_____
4 99204	_____
5 99205	_____

Examination. The patient has presented the physician with the **subjective** information regarding the complaint or problem in the history portion of the encounter; now the physician will do an examination of the patient to provide **objective** information (those findings observed by the physician) about the complaint or problem. The physician then documents the objective findings in the patient record.

Examination Levels. The examination levels have the same titles as the history levels—problem focused, expanded problem focused, detailed, and comprehensive. The four levels are used to indicate the extent and complexity of the patient examination.

EXAMINATION LEVELS

- Problem focused
- Expanded problem focused
- Detailed
- Comprehensive

1. **Problem focused:** Examination is limited to the affected body area or organ system identified by the chief complaint.
2. **Expanded problem focused:** A limited examination is made of the affected body area or organ system and other symptomatic or related body area(s)/organ system(s).
3. **Detailed:** An extended examination is made of the affected body area(s) and other symptomatic or related organ system(s).
4. **Comprehensive:** This is the most extensive examination; it encompasses a complete single-specialty examination or a complete multisystem examination.

Fig. 2–5 (on page 40) summarizes the elements required for each level of examination. These elements include various body areas (BAs) and organ systems (OSs). The elements also include an assessment of a patient's general condition, which is indicated by the patient's general appearance, vital signs, and the like. The three elements—constitutional, BAs, and OSs—are as follows:

Constitutional

- Blood pressure, sitting
- Blood pressure, lying
- Pulse

- Respirations
- Temperature
- Height
- Weight
- General appearance

Body Areas (BA)
- Head (including the face)
- Neck
- Chest (including breasts and axillae)
- Abdomen
- Genitalia, groin, buttocks
- Back
- Each extremity

Organ Systems (OS)
- Ophthalmologic (eyes)
- Otolaryngologic (ears, nose, mouth, throat)
- Cardiovascular
- Respiratory
- Gastrointestinal
- Genitourinary
- Musculoskeletal
- Integumentary (skin)
- Neurologic
- Psychiatric
- Hematologic/Lymphatic/Immunologic

EXERCISE 2-3 *Examination Levels*

Using the CPT manual, locate the Office or Other Outpatient Services subsection, New Patient category, to identify the examination levels for each of the following codes:

CODE	EXAMINATION LEVELS
1 99201	
2 99202	
3 99203	
4 99204	
5 99205	

The patient's medical record will reflect the number of systems examined in a brief statement of the findings. The examination would include the examination elements and the number and extent of elements required for the physician to arrive at the diagnosis. For example, if a patient came to a physician with the complaint of a small foreign object lodged in the eye, the physician would not need to do a cardiologic examination. The extent of the examination is based on what needs to be done to treat the patient.

Examination Elements

Constitutional
Blood pressure, sitting
Blood pressure, lying
Pulse
Respirations
Temperature
Height
Weight
General appearance

Body Areas (BA)
Head (including the face)
Neck
Chest (including breasts and axillae)
Abdomen
Genitalia, groin, buttocks
Back
Each extremity

Organ System (OS)
Ophthalmologic (eyes)
Otolaryngologic (ears, nose, mouth, throat)
Cardiovascular
Respiratory
Gastrointestinal
Genitourinary
Musculoskeletal
Integumentary (skin)
Neurologic
Psychiatric
Hematologic/Lymphatic/Immunologic

Elements Required for Each Level of Examination

	Problem Focused	Expanded Problem Focused	Detailed	Comprehensive
Examination	Limited to affected BA or OS	Limited to affected BA or OS and other related OS(s)	Extended of affected BA(s) and other related OS(s)	General multi-system or complete single OS
# of OS/BA	1	2-7 limited	2-7 extended	8+

FIGURE 2–5
Examination elements required for each level of examination.

Now you need to pull all the information on history and examination together so that it is usable information (abstract). What better way to do that than to use the information in the practical application of an exercise?

EXERCISE 2–4 *Examination Elements*

Label each of the following as body area (BA) or organ system (OS):

1 Skin _____   5 Nose _____

2 Head _____   6 Mouth _____

3 Eyes _____   7 Throat _____

4 Ears _____   8 Neck _____

9	Thorax, anterior and posterior _____	15	Vaginal _____
10	Breasts _____	16	Arm _____
11	Lungs _____	17	Musculoskeletal _____
12	Heart _____	18	Lymphatics _____
13	Abdomen _____	19	Psychiatric _____
14	Genitourinary _____	20	Neurologic _____

Read the following patient record:

21 A new patient, an 8-year-old female, is brought into the office by her mother, who states that the child has an earache in her right ear. Mother reports that the child has been complaining of aching and ringing in right ear of increasing severity for the past 2 days. Exam: Child appears to be in only minor distress. Vitals: Temperature, 101° F. HEENT: ears, eyes, and nose. Tympanic membrane red, fluid noted in right ear. PERRLA. Health history reviewed. Diagnosis: Otitis media.

From the patient record, we can identify the history elements—chief complaint (CC), history of present illness (HPI), past, family, and/or social history (PFSH), and review of systems (ROS)—as in the following:

HISTORY ELEMENTS	PATIENT RECORD
CC:	Earache in the right ear
HPI:	Aching and ringing in right ear of increasing severity for the past 2 days (Note: This HPI indicates location, quality, severity, and duration.)
PFSH:	Review of child's health history (The patient information form completed by the mother contains the information that the physician reviewed, along with questions to the patient.)
ROS:	Ears (one organ system, otolaryngologic)

In this case, the physician focused on the chief complaint and did a brief history centered on gathering information about the present illness. Referring to the description of history levels summarized in Fig. 2–4 or discussed in the E/M Guidelines, answer the following question:

a. What is the history level for this case? _____

Now let's establish the level of examination:

EXAMINATION	PATIENT RECORD
General Survey:	Child appears to be in only minor distress
Vital Signs:	Temperature, 101° F
Body Areas/Organ Systems	Ears and eyes (two organ systems)

In this case, the physician focused on constitutional (temperature) and two organ systems (eyes and ears). Referring to the description of examination levels summarized in Fig. 2–5 or discussed in the E/M Guidelines, answer the following question:

b. What is the examination level for this case? _____

That wasn't so difficult, was it? Okay, now you do one.

Read the following patient record:

22 A 68-year-old female established patient presents to the office today with a "cold" of 9 days' duration. Patient reports that she has had a dry, hacking cough and nasal congestion for the past 6 days and a fever for the past 3 days. She states that she is unable to sleep due to the cough,

fever, and aching. She appears to be in minor distress. Personal and family history are negative for respiratory problems. Temperature is 100° F; blood pressure 150/90; pulse 93 and regular. Lungs clear to percussion and auscultation. Examination of head and ears, normal; nose, mucous membranes inflamed with postnasal phlegm. Diagnosis: Sinusitis. Plan: Patient was advised to drink fluids, take aspirin as needed for pain, obtain bed rest, and to return if symptoms have not improved in 5 days.

Locate the information in the patient record that matches the history element and place the information on the lines provided:

HISTORY ELEMENTS   **PATIENT RECORD**

CC: _____

_____

_____

HPI: _____

_____

_____

PFSH: _____

_____

_____

ROS: _____

_____

_____

With the information you placed on the preceding lines, choose the correct history level:

   a. What is the history level for this case? _____

Locate the information in the patient record that matches the examination, and place the information on the lines provided:

EXAMINATION   **PATIENT RECORD**

General Survey: _____

Vital Signs: _____

_____

_____

_____

Body Areas/Organ Systems: _____

With the information you placed on the preceding lines, choose the correct examination level:

b. What is the examination level for this case? _____

Medical Decision Making. The key component of medical decision making (MDM) is based on the complexity of the decision the physician must make about the patient's diagnosis and care. Complexity of decision making is based on three elements:

1. Number of diagnoses or management options. The options can be minimal, limited, multiple, or extensive.

2. Amount or complexity of data to review. The data can be minimal or none, limited, moderate, or extensive.

3. Risk of complication or death if the condition goes untreated. Risk can be minimal, low, moderate, or high.

Levels. The extent to which each of these elements is considered determines the levels of MDM complexity.

MEDICAL DECISION MAKING COMPLEXITY LEVELS

■ Straightforward

■ Low

■ Moderate

■ High

1. **Straightforward decision making:** minimal diagnosis and management options, minimal or none for the amount and complexity of data to be reviewed, and minimal risk to the patient of complications or death if untreated.

2. **Low-complexity decision making:** limited number of diagnoses and management options, limited data to be reviewed, and *low* risk to the patient of complications or death if untreated.

3. **Moderate-complexity decision making:** multiple diagnoses and management options, moderate amount and complexity of data to be reviewed, and moderate risk to the patient of complications or death if untreated.

4. **High-complexity decision making:** extensive diagnoses and management options, extensive amount and complexity of data to be reviewed, and high risk to the patient for complications or death if the problem is untreated.

Management Options. According to the 1995 E/M Documentation Guidelines, documentation of management options in the medical record are as follows:

1. For each encounter, an assessment, clinical impression, or diagnosis should be documented. It may be explicitly stated or implied in documented decisions regarding management plans or further evaluation.

   ■ For a presenting problem with an established diagnosis, the record should reflect whether the problem is (a) improved, well controlled, resolving, or resolved; or (b) inadequately controlled, worsening, or failing to change as expected.

   ■ For a presenting problem without an established diagnosis, the assessment or clinical impression may be stated in the form of differential diagnoses or as a "possible," "probable," or "rule out" (R/O) diagnosis.

   ■ Note: Physician/Provider coders do not code "rule out," "possible," or "probable" diagnosis; rather they code the presenting symptoms.

2. The initiation of, or changes in, treatment should be documented. Treatment includes a wide range of management options, including patient instructions, nursing instructions, therapies, and medications.

3. If referrals are made, consultations requested, or advice sought, the record should indicate to whom or where the referral or consultation has been made or from whom the advice is requested.

Data to Be Reviewed. The following are some basic documentation guidelines for the amount and complexity of data to be reviewed:

1. If a diagnostic service (test or procedure) is ordered, planned, scheduled, or performed at the time of the E/M encounter, the type of service (e.g., laboratory or radiology) should be documented.

2. The review of laboratory, radiology, or other diagnostic tests should be documented. An entry in a progress note such as "WBC elevated" or "chest x-ray negative" is acceptable. Alternatively, the review may be documented by initialing and dating the report containing the test results.

3. A decision to obtain old records or to obtain additional history from the family, caregiver, or other source to supplement that obtained from the patient should be documented.

4. Relevant findings from the review of old records or the receipt of additional history from the family, caregiver, or other source should be documented. If there is no relevant information beyond that already obtained, that fact should be documented. A notation of "old records reviewed" or "additional history obtained from family" without elaboration is insufficient.

5. The results of discussion of laboratory, radiology, or other diagnostic tests with the physician who performed or interpreted the study should be documented.

6. The direct visualization and independent interpretation of an image, tracing, or specimen previously interpreted by another physician should be documented.

Risk. Some basic documentation guidelines for risk of significant complications, morbidity, or mortality include the following:

1. Comorbidities (secondary conditions), underlying diseases, or other factors that increase the complexity of medical decision making by increasing the risk of complications, morbidity, or mortality should be documented.

2. If a surgical or invasive diagnostic procedure is ordered, planned, or scheduled at the time of the E/M encounter, the type of procedure (e.g., laparoscopy) should be documented.

3. If a surgical or invasive diagnostic procedure is performed at the time of the E/M encounter, the specific procedure should be documented.

4. The referral for or decision to perform a surgical or invasive diagnostic procedure on an urgent basis should be documented or implied.

Examples of the levels of risk may be found in Table 2–1 (p. 46).

When you select one of the four types of complexity of medical decision making—straightforward, low, moderate, or high—the documentation in the medical record must support the selection in terms of the number of diagnoses or management options, amount and/or complexity of data to be reviewed, and risks. Two of the three elements in Fig. 2–6 must be met or exceeded to qualify for a level of medical decision making.

CODING SHOT When selecting an MDM level, the choice goes to the majority. For example, if the number of diagnosis management options is a level 2, the amount of data is a level 2, but the risk is a level 1, the MDM level is 2. Another example is if the number of management options is a level 1, the amount of data is a level 3, and the risk is a level 2, the history is a level 2. This is different than the history in which the lowest level directed the level choice; in the MDM the level is the highest two.

Refer to Fig. 2–6 (p. 46) for an overview of medical decision making. Given the information in the medical record, you would consider the information in the context of the complexity of the diagnosis and management options, data to be reviewed, and risks to the patient in order to choose the complexity of MDM. Let's look at an example of choosing the MDM level.

Example 1

An established patient's office medical record states the following: Female patient fell and scraped arm; problem focused history and examination were done. The patient states that she slipped on the ice on the walk outside her home approximately 3 hours earlier. The area of abrasion appears to be relatively clean, with no noted foreign materials imbedded. There appears to be only minimal cutaneous damage. The area was washed and a dressing applied.

1. **Diagnosis and management options** for an abrasion (clean and dress). (Options can be minimal, limited, multiple, or extensive.)

   As a coder, you think about how many various options are open to the physician to diagnose the problem and decide how to manage this patient's care—minimal, limited, multiple, extensive? The management of an abrasion is fairly clear—clean and dress the wound; therefore, the diagnosis and management options are minimal.

2. **Data to review** to provide service. (Data can be minimal/none, limited, moderate, or extensive.)

   As a coder, you think about how much and how complex would the information (data) be that the physician must obtain, review, and analyze to care for this patient—minimal/none, limited, moderate, or extensive? The amount of data to review would be minimal/none for the abrasion.

3. **Risk** of infection if not treated. (Risk can be minimal, low, moderate, or high.)

   As a coder, you think about how great a risk there is that the patient would die or encounter severe complications (e.g., infection), morbidity (additional diseases such as gangrene), or mortality (death) if the abrasion were not treated—minimal, low, moderate, or high? The risk of death or of complications is minimal.

The diagnosis and management options are minimal, data are minimal/none, and risk is minimal. Consideration of these three elements has placed this patient's care into a straightforward MDM complexity level.

The history level is stated to be problem focused and the examination level is problem focused. The patient was an established patient seen as an outpatient. Carefully look at each of the items set in boldface type in code 99212 below for an established patient. The place of service, type of service, type of history, type of examination, and complexity level of the MDM are identified in the description of the code.

99212　　**Office or other outpatient** visit for the evaluation and management of an **established patient** that requires at least two of these three key components:

   ▪ **a problem focused history**

   ▪ **a problem focused examination**

   ▪ **straightforward medical decision making**

CPT code 99212 is the correct code for this service.

TABLE 2–1

LEVELS OF RISK

Level of Risk	Presenting Problem or Problems
Minimal (Level 1)	One self-limited or minor problem (e.g., insect bite, tinea corporis)
Low (Level 2)	Two or more self-limited or minor problems One stable chronic illness (e.g., well-controlled hypertension or non–insulin dependent diabetes, cataract, benign prostatic hypertrophy) Acute, uncomplicated illness or injury (e.g., cystitis, allergic rhinitis, simple sprain)
Moderate (Level 3)	One or more chronic illnesses with mild exacerbation, progression, or side effects of treatment Two or more stable chronic illnesses Undiagnosed new problem with uncertain prognosis (e.g., lump in breast) Acute illness with systemic symptoms (e.g., pyelonephritis, pneumonitis, colitis)
High (Level 4)	One or more chronic illnesses with severe exacerbation, progression, or side effects of treatment Acute or chronic illnesses or injuries that pose a threat to life or body function (e.g., multiple trauma, acute myocardial infarction, pulmonary embolus, severe respiratory distress, progressive severe rheumatoid arthritis, psychiatric illness with potential threat to self or others, peritonitis, acute renal failure) An abrupt change in neurologic status (e.g., seizure, transient ischemic attack, weakness, or sensory loss)

Medical Decision-Making Elements

Number of Diagnoses or Management Options
Minimal
Limited
Multiple
Extensive

Amount or Complexity of Data to Review
Minimal/None
Limited
Moderate
Extensive

Risk of Complications or Death if Condition Goes Untreated
Minimal
Low
Moderate
High

Elements Required for Each Level of Medical Decision-Making

	Straightforward	Low	Moderate	High
Number of DX or management options	Minimal	Limited	Multiple	Extensive
Amount or complexity of data	Minimal/None	Limited	Moderate	Extensive
Risks	Minimal	Low	Moderate	High

FIGURE 2–6 Decision making elements required for each level of medical decision making complexity. Two of the three elements must be met or exceeded to qualify for a level of medical decision making.

Example 2

The patient's record states the following: Unknown (new) patient presenting in the office with chest pain. A comprehensive history was taken and a comprehensive examination immediately performed.

Again, the MDM complexity level must be chosen:

1. **Diagnosis and management options** for cardiac origin of possible myocardial infarction, angina, or heart block. Gastrointestinal origin could be reflux or an ulcer. Respiratory origin could be a pulmonary embolism or pleuritis. (Diagnosis and management options can be minimal, limited, multiple, or extensive.)

    What do you think it would take for the physician to decide on the diagnosis or management options for this patient? There are many possibilities of origin for the chest pain; therefore, the diagnosis and management options are extensive.

2. **Data to review** in order to provide service. (Data can be minimal/none, limited, moderate, or extensive.) How much data would the physician have to obtain through current tests on the patient and how much review and analysis of previous records would be necessary to provide services to the patient—minimal/none, limited, moderate, extensive? In this case, the patient's care requires moderate data review, including laboratory reports, radiology reports, and ECG. You very well may have chosen the data review level of extensive rather than moderate.

3. **Risk** if left untreated. (Risk can be minimal, low, moderate, or high.) If the patient's condition were untreated, what do you think the risk of death or serious complication would be—minimal, low, moderate, or high? This patient would have a high risk of death or of severe complications if untreated.

    The extensive diagnosis and management options and high risk to the patient if this condition is not treated mean that the necessary standard of two of the three elements being present has been met. So this patient's care is considered to have a high level of MDM complexity. A new patient with a comprehensive history and examination together with a high MDM complexity places this case in the category of 99205.

EXERCISE 2–5 *Medical Decision Making Complexity*

A patient's record states that an initial office visit was made for the evaluation and management of a 48-year-old male with recurrent low back pain from a herniated disk, with pain radiating to the leg. A detailed history was obtained from this new patient and a detailed physical examination was performed.

Using the information given for this patient, identify the following factors in the case:

1 Diagnosis and management options for recurrent low back pain radiating to the leg. (Options can be minimal, limited, multiple, or extensive.)

_____

2 Data to review in order to provide service. (Data can be minimal/none, limited, moderate, or extensive.) Current record available.

_____

3 Risk if left untreated. (Risk can be minimal, low, moderate, or high.)

_____

4 Two of the three elements have been met to qualify this patient for what level of MDM complexity? (Complexity can be straightforward, low, moderate, or high.)

_____

5 The patient record indicates that a detailed history was taken and a detailed examination was performed. When this is combined with the level of MDM complexity you arrived at for this patient, what is the correct CPT code for the case?

Code:_____

Now, let's look again at two cases for which you previously established the history and examination levels:

6 A new patient, an 8-year-old female, is brought into the office by her mother, who states that the child has an earache in the right ear. Mother reports that the child has been complaining of aching and ringing in the right ear of increasing severity for the past 2 days. Child appears to be in only minor distress. Temperature, 101° F. Examination: ears, eyes, and nose. Tympanic membranes red, fluid noted in right ear. Health history reviewed. Diagnosis: Otitis media.

What is the MDM level for this patient? _____

7 A 68-year-old female established patient presents to the office today with a "cold" of 9 days' duration. Patient reports that she has had a dry, hacking cough and nasal congestion for the past 6 days and a fever for the past 3 days. She states that she is unable to sleep due to the cough, fever, and aching. She appears to be in minor distress. Personal and family history are negative for respiratory problems. Temperature is 100° F; blood pressure 150/90; pulse 93 and regular. Lungs clear to percussion and auscultation. Examination of head and ears, normal; nose, mucous membranes inflamed with postnasal phlegm. Diagnosis: Sinusitis. Plan: Patient was advised to drink fluids, take aspirin as needed for pain, obtain bed rest, and return if symptoms have not improved in 5 days.

What is the MDM level for this patient? _____

There is certainly a great amount of information that must be considered in order to choose the correct E/M code! Only with practice can you expect to remember all of the various elements and levels within each component. Each medical facility has its own procedure for identifying the level of E/M service; some facilities require the physician to identify all the components of service, whereas other facilities require the component information to be abstracted from the medical record by support personnel. Either way, you need to be knowledgeable about all components of E/M codes.

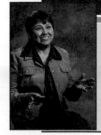

From the Trenches

"I tell people that while the study and practice of medicine is considered a science, the coding is an art. There are often varying ways to do things, dependent on different circumstances. Attention to detail is important, but flexibility is also necessary."

JOAN

 STOP *You have examined each of the three key components and seen how they apply to the assignment of a code. You will be referring to the information as you are presented with additional cases. Make note of the important points and remember that the information about the key components is in the E/M Guidelines at the beginning of the E/M section in the CPT manual.*

Now that you are familiar with the key components of history, examination, and medical decision making, let's review the contributory factors.

Contributory Factors

There are 3 contributory factors: counseling, coordination of care, and the nature of the presenting problem. Contributory factors are those conditions that help the physician to determine the extent of history, examination, and decision making (key components) necessary to treat the patient. Contributory factors may or may not be considered in every patient case.

CONTRIBUTORY FACTORS

- Counseling
- Coordination of care
- Nature of presenting problem

Counseling. Counseling is a service that physicians provide to patients and their families. It involves discussion of diagnostic results, impressions, and recommended diagnostic studies; prognosis; risks and benefits of treatment; instructions for treatment; importance of compliance with treatment; risk factor reduction; and patient and family education. Some form of counseling usually takes place in all physician-patient encounters, and this was factored into the codes when they were developed by the AMA. Only when counseling is the reason for the encounter or consumes most of the visit time (more than 50% of the total time) is counseling considered a component of code assignment. The following statement is made often within the codes in the E/M section:

Counseling and/or coordination of care with other providers or agencies are provided consistent with the nature of the problem(s) and the patient's and/or family's needs.

Coordination of Care. Coordination of care with other health care providers or agencies may be necessary for the care of a patient. In coordination of care, a physician might arrange for other services to be provided to the patient, such as arrangements for admittance to a long-term nursing facility.

Nature of the Presenting Problem. The presenting problem is the patient's chief complaint or the situation that leads the physician to determining the level of care necessary to diagnose and treat the patient. The CPT describes the **presenting problem** as a disease, condition, illness, injury, symptom, sign, finding, complaint, or other reason for the encounter, with or without a diagnosis being established at the time of the encounter. There are five types of presenting problems:

- Minimal
- Self-limited
- Low severity
- Moderate severity
- High severity

1. **Minimal:** A problem may not require the presence of the physician, but service is provided under the physician's supervision. A minimal problem is a blood pressure reading, a dressing change, or another service that can be performed without the physician's being immediately present.
2. **Self-limited:** Also called a minor presenting problem, a self-limited problem runs a definite and prescribed course, is transient (it comes and goes), and is not likely to permanently alter health status, or the presenting problem has a good prognosis with management and compliance.
3. **Low severity:** The risk of complete sickness (morbidity) without treatment is low, there is little or no risk of death without treatment, and full recovery without impairment is expected.

4. **Moderate severity:** The risk of complete sickness (morbidity) without treatment is moderate, there is moderate risk of death without treatment, and an uncertain prognosis or increased probability of impairment exists.

5. **High severity:** The risk of complete sickness (morbidity) without treatment is high to extreme, there is a moderate to high risk of death without treatment, or there is a strong probability of severe, prolonged functional impairment.

The patient's medical record should contain the physician's observation concerning the complexity of the presenting problem(s). Your responsibility is to identify the words that correctly indicate the type of presenting problem.

EXERCISE 2–6 *Presenting Problem*

Match the presenting problem to the severity level in the patient:

1 Four-year-old female established patient presents with slight pain in right ear, of 2 days' duration. Physician diagnosed a minor infection, prescribes antibiotic.

_____

2 Eighty-six-year-old woman who has a history of chronic obstructive pulmonary disease (COPD) and is oxygen-dependent comes in today because of dizziness and weakness. _____

3 Established patient, 71 years old, with shortness of breath on exertion and a history of left ventricular dysfunction with cardiomyopathy.

_____

4 Fourteen-year-old presents with moderate pain in left thumb after a fall from his skateboard. _____

5 Established patient, 34 years old, presents for a blood pressure check. _____

6 Physician recommends an over-the-counter medication. _____

a. minimal

b. self-limited

c. low

d. moderate

e. high

Time. Time was not included in the CPT manual before 1992 but was incorporated to assist with the selection of the most appropriate level of E/M services. The times indicated with the codes are only **averages** and represent a simple estimate of the possible duration of a service.

Direct face-to-face and **unit/floor time** are two measures of time. Outpatient visits are measured as direct face-to-face time. Direct face-to-face time is the time a physician spends directly with a patient during an office visit obtaining the history, performing an examination, and discussing the results. Inpatient time is measured as unit/floor time and is used to describe the time a physician spends in the hospital setting dealing with the patient's care. Unit/floor time includes care given to the patient at the bedside as well as at other settings on the unit or floor (e.g., the nursing station). It is an often-heard comment that physicians get paid a great deal of money just for stopping in to see a hospitalized patient. However, what is not realized is that the physician spends additional time reviewing the patient's records and writing orders for the patient's care.

Time in the E/M section is referred to in statements such as this one that is located with code 99203:

> *Usually, the presenting problem(s) is (are) of moderate severity. Physicians typically spend 30 minutes face to face with the patient and/or family.*

These statements concerning time are used when counseling or coordination of care represent more than **50% of the time spent with a patient.** The times referred to in these statements are the basis of the selection of the correct E/M code. For example: An established patient returns for an office visit to get the results of tests. The physician spends 25 minutes going over the unfavorable results of the tests. The physician discusses various treatment options, the prognosis, and the risks of treatment and of treatment refusal. The correct code would be 99214, in which the time statement is, "Physician typically spends 25 minutes face to face with the patient and/or family." The physician must either document the beginning and ending time in the patient's medical record or document the total time spent and how much was spent in counseling in order to be able to consider time in the code assignments.

AN E/M CODE EXAMPLE

With the CPT manual open to the first page of the E/M section, locate the notes above the 99201 code. These notes highlight the incidents in which codes in that particular category are appropriate for assignment. The notes above 99201 indicate that the codes that follow the notes are appropriate for use in coding services provided in a "physician's office or in an outpatient or other ambulatory facility."

The information also directs you to other code subsections if the patient classification is not correct. As an example of this directional feature, the notes above 99201 state, "For services provided by physicians in the Emergency Department, *see* 99281-99285."

Fig. 2–7 shows the first code for a new patient under the category New Patient under subsection Office or Other Outpatient Services. Review Fig. 2–7 carefully before continuing. Note the location of each important piece of information.

Locate the following items in Fig. 2–7:

1. Three key components
2. Three contributory factors
3. Number of key components required
4. Place of service
5. Category of the code
6. Code

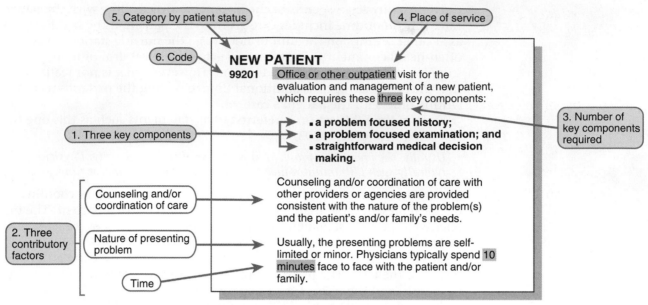

FIGURE 2–7 Code information.

USING THE E/M CODES

Now you are going to use the information you have learned about codes in the E/M services section as you continue to identify the differences among the code numbers.

Office and Other Outpatient Services

New Patient. The first subsection in the E/M section is Office and Other Outpatient Services, New Patient Category (99201-99205).

You will recall from information presented earlier that a new patient is defined as one who has not received any face-to-face professional services from the physician or another physician with the same specialty in the same group within the past 3 years. A physician must spend more time with a new patient—obtaining the history, conducting the examination, and considering the data—than with an established patient. Consider that the established patient is probably known to the physician, and the person's medical records are available. For these reasons, the cost of a new patient office visit is higher, so third-party payers reimburse the physician at a higher rate for new patient services than for the same type of service when it is provided to an established patient.

EXERCISE 2–7 *New Patient Services*

Using the CPT manual, fill in the blanks with the correct words:

1 For code 99203, the history level is _____, the examination is_____, and the MDM is of _____ complexity.

2 For code 99204, the history level is _____, the examination is _____, and the MDM complexity is _____.

3 For code 99205, the history level is _____, the examination is _____, and the MDM complexity is _____.

Code the following cases for new patients:

4 A 53-year-old new patient presents for an initial office visit to discuss a surgical vasectomy for sterilization. The history and examination are detailed and the MDM is of low complexity.

   Code: _____

5 A 4-year-old new patient presents for the removal of sutures made for an appendectomy 10 days earlier in another city. The physician conducts a brief history and examination prior to removing the stitches.

   Code: _____

6 A 23-year-old man who is a new patient has an initial office visit for severe depression that has led to frequent thoughts of suicide in the past several weeks and is acute today. More than an hour is spent discussing the patient's problems and options. Past medical history is negative. The social history reveals that the patient suffers from sleeplessness; smokes between two and two and a half packs of unfiltered cigarettes a day; drinks 10 to 12 cups of coffee; and denies current use of drugs. (The actual patient record continues and indicates that a comprehensive examination was conducted; high MDM complexity.)

   Code: _____

7 A new patient, a 10-year-old boy, is brought in by his father for a knee injury sustained in a hockey game. The knee is swollen and the patient is in apparent pain. A detailed history and examination are obtained. A diagnosis of probable meniscus tear is made. Low MDM complexity.

   Code: _____

8 A 41-year-old woman, new to the office, complains of headache and rhinitis of 4 days' duration. The patient states that she has had a problem with her allergies during this season for years. An expanded problem focused history and examination are done. Straightforward MDM complexity.

   Code: _____

Established Patient. The second category of codes in subsection Office and Other Outpatient Services is for the established patient in an outpatient setting (99211-99215). You will recall that the definition of an established patient is one who has received face-to-face professional services from the physician or another physician of the same specialty in the same group within the past 3 years.

Code 99211 is used to report services provided in the office for which the physician is not present during the service but is in the office suite and is immediately available. Further, the employee providing the service must have the credentials necessary to provide the service, and the service must be part of a documented treatment plan. The physician should sign the documentation of the service.

QUICK CHECK 2-4

Could a physician assign 99211 to report a patient encounter?
Yes or No?

EXERCISE 2–8 *Established Patient Services*

Fill in the blanks with information from codes in the Established Patient category:

1 99211: This minimal service level does not exist in the New Patient category because a new patient is seen by the physician. The established patient may or may not be seen by the physician. Read the description and information for code 99211 in the CPT manual. Would an established patient returning for a simple blood pressure check be appropriately reported as 99211?

   _____

2 A 42-year-old established patient presents for an office visit with complaints of severe vaginal itching and moderate pain. During the problem focused history, the patient states that several weeks earlier she had noted a slight itching, which has increased in severity. Yesterday, she noted a lesion on her genitalia. Burning and painful urination have increased over the past 5 days accompanied by rectal itching. She has tried a variety of over-the-counter ointments and creams, which induced no improvement. The patient states that she has had several yeast infections in the past that had been successfully treated by her previous physician. Personal history indicates several prior urinary infections. No discharge noted. A problem focused examination of the external genitalia reveals a lesion, which had previously ruptured, located on the vulva. Bacterial and viral smears are done. The MDM complexity is straightforward. The patient is advised that the smears would be back in 24 hours and that a treatment plan would be developed based on the reports. (The smear was positive for a bacterial infection, for which antibiotics were prescribed.)

   Code: _____

3 A 17-year-old football player comes to the clinic for a gold injection by the nurse. Only the nurse sees this established patient. (Code only the E/M service.)

   Code: _____

4 A 53-year-old established patient complains of frequent fainting. The history and examination are comprehensive, and the MDM is of high complexity.

   Code: _____

5 A 61-year-old established patient is seen for medication management of fatigue produced by hypertensive medication. An expanded problem focused history and examination are done, and the MDM is of moderate complexity.

Code: _____

6 An established 31-year-old patient presents with an irritated skin tag. A problem focused history and examination are done. MDM complexity is low.

Code: _____

7 A 48-year-old woman has had diarrhea for the past 5 days. Her temperature is 101° F. An expanded problem focused history and examination are done. MDM complexity is low.

Code: _____

STOP *Remember, it takes a lot of practice to learn to code. It is not a skill that is quickly acquired. You need to have patience and know that practice, practice, practice is the only thing that will make this skill yours.*

Hospital Observation Services

The codes in the Hospital Observation subsection (99217-99220) are used to identify initial observation care or observation discharge services. The services in the observation subsection are for patients who are in a hospital on observation status.

Observation is a status used for the classification of a patient who does not have an illness severe enough to meet acute inpatient criteria and does not require resources as intensive as an inpatient but does require hospitalization for a short period of time. Patients are also admitted to observation so further information can be obtained about the severity of the condition and so it can be determined whether the patient can be treated on an outpatient basis. In some hospitals in some parts of the country, observation status is conducted in the temporary care unit (TCU).

The observation codes are for new or established patients. There are no time components with observation codes, as codes are based on the level of service. Each code from the range 99218-99220 requires all three of the key components to establish a level of service.

If a patient is admitted to the hospital as an inpatient after having been admitted earlier the same day as an observation patient, you do not report the observation status separately. The services provided during observation become part of (are bundled into) the initial inpatient hospital admission code.

QUICK CHECK 2-5

Are observation codes 99218-99220 reported for inpatient or outpatient services? _____

Observation Care Discharge Services. The Observation Care Discharge Services code (99217) includes the final examination of the patient upon discharge from observation status. Discussion of the hospital stay, instructions for continued care, and preparation of discharge records are also bundled into the Observation Care Discharge Services code. The code is used only with patients who are discharged on a day that follows the first day of observation.

Initial Observation Care. Initial Observation Care codes (99218-99220) are used to designate the beginning of observation status in a hospital. Again, the hospital does not need to have a formal observation area, since the designation of observation status is dependent on the severity of illness of the patient. These codes also include development of a care plan for the patient and periodic reassessment while on observation status. Observation admission can be reported only for the first day of the service. If the patient is admitted and discharged on the same day, a code from the range 99234-99236, Observation or Inpatient Care Services, is used to report the service. If the patient is in the hospital overnight but remains there for a period that is **less than 48 hours**, the first day's service is coded with a code from the range 99218-99220, Initial Observation Care, and the second day's service is coded 99217, Observation Care Discharge Services. If the patient is on observation status for **longer than 48 hours**, the first day is coded with a code from the range 99218-99220, Initial Observation Care; the second day is coded with a code from the range 99212-99215, Established Office or Other Outpatient Services; and the third day is coded 99217, Observation Care Discharge Services.

Services performed in sites other than the observation area (e.g., clinic, nursing home, emergency department) and that precede admission to observation status are included in (bundled into) the Initial Observation Care codes and are not to be coded separately.

For example, an established patient was seen in the physician's office for frequent fainting of unknown origin. The history and examination were comprehensive and the MDM complexity was moderate. The code for the office visit would be 99215 (or if the patient were a Medicare patient, 99214). But the physician decided to admit the patient immediately on observation status until a further determination could be made as to the origin of the fainting. You would choose a code from the Hospital Observation Services subsection, Initial Observation Care subheading, in order to report the physician's service of admission on observation status (99219) and would not separately report the office visit (99215).

If a patient is admitted to observation status and then becomes ill enough to be admitted to the hospital, an Initial Hospital Care code (99221-99223), not an observation code, is used to report services.

CAUTION *Observation or Inpatient Care Services (including admission and discharge service), codes 99234-99236, have a very specific purpose: they report services to a patient who is admitted to and discharged from observation or inpatient status on the same day. All the services provided to the patient—same-day office services, observation care, and discharge—are covered by the use of one code from the 99234-99236 range.*

CODING SHOT When reporting physician services, Medicare requires a patient to be on observation status for more than 8 hours. A time period of 8 hours or less is reimbursed as initial observation status (99218-99220), even if the patient is discharged on the same date.

EXERCISE 2–9 *Hospital Observation Services*

Using the CPT manual, code the following:

1 A patient was in an automobile accident and is complaining of a minor headache and no other apparent injuries. History gathered from bystanders states that patient was not wearing a seat belt and hit his head on the windshield. A 15-minute loss of consciousness was noted. The patient was then admitted for 24-hour observation to rule out head injury. A comprehensive history and examination are done. The MDM is of moderate complexity.

Code: _____

Hospital Inpatient Services

Hospital Inpatient Services codes (99221-99239) are used to indicate a patient's status as an inpatient in a hospital or partial hospital setting and, therefore, to identify the hospital setting as the place where the physician renders service to the patient. An **inpatient** is one who has been formally admitted to an acute health care facility.

Note that within the subsection Hospital Inpatient Services, all the subheadings except Hospital Discharge Services are divided primarily on the basis of the three key components of history, examination, and MDM complexity. Further, within this subsection only Subsequent Hospital Care codes do not require all three key components to be at the level described in the code. For example, the key components for code 99222 are a comprehensive history, a comprehensive examination, and a moderate level of MDM complexity. If the case you are coding has a comprehensive history and a comprehensive examination but a low complexity of MDM, you cannot assign code 99222 to the case; instead, you would have to assign the lower level code of 99221, which has a low complexity of MDM.

The subsection of Hospital Inpatient Services is divided into three subheadings.

1. Initial Hospital Care
2. Subsequent Hospital Care
3. Hospital Discharge Services

Initial Hospital Care. Initial Hospital Care codes are used to code for the initial service of admission to the hospital by the admitting physician. Only the admitting physician can use the Initial Hospital Care codes. These codes reflect services in any setting (office, emergency department, nursing home) that are provided in conjunction with the admission to the hospital. For example, if the patient is seen in the office and subsequently is admitted to the hospital, the office visit is considered bundled into the initial hospital care service. All services provided in the office may be taken into account when selecting the appropriate level of hospital admission.

EXERCISE 2–10 *Initial Hospital Care*

Fill in the missing words or codes for the following:

1 Which Initial Hospital Care code has a comprehensive history with a straightforward or low complexity of MDM?

Code: _____

2 Which code has a time component of 70 minutes?

Code: _____

3 Code 99222 has a _____ history and examination level and a _____ MDM complexity.

4 An 80-year-old woman has inflammation of the kidneys and renal pelvic area. She is complaining of hematuria, dysuria, and pyuria. She is in good general health other than this condition. She has had some previous workup for this condition as an outpatient but is now being admitted for a cystoscopy. In the patient's history, the physician noted the patient's chief complaints and described the bright red nature of the hematuria, the severe discomfort associated with the dysuria, including burning and itching, and her other symptoms of frequency and urgency. The patient had stated that her symptoms had begun gradually over the past 2 weeks but had become more intense in the past 48 hours. The physician documented the patient's positive responses and pertinent negative responses in his review of her cardiovascular, respiratory, genitourinary, musculoskeletal, neurologic, and endocrine systems. Her past history relating to urinary and renal problems was reviewed. The physical examination noted the complete findings relative to her reproductive system as well as to her urinary system. An examination of her back and related musculoskeletal structures was included because she complained of mild back pain as well. After completing the detailed history and examination, the physician concluded with a provisional diagnosis of cystitis and pyelitis, possibly associated with endometritis. The MDM complexity was low. The patient was reassured and told to expect a short stay once the exact problem was pinpointed.

Code: _____

Subsequent Hospital Care. Subsequent Hospital Care codes (99231-99233) are the second subheading of codes in the Hospital Inpatient Services subsection. The Subsequent Hospital Care codes are used by physicians to report daily hospital visits while the patient is hospitalized.

The first Subsequent Hospital Care code is 99231. Typically, the 99231 level implies that the patient is in stable condition and is responding well to treatment. Subsequent codes in the subsection indicate (in the "Usually, the patient . . ." area) the status of the patient, such as stable/unstable or recovering/unresponding. Be certain to read the contributory factors area for each code in this subheading.

A general rule of thumb for subsequent hospital services is as follows:

Level 1 The patient is recovering and improving.

Level 2 The patient has a minor complication or inadequate response to the current therapy.

Level 3 The patient is unstable, has a significant complication, or has developed a new problem.

The patient's medical record should indicate the patient's progress from the status indicated in the previous note.

Several physicians, of different specialties, can use the subsequent care codes on the same day. This is called concurrent care. **Concurrent care** is being provided when more than one physician provides service to a patient on the same day for different conditions. An example of concurrent care is a circumstance in which physician A, a cardiologist, treats the patient for a heart condition and at the same time physician B, an oncologist, treats the patient for a cancer condition. The patient's attending (admitting) physician maintains the primary responsibility for the overall care of the patient, no matter how many other physicians are providing services to the patient, unless a formal transfer of care has occurred.

An **attending physician** is a doctor who, on the basis of education, training, and experience, is granted medical staff membership and clinical privileges by a health care organization to perform diagnostic or therapeutic procedures in the facility. An attending physician is legally responsible for the care and treatment provided to a patient. The attending physician may be a patient's personal physician or may be a physician assigned to a patient who has been admitted to a hospital through the emergency department. The attending physician is usually a provider of primary care, such as a family practitioner, internist, or pediatrician, but the attending physician may also be a surgeon or another type of specialist. In an academic medical center, the attending physician is a member of the academic or medical school staff who is responsible for the supervision of medical residents, interns, and medical school students and oversees the care the residents, interns, or students provide to the patients.

CODING SHOT Note that there is no comprehensive history or comprehensive examination level in the codes in the Subsequent Hospital Care subheading because the comprehensive level of service would have been provided at the time of admission.

Hospital Discharge Services. Inpatient Hospital Discharge Services (99238, 99239) are reported on the final day of services for a multiple-day stay in a hospital setting. The service reflects the final examination of the patient as appropriate, follow-up instructions to the patient, and arrangements for discharge, including completion of discharge records. The codes are based on the time spent by the physician in handling the final discharge of the patient and the time spent must be documented in the medical record.

The Hospital Discharge Services codes are not used if the physician is a consultant, unless the primary physician transfers complete care to the consultant. If a consulting physician is following the patient for a separate condition, those services would require a subsequent hospital care code. Only the attending physician, not the consultant, is responsible for completion of the final examination, follow-up instructions, and arrangements for discharge and discharge records. Because these additional services are included in the Hospital Discharge codes, only the attending physician's services can be reported using the codes.

QUICK CHECK 2-6

What is the one criterion for selecting a hospital discharge day management code?

_____

EXERCISE 2–11 *Hospital Discharge Services*

Fill in the blanks:

1 What are the times indicated for each of the Hospital Discharge Services codes?

_____

2 According to the category notes in Hospital Discharge Services, does the time spent by the physician arranging for the final hospital discharge of the patient have to be continuous?

_____

Consultation Services

We all need advice once in a while—maybe for a problem or situation that we cannot find a solution to. Perhaps we think we are doing the right thing but want another person's advice or view to make certain we are following the best course of action. Physicians need opinions and advice, too, and when they do, they ask another physician for an opinion or advice on the treatment, diagnosis, or management of a patient. The physician asking for the advice or opinion is making a **request for consultation** and is the **requesting** physician. The physician giving the advice is providing a consultation and is the **consultant.** Consultations can be done for both outpatients and inpatients. The CPT manual has different codes for each of the two types of patient consultation—outpatient and inpatient.

"Request for consultation" used to be termed "referral"; making a referral meant that the referring physician was asking for the advice or opinion of another physician (a consultation). However, some third-party payers have chosen to define **referral** to mean a total transfer of the care of a patient. In other words, if a patient is referred by physician A to physician B, physician A is expecting physician B to evaluate and treat the patient for the condition for which the patient is being referred. The services of physician B would **not** be reported using consultation codes. On the other hand, if physician A makes a **request for a consultation** to physician B, it is expected that physician B will provide physician A with his or her advice or opinion and that the patient will return to physician A for any necessary treatment. Physician B would then report his or her services using consultation codes. Although these semantics (uses of words) may seem unimportant, they make a difference in the codes you use to report the services.

QUICK CHECK 2-7

The criteria required to report a consultation include:

- _____ from the attending to the consultant to see the patient
- Evaluation of the patient by the consultant
- _____ back to the attending of the findings and recommendations of the consultant

In the Consultation subsection (99241-99255), there are two subheadings of consultations:

1. Office or Other Outpatient Consultations

2. Inpatient Consultations

These subheadings define the location in which the service is rendered; the patient is either an outpatient or an inpatient.

Only one initial consultation is reported by a consultant for the patient on each admission, and any subsequent service is reported using codes from the Subsequent Hospital Care codes (99231-99233) or Office or Other Outpatient Services, established patient (99211-99205). If more than one consultation is ordered on an inpatient, each consultant may report the initial consultation using the Inpatient Consultation codes (99251-99255).

A **consultation** is a service provided by a physician whose opinion or advice regarding the management or diagnosis of a specific problem has been requested. The consultant provides a written report of the opinion or advice to the attending physician and documents the opinion and services provided in the medical record; the care of the patient is thus complete. Sometimes the attending physician will request the consultant to assume responsibility for a specific area of the patient's care. For example, a consultant may be asked by the attending physician to see an inpatient regarding the care of the patient's diabetes while the patient is hospitalized for gallbladder surgery. After the initial consultation, the attending physician may ask the consultant to continue to monitor the patient's diabetic condition. The consultant assumes responsibility for management of the patient in the specific area of diabetes. Subsequent visits made by the consultant would then be coded using the codes from the subheading Subsequent Hospital Care or Subsequent Nursing Facility Care.

Documentation in the medical record for a consultation must show a request from a physician for an opinion or the advice of a consultant on a specific condition. Findings and treatments rendered during the consultation must be documented in the medical record by the consulting physician and communicated to the requesting physician. The consulting physician can order tests and services for a patient, but the medical necessity of all tests and services must be indicated in the medical record.

Office or Other Outpatient Consultations. The Office or Other Outpatient Consultations codes (99241-99245) are used to code consultative services provided to a patient in an office setting, including hospital observation services, home services, custodial care, and services that are provided in a domiciliary, rest home, or emergency department. Outpatient consultations include consultations provided in the emergency department because the patient is considered an outpatient in the emergency department setting. The codes are for both new and established patients. The codes in this subsection are of increasing complexity, based on the three key components and any contributory factors.

Inpatient Consultations. The codes in the Inpatient Consultations subheading (99251-99255) are used to report services by physicians in inpatient settings. This subheading is used for both new and established

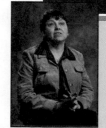

From the Trenches

"Keep the lines of communication open with fellow students, former instructors, co-workers, and the medical staff for whom you code. If you can establish yourself as someone who is dedicated to doing your work with integrity, interact with respect, and is always willing to help out, you will be successful."

JOAN

patients and can be reported only one time per patient admission, per consulting physician, per specialty.

After the initial consultation report, the subsequent hospital or nursing facility codes would be used to report services.

The office and inpatient consultation codes (99241-99255) require the documentation in the medical record to support all three of the key components listed in the code description. For example, 99243, office consultation, requires a detailed history and examination as well as a low level of medical decision making complexity. Let's say the documentation indicated a detailed history and examination, but only a straightforward level of medical decision making. Code 99243 could not be reported because only two of the three key components were at the correct level. The lower level code, 99242, would be assigned.

Various people request consultations on a recommended treatment or diagnosis. Insurance companies or other third-party payers may request a consultation regarding a diagnosis, prognosis, or treatment plan for a patient. These types of consultations are also coded based on the location of the service—office or inpatient. If the consultation is mandated, such as those required by an insurance company or a required school physical, add modifier -32 (Mandated Service) to the five-digit code. This modifier is only added if the consultation is mandated by an official body.

For office consultations, a letter stating the results is sent to the requesting physician. This is not necessary with an inpatient consultation because the physicians share the patient's medical record, and the inpatient consultant would dictate a consultation report to be included in the medical record.

QUICK CHECK 2-8

Can time be utilized to determine a consultation level of service rather than the key components?

Yes or No?

EXERCISE 2–12   *Consultation Services*

Using the CPT manual, code the visit in the following scenarios:

1 A 56-year-old female was sent by her primary care physician (PCP) to the oncologist for his opinion regarding the treatment options. The patient had had a right breast carcinoma 6 years earlier but over the past 4 months had developed progressively more painful back pain. In the physician's HPI it was noted that the pain was in the mid-back, with the patient rating it an 8 in intensity on a scale of 1 to 10. However, when the pain started, she thought it was about a 4 on the same scale. The pain has caused her to have neck and leg pains as well, as she has adjusted her walking stance in order to alleviate the pain. She responded to the physician's questions in the review of 10 of her organ systems. Her past medical and surgical history was noted, including the fact that her mother and one sister had also had breast cancer. A comprehensive history was taken. She had worked as a legal secretary up until 2 weeks earlier but is now on sick leave. The comprehensive physical examination performed by the physician was a complete multisystem review of 12 organ systems. The physician ordered a series of radiographic and laboratory tests and reviewed her recent spine x-ray series, which revealed multiple vertebral compression fractures. The MDM complexity was moderate.

Code: _____

2 A 45-year-old man was sent by his PCP to an orthopedic surgeon's office for acute pain and stiffness in his right elbow. In his problem focused history, the physician noted that the man was a farmer and used his right hand and arm repeatedly, lifting heavy objects. The patient had no other complaints and reported to be in otherwise excellent health. The patient described the pain as severe and unrelenting, and it prevented him from using his arm. The problem focused physical examination noted the man's slightly swollen right elbow, with marked pain on movement. No other problems were noted with his right upper extremity. The physician diagnosed the problem as elbow tendinitis and bursitis, recommended warm compresses, and gave the patient a prescription for an antiinflammatory medication. The MDM complexity was straightforward.

Code: _____

3 A 72-year-old man was seen in the internal medicine clinic as an outpatient for medical clearance prior to the replacement of his right knee. The patient had a history of essential hypertension and mild coronary artery disease. The internist noted, during the expanded problem focused history, that the patient had no complaints relative to his hypertension or heart disease. His blood pressure appeared to be controlled by his medication and low-salt diet. The patient denied any chest pain or discomfort either while working or at rest. In the physician's review, his cardiovascular and respiratory systems appeared to be negative. The physician performed an expanded problem focused physical examination of his head, neck, chest, and abdomen but found no major problems related to his cardiovascular or respiratory system. The internist confirmed the diagnoses previously established and made no changes in the management of either condition. The MDM complexity was straightforward.

Code: _____

4 A 52-year-old patient was sent to a surgeon for an office consultation concerning hemorrhoids. A problem focused history and examination were performed. The consultant recommended treating with medication after a straightforward MDM.

Code: _____

5 A 60-year-old man was seen in consultation by a cardiologist in the clinic for complaints of dyspnea, fatigue, and lightheadedness. His history included the insertion of a pacemaker 6 years earlier. He also had a history of mitral regurgitation. The cardiologist performed a comprehensive cardiology physical examination, including cardiac monitoring, pacemaker evaluation, and review of his associated respiratory status. Noted in the comprehensive history were a variety of complaints the patient had in addition to the past pacemaker insertion and mitral valve regurgitation diagnosed by cardiac catheterization. The physician reviewed the patient's medical history, from the first signs of problems 6 years earlier until the present. His review of systems elicited positive findings in the cardiovascular, respiratory, gastrointestinal, genitourinary, musculoskeletal, and neurologic systems. The other systems had negative responses. The physician had multiple management options concerning the pacemaker function but also had to consider new valvular problems that might have been present as well as related gastrointestinal symptoms. Extensive tests that had been performed recently were reviewed, and additional testing was ordered. The MDM complexity was moderate.

Code: _____

6 A 65-year-old man had recently undergone a prostatectomy for prostate cancer. Since the surgery, his previously controlled atrial fibrillation had become a problem again. A cardiologist was called in for an inpatient consultation; he reviewed the patient's present status, including the duration and severity of his symptoms. The cardiologist's review of systems related strictly to the cardiovascular system during an expanded problem focused history. The expanded problem focused physical examination concentrated on the man's neck, chest, and abdomen and attempted to elicit all cardiovascular pathology. The consultant suggested that the atrial fibrillation could be controlled better with a different medication. The MDM complexity was straightforward.

Code: _____

7 An internist requested an inpatient consultation from an orthopedic surgeon to evaluate and manage a 35-year-old female who had been in a motor vehicle accident. After reviewing the multiple x-ray reports and the documentation generated by the emergency department physicians, the paramedics' progress notes from the scene of the accident, and the history and physical examination produced by the internist, the orthopedist performed a complete review of systems; complete past, family, and social history; and extended details of the history of the present illness in a comprehensive history review. The comprehensive physical examination was a complete musculoskeletal and neurologic examination with a review of all other organ systems. Based on the patient's multiple fractures and internal injuries, the orthopedist concluded that the patient needed immediate surgery to repair and control the life-threatening conditions that existed. The MDM complexity was high. A neurosurgeon and a general surgeon were also asked to see the patient immediately and possibly to assist in surgery. (Code only the orthopedic consultation.)

Code: _____

8 A 55-year-old patient was injured at work when he fell from a house roof and struck his head. He was admitted for a right frontal parietal craniotomy with removal of a subdural hematoma. After 5 days of rapid recovery from this surgery, a consultation was requested regarding a drug reaction that produced a rash on his upper torso. The physician conducted a brief HPI during the expanded problem focused history, in addition to an ROS focused on the patient's condition. The expanded problem focused examination included three body areas and one organ system. The MDM complexity was straightforward.

Code: _____

9 A 10-year-old was admitted 4 days ago for tympanotomy. Postsurgically, the child developed fever and seizures of unknown origin. A pediatric consultation was requested. The HPI was extended with a complete ROS. A complete PFSH was elicited from the mother as part of a comprehensive history. A comprehensive examination was conducted on all body areas and organ systems. The MDM complexity was high.

Code: _____

10 A cardiologist was asked by a family practitioner to see an 80-year-old male inpatient a second time. One week prior, the patient, who had multiple other medical problems, had suffered an anterior wall myocardial infarction. Despite following the medical management suggested by the cardiologist, the patient continued to have angina and ventricular arrhythmias. The cardiologist closely examined all of the documentation and test results that had been generated in the past week and performed a complete ROS and an extended HPI during the detailed interval history. The detailed physical examination performed was a complete cardiovascular system examination. Based on the subjective and objective findings, the cardiologist concluded that more aggressive medical management was in order. Given the patient's multiple problems coupled with the new threat of cardiorespiratory failure, the patient was immediately transferred to the intensive care unit. The MDM was of high complexity.

Code: _____

11 The attending physician had requested an inpatient consultation on a 10-year-old admitted 7 days earlier for tympanotomy. Postsurgically, the patient developed fever and seizures. An initial consultation diagnosis was febrile seizure. Now, on day 7, the child's temperature had returned to normal but the child had had a recurrence of seizures of increased severity. A follow-up consultation was requested. The consultant performed a detailed history and physical examination. The MDM was of high complexity.

Code: _____

12 Dr. Jones asked Dr. Williams to confirm the diagnosis of tetralogy of Fallot in a 6-day-old male infant prior to cardiovascular surgery. The patient was seen in the office, where Dr. Williams performed an initial comprehensive history and physical examination on the infant and reviewed the results of the extensive tests already performed. The consultant concluded that the child's problem was of high severity and recommended immediate surgery. The MDM complexity was moderate.

Code: _____

13 The 45-year-old female's insurance company required a second opinion regarding the degenerative disk disease of her lumbar spine. One orthopedic surgeon had recommended a laminectomy. A second orthopedic surgeon was consulted in the office and performed an expanded problem focused history and physical examination, particularly of her musculoskeletal and neurologic systems. Based on his findings and the conclusive findings of a recent myelogram, the second orthopedic surgeon was quick to conclude that the laminectomy was a reasonable course to follow. The MDM complexity was straightforward.

Code: _____

14 A third-party payer sought consultation for confirmation about a patient's ability to return to work after the removal of a subdural hematoma 2 months previously. The patient's primary physician had stated that the patient was not yet able to return to his employment, and the third-party payer wanted a second opinion. The patient stated that he continued to have severe and incapacitating headaches and was unable to return to work. A comprehensive history and physical examination were performed in the office. The MDM was of moderate complexity, based on physician findings.

Code: _____

Emergency Department Services

Emergency Department Services codes (99281-99288) are used for new or established patients when services are provided in an emergency department that is a part of a hospital and available 24 hours a day. These patients are presenting for immediate attention. The codes are used for patients without appointments. Emergency Department Services codes are not used for patients at the hospital on observation status, even if the observation unit is located at or near the emergency department.

Codes 99281-99285 are based on the type of service the physician performs in terms of the history, the examination, and the complexity of the MDM. These codes require all three of the key components to be assigned. In addition to this information within each code, note that the paragraph at the end of each code that begins with "Usually, the presenting problem(s) are of . . ." identifies the immediacy of the care. For example, 99283 indicates that the presenting problem is of "moderate severity," whereas 99285 indicates that the presenting problem is of "high severity and poses an immediate significant threat to life . . ." Sometimes the patient's clinical condition poses an immediate threat to life, making it possible for the physician to use the higher level code even if it may not be possible to perform the required history and physical examination.

QUICK CHECK 2-9

1. What are the times associated with codes 99281-99285?

_____

2. If a patient presents to the emergency department in a clinically life-threatening state that prevents the physician from performing a complete history or physical examination, could the code 99285 still be reported?
Yes or No?

Critical care provided to a patient in the emergency department is reported using additional codes from the Critical Care Service code section, which we will discuss in another section.

If a patient initially treated in the emergency department requires admittance to the hospital, the patient's attending physician would serve as the admitting physician.

Emergency department codes can be used to report the services not only of the ED physician, but also of any physician who cares for a patient in the ED. For example, if the patient's primary care physician (PCP) meets the patient at the ED or is called into the ED, and the PCP cares for the patient in the ED, not admitting the patient to the hospital, then the PCP reports the services using ED codes.

Also, ED physicians do not admit patients to a hospital. If a patient is seen in the ED and has to be admitted to the hospital, the patient's PCP will admit the patient.

Other Emergency Department Services. The Other Emergency Department Services subheading is at the end of the Emergency Department Services subsection, and the code located there (99288) is used to report the services of a physician based at the hospital who provides two-way communication with the ambulance or rescue team. This physician provides direction and advice to the team as they attend the patient en route to the emergency department.

The subheading notes contain examples of the types of medical services the physician might direct. Be certain to read these notes so you understand the types of services the code refers to.

EXERCISE 2–13 *Emergency Department Services*

Use the information contained in the code descriptions in the Emergency Department Services subsection to answer the questions in this exercise.

1 The severity of the presenting problem for code 99281 would usually be

_____.

2 The severity of the presenting problem for code 99284 would usually be

_____.

3 The severity of the presenting problem for code 99283 would usually be

_____.

4 The severity of the presenting problem for code 99282 would usually be

_____.

Code the following:

5 A patient in the emergency department has extreme acute chest pains and goes into cardiac arrest. The emergency department physician is unable to obtain a history or perform a physical examination because the patient's condition is critical. The MDM is of high complexity.

Code(s): _____

6 A patient in the emergency department has a temperature of 105° F and is in acute respiratory distress. Symptoms include shortness of breath, chest pain, cyanosis, and gasping. The physician is unable to obtain a history or perform a comprehensive physical examination because the patient's condition is critical. The MDM complexity is high.

Code(s): _____

7 A child presents to the emergency department with his parents after being bitten by a dog. The child is in extreme pain and bleeding from a wound on the forearm. The animal has not been located to quarantine for rabies. An expanded problem focused history is obtained and an expanded problem focused physical examination is performed. The MDM complexity is moderate because of the possibility of rabies.

Code(s): _____

8 The physician directs the emergency medical technicians via two-way communications with an ambulance en route to the emergency department with a patient in apparent cardiac arrest.

Code(s): _____

Critical Care Services

Critical Care Services codes (99291-99292) are used to identify services that are provided during medical emergencies to patients over 24 months of age who are either critically ill or injured. These service codes require the physician to be constantly available to the patient and providing services exclusively to that patient. For example, a patient who is in shock or cardiac arrest would require the physician to provide bedside critical care services. Critical care is often, but not required to be, provided in an acute care setting of a hospital. Acute care settings are intensive care units, coronary care units, emergency departments, and similar critical care units of a hospital. Codes in this subsection are listed according to the time the physician spends providing critical care to the patient. The time calculation is not just the face-to-face time the physician spends with the patient. The review of records and diagnostic results at the time of the encounter should also be counted in determining the time spent in providing critical care to the patient. The time the physician spends in providing other procedures must be deducted from the total critical care time. For example, if an adult patient is intubated during critical care, the time spent on the intubation (31500) is deducted from the total critical care time.

The total critical care time, per day, the physician spends in care of the patient is stated in one amount of time, even if the time was not continuous. Code 99291 is used only once a day. Code 99291 is reported for the first 30 to 74 minutes of critical care, and code 99292 is used for the time beyond 74 minutes. If the critical care is less than 30 minutes, an E/M code would be used to report the service.

TOTAL DURATION OF CRITICAL CARE TIME	CPT CODES
Less than 30 minutes	Appropriate E/M code
30-74 minutes	99291
75-104 minutes	99291 and 99292
105-134 minutes	99291 and 99292 × 2
135-164 minutes	99291 and 99292 × 3
165-194 minutes	99291 and 99292 × 4
194 minutes or longer	99291 and 99292 × each additional 30 minutes over initial 74

As an example, if a physician sees a critical care patient for 74 minutes and then leaves and returns for 30 minutes of critical care at a later time in the same day, the coding would be for 104 minutes of care. The coding for 104 minutes would be:

99291 for the 74 minutes

99292 for the additional 30 minutes

CODING SHOT Most third-party payers will not pay for more than one physician at a time for critical care services.

There are service codes that are bundled into the Critical Care Services codes. These services are normally provided to stabilize the patient. An example of this bundling is as follows: A physician starts ventilation management (94002) while providing critical care services to a patient in the intensive care unit of a hospital. The ventilator management is not reported separately but, instead, is considered to be bundled into the Critical Care Services code. The notes preceding the critical care codes in the CPT manual list the services and procedures bundled into the codes. If the physician provided a service at the same time as critical care and that service is not bundled into the code, the service could be reported separately. Some third-party payers may require the use of modifier -25 with the critical care codes when reporting a service that is not bundled into the Critical Care Services. You will know what is bundled into the codes because this information is listed either in the extensive description of the code or in the notes preceding the code. Be certain to read these notes, as they contain many exclusions and inclusions for these codes.

If the patient is in a critical care unit but is stable, you report the services using codes from the Hospital Inpatient Services subsection, Subsequent Hospital Care subheading or from the Consultations subsection, Inpatient subheading.

QUICK CHECK 2-10

List two types of service and the CPT code for the service that are bundled into critical care services.

Such as: Gastric intubation (43752, 91105)

_____

_____

EXERCISE 2-14 *Critical Care Services*

Fill in the information for the following:

1 Critical care is provided to a 50-year-old patient for 70 minutes.

    🔗 Code(s): _____

2 Can code 99292 be reported without code 99291? _____

3 A physician is called to the intensive care unit to provide care for a 24-year-old patient who has received second-degree burns over 50% of his body. The physician provides support for 2 hours. After leaving the unit, the physician returns later that day to provide an additional hour of critical care support to the patient.

    🔗 Code(s): _____

Nursing Facility Services

A **nursing facility** is not a hospital but does have inpatient beds and a professional health care staff that provides health care to persons who do not require the level of service provided in an acute care facility.

A **skilled nursing facility** (SNF) is one that has a professional staff that often includes physicians and nurses. The patients of a skilled nursing facility require less care than that given in an acute care hospital, but more care than that provided in a nursing home. Skilled nursing facilities are also called skilled nursing units, skilled nursing care, or extended care facilities. Professional and practical nursing services are available 24 hours a day. Rehabilitation services, such as occupational therapy, physical therapy, and speech therapy, are available on a daily basis. A skilled nursing facility may previously have been called an extended care facility. Patients may stay for several weeks in a skilled nursing facility before returning home or being transferred to an intermediate care facility for long-term care. Skilled nursing facilities provide care for individuals of all ages, even though the majority of services are provided to geriatric patients.

An **intermediate care facility** provides regular, basic health services to individuals who do not need the degree of care or treatment provided in a hospital or a skilled nursing facility. Residents, because of their mental or physical conditions, require assistance with their activities of daily living, such as bathing, dressing, eating, and ambulating. Intermediate care facilities generally provide long-term care, usually over several years. Professional and practical nursing services are available on a 24-hour basis. Activities, social services, and dietary and other therapies are available on a daily basis. The majority of residents of intermediate care facilities are geriatric individuals or individuals of any age with mental retardation or developmental disabilities.

The phrase **long-term care facility** describes health and personal services provided to ill, aged, disabled, or retarded individuals for an extended period of time. Other types of facilities are better described as skilled or intermediate care facilities.

Four subheadings of nursing facility services are available: Initial Nursing Facility Care, Subsequent Nursing Facility Care, Nursing Facility Discharge Services, and Other Nursing Facility Services.

Initial Nursing Facility Care. Initial Nursing Facility Care codes (99304-99306) do not distinguish between new and established patients. These codes are used to report services provided by the physician at the time of admission or re-admission. Assessments by physicians play a central role in the development of the resident's individualized care plan. The care plan is developed by an interdisciplinary care team using the Resident Assessment Instrument (RAI) and the Minimum Data Set (MDS).

Subsequent Nursing Facility Care. Subsequent Nursing Facility Care codes (99307-99310) do not distinguish between a new and an established patient. These codes reflect services provided by a physician on a periodic basis when a resident does not need a comprehensive assessment. Typically, such a resident has not had a major change in his or her condition since the previous physician visit but requires ongoing management of a chronic condition or treatment of an acute short-term problem. The higher level codes are developed to address patients with new problems or significant changes in existing problems.

Nursing Facility Discharge Services. The Nursing Facility Discharge Services codes (99315, 99316) are used to report the services the physician renders to the patient on the day of discharge. The code is assigned based on the amount of time documented for discharge management. Code 99315 is assigned if 30 minutes or less or no time is documented. Code 99316 is reported for documented time of greater than 30 minutes. The time spent need not be continuous or spent entirely with the patient but must be documented. The physician may conduct a final physical examination, give instructions to the patient's caregivers, and prepare all necessary discharge documentation, referral forms, and medication orders.

Other Nursing Facility Services. Other Nursing Facility Services contains only one code, 99318, that is used to report the annual nursing facility assessment provided by the physician. By law, the nursing facility must conduct a comprehensive assessment of each resident at least once a year and if there is any significant change in the resident's physical or mental condition. As with many subheadings throughout the E/M section, if a patient is admitted to a nursing facility but the service was started elsewhere, such as a physician's office or emergency department, all the evaluation and management services provided to the patient are considered part of the nursing facility code. For example, a patient was seen in the hospital emergency department, where a comprehensive history and examination were performed for a condition that required high MDM complexity, coded 99285, Emergency Department Services. The physician made the decision to admit the patient to a nursing facility on the same day. Rather than coding the 99285 (Emergency Department Services), you would code the same level service from the subheading Initial Nursing Facility Care, code 99306.

Nursing Facility Services codes are also used for coding services in a type of place you would not think would apply—psychiatric residential treatment centers. The center must be a stand-alone facility or a separate part of a facility that provides group living facilities and it must have 24-hour staffing. Nursing Facility Services codes are used to identify evaluation and management services. If a physician also provides medical psychotherapy, you would code those services separately.

When a patient has been in the hospital and is discharged from the hospital to a nursing facility, all on the same day, you can code the hospital discharge (99238-99239) and the nursing facility admission (99304-99306) separately. This is also true for same-day services for patients who are discharged from observation status (99217) and admitted to a nursing facility (99304-99306).

EXERCISE 2–15 *Nursing Facility Services*

Answer the following:

1 According to the code description for 99305, the usual level of severity of the problem(s) that

required admission to the nursing facility is: _____

2 A 72-year-old male patient is transferred to a nursing facility from a hospital after suffering a cerebrovascular accident (stroke). The patient needs a comprehensive assessment before his active rehabilitation plan can be started. A comprehensive history is gathered by the internist, including the patient's chief complaint of paralysis and weakness, an extended HPI, and a complete ROS. Details of the patient's past, family, and social history add information to the care-planning process. The internist performs a comprehensive multisystem physical examination. After much deliberation with the multidisciplinary rehabilitation team, the physician determines that the patient is ready for active rehabilitation. The physician also writes orders to continue treatment of the patient's other medical conditions, including hypertension and diabetes. The MDM complexity is high.

⚙ Code(s): _____

Using the following information within the code descriptions in the Subsequent Nursing Facility Care subheading, match the medical decision making complexity in the description of the code with the code:

3 99307 _____   a. moderate

4 99308 _____   b. low

5 99309 _____   c. straight forward

Code the following:

6 Subsequent follow-up care is provided for a comatose patient transferred to a long-term care center from the hospital. The resident shows no signs of consciousness on examination but appears to have developed a minor upper respiratory tract infection with a fever and cough. The physician performs an expanded problem focused interval history (by way of nursing staff notes) and physical examination, including neurologic status, respiratory status, and status of related organ systems. Because the physician is concerned that the respiratory infection could progress to pneumonia, appropriate treatment is ordered. The MDM complexity is moderate.

⚙ Code(s): _____

| Domiciliary, Rest Home (e.g., Boarding Home), or Custodial Care Services | These codes (99324-99337) are divided into subheadings based on the patients' status as new or established service provided. The codes are arranged in levels based on the documentation in the patients' medical records. Time estimates are established for codes in this category. |

These codes are used for the evaluation and management of residents who reside in a domiciliary, rest home, or custodial care center. Generally, health services are not available on site, nor are any medical services included in the codes. These facilities provide residential care, including lodging, meals, supervision, personal care, and leisure activities, to persons who, because of their physical, mental, or emotional condition, are not able to live independently. Such facilities might include alternative living residences, assisted living facilities, retirement centers, community-based living units, group homes, or residential treatment centers. These facilities provide custodial care for residents of all ages.

Domiciliary, Rest Home (e.g., Assisted Living Facility), or Home Care Plan Oversight Services

Codes 99339-99340 apply to services provided to a patient who is being cared for at home and not enrolled with a home health care agency. These patients are being cared for by family members, health care professionals, and other types of caregivers. These codes are not reported if the patient is receiving his or her care from a home health agency, hospice program, or nursing facility. When reporting these codes the patient is not present, rather the physician is developing a care plan or overseeing the care of the patient. The physician's time may be reported if the time was over 15 minutes within a calendar month. Code 99339 reports 15-29 minutes, and 99340 reports 30 minutes or more. Again, these codes are only reported once for each calendar month.

Home Services

Health care services can also be provided to patients in their homes. Times have been established for this category of services. Note that there is a statement about typical time located under the code description in the paragraph that begins, "Usually, the presenting problem(s) is . . ." Never report a code based on time unless at least 50% of the time was spent on counseling/coordinating care. The codes (99341-99350) for these services are also divided into categories for new and for established patients.

From the Trenches

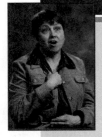

"I have found that there is definitely a sense of family among coders. Like all families, we don't always agree on everything, but we care about each other's thoughts and challenges . . . and know that there is always someone out there that can be there for you, whether it is a coding dilemma or a bigger, career-type decision."

JOAN

EXERCISE 2–16 *Home Services*

Code the following scenario:

1 A 64-year-old established female patient has diabetes mellitus and has been having problems adjusting her insulin doses. She has had an onset of dizziness and sensitivity to light. The physician makes a home visit during which he gathers a brief HPI and a problem-pertinent ROS during the problem focused history. The problem focused physical examination focuses on the body systems currently affected by the diabetes. The physician finds the patient's condition to be moderately severe and the MDM complexity is straightforward.

🌐 Code(s): _____

Prolonged Services

In the Prolonged Services subsection there are three subheadings:

- Prolonged Physician Service *With* Direct (Face-to-Face) Patient Contact
- Prolonged Physician Service *Without* Direct (Face-to-Face) Patient Contact
- Physician Standby Services

Prolonged Physician Services With or Without Direct Patient Contact. Prolonged Physician Services codes (99354-99359) are all add-on codes. Note the plus symbol (+) beside all codes in the range 99354 to 99359. Because add-on codes can be used only with another code, all Prolonged Physician Services codes are intended to be used only in addition to other codes to show an extension of some other service. The following example illustrates the use of these codes.

Example

An established patient with a history of COPD presents, in an office visit, with moderate respiratory distress. The physician conducts a problem focused history followed by a problem focused examination, which shows a respiratory rate of 30, and labored breathing and wheezing are heard in all lung fields. Office treatment is initiated; it includes intermittent bronchial dilation and subcutaneous epinephrine. The service requires the physician to have intermittent face-to-face contact with the patient over a 2-hour period. The MDM complexity is low.

The office visit service would be reported using the office visit code 99212; but the additional time the physician spent providing service to the patient over and above that which is indicated in code 99212 would have to be coded using a prolonged service code.

CAUTION *If you hadn't carefully read the notes preceding the Prolonged Services codes, you would not know that there are many rules that govern the calculation of time when determining the codes.*

As the notes indicate, the first 30 minutes of prolonged services are not even counted but are considered part of the initial service. So you cannot use a prolonged services code until after the first 30 minutes of the prolonged services have been provided. The physician, therefore, has to spend 30-74 minutes with the patient in prolonged services before it is possible to code for 30 minutes using code 99354. That takes care of 30-74 minutes of our physician's time for the case above. Now, what about the next hour?

Read the description for the indented code 99355. The description states that 99355 is to be used for each additional 30 minutes; but this is where the second time rule comes in. You can use 99355 only if the physician has spent at least 15 minutes providing service over and above the first 60 minutes. The physician in this example spent 1 hour beyond the first 60 minutes providing service, so we can claim 99355 twice. The coding for the case is 99212 for the office visit; 99354 for the first hour of prolonged services; and 99355 × 2 for the next hour.

The time the physician spends providing the prolonged services does not have to be continuous, as is the situation in this example; the physician monitored the patient on an intermittent basis, coming into the room to check on the patient and then leaving the room.

But let's change this case a bit and see how the coding changes. If the physician spent 70 minutes with the patient, you could code only the first hour at 99354. The additional 10 minutes beyond the first 60 are not coded separately. Remember that you would need at least 15 minutes beyond the first hour to code for the time beyond the first hour. For help in applying these codes, note the table preceding the codes; there you can locate the total time your physician spent with the patient and see an example of the correct coding.

The face-to-face Prolonged Physician Services codes describe services that require the physician to have **direct contact** with the patient; but the Prolonged Physician Services Without Direct (Face-to-Face) Patient Contact codes describe services during which the physician is not in direct contact with the patient. For example, a physician evaluates an established patient, a 70-year-old female with dementia, in an office visit. The physician then spends an extensive amount of time discussing the patient's condition, her treatment plan, and other recommendations with the daughter of the patient. The services would be reported by using an office visit code for the patient evaluation and the appropriate prolonged service without face-to-face contact code for the time spent with the daughter.

Prolonged Physician Services codes are most often used with the higher level E/M codes, which themselves carry longer time frames. According to the CPT notes for Prolonged Physician Services, these codes are add-on codes and are reported in addition to another E/M code.

Prolonged Physician Services With Direct Patient Contact codes are divided on the basis of whether the services were provided to an outpatient or an inpatient.

Physician Standby Services. The code (99360) for Physician Standby Services is used when a physician, at the request of the attending physician, is standing by in case his or her services are needed. The standby physician cannot be rendering services to another patient during this time. The standby code is reported in increments of 30 minutes. The 30-minute increments referred to here really mean from the 1st minute to the 30th minute and do not have any of the complicated rules for reporting time that exist for reporting prolonged or critical services.

An important note concerning the standby code is that this code is used only when **no service** is performed and there is **no face-to-face contact** with the patient. This code is not used when a standby status ends, and the physician is providing a service to a patient. The service the physician provides is reported as any other service would be, even though it began as a physician standby service.

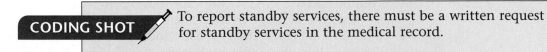

CODING SHOT To report standby services, there must be a written request for standby services in the medical record.

Read the notes before code 99360 before completing Exercise 2–17.

EXERCISE 2–17 *Prolonged and Physician Standby Services*

Using the notes in the subsections, answer the following:

1 Does the time the physician spends with the patient in prolonged, direct contact have to be continuous? _____

2 Can a code from the Prolonged Services subsection be reported alone? _____

3 If the prolonged contact with the patient lasts less than 30 minutes, is the time reported separately? _____

4 The codes in the Prolonged Physician Services With Direct Patient Contact subheading are based not only on the time the physician spends with the patient, but also on another factor. What is that other factor? _____

5 Are the codes in the subheading Prolonged Physician Services Without Direct Patient Contact categorized according to the place of service? _____

6 According to the notes in the Physician Standby Services subsection, can a physician report the time spent in proctoring (monitoring) another physician? _____

Case Management Services

The Case Management Services subsection (99363-99368) consists of codes used by physicians to report anticoagulant therapy and coordination of care services with other health care professionals.

EXERCISE 2–18 *Case Management Services*

Complete the following:

1 What is the time component specified in the Medical Team Conference codes from the Case Management Services subsection? _____

_____

2 What are the three Medical Team Conferences codes? _____

_____

Anticoagulant Management

The codes report anticoagulant services using warfarin/Coumadin. Anticoagulants inhibit coagulation of the blood and are prescribed to patients with various thromboembolic disorders. Patients on this medication are monitored by means of blood tests and adjustments are then made in the blood thinner dosage if the physician determines the clotting levels are not ideal. Codes 99363 and 99364 are used to report the monitoring sevices provided on an outpatient basis for the initial 90 days of therapy (with a minimum of 8 assessments) and each subsequent 90 days of therapy (with at least 3 assessments). Any period less than 60 days is not reported and only outpatient anticoagulant management is reported.

Medical Team Conferences

The medical team must include at least three qualified health care professionals that are from different specialties. The team members must have all performed a face-to-face evaluation or treatment of the patient within the previous 60 days. Codes 99366-99368 are divided based on if the patient and/or family is/are present in the conference and with the participation of the physician or a nonphysician health care professional.

Care Plan Oversight Services

At times, a physician is asked to manage a complex case that involves an individual such as a hospice patient or a patient who is homebound and receives the majority of his or her health care from visiting nurses. When regular communication is necessary between the nurses and the physician to discuss revising the care plan, coordinating the treatment plan with other professionals, or adjusting the therapies, codes from the Care Plan Oversight Services subsection (99374-99380) may be used to report these additional services. The codes are divided according to whether the physician is supervising a patient being cared for by home health workers or a patient in a hospice or nursing facility. The codes are also divided based on the length of time of the service—either 15 to 29 minutes or 30 minutes or more. Reporting is by time over a month-long period.

Preventive Medicine Services

Use Preventive Medicine Services codes (99381-99429) to report the routine evaluation and management of a patient who is healthy and has no complaint. The codes in this subsection would be used to report a routine physical examination done at the patient's request, such as a well-baby check-up. Preventive Medicine codes are intended to be used to identify comprehensive services, not a single system. The codes are used for infants, children, adolescents, and adults; they differ according to the age of the patient and whether the patient is a new or an established patient.

CODING SHOT

If the physician should encounter a problem or abnormality during the course of a preventive service, and the problem or abnormality requires significant additional service, you can also code an office visit code with a modifier -25 added. The modifier -25 is used to indicate that a significant, separately identifiable E/M service was performed by the physician on the same day as the preventive medicine service. If you did not add the modifier -25, the third-party payer would think that you had made an error and were reporting both a preventive medicine service code and an office visit code for the same service. Only with the use of the modifier -25 can you convey that the services were indeed separate.

Note that in the code descriptions for both the New Patient and the Established Patient categories, the terms "comprehensive history" and "comprehensive examination" are used. These terms are not the same as the ones used with other E/M codes (99201-99350). Here, "comprehensive" means a complete history and a complete examination, as is conducted during an annual physical. The comprehensive examination performed as part of the preventive medicine E/M service is a multisystem examination, but the extent of the examination is determined by the age of the patient and the risk factors identified for that individual.

EXERCISE 2-19 *Preventive Medicine Services*

Complete the following:

1 According to the notes in the Preventive Medicine Services subsection, the extent and focus of the services provided, whether to a new or to an established patient, will depend largely upon

what factor? _____

2 If, during the preventive medicine evaluation, a problem is encountered that requires the physician to perform a problem focused E/M service, what modifier would be appended to the

code? _____

Counseling Risk Factor Reduction and Behavior Change Intervention. These codes (99401-99429) are for both new and established healthy patients. The services are based on whether individual or group counseling is provided to the patient and on the amount of time the service requires. Codes in this category would be used to report a physician's services to a patient for risk factor interventional counseling, such as a diet and exercise program, smoking cessation, or contraceptive management.

Non-Face-to-Face Physician Services

These codes are divided into Telephone Services (99441-99443) and On-Line Medical Evaluation (99444) and are used to report services provided by a physician. To report these same services provided by a nonphysician, use Medicine codes 98966-98969. The notes and the code descriptions for these codes indicate that the telephone or online service cannot originate from a related assessment that was provided within the previous seven days or result in an appointment within the next 24 hours or the soonest available appointment. The telephone services are reported based on the documented time, and the online service is per incident.

Special Evaluation and Management Services

The codes in this subsection (99450-99456) are used to report evaluations for life or disability insurance baseline information. The services can be performed in any setting for either a new or an established patient. The codes vary, based on whether the service is for an examination for life or disability insurance and whether the examination is done by the physician treating the patient's disability or by someone other than the treating physician.

EXERCISE 2-20 *Special Evaluation and Management Services*

Answer the following:

1 An insurance examination was conducted by the physician for a new patient for a term life insurance policy. From what subheading would you select a code to report this service?

_____

2 A 50-year-old man was referred for a disability examination. The patient had been injured at work when he slipped off a ladder and fell from a height of 10 feet, landing on his back. He has not returned to work since that time 6 months ago. The patient had been under the care of a physician from another state and was referred by the insurance company for the assessment of the patient's ability to return to work. His primary physician had stated that this patient will be unable to return to his previous work as a bricklayer. From what subheading would you select a code to report

this service? _____

3 What is the difference between the two codes in the Work Related or Medical Disability Evaluation

Services codes? _____

_____

_____

4 A 58-year-old man was seen by his private physician for an examination as part of his claim for long-term medical disability. The patient has chronic obstructive lung disease with severe emphysema and has been unable to work during the past year. The physician completed all the necessary documentation required by the insurance company, including his opinion that the patient would be unable to work in the future, as his pulmonary function is markedly impaired, in spite of continual respiratory and pharmacologic therapy.

Code: _____

Newborn Care Services

Newborn Care Services codes 99460 through 99465 report services provided to normal newborns from birth through 28 days of age. There are three history and examination codes; one is specifically for a newborn assessment and discharge from a hospital or birthing center on the same date (99463), one is for initial assessment **in** a hospital or birthing center (99460), and one is for initial assessment **in other** than a hospital or birthing center (99461). All of the codes report a "per day" service, which is a 24-hour period. Subsequent services are reported with 99462, also a per day service. If the physician provides a discharge service to a newborn on a date that is subsequent to the admission date, you would assign a code from the Hospital Inpatient Services, Hospital Discharge Services (99238, 99239).

Delivery/Birthing Room Attendance codes 99464 and 99465 report the attendance of a physician, at the request of the delivering physician, to provide the initial stabilization of a newborn or for the resuscitation/ventilation of the newborn. The request for physician's attendance must be documented in the patient's medical record. These attendance codes are reported in addition to the other services provided. For example, a physician is requested to be in attendance at the time of delivery to provided newborn resuscitation (report 99465). The physician also performs an emergency endotracheal intubation (report 31500).

Inpatient Neonatal Intensive Care Services and Pediatric and Neonatal Critical Care Services

Pediatric Critical Care Patient Transport. Codes 99466 and 99467 report face-to-face physician services provided to a pediatric patient (24 months of age or less). During the provision of these services, the patient is being transported from one facility to another and the physician is in direct contact with the patient during the transport. The codes are time-based and time less than 30 minutes is not reported with these transport codes. The codes are divided on the first 30 to 74 minutes and each additional 30 minutes beyond 74. Bundled into the codes are routine monitoring evaluations, such as heart rate and blood pressure. Other services provided by the physician before transport and nonroutine services provided during transport may be reported separately.

Inpatient Neonatal and Pediatric Critical Care. Critical care inpatient services provided to neonates (28 days or less) are reported with 99468 and 99469. Critical care inpatient services provided to pediatric patients (29 days through 24 months) are reported with 99471/99472 and pediatric patients 2 through 5 years of age are reported with 99475/ 99476. Critical care provided to pediatric patients 6 years of age and older is reported with the adult critical care codes 99291/99292.

The name of the intensive care unit does not matter in the assignment of these codes. The services can be provided in a pediatric intensive care unit, neonatal critical care unit, or any of the many other names of these intensive care units. Bundled into the codes are many services you would anticipate would be provided in support of a critically ill neonate/pediatric patient (for example, arterial catheters, nasogastric tube placement, endotracheal intubation, and invasive electronic monitoring of vital signs). The notes preceding the codes detail the bundled services, such as 31500, endotracheal intubation, that are bundled into the codes and not reported separately. To ensure that you do not unbundle, refer back to the list of bundled services when assigning these codes. If the physician performed a service not listed as a bundled service, report the service separately. The bundled services also include those procedures listed as bundled for the critical care codes 99291 and 99292. For example, gastric intubation (43752, 91105) is bundled into critical care codes 99291 and 99292 and is therefore bundled into the neonate/pediatric critical care codes.

Initial and Continuing Intensive Care Services. When a neonate or infant is not considered critically ill but still needs intensive observation and other intensive care services, the Initial and Continuing Intensive Care Services codes (99477-99480) are reported. All of these codes, except for 99477, are not based on the age of the patient, but are based on the weight of the infant:

- Very low birth weight (VLBW) is less than 1500 grams (less than 3.3 pounds)

- Low birth weight (LBW) is 1500-2500 grams (3.3-5.5 pounds)

- Normal birth weight is 2501-5000 grams (5.51-11.01 pounds)

The assignment of these codes changes as the weight of the neonate/infant changes. The codes are reported only once per day (24-hours). If the neonate or pediatric patient receives the service in an outpatient setting, critical care codes 99291 and 99292 are reported because 99468-99476 codes are only reported for inpatients.

EXERCISE 2–21 *Newborn Care and Neonatal/Pediatric Critical Care Services*

Answer the following:

1. What does the abbreviation VLBW mean?_____

2. What code would you assign to report the face-to-face service provided by a physician during an interfacility transport of a critically ill patient who is 16 months of age? The service was for

   60 minutes. _____

3. A normal newborn was admitted to the hospital on Saturday morning and was discharged Saturday evening. The physician provided evaluation and management services including the admission and the discharge. What code would you assign to report the physician service?

   _____

4. The physician provided a subsequent inpatient service to a 3-year-old critically ill patient.

   🖜 Code: _____

5. The physician provided an intensive care inpatient service to an infant of very low birth weight on the patient's second day of the hospital stay.

   🖜 Code: _____

Other Evaluation and Management Services

Other Evaluation and Management Services (99499) is the last subsection in the E/M section. Code 99499 is an unlisted code that is used to indicate that there is no other code that accurately represents the services provided to the patient. A special report would accompany the unlisted E/M service code.

Coding Practice

CONGRATULATIONS! Good job! You have been through all of the E/M codes and are now familiar with the basics of CPT code arrangement. Can you imagine how well you would know your favorite novel if you read it several times a month? Well, coders use their CPT manuals every day and become very familiar with the information in the guidelines, notes, and descriptions of the codes. Please be sure to locate the code in the CPT manual and read all notes, guidelines, and descriptions about each code you work with. In this way, you will build a solid knowledge foundation.

Now let's begin to do some coding that will require you to combine all the information you have learned in Chapters 1 and 2 as you begin to code patient cases.

EXERCISE 2-22 *Coding Practice*

Code the following:

1 A new patient is seen in the office for an earache (otalgia). The history and examination are problem focused and the MDM complexity is straightforward.

☥ Code(s): _____

2 An established patient is seen in the office of an ENT (ear-nose-throat) specialist with the chief complaint of otalgia. The physician completes a problem focused history and physical examination of the head, eyes, ears, nose, and throat. To the physician, this is a straightforward case of acute otitis media, and prescription medications are ordered. The MDM complexity is straightforward.

☥ Code(s): _____

3 An established patient is seen in the office for a blood pressure check, which is done by the physician's nurse.

☥ Code(s): _____

4 Lilly Wilson, a new patient, is seen by the physician in the skilled nursing facility for an initial nursing facility assessment. Mrs. Wilson recently suffered a cerebral thrombosis with residual dysphagia and paresis of the left extremities. She was transferred from the acute care hospital to the skilled nursing facility for concentrated rehabilitation. Mrs. Wilson also has arteriosclerotic heart disease with a permanent pacemaker in place, rheumatoid arthritis, urinary incontinence, and macular degeneration in her right eye. The physician, who did not know Mrs. Wilson prior to her transfer, performs a comprehensive history and physical examination. Given the patient's multiple diagnoses and the moderate amount of data the physician has to review, the MDM is of a high level of complexity.

☥ Code(s): _____

5 John Taylor is a 16-year-old outpatient who is a new patient to the office. John complains of severe facial acne. The history and physical examination are expanded problem focused. The physician must consider related organ systems in addition to the integumentary system in order to treat the condition properly. With the minimal number of diagnoses to consider and the minimal amount of data to review, the physician's decision making is straightforward with regard to the plan of care.

☥ Code(s): _____

6 Jan Sharp, an established patient, has an office appointment because she needs a new dressing on the laceration on her arm. The physician's nurse changes the dressing.

☥ Code(s): _____

7 Anna Rall is seen in the emergency department, complaining of pressure in her chest and the feeling that her heart is racing. After her vital signs are taken, an immediate electrocardiogram is performed, and her heart rate is found to be in excess of 160 beats per minute, with increased activity at the atrioventricular junction. After performing a comprehensive history and physical examination, the physician continues to evaluate the patient, who has been placed on continuous electrocardiographic monitoring. The emergency department physician considers the diagnosis of paroxysmal nodal tachycardia and calls a cardiologist for a consultation and possible admission of the patient to the hospital. Given the uncertainty of the diagnosis and the various other possible options, the physician's decision making is at a highly complex level. (Code only the emergency department physician's services.)

☥ Code(s): _____

8 A physician is called to the intensive care unit at the local hospital to care for Joe West, a patient in coronary crisis. The physician spends an hour at the patient's bedside, stabilizing him.

 Code(s): _____

9 The physician is preparing to leave the hospital after seeing Joe West but is called back to the intensive care unit to see and stabilize another patient, Ted Keel. The service to the patient takes $1\frac{1}{2}$ hours.

 Code(s): _____

10 An established patient, Harriet Turner, comes into the office for a follow-up visit. She had been prescribed medication for her recent onset of depression, but since her last visit, when the dosage was increased, she has felt that the medication is making her sleepy and lethargic. Considering the other factors such as other medical problems and drug interactions, the physician spends 25 minutes with the patient performing a detailed history and physical examination. After reviewing the details as well as recent laboratory work, the physician concludes that a different medication should be prescribed. The physician's decision making is moderately complex, given the possible medical complications that could arise.

 Code(s): _____

11 Dr. Welton calls Dr. Stouffer to perform a consultation on Carol Jones for advice on the management of her diabetes. Mrs. Jones is hospitalized for a hysterectomy, which had been an uncomplicated procedure, but is experiencing a slow recovery 4 days post op. Her abdominal wound does not appear to be healing well and her blood sugar has been fluctuating each day. Dr. Stouffer, who has never met Mrs. Jones before, performs a comprehensive, multisystem physical examination and completes a comprehensive history with a complete review of systems and extensive past medical history review. Dr. Stouffer recommends a new insulin regimen in addition to other medications to manage what might be a postoperative wound infection. Dr. Stouffer's medical decision making is of moderate complexity because he has to consider multiple diagnoses, a moderate amount of data, and the moderate risk of complications that Mrs. Jones could develop.

 Code(s): _____

CONGRATULATIONS! Now you're coding! Be sure to check your answers as you complete each activity. If you identify a code incorrectly, go back and read the CPT manual information again.

DOCUMENTATION GUIDELINES

Medicare recipients account for the majority of patients receiving services in the American health care system. Thus, any change by the third-party payer, Medicare, has dramatic effects on the health care system. One such change that currently is in development is the documentation necessary when submitting a claim for Evaluation and Management services provided to a Medicare patient. The Medicare program is the responsibility of the Centers for Medicare and Medicaid Services (CMS), formerly the Health Care Financing Administration (HCFA). Several years ago, CMS determined that there should be a nationally uniform requirement for documentation contained in the patient record when submitting charges for E/M services. The CMS developed a set of standards for documentation of E/M services. The standards are informational items that must be in the patient record to substantiate a given level of service. The standards are called the **Documentation Guidelines**. These guidelines apply only to E/M services and only to patients covered by Medicare and Medicaid. E/M services represent 50% of all services provided to these patients. The importance of the guidelines cannot be underestimated. Whatever guidelines the CMS institutes for patients have a dramatic effect on the systems in health care and will soon spread to other third-party payers, who will then begin to require the same or similar documentation.

History of the Development of Guidelines

The CMS published the first set of documentation guidelines in 1995, but did not require compliance for payment of claims. The 1995 Documentation Guidelines are displayed in **Appendix C** of this text. The 1995 guidelines are easier to understand because they are not lengthy or complex. The documentation guidelines (DG) present information about what must be contained in the medical record for that information to "qualify" as documentation. For example, one DG states, "The CC, ROS and PFSH may be listed as separate elements of history, or they may be included in the description of the history of the present illness." This means that the location in the documentation of the chief complaint; review of systems; and past, family, or social history is not important, but what is important is that each of these items is documented in the record. Another example of the content of the 1995 guidelines is a DG for a general multi-system examination as: "The medical record for a general multi-system examination should include findings about 8 or more of the 12 organ systems." The documentation guidelines provide further clarification as to the documentation required to assign a level to the history, examination, and medical decision making as stated in the medial record.

A new set of guidelines was published in July 1997 for implementation January 1, 1998. The 1997 set of guidelines was intended to be the standard used when reviewing claims for payment and are located in Appendix D of this text. If the physician did not have the documentation required in the guidelines, payment would be adjusted based on what was actually in the medical record. The guidelines were so complex and required such extensive revision of medical record-keeping practices that the AMA (American Medical Association), on behalf of its physician members, requested an extension of the implementation date to allow time for education about the guidelines and for the CMS to meet with representatives of the AMA to reconsider the guidelines. Although the CMS rescinded the requirement for strict compliance with the guidelines, they continue random review of claims, based on whichever set of guidelines (1995 or 1997) the provider has elected to use.

The 1997 Documentation Guidelines specify the information that must be documented in the medical record for an E/M service to qualify for a given level of service. Fig. 2–8 illustrates the examination requirements for a general multisystem examination under the 1997 Documentation Guidelines. Note that for an examination to qualify as an expanded problem focused examination, the medical record must document that the physician performed at least six of the elements identified by a bullet (•) in Fig. 2–9. If the medical record documents that only five of the elements identified by a bullet were performed, the ex/amination would have to be reported at the lower problem focused examination level.

A revised set of guidelines, published in 2000, took into consideration some of the suggestions put forth by the AMA. At the time of the publication of this text, the CMS and the AMA were still in discussions regarding which set of documentation guidelines would become the standard for documenting E/M services.

GENERAL MULTISYSTEM EXAMINATION

To qualify for a given level of multisystem examination, the following content and documentation requirements should be met:

- **Problem Focused Examination**—should include performance and documentation of one to five elements identified by a bullet (•) in one or more organ system(s) or body area(s).

- **Expanded Problem Focused Examination**—should include performance and documentation of at least six elements identified by a bullet (•) in one or more organ system(s) or body area(s).

- **Detailed Examination**—should include at least six organ systems or body areas. For each system/area selected, performance and documentation of at least two elements identified by a bullet (•) is expected. Alternatively, a detailed examination may include performance and documentation of at least twelve elements identified by a bullet (•) in two or more organ systems or body areas.

- **Comprehensive Examination**—should include at least nine organ systems or body areas. For each system/area selected, all elements of the examination identified by a bullet (•) should be performed, unless specific directions limit the content of the examination. For each area/system, documentation of at least two elements identified by a bullet is expected.

FIGURE 2–8 Documentation Guidelines for general multisystem examination requirements. (Courtesy U.S. Department of Health and Human Services, Centers for Medicare and Medicaid Services.)

General Multisystem Examination

System/Body Area	Elements of Examination
Constitutional	• Measurement of **any three of the following seven** vital signs: (1) sitting or standing blood pressure, (2) supine blood pressure, (3) pulse rate and regularity, (4) respiration, (5) temperature, (6) height, (7) weight (may be measured and recorded by ancillary staff) • General appearance of the patient (e.g., development, nutrition, body habitus, deformities, attention to grooming)
Eyes	• Inspection of conjunctivae and lids • Examination of pupils and irises (e.g., reaction to light and accommodation, size and symmetry) • Ophthalmoscopic examination of optic disks (e.g., size, C/D ratio, appearance) and posterior segments (e.g., vessel changes, exudates, hemorrhages)
Ears, Nose, Mouth, and Throat	• External inspection of ears and nose (e.g., overall appearance, scars, lesions, masses) • Otoscopic examination of external auditory canals and tympanic membranes • Assessment of hearing (e.g., whispered voice, finger rub, tuning fork) • Inspection of nasal mucosa, septum, and turbinates • Inspection of lips, teeth, and gums • Examination of oropharynx: oral mucosa, salivary glands, hard and soft palates, tongue, tonsils, and posterior pharynx
Neck	• Examination of neck (e.g., masses, overall appearance, symmetry, tracheal position, crepitus) • Examination of thyroid (e.g., enlargement, tenderness, mass)

FIGURE 2–9 1997 Documentation Guidelines of the general multisystem elements. (Courtesy U.S. Department of Health and Human Services, Centers for Medicare and Medicaid Services.)

CHECK THIS OUT 🖙 The CMS has its own website: www.cms.hhs.gov. You will find many articles regarding documentation guidelines for E/M services if you do a search of the CMS website.

Although the guidelines will continue to be revised, documentation guidelines will be a part of the standard for the medical record now and in the future for Medicare and Medicaid patients. You can anticipate that, as a coder, you will be required to learn about and follow these documentation guidelines.

CHAPTER REVIEW

CHAPTER 2, PART I, THEORY

Without using the CPT manual, complete the following:

1 Is examination of the back an organ system or body area examination?

_____

2 The four types of patient status are

_____, _____,

_____, and

_____.

3 The first outpatient visit is called the

_____ visit, and the second visit

is called the _____ visit.

4 The first three factors a coder must consider when coding are patient

_____, _____,

and _____.

5 How many types of histories are there?

_____

6 Which history is more complex: the problem focused history or the expanded problem

focused history? _____

7 The four types of examinations, in order of difficulty (from least difficult to most difficult), are as follows:

a. _____

b. _____

c. _____

d. _____

8 The examination that is limited to the affected

body area is the _____.

9 What does VLBW stand for?

_____

10 What medical decision making involves a situation in which the diagnosis and management options are minimal, data amount and complexity that must be reviewed are minimal/none, and there is a minimal risk to the patient of complications or death?

_____

11 What term is used to describe a patient who has been formally admitted to a hospital?

_____

CHAPTER 2, PART II, PRACTICAL

Using the CPT manual, identify the codes for the following cases:

12 The physician provides initial intensive care service for the evaluation and management of a critically ill newborn (5 days old) inpatient for 1 day.

   ◉ Code(s): _____

13 A 55-year-old man is seen by the dermatologist for the first time and complains of two cystic lesions on his back. Considering that the patient is otherwise healthy and has a primary care physician caring for him, the dermatologist focuses the history of the present illness on the skin lesions (problem focused history) and focuses the problem focused physical examination on the patient's trunk. The physician concludes with straightforward decision making that the lesions are sebaceous cysts. The physician advises the patient that the lesions should be monitored for any changes but that no surgical intervention is warranted at this time.

   ◉ Code(s): _____

14 A 68-year-old woman visits her internist again complaining of angina that seems to have worsened over the past 3 days. The patient had had an acute anterior wall myocardial infarction (MI) 2 months earlier. One month after the acute MI, she began to have angina pectoris. The patient also states that she thinks the medications are causing her to have gastrointestinal problems while not relieving her symptoms. She had refused a cardiac catheterization after her MI to evaluate the extent of her coronary artery disease. The physician performs a detailed history and a detailed physical examination of her cardiovascular, respiratory, and gastrointestinal systems. The physician indicates that the decision making process is moderately complex, given the number of conditions it is necessary to consider.

   ◉ Code(s): _____

15 A 22-year-old woman visits the gynecologist for the first time since relocating from another state last year. The patient wants a gynecologic examination and wants to discuss contraceptive options with the physician (think Preventive Medicine Services!). The physician collects pertinent past and social history related to the patient's reproductive system and performs a pertinent systems review extended to a limited number of additional systems. The physician completes the history with an extended history of her present physical state. A physical examination includes her cardiovascular and respiratory systems with an extended review of her genitourinary system. Given the patient's history of not tolerating certain types of oral contraceptives in the past, the physician's decision making involves a limited number of management options, all with low risk of morbidity to the patient.

   ◉ Code(s): _____

16 An established patient is admitted on observation status for influenza symptoms and extreme nausea and vomiting. The patient is severely dehydrated and has been experiencing dizziness and mental confusion for the past 2 days. Prior to this episode the patient was well but became acutely ill overnight with these symptoms. Given the abrupt onset of these symptoms, the physician has to consider multiple possible causes and orders a variety of laboratory tests to be performed. The patient is at risk for a moderate number of complications. The MDM complexity is moderate. A comprehensive history is collected, and a comprehensive head-to-toe physical examination is performed.

   ◉ Code(s): _____

17 A physician visits another patient on observation status who has severe influenza. The decision is made to admit the patient, whose condition has worsened and who is not responding to the therapy initiated on the observation unit. The physician performs a detailed history and a detailed physical examination to reflect the patient's current status. The patient's problem is of low severity but requires ongoing active management, with possible surgical consultation. The MDM complexity is low.

   ◉ Code(s): _____

18 An 8-month-old infant, who is a new patient, is brought in by her mother for diaper rash. The physician focuses on the problem of the diaper rash for the problem focused history and examination. The MDM complexity is straightforward.

 Code(s): _____

19 A 33-year-old man is brought to his private physician's office by his wife. The man, who is an established patient, has been experiencing severe leg pain of 2 weeks' duration. In the past 2 days, the patient has experienced fainting spells, nausea, and vomiting. The patient has had multiple other vague complaints over the past month that he dismissed as unimportant, but his wife is not so sure, and she describes his general health as deteriorating. The physician performs a comprehensive multisystem physical examination after performing a complete review of systems and a complete past medical, family, and social history, with an extended history of the present illness (comprehensive history). The physician has to consider an extensive number of diagnoses, orders a variety of tests to be performed immediately, and indicates the MDM complexity to be high.

Code(s): _____

20 A 42-year-old woman, who is an established patient, visits her family practitioner with the chief complaint of a self-discovered breast lump. She describes a feeling of fullness and tenderness over the mass that has become more pronounced in the past 2 weeks. Because the patient is otherwise healthy and has had a physical within the past 6 months, the physician focuses his attention on the breast lump during the taking of a problem focused history and the performance of a problem focused physical examination. The physician orders an immediate mammography to be performed nd a follow-up appointment in 5 days. The physician has given the patient no other options and indicates that the MDM complexity is straightforward.

Code(s): _____

QUICK CHECK ANSWERS

QUICK CHECK 2-1
exceed, three

QUICK CHECK 2-2
True

QUICK CHECK 2-3
e. All of the above

QUICK CHECK 2-4
Yes

QUICK CHECK 2-5
outpatient

QUICK CHECK 2-6
Time

QUICK CHECK 2-7
Request, Report

QUICK CHECK ANSWERS

QUICK CHECK 2-8
Yes

QUICK CHECK 2-9
1. None
2. Yes

QUICK CHECK 2-10
1. Any two of:
   - Interpretation of cardiac output measure (93561-93562)
   - Chest x-rays (71010, 71015, 71020)
   - Pulse Oximetry (94760, 94761, 94762)
   - Blood gases and information data in computers (e.g., ECGs, blood pressures, hematologic data) 99090
   - Gastric intubation (43752, 91105)
   - Temporary transcutaneous pacing (92953)
   - Ventilation management (94002-94004, 94660, 94662)
   - Vascular access procedures (36000, 36410, 36415, 36591, 36600)

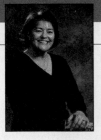

"I have a suspicion that many of us are drawn to the health care profession to begin with because we have 'care-taking' personality traits. Coding allowed me to take my natural talents and abilities for teaching and communication and apply them to my field in a compassionate and meaningful way."

Jane A. Tuttle CPC-I, CCS-P
Coding Education Endeavors
Westford, Massachusetts

Anesthesia Section and Modifiers

Chapter Topics

Learning Objectives

After completing this chapter, you should be able to

1 Define types of anesthesia.
2 Explain the format of the Anesthesia section and subsections.
3 Understand the anesthesia formula.
4 Demonstrate ability to code anesthesia services.
5 Recognize HCPCS modifiers.
6 Understand the purpose of CPT modifiers.
7 Assign CPT modifiers.

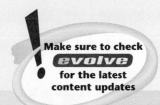

Make sure to check **evolve** for the latest content updates

PART I ■ *Learning about the Anesthesia Section*

TYPES OF ANESTHESIA

The Anesthesia section is a specialized section that is used by an anesthesiologist, anesthetist, or other physician to report the provision of anesthesia services, usually during surgery. **Anesthesia** means induction or administration of a drug to obtain partial or complete loss of sensation. **Analgesia** (absence of pain) is achieved so that a patient may have surgery or a procedure performed without pain. Types of anesthesia may be general, regional, and local, or moderate (conscious) sedation.

The practice of anesthesiology is not limited to administration of anesthesia for the surgical patient. The American Society of Anesthesiologists (ASA) defines the practice of anesthesiology as follows:

■ The management of procedures for rendering a patient insensible to pain and emotional stress during surgical, obstetrical, and other diagnostic and therapeutic procedures.

■ The evaluation and management of essential physiologic functions under the stress of anesthetic and surgical manipulations.

■ The clinical management of the patient unconscious from whatever cause.

■ The evaluation and management of acute or chronic pain.

■ The management of problems in cardiac and respiratory resuscitation.

■ The application of specific methods of respiratory therapy.

■ The clinical management of various fluid, electrolyte, and metabolic disturbances.*

Take a moment and consult a good medical dictionary under the entry "anesthesia." You will see that besides the definition of the term anesthesia, a wide variety of anesthesias are defined. Some types of anesthesia are named for the site of the anesthesia administration, such as sacral, lumbar, and caudal. Other types of anesthesia are named for the category of anesthesia, such as frost for cryoanesthesia. Some of the more commonly used anesthesia terms are endotracheal, epidural, regional, and patient-controlled.

Endotracheal anesthesia is accomplished by inserting a tube into the nose or mouth and passing the tube into the trachea for ventilation, as illustrated in Fig. 3–1. **Epidural** anesthesia is the injection of an anesthetic agent into the epidural spaces between the vertebrae, also known as peridural anesthesia, epidural, epidural block, and intraspinal anesthesia. **Spinal** anesthesia generally applies to all anesthesia procedures applied in the spinal cord area, outside of or inside of the dura mater. **General** anesthesia is a state of unconsciousness that is accomplished by the use of a drug administered by inhalation, intramuscularly, rectally, or intravenously. **Regional** anesthesia is used to interrupt the sensory nerve conductivity in a region of the body and is produced by a field block (forming a wall of anesthesia around the site by means of local injections) or nerve block (injection of the area close to the site), also known as block, block anesthesia, or conduction anesthesia. Although not a type of anesthesia, a procedure used by anesthesiologists is a **blood patch**, a procedure in which a cerebrospinal fluid leak is closed by means of an injection of the patient's blood into the area that was used during spinal anesthesia. **Local** anesthesia can be accomplished by means of application of an anesthetic agent such as lidocaine directly to the area involved (**topical** anesthesia) or local

---

*Definitions excerpted from the *2008 Relative Value Guide*, American Society of Anesthesiologists, p. v. A copy of the full text can be obtained from ASA, 1501 M Street NW, Suite 300, Washington, DC 20005.

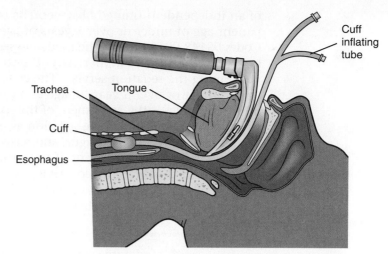

Cuff
inflating
tube

Trachea   Tongue

Cuff

Esophagus

FIGURE 3–1 Placement of the endotracheal tube for administration of anesthesia.

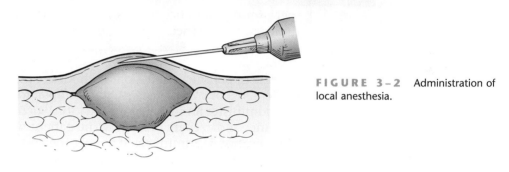

FIGURE 3–2 Administration of local anesthesia.

infiltration through subcutaneous injection of an anesthetic agent; lidocaine could be subcutaneously injected, as illustrated in Fig. 3–2.

Patient-controlled analgesia (PCA) is a system that allows the patient to administer an analgesic drug such as morphine to control pain. A handheld device is attached to a pump holding the drug and the patient can depress a button to administer a dose of the drug. In this way, the patient can control the amount of the drug and the frequency of administration. One use of the system is for patients with chronic pain.

QUICK CHECK 3-1

In the index of the CPT, you would reference this main term and these two subterms to locate a blood patch code.

_____

Moderate (Conscious) Sedation

Moderate or conscious sedation is a type of sedation that can be provided by a physician performing a procedure; it provides a decreased level of consciousness that does not put the patient completely to sleep. This level of consciousness allows the patient to breathe without assistance and to respond to stimulation and verbal commands. A trained observer is often present during the use of the conscious sedation to assist the physician in monitoring the patient. The codes used to report this type of conscious sedation are located in the Medicine section (99143-99150), not in the Anesthesia section. Codes 99143-99145 are used to report the moderate sedation services when the service is provided by the same physician performing the diagnostic or therapeutic service and requires the presence of an independent trained observer. The codes are divided based on the patient age of under or over 5 years of age and the duration of the service. Codes 99148-99150 report the moderate sedation services when the anesthesia service is provided by a physician other than the health care professional performing the sedation service. The codes are divided based on the patient age of under or over 5 years of age and the duration of the service. Bundled into these codes is the assessment of the patient, establishment of intravenous access, administration of the sedation agent, sedation maintenance, monitoring of patient vital signs, and recovery. The time the physician spends with the patient in assessment of the patient prior to administration of the sedation and the time in recovery is not included in the intraservice time because the intraservice time begins with the administration of the sedation agent and ends at the conclusion of the physician contact with the patient.

CODING SHOT Moderate (conscious) sedation codes 99143-99145 from the Medicine section are used only when the physician performing the procedure administers the sedation and an independent trained observer assists.

Moderate or conscious sedation methods are much less invasive than is the complete loss of consciousness. For example, for a colonoscopy, a physician could administer an intravenous sedation, such as meperidine (Demerol), morphine, or diazepam (Valium). The patient would be monitored closely as the medication is administered so that the appropriate level of sedation is reached. After the procedure, the physician may administer a drug such as naloxone (Narcan) intravenously to reverse the effects of the sedation. The patient would have this procedure in an outpatient setting and be able to go home after the procedure.

ANESTHESIA SECTION FORMAT

Anesthesia procedure codes are divided first by anatomic site and then by specific type of procedure, as shown in Fig. 3–3.

More than one CPT procedure code may be represented by one anesthesia code. For example, anesthesia code 00566, Anesthesia for direct coronary artery bypass grafting without pump oxygenator, is used to report the anesthesia services provided during direct coronary artery bypass grafting procedures performed without pump oxygenator (off pump), such as 33510-33536.

The last four subsections in Anesthesia—Radiologic Procedures (01916-01936), Burn Excisions or Debridement (01951-01953), Obstetric (01958-01969) and Other Procedures (01990-01999)—are *not* organized by anatomic division. The CPT codes in the Radiologic Procedures subsection are used to report anesthesia service when radiologic services are provided to the patient for diagnostic or therapeutic reasons.

Example		
Therapeutic reason:	01925	Anesthesia for therapeutic interventional radiological procedures involving the carotid and coronary
Diagnostic reason:	01922	Anesthesia for non-invasive imaging or radiation therapy

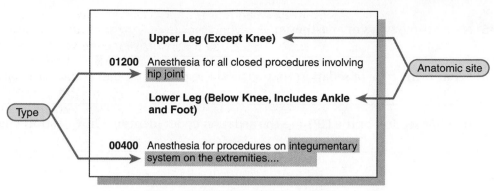

FIGURE 3-3 Anatomic divisions in Anesthesia section.

EXERCISE 3-1 *Anesthesia Format*

Complete the following exercise:

1 Using the CPT manual, list each subsection in the Anesthesia section.

_____

_____

_____

_____

_____

_____

_____

_____

_____

_____

_____

_____

_____

_____

_____

_____

_____

_____

_____

_____

_____

2 Which subsections are *not* divided by anatomic site? _____

3 What is analgesia? _____

4 What is anesthesia? _____

5 Name three types of anesthesia: _____, _____, and
_____

6 What is the type of sedation that enables the patient to maintain breathing for himself/herself?
_____

7 In what section of the CPT are the sedation codes identified in Question 6 located?
_____

FORMULA FOR ANESTHESIA PAYMENT

When an anesthesiologist provides an anesthesia service to a patient, the preoperative, intraoperative (care during surgery), and postoperative care are all included in the CPT code. These services include the usual preoperative and postoperative visits to the patient by the anesthesiologist; the routine intraoperative care, such as administration of fluids and/or blood; and the usual monitoring services. The care also includes the patient's history taken by the anesthesiologist, ventilation establishment, and administration of preoperative and postoperative medications. Monitoring services include blood pressure, temperature, arterial oxygen levels (oximetry), exhalation of carbon dioxide (capnography), and spectrometry (blood analysis). The intraoperative care includes intubation and placement of the tubes to administer anesthesia. Postoperative care usually includes pain management. Some pain management is reported separately, e.g., spinal injection for significant pain. If the anesthesiologist provides care that is unusual or beyond that which would usually be provided, these services can be reported in addition to the base anesthesia service. For example, if the patient requires intraoperative cardiac monitoring, the anesthesiologist might insert a Swan-Ganz catheter, as illustrated in Fig. 3–4.

A Swan-Ganz catheter is not a normal service provided during a surgery, so it could be reported using a code from the Medicine section for placement of a flow-directed catheter (93503). The time necessary to insert the catheter is not counted in the anesthesia time because the service of the insertion is reported separately. Reporting the insertion time separately would result in additional payment.

QUICK CHECK 3-2

Where in CPT is much of the information regarding what is included in an anesthesia service located?

_____

What makes anesthesia coding different from any other coding is the way in which anesthesia services are billed. There is a standard formula for payment of anesthesia services that is, for the most part, nationally accepted. The formula is base units + time units + modifying units (B + T + M) × conversion factor. Let's look at each of these elements in more detail.

B Is for Base Unit

The ASA publishes a *Relative Value Guide* (RVG), which contains codes for anesthesia services. The CPT manual also contains these anesthesia service codes in the Anesthesia section. Italicized comments appear in the

American Society of Anesthesiologists' *Relative Value Guide*™ to clarify code assignment as illustrated in Figure 3–5. These italicized comments are not part of the CPT.

CMS's Base Units The RVG is not a fee schedule (a list of the charges for services) but instead compares anesthesia services with each other. For example, anesthesia services provided for a biopsy of a sinus are less complicated than services provided for a radical sinus surgery. A team of physicians with expertise in anesthesiology developed the comparisons and assigned numerical values to each service, termed the **base unit value** (Fig. 3–6). Annually, CMS publishes a list of the base unit values for the codes, as illustrated in Figure 3–7.

The ASA's base unit value is accepted as the standard in the United States.

One coding circumstance unique to anesthesia coding occurs when multiple surgical procedures are performed during the same session. In this case the procedure with the highest unit value is the base unit value. For example, if during the same surgical procedure session a clavicle biopsy (base unit value of 3) and a radical mastectomy (base unit value of 5) are done, the base unit value for both procedures becomes 5. The anesthesia service is then reported with only the code of the higher base unit value.

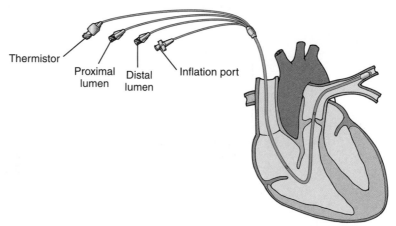

FIGURE 3–4 Swan-Ganz catheter is the most commonly used central venous catheter.

INTRATHORACIC

00500	Anesthesia for all procedures on esophagus..	15 + TM
00520	Anesthesia for closed chest procedures; (including bronchoscopy) not otherwise specified.. *(For transvenous pacemaker insertion, report 00530.)*	6 + TM

FIGURE 3–5 The ASA's *Relative Value Guide* contains italicized comments that do not appear in the code description in the CPT. (Excerpted from 2008 Relative Value Guide, © 2007 of the American Society of Anesthesiologists. All Rights Reserved. *Relative Value Guide is a registered trademark of the American Society of Anesthesiologists.* A copy of the full text can be obtained from ASA, 520 N. Northwest Highway, Park Ridge, IL, 60068-2573.)

Base unit value

LOWER LEG (BELOW KNEE, INCLUDES ANKLE AND FOOT)
(For procedures on integumentary system, report code 00400.)

01462   Anesthesia for all closed procedures on lower leg, ankle, and foot .... 3 + TM

01464   Anesthesia for arthroscopic procedures of ankle and/or foot .... 3 + TM

01470   Anesthesia for procedures on nerves, muscles, tendons, and fascia of
          lower leg, ankle, and foot; not otherwise specified .... 3 + TM

01472   repair of ruptured Achilles tendon, with or without graft .... 5 + TM

01474   gastrocnemius recession (eg, Strayer procedure) .... 5 + TM

FIGURE 3–6   The ASA's *Relative Value Guide* lists the base unit value for the codes.
(Excerpted from 2008 Relative Value Guide, © 2007 of the American Society of Anesthesiologists.
All Rights Reserved. *Relative Value Guide is a registered trademark of the American Society of
Anesthesiologists.* A copy of the full text can be obtained from ASA, 520 N. Northwest Highway,
Park Ridge, IL, 60068-2573.)

Code	Base Unit Value
00100	5
00102	6
00103	5
00104	4
00120	5
00124	4
00126	4
00140	5
00142	4
00144	6
00145	6
00147	4
00148	4
00160	5
00162	7
00164	4
00170	5
00172	6
00174	6
00176	7
00190	5
00192	7
00210	11

FIGURE 3–7   CMS's annual list of base units. (Courtesy U.S. Department of Health and
Human Services, Centers for Medicare and Medicaid Services.)

CODING SHOT For Medicare, the pricing for add-on anesthesia codes is different than most CPT codes because only the base unit value of the add-code is allowed and all anesthesia time is reported with the primary anesthesia code. There is an exception to this rule when reporting obstetrical anesthesia in which both the base unit value and time units for the primary and add-on codes are reported.

From the Trenches

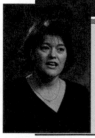

"Learning to use the CPT book effectively as a tool is one of the best skills I can teach my students to develop . . . I always advise them to start with a strong foundation by taking classes in medical terminology and anatomy and physiology."

JANE

T Is for Time

Anesthesia services are provided based on the time during which the anesthesia was administered, in total minutes. The timing is started when the anesthesiologist begins preparing the patient to receive anesthesia, continues through the procedure, and ends when the patient is no longer under the personal care of the anesthesiologist. The minutes during which anesthesia was administered are recorded in the patient record. Carriers independently determine the amount of time in a unit. Often, 30 minutes equal a unit but for some carriers, 1, 10, 15, or 30 minutes equal a unit.

CODING SHOT When a physician and a certified registered nurse anesthetist (CRNA) are involved in one anesthesia case and the services of both are medically necessary, report the physician services with -AA (anesthesia services performed personally by anesthesiologist) and the CRNA services with -QZ (CRNA services without medical direction by a physician).

M Is for Modifying Unit

As the name implies, modifying units reflect circumstances or conditions that change or modify the environment in which the anesthesia service is provided. There are two basic modifying characteristics: qualifying circumstances and physical status modifiers.

Qualifying Circumstances. At times, anesthesia is provided in situations that make the administration of the anesthesia more difficult. These types of cases include those that are performed in emergency situations and those dealing with patients of extreme age; they also include services performed during the use of controlled hypotension or the use of hypothermia. The Qualifying Circumstances codes begin with the number 99 and are considered **adjunct codes,** which means that the codes cannot be used alone but must be used in addition to another code and are used to provide additional information only. A Qualifying Circumstances code is used in addition to the anesthesia procedure code. Qualifying Circumstances codes are located in two places in the CPT manual: the Medicine section and the Anesthesia section guidelines. In both locations the plus symbol is located next to the codes (99100-99140), indicating their status as add-on codes only.

STOP *You were just presented with some very important information about the use of certain codes in the CPT manual. The plus (+) symbol next to any CPT code—not just next to Qualifying Circumstances codes—indicates that that code cannot be used alone. Throughout the remaining sections of the CPT manual, the plus symbol will appear to caution you to use the code only as an adjunct code (with other codes).*

When used, the Qualifying Circumstances code is listed separately in addition to the primary anesthesia procedure code. For example, if anesthesia was provided for an 80-year-old patient during a corrective lens procedure, the coding would be:

00142   Anesthesia for procedure on eye; lens surgery

99100   Anesthesia for 80-year-old patient

The RVG lists the qualifying circumstances along with the relative value for each code (Fig. 3–8).

The CPT index lists the qualifying circumstances coded under Anesthesia, Special Circumstances.

Physical Status Modifiers. The second type of modifying unit used in the Anesthesia section is the physical status modifier. These modifiers are used to indicate the patient's condition at the time anesthesia was administered. The physical status modifier not only indicates the patient's condition at the time of anesthesia but also serves to identify the level of complexity of the services provided to the patient. For instance, anesthesia service to a gravely ill patient is much more complex than the same type of service to a normal, healthy patient. The physical status modifier is not assigned by the coder but is determined by the anesthesiologist and documented in the anesthesia record. The physical status modifier begins with the letter "P" and contains a number from 1 to 6 (Fig. 3–9).

Note that the base unit value for P1, P2, and P6 is zero because these conditions are considered not to affect the service provided. A physical status modifier is used after the five-digit CPT code and is illustrated in Fig. 3–10.

V. Qualifying Circumstances (more than one may be reported)

		Base Unit Value
+99100	Anesthesia for patient of extreme age, younger than 1 year and older than 70	1
+99116	Anesthesia complicated by utilization of total body hypothermia	5
+99135	Anesthesia complicated by utilization of controlled hypotension	5
+99140	Anesthesia complicated by emergency conditions (specify)	2
	(An emergency is defined as existing when delay in treatment of the patient would lead to a significant increase in the threat to life or body part.)	

FIGURE 3–8 Qualifying Circumstances with relative value. (Excerpted from 2008 Relative Value Guide, © 2007 of the American Society of Anesthesiologists. All Rights Reserved. *Relative Value Guide is a registered trademark of the American Society of Anesthesiologists.* A copy of the full text can be obtained from ASA, 520 N. Northwest Highway, Park Ridge, IL, 60068-2573.)

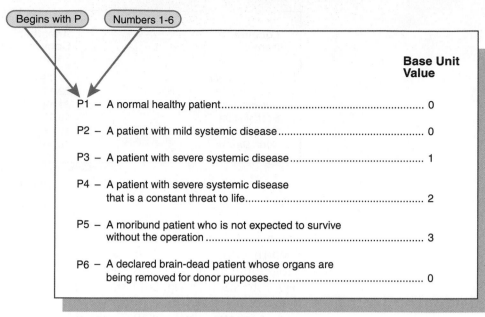

	Base Unit Value
P1 – A normal healthy patient	0
P2 – A patient with mild systemic disease	0
P3 – A patient with severe systemic disease	1
P4 – A patient with severe systemic disease that is a constant threat to life	2
P5 – A moribund patient who is not expected to survive without the operation	3
P6 – A declared brain-dead patient whose organs are being removed for donor purposes	0

FIGURE 3–9 Physical status modifiers. (Excerpted from 2008 Relative Value Guide, © 2007 of the American Society of Anesthesiologists. All Rights Reserved. *Relative Value Guide is a registered trademark of the American Society of Anesthesiologists.* A copy of the full text can be obtained from ASA, 520 N. Northwest Highway, Park Ridge, IL, 60068-2573.)

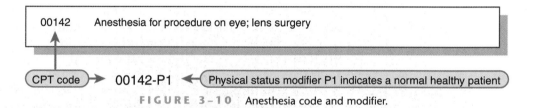

FIGURE 3–10 Anesthesia code and modifier.

Summing It Up!

Most health care facilities have software that does the conversion calculations because of the various conversion factors and unit designations. However, you still need to understand the process used to convert the anesthesia formula into the anesthesia payment. Let's put the elements of the equation to practical use by applying the equation (B + T + M) to a specific case.

An 84-year-old female (qualifying circumstance for extreme age, value 1) with severe hypertension has a 4-cm malignant lesion removed from her right knee (base value of 3). The total time of anesthesia service was 60 minutes and the carrier indicates a unit is 15 minutes (4 units). The anesthesiologist indicates in the medical record that the patient's physical status at the time of the procedure was P3 for a severe systemic disease (relative value of 1).

3   base value

4   time units

2   modifiers: physical status = 1; extreme age = 1

------

9   total units

The coding that identifies all elements of this case would be:

00400-P3	Anesthesia for procedure of integumentary system of knee with severe systemic disease
99100	Anesthesia for an 84-year-old patient
9	Units at the third-party payer established rate per unit

Locality Name	Anesthesia Conversion Factor
Manhattan, NY	20.03
NYC suburbs/Long I., NY	22.18
Queens, NY	21.69
Rest of state	19.09
North Carolina	19.23
North Dakota	18.86

FIGURE 3–11 2008 CMS Anesthesia Conversion Factors.

Conversion Factors. A conversion factor is the dollar value of each unit. Each third-party payer issues a list of conversion factors. The lists vary with geographic location because the cost of practicing medicine varies from one region to another. Fig. 3–11 shows an example of a third-party payer's (CMS) anesthesia conversion factors. Note that North Dakota is $18.86 per unit and Manhattan, NY, is $20.03 per unit, as it is much less expensive to provide anesthesia services in Grand Forks, ND, than it is to provide the same services in Manhattan, NY.

The conversion factor for the locale is multiplied by the number of units in the procedure. For example, the previous case has 9 units. If the anesthesiologist were located in Manhattan, NY, which has a conversion factor of $20.03, the total for the procedure would be $180.27 (9 × $20.03). If the same services were provided in North Dakota, with the conversion factor of $18.86, the total for the procedure would be $169.74 (9 × $18.86).

Multiple Procedures

When multiple surgical procedures are performed during a single anesthetic administration, the anesthesia code that represents the most complex procedure is reported. The time reported is the combined total for all procedures.

CODING SHOT According to Medicare rules, when reporting bilateral procedures, the coder is to report the anesthesia procedure with the highest base unit value with modifier -50.

EXERCISE 3-2 *Modifiers in Anesthesia*

Complete the following:

1 If the anesthesia service was provided to a patient who had mild systemic disease, what would the physical status modifier be likely to be? _____

2 If the same service was provided to a patient who had severe systemic disease, what would the physical status modifier be likely to be? _____

3 Anesthesia complicated by utilization of total body hypothermia

   Code(s): _____

Concurrent Care Modifiers

Some third-party payers require additional modifiers to indicate how many cases an anesthesiologist is performing or supervising at one time. Certified registered nurse anesthetists (CRNAs) may administer anesthesia to patients under the direction of a licensed physician, or they may work independently. An anesthesiologist may medically direct multiple cases at the same time (concurrently). Medically directing means the physician is present at the induction and emergence from anesthesia and is immediately available in case of an emergency. The CRNA would be with the patient the majority of the time.

When medical direction occurs, certain documentation must be submitted for services for Medicare patients. The documentation supports that certain services were personally performed by the physician; These include:

1. Pre-anesthesia examination and evaluation

2. Prescription of an anesthesia plan

3. Personal participation in the most demanding procedures in the anesthesia plan, including induction and emergence

4. Ensures that any procedures in the anesthesia plan that he or she does not perform are performed by a qualified anesthetist

5. Monitors the course of anesthesia administration at frequent intervals

6. Remains physically present and available for immediate diagnosis and treatment of emergencies

7. Provides indicated postanesthesia care

Additional modifiers that define the types of providers involved in the case are:

AA	Anesthesia services performed personally by an anesthesiologist
AD	Medical supervision by a physician; more than 4 concurrent anesthesia procedures
G8	Monitored anesthesia care (MAC) for deep complex complicated, or markedly invasive surgical procedures
G9	Monitored anesthesia care for patient who has a history of severe cardiopulmonary condition
QK	Medical direction of two, three, or four concurrent anesthesia procedures involving qualified individuals
QS	Monitored anesthesia care service
QX	Certified registered nurse anesthetist (CRNA) service, with medical direction by a physician
QY	Medical direction of one certifed registered nurse anesthetist by an anesthesiologist
QZ	CRNA service, without medical direction by a physician

These modifiers are not CPT modifiers but HCPCS modifiers. These modifiers further define the services provided. As a coder, you will need to become familiar with numerous coding systems that are used in addition to the CPT codes.

QUICK CHECK 3-3

What is the difference between modifiers QX and QY?

EXERCISE 3–3 *Modifiers*

Using Appendix A of the CPT manual, identify the following CPT modifiers:

1 Increased Procedural Services _____

2 Unusual Anesthesia _____

Using the descriptions for the preceding modifiers, answer the following questions. Which modifier would be used to identify

3 A service greater than that usually provided? _____

4 A service that required general anesthesia when usually a local anesthesia would be used?

_____

UNLISTED ANESTHESIA CODE
In the Anesthesia section, an unlisted procedure code is available and is located under the Other Procedures subsection in the Anesthesia section. When a new surgical procedure is used, there is no CPT code to indicate the surgical procedure or the anesthesia services provided during the procedure. The anesthesia services are reported using the lone unlisted anesthesia code —01999.

EXERCISE 3–4 *Anesthesia Codes*

Complete the following:

1 What is the unlisted anesthesia procedure code?

   Code: _____

Locate anesthesia procedures in the CPT manual index under the entry "Anesthesia" and then subtermed by the anatomic site. Write the CPT index location on the line provided (e.g., Anesthesia, Thyroid). Then locate the code(s) identified in the Anesthesia section of the CPT manual. Choose the correct code(s) and write the code(s) on the line provided.

2 Needle biopsy of the thyroid (neck)

   Index location: _____

   Code(s): _____

3 Cesarean section, delivery only

   Index location: _____

   Code(s): _____

4 Transurethral resection of the prostate

   Index location: _____

   Code(s): _____

5 Repair of cleft palate

   Index location: _____

   Code(s): _____

6 Repair of ruptured Achilles tendon without graft

Index location: _____

Code(s): _____

Using the following information and the B + T + M formula, calculate the payment for the anesthesia services.

For the following questions a time unit will be 15 minutes. Base unit value for each case is provided within the questions. Refer to Fig. 3–11 for the conversion factors used in these questions; to Fig. 3–8 for the value of the Qualifying Circumstances; and to Fig. 3–9 for the value of the Physical Status Modifiers.

7 A needle biopsy lasting 15 minutes was conducted in North Dakota on a normal healthy 75-year-old patient. The base unit value for the service is 3.*

Anesthesia payment: _____

8 A patient with diabetes mellitus, controlled by diet and exercise, undergoes a 60-minute anesthesia period for a transurethral resection of the prostate (base unit value of 5).* Calculate the anesthesia rate if the procedure were performed in the following locales:

a. Manhattan _____

b. North Carolina _____

9 A cesarean section was conducted in Alfred, NY, on a patient with preeclampsia (1 modifying unit). The base unit value for the service is 7.* Calculate the anesthesia rates for procedures lasting two different lengths of time (refer to Fig. 3–11 on p. 100 for conversion rates):

a. 30-minute procedure _____

b. 45-minute procedure _____

*Excerpted from the *2008 Relative Value Guide,* American Society of Anesthesiologists, 1501 M Street NW, Suite 300, Washington, DC 20005.

If a patient is returned to the operating room on the same day for the same or a related procedure, and the same physician is performing the second procedure, report the service with modifier -76. For example, the anesthesiologist provides the service for an upper gastrointestinal endoscopic procedure and reports the service 00740-AA. Later that day, the patient is returned for a lower intestinal endoscopic procedure. The second service would be reported 00810-AA-76. If that second procedure was performed by another anesthesiologist, the second service would be reported 00810-AA-77.

If the pre-anesthetic examination was provided by an anesthesiologist to a patient who did not undergo surgery, the service would be reported for consideration for reimbursement. If a CRNA provided the service, report the service with subsequent hospital care codes (99231-99233).

The Anesthesia section is a very specialized section used to report anesthesia services provided to patients.

You learned about a few modifiers that are used with anesthesia codes. Now it is time to expand your knowledge of the use of modifiers. Modifiers are very important in coding, and a skilled coder knows when and how to apply them. In Part II of this chapter you will learn the basics of modifiers, so if you are ready, let's begin.

PART II ■ *Modifiers*

THE CPT MODIFIERS

Modifiers are used to inform third-party payers of circumstances that may affect the way payment is made. The CPT manual's Appendix A lists all modifiers and the circumstances for their use.

Modifiers are used to indicate the following types of information:

■ altered service

   prolonged service
   service greater than usually required
   unusual circumstances
   part of a service

■ bilateral procedure

■ multiple procedures

■ professional part of the service/procedure only

■ more than one physician/surgeon

The CPT modifiers are shown in Fig. 3–12.

-21, Prolonged Evaluation and Management Services

Deleted in 2009

As is indicated by the title of modifier -21, the purpose of this modifier is to indicate an extended E/M service, and it is not used with codes other than E/M codes. The full description of the modifier is as follows:

When the face-to-face or floor/unit service(s) provided is prolonged or otherwise greater than that usually required for the highest level of E/M service within a given category, it may be identified by adding modifier -21 to the E/M code number. A report may also be appropriate.

✋ **CAUTION** *Modifier -21 should be used only with the highest level E/M code. For example, 99205 is the highest level for a new patient office visit. If an extended service (more than 50% of the time was spent in counseling/ coordination or there was a comprehensive history, examination, and a high complexity of medical decision making) above that described in 99204 were provided, you would move up to code 99205 to report the service. Therefore, it is never correct to report modifier -21 with anything but the highest level code. This rule applies to both outpatient and inpatient services.*

CPT Modifiers

-21	-50	-58	-79
-22	-51	-59	-80
-23	-52	-62	-81
-24	-53	-63	-82
-25	-54	-66	-90
-26	-55	-76	-91
-32	-56	-77	-92
-47	-57	-78	-99

FIGURE 3–12 CPT Modifiers.

The assignment of modifier -21 in the E/M section is limited to some of the codes in the range 99205-99397. Codes in the range 99291-99292 (critical care) are based on time units, so additional time would be reported by using additional codes or units rather than by adding the prolonged service modifier -21.

For an example of the use of modifier -21, review the following case:

Example

A 34-year-old male patient is admitted to the hospital with acute chest pains. The physician conducts a comprehensive history and examination. The decision making complexity is high. The physician spends 90 minutes at the bedside of the patient on the unit, with the patient's family, and in the development of a plan for the patient's care.

You would code this case as a 99223, initial hospital care, the highest level code available. But the code description indicates that the typical time for a 99223 is 70 minutes. To fully describe the service provided to this patient you would have to add modifier -21. The code for the service would be 99223-21.

CODING SHOT Modifier -21 is not used with prolonged services (99354-99357) because the prolonged service codes report the additional services.

The use of the modifier -21 does not always have an effect on third-party reimbursement. For example, Medicare does not pay additionally for the use of modifier -21. But you still want to be as specific as possible when coding all services, and this includes the use of modifiers to fully explain a service.

-22, Increased Procedural Services

Modifier -22 indicates that a service was provided that was greater than usual, and a special report would accompany the use of the code to explain exactly in which ways the service was greater. A description of modifier -22 is as follows:

> When the work required to provide a service is substantially greater than typically required, it may be identified by adding modifier -22 to the usual procedure code. Documentation must support the substantial additional work and the reason for the additional work (i.e., increased intensity, time, technical difficulty of procedure, severity of patient's condition, physical and mental effort required). **Note:** This modifier should not be appended to an E/M service.

The use of modifier -22 indicates that the service provided was significantly greater than the service described in the CPT code. A few additional minutes spent on a procedure do not warrant the use of this modifier. The medical record must contain documentation that substantiates the claim that the service was unusual in some way, such as statements about the increased risk to the patient, the difficulty of the procedure, excessive blood loss, or other statements to indicate the occurrence of an unusually difficult situation. Modifier -22 is overused, so it comes under particularly close scrutiny by third-party payers, especially as there is a payment increase of 20% to 30% for services that qualify for the use of modifier -22. So when using it, you have to be sure that you have the documentation to support the claim. When the third-party payer receives a claim that includes a service to which modifier -22 has been added, the claim is sent to an individual who reviews the claim. Appropriate documentation must, therefore, accompany the claim—an operative report, a pathology report, office notes, hospital chart notes, and so forth.

CODING SHOT When using modifier -22, additional charges are added by the physician, and documentation that supports the higher charge is contained in the medical record.

-23, Unusual Anesthesia

Modifier -23 is used by an anesthesiologist to indicate a service for which general anesthesia was used when normally the anesthesia would have been local or regional. The description of the modifier is as follows:

> *Occasionally, a procedure, which usually requires either no anesthesia or local anesthesia, because of unusual circumstances must be done under general anesthesia. This circumstance may be reported by adding modifier -23 to the procedure code of the basic service.*

This modifier can be used only with codes in the Anesthesia section (00100-01999) and only by the physician providing the general anesthesia, usually provided by an anesthesiologist. When the modifier is used, the claim must be accompanied by a written report explaining the circumstance that required general anesthesia instead of the normally used local or regional anesthesia.

QUICK CHECK 3-4

Which of the following may be an example of "unusual anesthesia" circumstances?

a. Open wound repair on the face of a 2-year-old
b. Pelvic exam on a developmentally challenged woman
c. Cast application for fracture care of an Alzheimer's patient
d. All of the above

-24, Unrelated Evaluation and Management Service by the Same Physician During a Postoperative Period

Modifier -24 is used only with E/M codes. The full description of the modifier is as follows:

> *The physician may need to indicate that an evaluation and management service was performed during a postoperative period for a reason(s) unrelated to the original procedure. This circumstance may be reported by adding modifier -24 to the appropriate level of E/M service.*

Modifier -24 is used to report services that were performed during a postoperative period. As you will learn in Chapter 4, surgical procedures come with a package of services, such as preoperative, the procedure, and normal follow-up care. If an E/M service unrelated to the surgical procedure is provided to a patient during the postoperative period, the third-party payer would think that the service was part of the surgical care. Modifier -24 is added to indicate that the E/M service was not part of the surgical care but was an unrelated service. The postoperative period of a major surgical procedure is usually 90 days; of minor surgery, 10 days. Payment for the surgical procedure includes postoperative care of the patient during these periods.
  You can also use modifier -24 with the General Ophthalmological Services codes 92002-92014, even though these codes are located in the Medicine

section. Ophthalmologists report their new and established patient services for medical examination using these service codes.

CODING SHOT ✎ Modifier -24 requests payment for an unassociated E/M within a global period.

-25, Significant Separately Identifiable E/M Service by the Same Physician on the Same Day of the Procedure or Other Service

Modifier -25 is used to report an E/M service on a day when another service was provided to the patient by the same physician. The description of the modifier is as follows:

It may be necessary to indicate that on the day a procedure or service identified by a CPT code was performed, the patient's condition required a significant, separately identifiable E/M service above and beyond the other service provided or beyond the usual preoperative and postoperative care associated with the procedure that was performed. A significant, separately identifiable E/M service is defined or substantiated by documentation that satisfies the relevant criteria for the respective E/M service to be reported. (See Evaluation and Management Services Guidelines for instructions on determining level of E/M service.) The E/M service may be prompted by the symptom or condition for which the procedure and/or service was provided. As such, different diagnoses are not required for reporting of the E/M services on the same date. This circumstance may be reported by adding modifier -25 to the appropriate level of E/M service. Note: This modifier is not used to report an E/M service that resulted in a decision to perform surgery. See modifier -57. For significant, separately identifiable non-E/M services, see modifier -59.

CODING SHOT ✎ If reporting services for a Medicare patient, modifier -25 could be added to an E/M code when a decision for surgery was made on the same day as a procedure with a global surgical package of 0-10 days. Modifier -57 would be added to an E/M code when the service resulted in a decision for surgery on the day before or the day of a procedure with a global surgical package of 90 days.

For modifier -25 to be used correctly, there must be a medical necessity to provide a separate, additional E/M service on the same day a procedure was performed or another service was provided. The medical necessity for this additional E/M service must be documented in the patient's medical record. If you do not add the modifier -25 to the separate, additional E/M code for service on the day of a procedure, the third-party payer would disallow the charge because it would be thought to be the evaluation/management portion of the procedure. By adding modifier -25, you are stating that the service was separate from the procedure or original service and are thereby increasing the potential of receiving payment for the service. For example, if a physician provided a dialysis service to a hospital inpatient and then, in addition, provided a separate E/M service for that patient for something not related to the dialysis, you would report the dialysis service (the procedure) and also report an inpatient service (E/M service), adding the modifier -25. The use of modifier -25 is not limited to E/M services that have been provided in addition to a procedure; the modifier can also be used when other E/M services are provided on the same day to the same patient. For example, if a patient came into the office for a visit early in the day and then later in the day needed to return for a separate service, you would report both services using E/M codes and add modifier -25 to the second code.

> **CODING SHOT** ✎ Modifier -25 requests payment for both E/M and a minor procedure or two E/M services on same day.

-26, Professional Component

Modifier -26 is used to designate a physician (professional) component of a service. The description of modifier -26 is as follows:

Certain procedures are a combination of a physician component and a technical component. When the physician component is reported separately, the service may be identified by adding modifier -26 to the usual procedure number.

Modifier -26 is usually used with radiology service. An example of the technical component is an independent radiology facility that takes the x-rays (the technical component) and sends them to a private radiologist who reads the x-rays and writes a report of the findings (the professional component). The physician's services would be reported with the modifier -26 added to the code for the x-ray, indicating that only the professional component of the x-ray service was provided, as in the following:

Radiology Report

Two Views of Left Knee: Findings: This examination is compared to an AP view of both knees dated 03/28/xx, performed at the Manytown Clinic. The visualized bony structures appear demineralized. No evidence for fracture, dislocation or loosening of arthroplasty is seen. There is degenerative change involving the patellofemoral joint seen on this examination. Surgical skin staples and a surgical drain are noted to be present.

Impression: Status postmedical hemiarthroplasty of the left knee.

Code 73560-26

> **CODING SHOT** ✎ Modifier -26 requests payment for the professional component percentage only.

-22 through -26 (handwritten)

EXERCISE 3-5 Modifiers -21 through -26

Using the CPT manual, code the following:

1 The surgeon performed a repair of an enterocele using an abdominal approach (57270) on a morbidly obese patient, and because of the patient's obesity the procedure took a significant amount of additional time to perform.

   Code(s) and/or modifier(s): _____

2 During a radical orchiectomy for an extensive tumor (54535), the patient began to hemorrhage. After considerable time and effort, the hemorrhage was controlled.

   Code and/or modifier(s): _____

3 An extremely anxious elderly man presented to the outpatient same-day surgery unit for a gastroscopy. The patient was unable to cooperate. The physician determined that, because of the patient's advanced dementia, general anesthesia during this procedure, which usually does not require anesthesia, was the best approach to use with the patient. What modifier would you use when coding this case?

Modifier: _____

4 Dr. Foster admitted a patient to a skilled nursing facility because of the patient's advanced dementia (during the global period for a herniorrhaphy that Dr. Foster performed). What modifier would be added to the admission service?

Modifier: _____

5 A patient came to the office twice in one day to see the same physician for unrelated problems. What modifier would be added to the code for the second office visit?

Modifier: _____

6 A 60-year-old female patient is referred to a radiology laboratory by her general physician. The laboratory takes the x-rays requested and sends them on to a radiologist to interpret and to develop the written report that is sent to the general physician. If you were coding for the radiologist, what modifier would you use to indicate the service provided by the radiologist?

Modifier: _____

-32, Mandated Services

Modifier -32 indicates a service that was required by some entity. The description of the modifier is as follows:

> *Services related to* mandated *consultation and/or related services (e.g., third-party payer, governmental, legislative or regulatory requirement) may be identified by adding modifier -32 to the basic procedure.*

This modifier is **not** used to indicate a second opinion requested by a patient, a family member, or another physician. Modifier -32 is used only when a service is required. For example, the police require a suspected rape or abuse victim to have certain tests. Another common use of modifier -32 is to indicate that a third-party payer or Workers' Compensation mandated a physical examination of a covered patient. The third-party payer usually waives the deductible and copayment for the patient and usually pays 100% of the service.

-47, Anesthesia by Surgeon

Modifier -47 is used to report a surgical procedure in which the surgeon administered regional or general anesthesia to the patient. The description of the modifier is as follows:

> *Regional or general anesthesia provided by the surgeon may be reported by adding modifier -47 to the basic service. (This does not include local anesthesia.) Note: Modifier -47 would not be used as a modifier for the anesthesia procedures.*

There are times, although they occur infrequently, when a physician acts as both the anesthesiologist and the surgeon. This usually occurs during procedures that require a regional anesthetic and is not used to describe moderate (conscious) sedation. For example, a surgeon places a tourniquet on an arm, administers a regional anesthetic, and performs a surgical procedure. The physician is acting as the anesthesiologist and would report the time spent administering the block (regional anesthetic). If the third-party payer allowed payment for modifier -47, payment would be made based on the **time** spent administering the regional anesthetic. Modifier -47 is added **only to surgery codes** and is never added to anesthesia codes. The surgeon acting as anesthesiologist would therefore report modifier -47 added to a surgery code.

-50, Bilateral Procedures

If the same procedure is performed on a mirror-image part of the body, modifier -50, indicating a bilateral procedure, would be submitted. The description of the modifier is as follows:

Unless otherwise identified in the listings, bilateral procedures that are performed at the same operative session should be identified by adding the modifier -50 to the appropriate five-digit code.

For example, an arthroplasty (total knee replacement, 27447 and 27447-50) for both left and right knees at the same operative session would be coded using the modifier -50.

Another example in which the same services may be performed on two sides would be a bilateral breast procedure (e.g., bilateral, simple complete mastectomy, 19303 and 19303-50).

CODING SHOT It is very important to determine how the third-party payer wants bilateral procedures submitted on the claim form, on a single line or multiple lines. One payer may require two codes to be displayed for the bilateral procedure (such as 27447 and 27447-50) for which they would reimburse 100% for the first code and 50% for the second code. If you submit only one code (27447-50), the payer would reimburse 50%, based on their rules for submission. Another payer may require that bilateral procedures be reported with only one code (27447-50) and would reimburse 150% based on that one code with modifier -50 representing two services.

Be sure to find out whether your third-party payer wants the surgical code to be used once with the modifier (code plus modifier -50) or used twice (code alone and code plus modifier -50) or whether the procedure should be listed twice. For hospital outpatient coding, the code is usually listed twice, without modifier. As of 1999, some modifiers were allowed for hospital outpatient coding. Appendix A of the CPT manual contains a section that lists all modifiers approved for hospital outpatient coding.

 CAUTION *Some CPT codes are for bilateral procedures and do not require a bilateral modifier. For example, 27395 is for a bilateral lengthening of the hamstring tendon, and it would be incorrect to place a bilateral modifier on the code.*

-51, Multiple Procedures

During any given operative session, more than one procedure may be performed. This is referred to as "multiple procedures" and is indicated by modifier -51. The description of the modifier is as follows:

When multiple procedures, other than E/M services, physical medicine and rehabilitation services, or provision of supplies (e.g., vaccines), are performed at the same session by the same provider, the primary procedure or service may be reported as listed. The additional procedure(s) or service(s) may be identified by appending modifier -51 to the additional procedure or service code(s). Note: This modifier should not be appended to designated "add-on" codes. See Appendix D.

What is the symbol in the CPT that directs modifier -51 should not be used?

_____

✋ **CAUTION** *You have to be careful when coding multiple procedures because CPT codes include many different procedures bundled together in one code. For example, code 58200 is a total abdominal hysterectomy, but it also includes a partial vaginectomy (removal of the vagina) with para-aortic and pelvic lymph node sampling, with or without removal of tube(s), and with or without removal of ovary(ies). It would be incorrect to code separately for each service because they are included (bundled) in the description for code 58200. Listing the subsequent procedures separately (unbundling) is considered fraud by a third-party payer. Unbundling is assigning multiple codes when one code would fully describe the service or procedure. The assigning of multiple codes results in increased reimbursement.*

However, if one code does not describe all of the procedures performed, and the secondary procedure is not considered a minor procedure that is incidental to the major procedure, each additional procedure may be reported by using the multiple procedure modifier (-51). For example, if a patient has a laminectomy with lumbar disk removal (for a herniated disk) code 63030 and also has an arthrodesis (stabilization of the area where the disk was removed) code 22612 they are multiple procedures. Both services would be coded, and modifier -51 would be used after the lesser of the two codes (services).

There are three significant times when multiple procedures are coded:

1. Same Operation, Different Site
2. Multiple Operation(s), Same Operative Session
3. Procedure Performed Multiple Times

Same Operation, Different Site. Multiple procedures are coded using modifier -51 when the same procedure is performed on different sites. For example, a patient has an excision of a 1.5-cm benign lesion from the forearm and at the same time has an excision of a 3-cm benign lesion from the neck. In this case the coding would be 11423 for the 3-cm lesion and 11402-51 for the 1.5-cm lesion. The code after which you place the -51 modifier is very important because the third-party payer usually pays for the second procedure at 50% of the usual full cost of the procedure. Always list the most resource-intensive (expensive) procedure first, without a modifier.

Multiple Operation(s), Same Operative Session. Multiple procedures (-51) are also coded when more than one procedure is performed during the same operative session.

The primary procedure during the surgical session would be paid at the full fee, the second procedure during the same session would usually be paid at 50% of the fee, and the third procedure would usually be paid at 25% of the fee. Therefore, when you are coding procedures for payment, it is important that you put the most resource-intensive procedure first, without a modifier, and then list the subsequent procedures in order of complexity, remembering to use the -51 modifier for all subsequent procedures. This process of assigning the -51 modifier helps to ensure that optimal reimbursement occurs. For example, an abdominal hysterectomy (58150) may be performed along with a posterior (rectocele) repair (57250-51). The hysterectomy is the most resource-intensive procedure, so it is listed first, without the modifier, to be paid at the full fee. The posterior repair is less resource intensive so it is listed second, with the modifier, to be paid at 50% of the fee.

> **CODING SHOT** ✎ Modifier -51 is an indication to the payer that a discount should be taken on procedures other than the most resource-intensive procedure performed on the same day.

Procedure Performed Multiple Times. Multiple procedures are also coded when the same procedure code is used to identify a service performed more than once during a single operative session. There are two ways to report procedures performed multiple times, depending on the requirements of the third-party payer. One way is to use the code number only once but to list the number of times it is performed (number of units). For example, if a patient needs a repair of two flexor tendons of the leg, you would report 27658 × 2 units. Units are identified because the code description states "each" tendon, and two tendons were repaired. The other way to code this would be to list 27658 once without a modifier and again with modifier -51 (i.e., 27658-51).

Third-party payers require submission of codes in various formats. HCPCS (Healthcare Common Procedure Coding System) has modifiers that indicate the right side (-RT) and left side (-LT) and modifiers that indicate the digits of the foot and hand:

-FA	Left hand, thumb	-TA	Left foot, great toe
-F1	Left hand, second digit	-T1	Left foot, second digit
-F2	Left hand, third digit	-T2	Left foot, third digit
-F3	Left hand, fourth digit	-T3	Left foot, fourth digit
-F4	Left hand, fifth digit	-T4	Left foot, fifth digit
-F5	Right hand, thumb	-T5	Right foot, great toe
-F6	Right hand, second digit	-T6	Right foot, second digit
-F7	Right hand, third digit	-T7	Right foot, third digit
-F8	Right hand, fourth digit	-T8	Right foot, fourth digit
-F9	Right hand, fifth digit	-T9	Right foot, fifth digit

For all Medicare claims, the digit-specific modifiers must be used. You will learn more about HCPCS in Chapter 13 of this text. You will find some of the more common HCPCS modifiers on the front inside cover of the Professional Edition of the CPT manual and in Appendix A of the CPT manual. HCPCS modifiers add specificity and, for that reason, are required by many payers.

All of the variations in format can be a bit confusing when you begin coding, so let's stop here for a moment and review a few of the more common configurations that affect -50, -51, and the times symbol.

Example

MODIFIER -50 (BILATERAL)

The physician performs a surgical sinus endoscopy with total ethmoidectomy, 31255, on the left and right ethmoid sinuses (bilateral).

1. Using modifier -50, the service would be usually reported:
      31255 and 31255-50
2. Using the Medicare modifiers for sides, (-LT, left side and -RT, right side) the service would be reported:
      31255-LT and 31255-RT
3. Using the one line format, the service would be reported:
      31255-50

The most specific method of reporting is the second format, as it indicates not only the number of procedures, but also the side of the body.

Example

MODIFIER -51 (MULTIPLE)

The physician percutaneously repairs a distal phalangeal fracture of the second and third fingers of the left hand, with skeletal fixation (26756).

1. Using modifier -51, the service would be reported:
      26756 and 26756-51
2. Using the HCPCS modifiers for fingers (-F1, left hand, second digit, and F2, left hand, third digit) the service would be reported:
      26756-F1 and 26756-F2
3. Using the times symbol, the service would be reported:
      26756 × 2

You can see that the most specific method of reporting is again the second format, as it indicates the procedure, hand, and digit.

The use of the times symbol is another area of confusion when you first begin coding.

TIMES SYMBOL (×) EXAMPLE

The physician performs a skin biopsy on five skin lesions.
    11100 (first lesion) and 11101 × 4 (second-fifth lesions)

Look for the word "**each**" in the code description as a hint to use the times symbol. The code description for 11101 states "**each** separate/additional lesion . . . ," with the "each" being the hint to use the times symbol.

Another example of the use of the times symbol is in pathology codes because some pathology payers want multiple specimens reported in units. For example, the pathologist examines three specimens of tissue.
    88302 (first specimen) and 88302 × 2 (second and third specimens)

The number of units is placed in Block 24G (Units) on the CMS-1500 form.

> ✋ **CAUTION** *Modifier -51 is not used with add-on codes that specify "each additional. . . ." For example, 19290 is for the placement of one wire into a breast lesion. If two wires were placed, the first wire would be coded 19290 from the subheading Breast and the category Introduction, and the second wire would be coded 19291 for an additional wire.*

CODING SHOT

As always, be aware that the payers dictate how providers are to submit for payment of services. For example, some payers may not want providers to submit modifier -51 for the same operation performed on different sites but instead, modifier -59 (Distinct Procedural Service). Usually, however, the standard is to require -51 for the three significant times when multiple procedures are provided.

-52, Reduced Services

Modifier -52 is used to indicate that a service was provided but was reduced in comparison to the full description of the service. The description of the modifier is as follows:

> *Under certain circumstances a service or procedure is partially reduced or eliminated at the physician's discretion. Under these circumstances the service provided can be identified by its usual procedure number and the addition of modifier -52, signifying that the service is reduced. This provides a means of reporting reduced services without disturbing the identification of the basic service. Note: For hospital outpatient reporting of a previously scheduled procedure/service that is partially reduced or canceled as a result of extenuating circumstances or those that threatened the well-being of the patient prior to or after administration of anesthesia, see modifiers -73 and -74 (see modifiers approved for ASC hospital outpatient use).*

An example of a circumstance in which modifier -52 would be used is a surgical procedure for the removal of an abdominal carcinoma in which the patient was anesthetized and the excision begun but then terminated by the physician because the metastasis was too far advanced. When modifier -52 is used, additional documentation, such as operative reports and/or physician explanation of the reason for the reduced service, will facilitate the reimbursement process, as the third-party payer usually wants to know the reason for the reduction before making payment.

CODING SHOT

Modifier -52 may or may not affect reimbursement. Some payers decrease the payment if the procedure was not completed, and others pay in full if anesthesia was provided.

EXERCISE 3–6 *Modifiers -32 through -52*

Using the CPT manual, code the following:

1 Workers' compensation referred a patient to a physician for a mandatory examination to determine the legitimacy of a claim. What modifier would be added to the code for the examination service? _____

2 Dr. Ramus administers regional anesthesia by intravenous injection (a.k.a. Bier's local anesthesia) for a surgical procedure on the patient's lower arm. Dr. Ramus then performs the surgical procedure. What modifier would be added to the surgical code? _____

3 A patient underwent bilateral carpal tunnel surgery. When you assign a code, what modifier would you be certain to use? _____

4 Destruction of malignant lesion of neck (most resource-intensive), 4 cm in diameter (17274), with destruction of malignant lesion of arm, 4 cm in diameter (17264).

Code (s) and Modifier: _____

5 Two bilateral supratentorial burr holes (each, 61250)

Code and Modifier: _____

6 Treatment of two tarsal bone fractures, without manipulation (each 28450)

Code and Modifier: _____

7 What is the code for a bilateral total knee replacement (arthroplasty)?

Code(s) and Modifier: _____ and _____

8 What are the codes for bilateral arthrotomy of the elbows (24006)?

Code(s) and Modifier: _____

9 The code for a radical mastectomy is 19305. List two ways the bilateral modifier could be used to indicate that a bilateral procedure was performed, depending on the third-party payer's preferences.

Code(s) and Modifier: _____ or _____ and _____

10 Which modifier describes a procedure that was reduced at the direction of the physician?

_____

-53, Discontinued Procedure

Modifier -52 is used to describe circumstances in which services were reduced at the direction of the physician, whereas modifier -53 describes circumstances in which a procedure was stopped because of the patient's condition.

The description of the modifier is as follows:

Under certain circumstances, the physician may elect to terminate a surgical or diagnostic procedure. Due to extenuating circumstances or those that threaten the well-being of the patient, it may be necessary to indicate that a surgical or diagnostic procedure was started but discontinued. This circumstance may be reported by adding modifier -53 to the code reported by the physician for the discontinued procedure. Note: This modifier is not used to report the elective cancellation of a procedure prior to the patient's anesthesia induction and/or surgical preparation in the operating suite. For outpatient hospital/ambulatory surgery center (ASC) reporting of a previously scheduled procedure/service that is partially reduced or canceled as a result of extenuating circumstances or those that threaten the well-being of the patient prior to or after administration of anesthesia, see modifiers -73 and -74 (see modifiers approved for ASC hospital outpatient use).

An example of the correct use of modifier -53 is a situation in which a patient was undergoing a surgical procedure and during the procedure developed arrhythmia that could not be controlled. The physician discontinued the procedure because of the risk continuation presented to the patient. The code for the surgical procedure would be reported along with modifier -53 to indicate that although the procedure was begun, it was discontinued. The key to proper use of modifier -53 is that the patient has been prepared for surgery and anesthetized.

Modifier -53 is **not** used to report services

■ when the patient cancels the procedure

■ with E/M codes

■ with any code that is based on time (e.g., critical care codes)

Modifiers -54, -55, and -56

There may be times when a surgeon performs the surgery only (modifier -54) and asks another physician to perform the preoperative evaluation (modifier -56) and/or the postoperative care (modifier -55). When reporting his or her own individual services, each physician would use the same procedure code for the surgery, letting the modifier indicate to the third-party payer the part of the surgical package that each personally performed.

Example

19303	Mastectomy, simple, complete
19303-54	Mastectomy, simple, complete, surgery only
19303-56	Mastectomy, simple, complete, preoperative evaluation only
19303-55	Mastectomy, simple, complete, postoperative care only

---

-54, Surgical Care Only

Modifier -54 is used to indicate the surgical care portion of a surgical procedure (intraoperative). Use modifier -54 only with codes from the Surgery section (10021-69990). The description of the modifier is as follows:

When one physician performs a surgical procedure and another provides preoperative and/or postoperative management, surgical services may be identified by adding modifier -54 to the usual procedure number.

Modifier -54 is used correctly only when there has been a transfer of responsibility for care from one physician to another. This transfer takes place by means of a transfer order that is signed by both physicians and kept in the patient's medical record. Modifier -54 is not used for minor surgical procedures but for major procedures that involve follow-up care as a part of the service of the surgery (a surgery package). Although third-party payers vary, the payment for only the surgical procedure is usually about 70% of the total payment for the procedure, with 10% going to the physician who provides the preoperative service, and 20% to the physician who provides the postoperative care.

CODING SHOT Modifier -54 should result in reimbursement to the surgeon of the intraoperative percentage of the global package payment. Some providers also include the preoperative service as a part of the intraoperative care portion.

-55, Postoperative Management Only

Another part of a surgical package is the postoperative care. The amount of postoperative care that is considered part of a surgery varies according to the complexity of the surgery, with 0, 10, or 90 days being the most commonly used number of postoperative days. The description of modifier -55 is as follows:

When one physician performed the postoperative management and another physician performed the surgical procedure, the postoperative component may be identified by adding modifier -55 to the usual procedure number.

Modifier -55 is used only for services provided to the patient after discharge from the hospital. To report services by another physician provided while the patient is still in the hospital, you would use E/M codes because the payment to the operating physician (70%) assumes that the operating physician provides the care until the patient is discharged from the hospital.

You report the postoperative services by adding modifier -55 to the surgical code. For example, a patient had a nephrolithotomy (calculus removed from kidney), coded 50060, and the operating physician transferred to a second physician the postoperative care after the patient's discharge from the hospital. The operating physician would report services using 50060-54, and the physician providing the postoperative care would report 50060-55. The physicians use the same surgery code (50060) and also report the date of service as the date of the surgical procedure. In this way, the third-party payer knows that the two physicians are splitting the care of the patient into surgical care and postoperative care after discharge.

CODING SHOT Modifier -55 should result in reimbursement of the post-operative percentage for the global package. This percentage is based on how many days had passed after the operation before the care was transferred from the first physician to the second physician.

✋ **CAUTION** *For Medicare patients, care must be officially transferred from the physician providing the surgical care to the physician providing the postoperative care by way of a transfer order that is kept in the medical record.*

-56, Preoperative Management Only

The third part of a surgical service is the preoperative care. If a physician provides only the preoperative management to a patient in preparation for surgery, the service is reported with modifier -56 added to the surgical code. The description of the modifier is as follows:

When one physician performed the preoperative care and evaluation and another physician performed the surgical procedure, the preoperative component may be identified by adding modifier -56 to the usual procedure number.

Before a patient undergoes surgery, a physical examination is performed to determine whether the patient is physically able to withstand the surgery. This examination is the preoperative workup. When one physician performs the preoperative workup and another physician performs the surgery, both physicians report the services by using the surgical procedure code and adding the correct modifier. For example, in preparation for a nephrolithotomy, a physician at the Mayo Clinic provided the preoperative care (50060-56) and the patient was referred to his hometown surgeon for surgery (50060-54).

⬣ **STOP** *Modifier -56 is never used for services reported to Medicare, as Medicare considers the preoperative service to be part of the surgery.*

-57, Decision for Surgery

Modifier -57 is used with an E/M code to indicate the day the decision to perform a major surgery was made. The description of the modifier is as follows:

An E/M service that resulted in the initial decision to perform the surgery may be identified by adding modifier -57 to the appropriate level of E/M service.

Modifier -57 can be used not only with E/M codes (99201-99499) to indicate the initial decision to perform a procedure or service but also with the ophthalmologic codes (92002-92014) located in the Medicine section. Modifier -57 requests payment for an E/M service outside of the global package for a major procedure when the decision to perform the surgery was made during the E/M service.

At the present time, not all modifiers are recognized by all third-party payers. Some third-party payers have agreed to pay a physician separately from the surgical package for the initial evaluation of a condition during which the decision to perform surgery was made. Modifier -57 is used to let the payer know that payment for this initial evaluation should be made in addition to payment for surgery. E/M services provided the day before or on the day of a major surgery, or on the day of a minor procedure, are included in the global package unless it is the patient's initial visit to the physician or if the decision to perform surgery is made during the visit. To receive payment for these initial visits, modifier -57 is used to indicate the day before or the day of the **major** procedure and modifier -25 is used to indicate the day of the **minor** procedure.

✋ **CAUTION** *Don't make the all too common mistake of adding -57 to codes from the Surgery section. Modifier -57 is never added to surgical codes; rather, it is added only to E/M codes.*

CODING SHOT Note that the description of modifier -57 does not indicate whether the decided-upon procedure is diagnostic or therapeutic, minor or major. But Medicare guidelines direct that modifier -57 be used only with E/M or ophthalmologic codes to indicate when the decision to perform a major procedure was made.

-58, Staged or Related Procedure or Service by the Same Physician During the Postoperative Period

Modifier -58 explains that the subsequent surgery was planned or staged at the time of the first surgery. The description of the modifier is as follows:

It may be necessary to indicate that the performance of a procedure or service during the postoperative period was: a) planned or anticipated (staged); b) more extensive than the original procedure; or c) for therapy following a surgical procedure. This circumstance may be reported by adding modifier -58 to the staged or related procedure. Note: For treatment of a problem that requires a return to the operating or procedure room (e.g., unanticipated clinical condition), see modifier -78.

The procedure as a whole must have been intended to include the original procedure plus one or more subsequent procedures. For example, multiple skin grafts are often done in stages to allow adequate healing time between procedures. Modifier -58 can also be used if a therapeutic procedure is performed because of the findings of a diagnostic procedure. For example, a patient may have a surgical breast biopsy, and if the pathology report indicates that the specimen is malignant, the patient may elect to have an immediate radical mastectomy. The mastectomy may be performed during the postoperative period of the biopsy. Modifier -58 indicates to the third-party payer that the second surgery was therapeutic treatment that followed the original diagnostic procedure, and full payment would usually be made for the mastectomy. A new postoperative period would start after the mastectomy, and any postoperative care provided to the patient would be part of the surgical package for the mastectomy.

Modifier -58 requests full payment for a subsequent procedure that may have been planned in follow-up, at the time of the first surgery, or performed as a more extensive procedure subsequent to the first surgery. A new global period will begin with each subsequent procedure modified with -58.

-59, Distinct Procedural Service

Modifier -59 is used to indicate that services that are usually bundled into one payment were provided as separate services. The description of the modifier is as follows:

Under certain circumstances, it may be necessary to indicate that a procedure or service was distinct or independent from other non-E/M services performed on the same day. Modifier -59 is used to identify procedures or services, other than E/M services, that are not normally reported together, but are appropriate under the circumstances. Documentation must support a different session, different procedure or surgery, different site or organ system, separate incision or excision, separate lesion, or separate injury (or area of injury in extensive injuries) not ordinarily encountered or performed on the same day by the same individual. However, when another already established modifier is appropriate, it should be used rather than modifier -59. Only if no more descriptive modifier is available, and the use of modifier -59 best explains the circumstances, should modifier -59 be used. Note: Modifier -59 should not be appended to an E/M service. To report a separate and distinct E/M service with a non-E/M service performed on the same date, see modifier -25.

As the code description notes, modifier -59 is used to identify the following:

- Different session
- Different procedure or surgery
- Different site or organ system
- Separate incision/excision
- Separate lesion
- Separate injury or area of injury in extensive injuries

Modifier -59 is used with codes from all sections of the CPT manual except E/M codes. Medicare has lists of codes that cannot be reported together; they are called edits. These edits have been established to ensure that providers do not report services that are included in the bundle for a given code. For example, the same physician would not report a standard preoperative visit related to a major surgical procedure and report separately the surgery and follow-up care. All three services—preoperative, intraoperative, postoperative— are packaged together in one major surgical CPT code. The use of modifier -59 indicates that the service was not a part of another service but, indeed, was a distinct service. For example, a colonoscopy utilizing a snare (45385) and a colonoscopy with hot biopsy forceps (45384) would usually not be reported together as they would be in the edits, but if -59 is appended to 45384, the surgeon is indicating these were distinct services.

CODING SHOT ✎ Modifier -59 requests payment for a procedure performed on the same day as another procedure that normally would not be reimbursed separately, e.g., a biopsy of one site and an excision of another site.

EXERCISE 3-7 *Modifiers -53 through -59*

Using the CPT manual, code the following:

1 Mrs. Knight has a diagnostic surgical biopsy of deep cervical lymph nodes on May 8, and the pathology report comes back showing malignancy. Mrs. Knight elects to have a lymphadenectomy on May 11. What modifier would be used with the lymphadenectomy code?

 Modifier: _____

2 The surgical care only for a total esophagectomy without reconstruction (43124)

 Code(s) and Modifier: _____

3 The postoperative care only for a radical mastectomy including pectoral muscles, axillary, and internal mammary lymph nodes (19306)

 Code(s) and Modifier: _____

4 The procedure in question 3 when the preoperative service only is provided _____

-62, Two Surgeons

Modifier -62 is used to indicate that two surgeons acted as co-surgeons. The description of the modifier is as follows:

> *When two surgeons work together as primary surgeons performing distinct part(s) of a procedure, each surgeon should report his/her distinct operative work by adding modifier -62 to the procedure code and any associated add-on code(s) for that procedure as long as both surgeons continue to work together as primary surgeons. Each surgeon should report the co-surgery once using the same procedure code. If additional procedure(s), including add-on procedure(s), are performed during the same surgical session, separate code(s) may also be reported with modifier -62 added. Note: if a co-surgeon acts as an assistant in the performance of additional procedure(s) during the same surgical session, those services may be reported using separate procedure code(s) with the modifier -80 or modifier -82 added, as appropriate.*

From the Trenches

"As you develop your skills, you can move into dozens of different areas of specialization. Pay close attention to the areas of your work where you feel most inclined to excel and explore. You're likely to be very happy there!"

JANE

To use modifier -62 correctly, two physicians of different specialties must have worked together as co-surgeons. Each co-surgeon must dictate his/her own operative report. If one physician assists another physician, the service cannot be reported using modifier -62. The co-surgeons use different skills during the surgery. Many third-party payers require documentation showing the medical necessity of co-surgeons. The operative reports, one supplied by each surgeon documenting their participation, should clearly show the distinct services each surgeon provided. Modifier -62 is correctly used when two physicians are necessary to complete one surgical procedure, each completing a distinct portion of the procedure. For example, a cardiologist and a general surgeon may install a pacemaker, with the general surgeon preparing the implantation site, the cardiologist inserting and activating the pacemaker, and the general surgeon closing the site. Each physician would report his/her service using the pacemaker insertion code with the modifier -62 added.

CODING SHOT Modifier -62 will usually cue the payer to reimburse at 125% of the fee schedule, which is then divided, half for each surgeon.

-63, Procedure Performed on Infants Less than 4 kg

Modifier -63 is used to identify procedures provided to a neonate or infant up to 4 kg (8.8 lb). The description of the modifier is as follows:

Procedures performed on neonates and infants up to a present body weight of 4 kg may involve significantly increased complexity and physician work commonly associated with these patients. This circumstance may be reported by adding modifier -63 to the procedure number. Note: Unless otherwise designated, this modifier may only be appended to procedures/services listed in the 20000-69990 code series. Modifier -63 should not be appended to any CPT codes listed in the E/M, Anesthesia, Radiology, Pathology/Laboratory, or Medicine sections.

The Integumentary System subsection is the only Surgery section of codes with which modifier -63 cannot be used. Procedures on neonates or infants with a body weight of less than 4 kg are more complex than procedures that are performed on neonates or infants with a body weight of more than 4 kg.

QUICK CHECK 3-6

Would modifier -63 be reported with codes 49491-49496? Why or why not?

_____

-66, Surgical Team

Modifier -66 is used with very complex surgical procedures that require several physicians, usually of different specialties, to complete the procedure. The description of the modifier is as follows:

Under some circumstances, highly complex procedures (requiring the concomitant services of several physicians, often of different specialties, plus other highly skilled, specially trained personnel, various types of complex equipment) are carried out under the "surgical team" concept. Such circumstances may be identified by each participating physician with the addition of modifier -66 to the basic procedure number used for reporting services.

A surgical team consists of physicians, technicians, and other trained personnel who function together to complete a complex procedure. Teams are usually used in organ transplant surgeries, with each member of the team completing the same function at each surgery. Each physician would report the procedure code with modifier -66 added. Third-party payers will often increase the total reimbursement for a team. The reimbursement is then divided among the physicians on the basis of a prearranged agreement.

> **CODING SHOT** Modifier -66 will cue the payer that payment for a procedure should be increased by whatever the contract allows to be divided by all surgeons involved.

-76, Repeat Procedure or Service by Same Physician

Modifier -76 is used to report services or procedures that are repeated and are provided by the same physician. The description of the modifier is as follows:

> *It may be necessary to indicate that a procedure or service was repeated subsequent to the original procedure or service. This circumstance may be reported by adding modifier -76 to the repeated procedure/service.*

The modifier is used to indicate to third-party payers that the services are not duplicate services and, therefore, the bill is not a duplicate bill. Sometimes these repeat services are provided on the same day as the previous service, and without the use of modifier -76, the third-party payer would assume a duplicate bill had been submitted. When modifier -76 has been used, documentation must accompany the claim in order to establish medical necessity.

> **CODING SHOT** Modifier -76 requests payment for a service that was repeated. If the modifier was not used, the subsequent service would be denied as a duplicate service.

-77, Repeat Procedure by Another Physician

Modifier -77 is used to report services or procedures that are repeated and are provided by a physician other than the physician who originally provided the service or procedure. The description of the modifier is as follows:

> *The physician may need to indicate that a basic procedure or service performed by another physician had to be repeated. This situation may be reported by adding modifier -77 to the repeated procedure/service.*

The modifier is used to indicate to third-party payers that the services are not duplicate services and, therefore, the bill is not a duplicate bill. Sometimes these repeat services are provided on the same day as the original service or during the postop period. Without the use of modifier -77, the third-party payer would assume a duplicate bill had been submitted. If only a portion of the original service or procedure is repeated, you would use modifier -52 to indicate a reduced service. When modifier -77 has been used, documentation must accompany the claim in order to establish medical necessity.

> **CODING SHOT** Modifier -77 requests payment for a service that was repeated. If the modifier was not used, the subsequent service would be denied as a duplicate service.

-78, Unplanned Return to the Operating/ Procedure Room by the Same Physician Following Initial Procedure for a Related Procedure During the Postoperative Period

Modifier -78 is used to explain a circumstance in which a patient is returned to the operating room for surgical treatment of a complication resulting from the first procedure. The description of the modifier is as follows:

It may be necessary to indicate that another procedure was performed during the postoperative period of the initial procedure (unplanned procedure following initial procedure). When this procedure is related to the first and requires the use of an operating or procedure room, it may be reported by adding modifier -78 to the related procedure. (For repeat procedures on the same day, see modifier -76.)

Modifier -78 is placed after the subsequent procedure code to indicate to the third-party payer that the second surgery was necessary because of complications resulting from the first operation. For many third-party payers, only the surgery portion (intraoperative) of the surgical package is paid when the -78 modifier is used. The patient remains within the postoperative period of the first operation for any further preoperative or postoperative care. For example, if the patient were to develop a second set of complications stemming from the original surgery, you would again report the procedure performed to treat the second complication and add modifier -78 to the code. In this way, the third-party payer continues to know that the complication requiring surgery originated from the original surgery.

✋ **CAUTION** *If there were a complication, you would report -78 (Unplanned Return to the Operating Room) and -76 (Repeat Procedure Or Service By Same Physician). For example, a patient who has an open heart coronary artery bypass graft procedure (Session 1) returns to the operating room for tamponade (fluid accumulation in the pericardium) twice on the same day (Sessions 2 and 3).*

Session 1
33510   Coronary artery bypass graft

Session 2
35820-78   Exploration for postoperative hemorrhage, chest

Session 3
35820-76-78   Repeat exploration for postoperative hemorrhage
                 of chest

Sessions 2 and 3 should be reimbursed at the intraoperative rate and the global period would not start over again.

CODING SHOT 🖊 Modifier -78 will cue the payer to reimburse the procedure at the intraoperative percent of the service. The patient remains in the global period for the initial surgery.

-79, Unrelated Procedure or Service by the Same Physician During the Postoperative Period

Modifier -79 is used to explain that a patient requires surgery for a condition totally unrelated to the condition for which the first operation was performed. The description of the modifier is as follows:

The physician may need to indicate that the performance of a procedure or service during the postoperative period was unrelated to the original procedure. This circumstance may be reported by using modifier -79. (For repeat procedures on the same day, see modifier -76.)

For example, the patient may have had an appendectomy and 2 weeks later has a gallbladder episode that necessitates removal of the gallbladder. The modifier -79 would be placed on the cholecystectomy code, indicating that the subsequent procedure was unrelated to the first procedure. The diagnosis codes for the two procedures would also be different, thus substantiating that the two procedures were unrelated.

 CAUTION *Do not use modifier -79 with staged procedures (use modifier -58) or with procedures that are related to the original procedure. If the service is provided during the postoperative period of a major surgical procedure, billing separately for services included in the surgical package is fraudulent.*

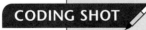 **CODING SHOT** Modifier -79 requests payment for the full fee of the subsequent service because it was unassociated with the first procedure. A new global period should start when this modifier is used.

-80, Assistant Surgeon

A surgical assistant is one who provides service to the primary surgeon during a surgical procedure. The description of the modifier is as follows:

Surgical assistant services may be identified by adding modifier -80 to the usual procedure number(s).

The assistant surgeon's services are reported using the same code as the primary surgeon's, but modifier -80 is added to alert the third-party payer to the assistant surgeon status. Usually, the assistant receives only 15% to 30% of the usual charge for a surgery when acting in the assistant capacity. Not all payers allow for a surgical assistant on all procedures. The preauthorization for surgery that would be completed before surgery should indicate whether the payer will consider reimbursement for a surgical assistant.

CODING SHOT Preauthorization does not guarantee payment, as the payer can always deny the approval upon review.

-81, Minimum Assistant Surgeon

Modifier -81 is used to indicate an assistant surgeon who provides services that are less extensive than those described by modifier -80. The description of the modifier is as follows:

Minimum surgical assistant services are identified by adding modifier -81 to the usual procedure number.

Some procedures require **more than one assistant.** Those additional assistant services are reported by using the surgical procedure code with modifier -81 added. In other instances, the first assistant is required to be in attendance for only a portion of the procedure, and this lesser service would be reported by using modifier -81. Many third-party payers do not pay for a minimum assistant surgeon. For example, Medicare will pay for a minimum assistant only on rare occasions in which medical necessity can be proven. Usually, the minimum assistant surgeon receives 10% of the usual charge for a surgery.

 CAUTION *Do not use modifier -81 to report nonphysician service assistance during a surgical procedure. Modifier -81 is limited to a physician serving in the capacity of an assistant.*

-82, Assistant Surgeon (When Qualified Resident Surgeon Not Available)

Modifier -82 is used when the hospital in which the procedure was performed has an affiliation with a medical school and has a residency program, but no resident was available to serve as an assistant surgeon. Residents are medical students who are completing a required surgical training period in the hospital. The description of the modifier is as follows:

The unavailability of a qualified resident surgeon is a prerequisite for use of modifier -82 appended to the usual procedure code number(s).

Do not confuse modifier -80 with -82 when reporting services. Medicare does not pay for an assistant surgeon if the hospital has a residency program because the residents serve as employees of the hospital who are there to receive training and provide assistance to physicians as part of the hospital's agreement with the medical school. Hospitals that have affiliations with medical schools are considered teaching facilities. Modifier -82 has very limited use and requires supporting documentation that the patient's condition was so severe that it required an assistant and that a qualified resident was not available.

CODING SHOT Modifiers -80, -81, and -82 will cue the payer to reimburse on a previously established percentage of the global payment for the service.

EXERCISE 3-8 Modifiers -62 through -82

Using the CPT manual, code the following:

1 Dr. Edwards, a cardiologist, and Dr. Mathews, a general surgeon, worked together as primary surgeons on a complex surgical case. What modifier would be added to the CPT surgery codes for the services of both Dr. Edwards and Dr. Mathews? _____

2 A team of physicians with different specialties, along with a highly skilled team of technical personnel, performed a liver transplant. Using which modifier would indicate the surgical team concept? _____

3 Dr. Stenopolis served as a surgical assistant to Dr. Edwards in a quadruple bypass procedure. Dr. Stenopolis' services were reported by using this modifier: _____

4 In the middle of the bypass procedure in Question 3, the patient experienced severe complications. Dr. Edwards asked Dr. Loren to come into the operating room to temporarily assist in stabilizing the patient. What modifier would be used when reporting the service Dr. Loren provided? _____

5 A patient has a hernia repair and 2 days later must be returned to the operating room for a related repair. When coding the secondary hernia repair, which modifier would you add onto the surgical code? _____

6 If Mr. Smith undergoes an appendectomy on June 8, and then a cholecystectomy is performed on August 16 by the same surgeon, what modifier would be placed on the cholecystectomy code? _____

7 What modifier would you add to a code to indicate that a basic procedure performed by another physician was repeated? _____

-90, Reference (Outside) Laboratory

Modifier -90 is used to indicate that services of an outside laboratory were used. The description of the modifier is as follows:

When laboratory procedures are performed by a party other than the treating or reporting physician, the procedure may be identified by adding modifier -90 to the usual procedure number.

This modifier is used with codes in the Pathology and Laboratory section to report that the procedures were performed by someone other than the treating or reporting physician. Medicare does not allow physicians to bill for outside laboratory services and then reimburse the outside laboratory for those services. If the outside laboratory provides the services, the outside laboratory must report the services.

-91, Repeat Clinical Diagnostic Laboratory Test

Modifier -91 is used to report a laboratory test that was performed on the same day as the original laboratory test. The description of the modifier is as follows:

In the course of treatment of a patient, it may be necessary to repeat the same laboratory test on the same day to obtain subsequent (multiple) test results. Under these circumstances, the laboratory test performed can be identified by its usual procedure number and the addition of modifier -91. Note: This modifier may not be used when tests are rerun to confirm initial results; due to testing problems with specimens or equipment; or for any other reason when a normal, one-time, reportable result is all that is required. This modifier may not be used when other code(s) describe a series of test results (e.g., glucose tolerance tests, evocative/suppression testing). This modifier may only be used for laboratory test(s) performed more than once on the same day on the same patient.

This modifier is correctly used when a laboratory test has been repeated so as to produce multiple test results. It cannot be used if the equipment malfunctioned or if there was a problem with the specimen, which would result in third-party payers' paying for laboratory errors. Nor can you use the modifier to report services performed because a subsequent test was done to confirm the results of the initial test. The modifier cannot be used when there is a series of test results, such as those found in allergy testing.

-92 Alternative Laboratory Platform Testing

Modifier -92 is used to report those incidents when a kit or transportable instrument is used in a laboratory test. For example, a single use, disposable HIV kit (86701-86703).

When laboratory testing is being performed using a kit or transportable intrument that wholly or in part consists of a single use, disposable analytical chamber, the service may be identified by adding modifier -92 to the usual laboratory procedure code (HIV testing 86701-86703). The test does not require permanent dedicated space; hence by its design it may be hand carried or transported to the vicinity of the patient for immediate testing at that site, although location of the testing is not in itself determinative of the use of this modifier.

24. A. DATE(S) OF SERVICE						B. PLACE OF SERVICE	C. EMG	D. PROCEDURES, SERVICES, OR SUPPLIES (Explain Unusual Circumstances)		E. DIAGNOSIS POINTER
From			To					CPT/HCPCS	MODIFIER	
MM	DD	YY	MM	DD	YY					
								19306		

FIGURE 3–13 Multiple modifiers on CMS-1500 (08/05).

-99, Multiple Modifiers

Modifier -99 is needed only if the third-party payer does not accept the addition of multiple modifiers to a code. This is the case with some computerized insurance submissions. The description of the modifier is as follows:

> Under certain circumstances two or more modifiers may be necessary to completely delineate a service. In such situations modifier -99 should be added to the basic procedure, and other applicable modifiers may be listed as part of the description of the service.

On the CMS-1500 (08/05) there is space for multiple modifiers (Fig. 3–13). Third-party payers vary in terms of how they require multiple modifiers to be reported, so be certain to check with the payer before submitting multiple modifiers.

EXERCISE 3-9   *Modifiers -90 through -99*

Using the CPT manual, code the following:

1 What is the modifier that indicates that multiple modifiers apply? _____

2 What modifier would be added to the laboratory procedure code to indicate testing by an outside laboratory? _____

3 The medical record indicated that the physician had an established patient go to the lab for a blood panel in the morning, and in the afternoon had the patient return to the lab for another blood panel so as to produce multiple test results. What modifier would you add to the code for the panel? _____

CHAPTER REVIEW

CHAPTER 3, PART I, THEORY

Complete the following:

1 Anesthesia services are based on _____ time the patient is under the anesthesiologist's care. Calculation of units of time is determined by the third-party payer.

2 Anesthesia time begins when the

anesthesiologist _____,

continues _____ the procedure,

and ends when _____.

3 According to the Anesthesia Guidelines, what is the one modifier that is not used with

anesthesia procedures? _____

4 "P1" is an example of what type of modifier?

_____

5 What word means "in a dying state"?

_____

6 What word means "affecting the body as a

whole"? _____

7 The letter "P" in combination with what number indicates a brain-dead patient?

_____

8 What type of circumstance identifies a component of anesthesia service that affects

the character of the service? _____

_____

9 Anesthesia procedures are divided by what type

of site? _____

10 When several physicians, with technicians and specialized equipment, work together to complete a complicated procedure and each physician has a specific portion of the surgery to complete, they are termed what?

_____

11 Is it true that a physician who personally administers the anesthesia to the patient upon whom he or she is operating cannot bill the

third-party payer? _____

12 What is the name of the guide that is published by the American Society of Anesthesiologists and provides the weights of various anesthesia services?

_____

_____

CHAPTER 3, PART II, PRACTICAL

Using your CPT manual, identify the modifier for the following descriptions:

13 Repeat procedure or service by same physician

_____

14 Two surgeons _____

15 Professional component _____

16 Multiple modifiers _____

17 Distinct procedural service

_____

18 Mandated service _____

19 ~~Prolonged E/M service~~ *Increased Procedure Service* _____

20 Minimum assistant surgeon

_____

21 Repeat procedure by another physician

_____

22 Unrelated procedure or service by the same physician during the postoperative period

_____

23 Unusual anesthesia _____

24 Unplanned return to the operating room for a related procedure during the postoperative period _____

25 Surgical care only _____

26 Reduced service _____

27 Surgical team _____

QUICK CHECK ANSWERS

QUICK CHECK 3-1
In the CPT index, locate the main term "Injection," subterm "Spinal Cord," then subterm "Blood" for code 62273.

QUICK CHECK 3-2
Anesthesia Guidelines

QUICK CHECK 3-3
QX: indicates direction is by a physician other than an anesthesiologist, such as a surgeon
QY: indicates direction is by an anesthesiologist

QUICK CHECK 3-4
d. All of the above

QUICK CHECK 3-5
⊘ Symbol preceding a code indicates it is modifier -51 exempt.

QUICK CHECK 3-6
No. Parenthetical notes following codes indicate modifier -63 is not reported with these codes.

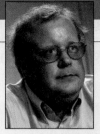

"Get all the codes in correct up front . . . It sets the stage for anything you have to do with the insurance companies."

Christopher P. Galeziewski, CPC
Coding Compliance Specialist
Coding Compliance Department
Kelsey-Seybold Clinic
Houston, Texas

Introduction to the Surgery Section and Integumentary System

Chapter Topics

PART I: *Introduction to the Surgery Section*

Format

Separate Procedures

Surgical Package

PART II: *General and Integumentary System Subsections*

General Subsections

Format

Skin, Subcutaneous, and Accessory Structures

Nails

Repair (Closure)

Burns

Destruction

Breast Procedures

Chapter Review

Quick Check Answers

Learning Objectives

After completing this chapter, you should be able to

1   Understand the Surgery section format.

2   Locate notes and Guidelines in the Surgery section.

3   Identify the text-change symbol used in the CPT manual.

4   State the use of the unlisted procedure codes.

5   Examine the separate procedure designation.

6   Analyze the contents of a surgical package.

7   Understand what is meant by a surgical tray.

8   Distinguish between professional and facility services.

9   Identify the elements of coding Skin, Subcutaneous, and Accessory Structures services.

10 Review the main services in Nails and Introductions.

11 Identify the major factors in wound repair.

12 State the important coding considerations in destruction, Mohs' micrographic surgery, and breast procedures.

13 Demonstrate the ability to code integumentary services and procedures.

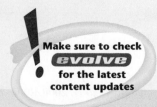

Make sure to check **evolve** for the latest content updates

PART I ■ *Introduction to the Surgery Section*

FORMAT The Surgery section is the largest in the CPT manual. The codes range from 10021 to 69990. Surgery is divided into 19 subsections. Most Surgery subsections are defined according to medical specialty or body system (e.g., integumentary or respiratory).

EXERCISE 4–1 *The Section Format*

To help you become familiar with the format of the Surgery section, write the names of the Surgery subsections on the lines provided in the order in which they are found in the CPT manual.

List the Surgery subsections:

1 _____

2 _____

3 _____

4 _____

5 _____

6 _____

7 _____

8 _____

9 _____

10 _____

11 _____

12 _____

13 _____

14 _____

15 _____

16 _____

17 _____

18 _____

19 _____

Within the Surgery section, some of the more complex subsections are the Integumentary, Musculoskeletal, Respiratory, Cardiovascular, Digestive, and Female Genital subsections. These subsections have extensive notes, and each is covered in this text. Before we get into the details of the subsections, let's look at the general information that is pertinent to the entire Surgery section.

Notes and Guidelines Guidelines are found at the beginning of each of the CPT sections. The section Guidelines define terms that are necessary for appropriately interpreting and reporting the procedures and services contained in that section. For example, the Surgery Guidelines contain the following information:

- Physicians' Services: a reference explaining how to use the E/M service codes when appropriate
- CPT Surgical Package Definition: defines what is included in the surgical procedure
- Follow-up Care for Diagnostic Procedures: defines follow-up care for diagnostic services
- Follow-up Care for Therapeutic Surgical Procedures: defines follow-up care for therapeutic services
- Materials Supplied by Physician: describes how and when to code for supplies
- Reporting More Than One Procedure/Service: identifies situations in which it may be appropriate to use modifiers for multiple services on the same day
- Separate Procedure: how to use codes with this designation
- Subsection Information: lists subsections that have instructional notes
- Unlisted Service or Procedure: unlisted service codes from the Surgery section
- Special Reports: what to include in and when to submit a special report
- Surgical Destruction: clarifies that destruction can be accomplished by any method, and that there are limited exceptions when the method is specifically coded

The **Guidelines** contain information that you will need to know in order to correctly code in the section, and most of the information is not repeated elsewhere in the section. So always review the Guidelines before coding in the section. Remember that with each new edition of the CPT manual, you will need to review the Guidelines for any changes. The changes are indicated by the "New or Revised Text" symbols used throughout the CPT manual (Fig. 4–1).

Common throughout the CPT manual are notes. Notes may appear before subsections (Fig. 4–2), subheadings (Fig. 4–3), categories (Fig. 4–4), and subcategories (Fig. 4–5).

The information in the notes indicates the special instructions unique to particular codes or unique to particular groups of codes. The notes are extremely important because the information contained in them is not usually available in the Guidelines of the CPT manual. Always make it a practice to read any notes available before coding. If notes are present, they must be followed if the coding is to be accurate.

Reporting More Than One Procedure/Service

▶ When a physician performs more than one procedure/service on the same date, during the same session, or during a postoperative period (subject to the "surgical package" concept), several CPT modifiers may apply. (See Appendix A for definition.) ◀

New or revised text symbol

FIGURE 4–1 New or revised text symbol.

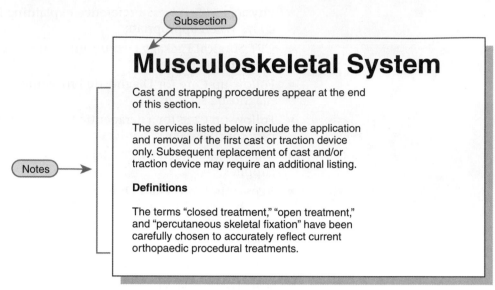

FIGURE 4-2   Subsection notes.

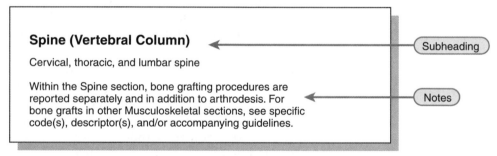

FIGURE 4-3   Subheading notes.

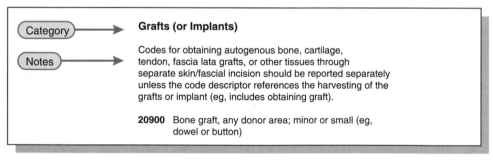

FIGURE 4-4   Category notes.

Additional information is enclosed in parentheses. Called parenthetical phrases, they sometimes follow the code or group of codes, and they provide further information about codes that may be applicable. For example, 42120, for the resection of the palate or extensive resection of a lesion, is followed by information about the codes you would use if reconstruction of the palate followed the resection (Fig. 4–6).

Deleted codes are also indicated in the CPT manual, enclosed in parentheses. Often the code that is to be used in place of the deleted code will be listed (Fig. 4–7).

Also note in Fig. 4–7 that the arrows at the beginning and end of the information indicate that the information is new or has been revised for the current edition.

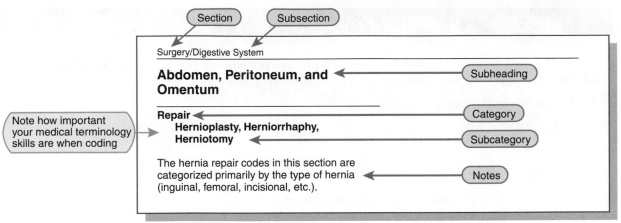

Section   Subsection

Surgery/Digestive System

Abdomen, Peritoneum, and Omentum ← Subheading

Note how important your medical terminology skills are when coding →

Repair ← Category
   Hernioplasty, Herniorrhaphy, Herniotomy ← Subcategory

The hernia repair codes in this section are categorized primarily by the type of hernia (inguinal, femoral, incisional, etc.). ← Notes

FIGURE 4–5   Subcategory notes.

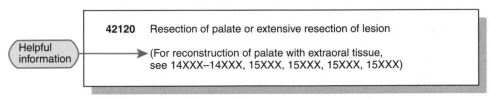

42120   Resection of palate or extensive resection of lesion

Helpful information → (For reconstruction of palate with extraoral tissue, see 14XXX–14XXX, 15XXX, 15XXX, 15XXX, 15XXX)

FIGURE 4–6   Additional helpful information.

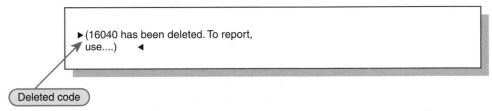

▶ (16040 has been deleted. To report, use....)   ◀

Deleted code

FIGURE 4–7   Deleted codes.

Unlisted Procedures

The Surgery Guidelines contain many unlisted procedure codes, presented by anatomic site. These unlisted codes are presented in alphabetical order by their location in the Surgery section and in the subsections by body system. For example, the unlisted procedure code for procedures of the forearm or wrist, 25999, is located at the end of the subheading Forearm and Wrist. The unlisted codes are used to identify procedures or services throughout the Surgery section for which there is no CPT code. If a Category III code is available for the unlisted service you are reporting, you must use the Category III code, not the unlisted Category I code.

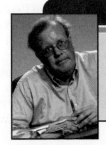

From the Trenches

"Learn as much as you can about human anatomy . . . Learn as much as you can about operative procedures. It speeds up the learning time 200-fold."

CHRIS

EXERCISE 4–2 *Unlisted Procedures*

Using the CPT manual, locate the unlisted procedure codes in the Surgical Guidelines, and identify the unlisted procedure codes for the following anatomic areas:

1 Musculoskeletal system, general

Code: _____

2 Inner ear

Code: _____

3 Skin, mucous membranes, and subcutaneous tissue

Code: _____

4 Leg or ankle

Code(s): _____

5 Nervous system

Code: _____

6 Eyelids

Code: _____

Special Reports

When using an unlisted procedure code for surgery, a special report describing the procedure must accompany the claim. According to the CPT manual, "Pertinent information [in the special report] should include an adequate definition or description of the nature, extent, and need for the procedure, and the time, effort, and equipment necessary to provide the service." Unlisted codes are used only after thorough research fails to reveal an existing code.

Example

When the first total arthroplasty (artificial disc) was performed there was no code to report the service, so a special report would have to be submitted. The report contained a detailed description of the procedure, why it was being performed, the extent of the procedure, the length of time the procedure required, and the equipment necessary. There is now a Category III code to describe this procedure (0090T).

SEPARATE PROCEDURES

Some procedure codes will have the words "separate procedure" after the descriptor. This term, "separate procedure," does not mean that the procedure was the only procedure that was performed; rather, it is an indication of how the code can be used. Locate code 19100 in the CPT manual. The breast biopsy code 19100 has the words "separate procedure" after the description. Procedures followed by the words "separate procedure" (in parentheses) are **minor** procedures that are coded only when they are the only services performed or when they are performed with another major procedure but at a different site or unrelated to the major procedure. When the same minor procedure is performed in conjunction with a related major procedure, the minor procedure is considered incidental and is bundled into the code with the major procedure.

Example

Separate procedure bundled into the major procedure: Breast biopsy (19100) has "separate procedure" after it. If a breast biopsy was performed in conjunction with a modified radical mastectomy (19307), only the mastectomy would be coded. Because the breast biopsy and the mastectomy were conducted on the same body area, the breast biopsy would be considered a minor procedure that was incidental and would be bundled into the major procedure of the mastectomy.

Example

Two separate procedures: If a breast biopsy (19100 a separate procedure) was performed in conjunction with an esophagoscopy (43200), both the breast biopsy and the esophagoscopy would be reported. The breast biopsy and the esophagoscopy were performed on different body areas and as such, the breast biopsy would not be bundled into the other procedure.

Example

Separate procedure bundled into the major procedure. Salpingo-oophorectomy (58720— removal of tubes and ovaries) has "separate procedure" after it. If a salpingo-oophorectomy was performed in conjunction with an abdominal hysterectomy (removal of the uterus, 58150), only the hysterectomy would be coded. Because the salpingo-oophorectomy and the abdominal hysterectomy were conducted on the same body area, the salpingo-oophorectomy would be bundled into the more major procedure of the hysterectomy. When performed as the only procedure, a salpingo-oophorectomy has a 90-day postoperative global period as is assigned to other major procedures.

Example

Two separate procedures: If a salpingo-oophorectomy (58720—separate procedure) was performed in conjunction with an esophagoscopy (43200), both the salpingo-oophorectomy and the esophagoscopy would be coded. Because the salpingo-oophorectomy and the esophagoscopy were conducted on different body areas, the salpingo-oophorectomy is considered a separate procedure, not a minor procedure incidental to a major procedure.

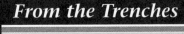

From the Trenches

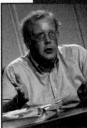

"Find a subspecialty you like . . . [and] if it's a surgical subspecialty, get as many operative reports as you can. Read them. Compare the codes in the book to what's on the operative report. See if you can get into the operating room with the doctors . . . [and] know your sterile field techniques so you know what NOT to touch!"

CHRIS

SURGICAL PACKAGE   Often, the time, effort, and services rendered when accomplishing a procedure are bundled together to form a surgical package. Payment is made for a package of services and not for each individual service provided within the package. The CPT manual describes the surgical package as including the operation itself, local anesthesia, and "typical follow-up care, one related E/M encounter prior to the procedure, and immediate follow-up care, including written orders."

Local anesthesia is defined as local infiltration, metacarpal/digital block, or topical anesthesia. The CPT manual further states that follow-up care for complications, exacerbations (a worsening), recurrence, and the presence of other diseases that require additional services is not included in the surgical package. General anesthesia for surgical procedures is not part of the surgical package; general anesthesia services are reported and billed separately by the anesthesiologist.

Third-party payers have varying definitions of what constitutes a surgical package and varying policies about what is to be included in the surgical package. Surgical packages also define the services for which you can or cannot submit additional charges because the rules of the surgical package define what is and is not included with the surgical procedure. Included in the definition of the surgical package are routine preoperative and postoperative care—including usual complications—and up to a predefined number of days before and after the surgery. Reimbursement policies vary from payer to payer because of the way each payer defines the costs that are in the surgical bundle. For instance, Medicare states that they averaged the costs associated with additional services for complications and added payments for those services into the surgical payment. Other commercial payers determine the reimbursement based on services associated only with performing the surgery and choose to let costs for services for complications be reported separately. The period of time following each surgery that is included in the surgery package is established by the third-party payer and is referred to as the **global (postoperative) surgery** period. The global surgery period is usually **90** days for major surgery and **10** days for minor surgery.

Fig. 4–8 shows CPT codes 10080 and 10081 for incision and drainage of a pilonidal cyst. The third-party payer may indicate that code 10080 has zero days for the global surgical package, so you would charge for any additional services that were provided in addition to the incision and drainage itself. The payer may indicate that 10081 has 10 days for the global surgical package that would include routine follow-up care and services (such as removal of sutures) at no charge.

One last coding guideline that you have to know before you begin to code surgical procedures pertains to materials and supply codes. When **materials or supplies** over and above those usually used in an office visit have been used, you code and charge for these materials and supplies in addition to charging for the office visit or procedure. For example, when a physician does a wound repair during an office visit and uses a surgical tray, the surgical tray is identified by CPT code 99070. Code 99070 is listed in the Medicine section, Special Services, Procedures, and Reports subsection, Miscellaneous subheading.

CODING SHOT HCPCS code A4550 is also used to report the use of a surgical tray. Third-party payers who pay separately for a surgical tray usually want the HCPCS "A" code to be used to report the tray. Many third-party payers do not pay separately for a surgical tray. Medicare, however, does pay separately for a surgical tray for a limited number of surgical procedures.

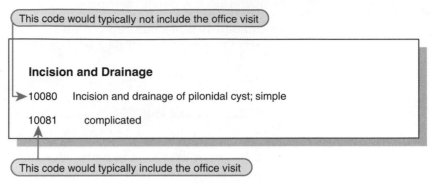

FIGURE 4–8 Surgery package.

The following examples recap the major guidelines concerning surgical packages:

1. Surgical packages for procedures usually include the preoperative service, the procedure, related services, and routine postoperative services. Payers vary in their interpretation of the global surgical package. Although most follow the CPT guidelines, some payers, such as Medicare, expand the services that are included in the surgical package to include treatment of complications by the same physician.

Example

An established patient, Mary Smith is referred to a surgeon for excessive bleeding. The surgeon decides a hysterectomy is necessary and schedules the surgical procedure for 2 weeks later. The surgeon plans to recheck Mary in the office the day before surgery. The initial visit, at which the decision is made to perform surgery, is billable, but the preoperative visit on the day before surgery is bundled into the surgical package, as is the procedure itself and any routine follow-up.

2. Complications are usually added on a service-by-service basis.

Even though the routine follow-up care is not billed for, the service is still coded to indicate that the service was provided. The CPT code 99024 (Postoperative follow-up visit, included in global service) alerts the third-party payer that the services were rendered to the patient but the services were included in a surgical package and not charged for.

Example

A patient undergoes a wound repair that is coded 12014 (The third-party payer indicated that there was a 10 day surgical package for this code.) and 5 days afterwards sees the physician for routine follow-up care. The fee statement for the office visit at which the routine follow-up care is provided would be:

99024   Postoperative follow-up visit   No charge

However, if the patient returned during the global period because of a breakdown in the skin around the surgical wound (dehiscence) but with no signs of infection, and the patient was returned to the operating room at which time the physician trimmed the skin margins around the wound and resutured the wound, you would report this complication during the global period with:

12020-78   Dehiscence, simple closure $xx.xx

But if a patient undergoes the repair of a 7.9-cm wound that is coded 12004 (the third-party payer indicated that there was no surgical package for this code) and sees the physician a few days later for routine follow-up care, the service is coded and charged for.

12004	Wound repair, 7.9 cm	$xx.xx
99070	Surgical tray	$xx.xx
99212	Office visit	$xx.xx

Inclusion or exclusion of a procedure in the CPT manual does not imply any health insurance coverage or reimbursement policy. Although the CPT manual includes guidelines on usage, third-party payers may interpret and accept the use of CPT codes and the guidelines in any manner they choose.

EXERCISE 4–3 *Surgical Package*

Answer the following:

1 What are the three things bundled into a surgical package?

a _____

b _____

c _____

2 Is general anesthesia included in the surgical package? _____

3 Do all third-party payers follow the same reimbursement guidelines for the global packages?

_____

PART II ■ *General and Integumentary System Subsections*

GENERAL SUBSECTIONS

The General subsection contains codes for fine needle aspirations (10021-10022), excluding bone marrow aspirations (see code 38220). The codes are divided based on whether **imaging guidance** was used during the aspiration. A **fine needle biopsy** is used to withdraw fluid that contains individual cells. The needle is inserted into the area being biopsied and moved several times to take multiple samples without withdrawing the needle. The aspirated cells are then examined by a pathologist using a microscope (88172 or 88173). This type of biopsy is not to be confused with a needle core biopsy, such as that identified by 19100, percutaneous breast biopsy using a **needle core**, in which a core of suspicious tissue is removed for examination or the biopsy represented in 19101, breast biopsy using an open incision, which reports a procedure in which the biopsy site is exposed to the surgeon's view and a sample of the lesion is removed. Notes following codes 10021-10022 indicate several other codes that are used to report percutaneous needle biopsies.

Integumentary System

The Integumentary System subsection includes codes used by many different physician specialties. There is no restriction on who uses the codes from this or any other subsection. You may find a family practitioner using the incision and drainage, debridement, or repair codes; a dermatologist using excision and destruction codes; a plastic surgeon using skin graft codes; or a surgeon using breast procedure codes.

You will learn about the Integumentary System subsection by first reviewing the subsection format and then learning about coding the services and procedures in the subsection.

QUICK CHECK 4-1

Dermatologists are the only providers who utilize the codes in the Integumentary System subsection of CPT.

True or False?

FORMAT

The subsection is formatted on the basis of anatomic site and category of procedure. For example, an anatomic site is "neck" and a category of procedure is "repair."

The subsection Integumentary contains the subheadings:

- Skin, Subcutaneous, and Accessory Structures
- Nails
- Pilonidal Cyst
- Introduction
- Repair (closure)
- Destruction
- Breast

Each subheading is further divided by category. For example, the subheading Skin, Subcutaneous and Accessory Structures is divided into the following categories:

- Incision and Drainage
- Excision—Debridement
- Paring or Cutting
- Biopsy
- Removal of Skin Tags
- Shaving of Epidermal or Dermal Lesions
- Excision—Benign Lesions
- Excision—Malignant Lesions

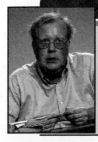

From the Trenches

"[Documentation] comes down to semantics. Certain words mean certain things . . . That's what insurance companies look for to describe what type of test or work effort was done to determine the patient's illness."

CHRIS

SKIN, SUBCUTANEOUS, AND ACCESSORY STRUCTURES

Incision and Drainage

Incision and Drainage (I&D) codes (10040-10180) are divided according to the condition for which the I&D is being done. Acne surgery, abscess, carbuncle, boil, cyst, hematoma, and wound infection are just some of the conditions for which a physician uses I&D. The physician opens the lesion, cutting into it to allow drainage. Also included under this heading is a **puncture aspiration** code (10160), which describes inserting a needle into a lesion and withdrawing the fluid (aspiration). Whichever method is used—incision or aspiration—the contents of the lesion are drained. Packing material may be inserted into the opening or the wound may be left to drain freely. A tube or strip of gauze, which acts as a wick, may be inserted into the wound to facilitate drainage.

The I&D codes are first divided according to the condition and then according to whether the procedure was simple or complicated/multiple. The medical record would indicate the condition and complexity of the I&D. Verify the body area where the incision and drainage is performed for any specific CPT that could be assigned outside of the range 10040-10180. For example, a simple finger abscess would be reported with an incision and drainage code (26010, 26011) from the Hand and Finger, Incision codes.

Excision–Debridement

Codes in this category (11000-11044) describe services of debridement based on depth, body surface, condition, and for 11004-11006 by location. **Debridement** is the cleaning of an area or wound. The first debridement codes (11000 and 11001) are used for eczematous debridement. **Eczema** is a skin condition that blisters and weeps, as illustrated in Fig. 4–9.

The dead tissue may have to be cut away with a scalpel or scissors or, in less severe cases, washed with saline solution. Code 11000 is used to report debridement of 10% of the body surface or less, and add-on code 11001 is used to report each additional 10% or part thereof.

Example

A patient presents for a debridement of 30% of the body surface. The service is reported: 11000, 11001 × 2. Code 11000 reports the first 10% and 11001 × 2 reports the remaining 20%.

Debridement cleans surface areas and removes necrotic tissue. Some codes in this category are based on the extent of the cleansing—skin, subcutaneous tissue, muscle fascia, muscle, or bone.

CODING SHOT Some surgical procedure codes include debridement as a part of the service. You may report a debridement as a separate service when the medical record indicates that a greater than usual debridement was provided. For example, if an extensive debridement was done when usually a simple debridement would be done, you would report the additional service using a debridement code from the 11040-11044 range.

Introduction to Lesions

Before you learn about coding the various methods of lesion destruction and excision, you need to review a few rules that apply broadly to this commonly performed procedure. After you have learned the general lesion information, you will review each of the destruction and excision methods.

Lesion Excision and Destruction. There are many types of lesions of the skin (Fig. 4–10) and many types of treatment for lesions. Types of treatment include **paring** (peeling or scraping), **shaving** (slicing), **excision** (cutting removal), and **destruction** (ablation). To code these procedures properly, you must know the **site, number,** and **size** of the excised lesion(s), as well as whether the lesion is malignant or benign.

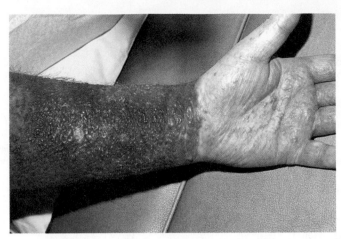

FIGURE 4–9 Eczematous dermatitis. (From Kumar V, et al: *Robbins & Cotran: Pathologic Basis of Disease,* ed 7, Philadelphia, 2005, Saunders.)

Prior to excision, the greatest diameter of the lesion is measured. The measurement includes the margin (extra tissue taken from around the lesion) at its narrowest part. The size of the margin necessary to completely remove the lesion is based on the physician's judgment. The pathology report is used to identify the size of the lesion only if no other record of the size can be documented.

All lesions that are excised will have a pathology report for diagnosing the removed tissue as malignant or benign; since the codes are divided based on whether the excised lesion is malignant or benign, the billing for the excision is not submitted to the third-party payer until the pathology report has been completed.

CAUTION *Destruction of lesions destroys the lesion, leaving none available for biopsy; therefore, there will be no pathology report for lesions that have been destroyed by laser, chemicals, electrocautery, or other methods. In these cases you will have to take the type of the destroyed lesion from the physician's notes only, as there is no pathology report.*

Codes in the Integumentary System subsection differ greatly in their descriptions. Some codes indicate only one lesion per code, others are for the second and third lesions only, and still others indicate a certain number of lesions (e.g., up to 15 lesions). When coding multiple lesions, you must read the description carefully to prevent incorrect coding.

If multiple lesions are treated, code the **most complex lesion procedure first and the others using modifier -51** to indicate that multiple procedures were performed. Remember that the third-party payer will usually reduce the payment for the services identified with modifier -51; so you want to be certain that you place the service with the highest dollar cost first, without the modifier. If the code description includes multiple lesions (a stated number of lesions), the -51 is not necessary.

Closure of Excision Sites. Included in the codes for lesion excision is the direct, primary, or simple closure of the operative site. The notes following the category for the excision of a benign lesion define a **simple excision** as being **full thickness** (through the dermis) and a **simple closure** as one that is nonlayered (Fig. 4–11).

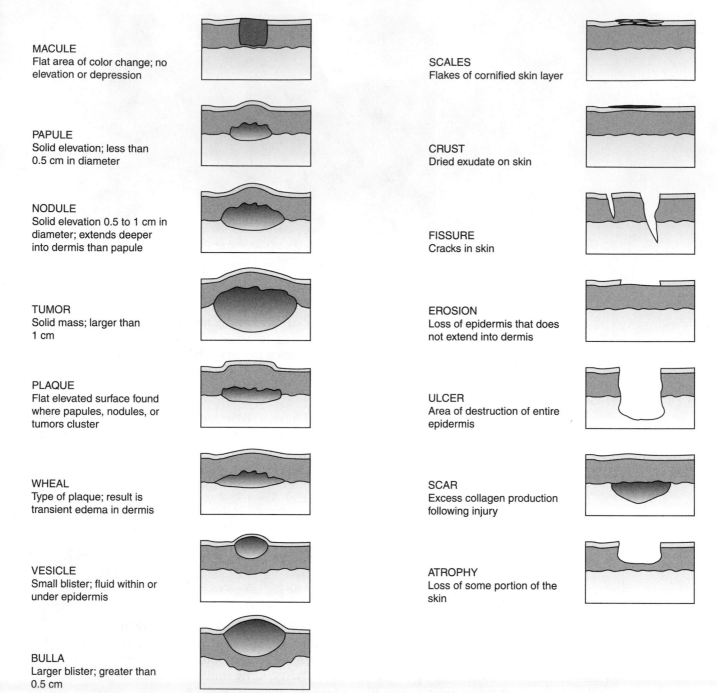

MACULE
Flat area of color change; no elevation or depression

PAPULE
Solid elevation; less than 0.5 cm in diameter

NODULE
Solid elevation 0.5 to 1 cm in diameter; extends deeper into dermis than papule

TUMOR
Solid mass; larger than 1 cm

PLAQUE
Flat elevated surface found where papules, nodules, or tumors cluster

WHEAL
Type of plaque; result is transient edema in dermis

VESICLE
Small blister; fluid within or under epidermis

BULLA
Larger blister; greater than 0.5 cm

SCALES
Flakes of cornified skin layer

CRUST
Dried exudate on skin

FISSURE
Cracks in skin

EROSION
Loss of epidermis that does not extend into dermis

ULCER
Area of destruction of entire epidermis

SCAR
Excess collagen production following injury

ATROPHY
Loss of some portion of the skin

FIGURE 4–10 Lesions of the skin.

Closures can also be **intermediate** (layered; Fig. 4–12) or **complex** (greater than layered). The local anesthesia is also included in the excision codes. Any closure other than a simple closure can be reported separately.

There are several codes at the end of the category (11450-11471) for excision of the skin and subcutaneous tissue in cases of **hidradenitis**, which is the chronic abscessing and subsequent infection of a sweat gland. The abscess is excised and the wound left open to heal. The hidradenitis codes are based on the abscess location (axillary, inguinal, perianal, perineal, or umbilical) and the complexity of the repair (simple, intermediate, or complex).

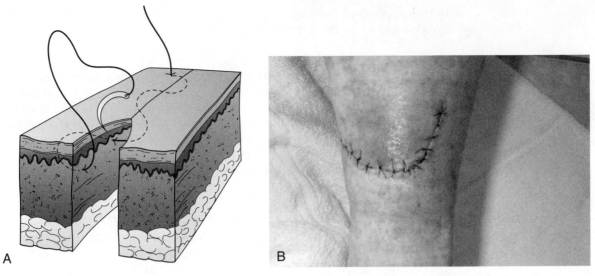

FIGURE 4–11 **A** and **B**, Simple subcuticular closure. (**B** courtesy Mary Garden.)

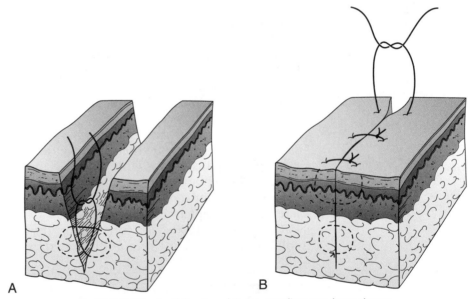

FIGURE 4–12 **A** and **B**, Intermediate two-layer closure.

Three final notes on treatment of lesions:

1. The shaving of lesions requires no closure because no incision has been made.

2. Excision includes simple closure but may require more complex closure. If more complex closure is required, follow the notes in the CPT manual to appropriately code for these services.

3. Destruction may be by any method, including freezing, burning, chemicals, and so on.

Paring or Cutting   Paring or Cutting codes (11055-11057) are used to report the services provided when a physician removes a benign hyperkeratotic skin lesion such as a callus or corn. Paring codes include removal by peeling or scraping. A small ring-shaped instrument (curette), blade, or similar sharp instrument is used for paring. Bleeding is usually controlled by a chemical that is applied to the surface after removal of the lesion. The codes are divided based on the number of lesions removed.

Biopsy

"Biopsy" is a term applied to the procedure of removing some or all of the tissue of a lesion for histopathology. Removing a tissue sample of a lesion may be by needle aspiration, incisional biopsy (open, sharp, and partial removal), or by excisional biopsy (complete removal). You would not report *both* a biopsy and an excision, as the biopsy is bundled into the excision service. In a biopsy, only a portion of the lesion and some of the surrounding tissue is removed. The section of surrounding tissue (margin) is included so the pathologist can compare the normal tissue to the lesion tissue and note differences.

CODING SHOT Included in the Biopsy codes are codes that are to be used for biopsies of mucous membranes. A mucous membrane is tissue that covers a variety of body parts, such as the tongue and the nasal cavities.

Many methods are used to obtain biopsies; the method chosen is determined by the size and type of the lesion and the physician's preference. Common biopsy methods are scraping, cutting, and the punch. A punch biopsy is illustrated in Fig. 4–13; it is used to excise a disk of tissue. A punch can also be used in the excision of the entire lesion, so just because the medical record refers to the use of a punch, it does not necessarily mean that only a biopsy was done.

Biopsy sites do not necessarily have to be closed; some are so small that they will close readily by themselves. Other sites are large enough that closure is required, and simple closure is included in the biopsy codes. If closure of the biopsy site is more than a simple closure, you would code separately for the more extensive closure. You will learn more about closure later in this chapter.

On the CMS-1500 claim form, report the number of lesions treated in column 24G, Days or Units, as illustrated in Fig. 4–14.

CAUTION *Do not use modifier -51 with these biopsy codes, as 11100 is used to report a single lesion, and 11101 is used to report two or more lesions. The correct coding for three lesions would be to use 11100 for lesion number one and 11101 × 2 for lesions two and three.*

Skin Tags

Skin tags are flaps of skin (benign lesions) that can appear anywhere, but most often appear on the neck or trunk, especially in older people (Fig. 4-15, *A*). Skin tags are removed in a variety of ways—scissors, blades, ligatures, electrosurgery, or chemicals. **Scissors removal** is illustrated in Fig. 4–15, *B*.

Scissoring is often used for tissue column lesions. The forceps grasps the column, and the physician snips the lesion off at its base. Closure is achieved by using sutures or an aluminum chloride solution. In **ligature strangulation**, a thread is tied at the base of the lesion and left there until the tissue dies. The lesion then drops off. Whatever method of removal is used, simple closure is included in the skin tag codes, as is any local anesthesia that is used. Also, note that the codes (11200, 11201) are based on the first 15 lesions and then on each additional 10 lesions or part thereof after the first 15.

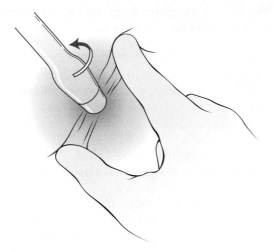

FIGURE 4-13 Punch biopsy.

F.		G.	H.	I.	
		DAYS OR	EPSDT Family	ID.	
$ CHARGES		UNITS	Plan	QUAL.	
28. TOTAL CHARGE			29. AMOUNT PAID		
$			$		

FIGURE 4-14 Units column (G) of the CMS-1500. (Courtesy U.S. Department of Health and Human Services, Centers for Medicare and Medicaid Services.)

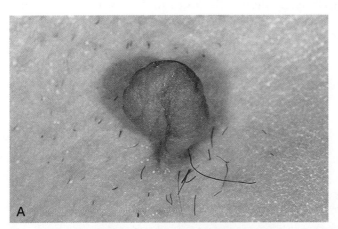

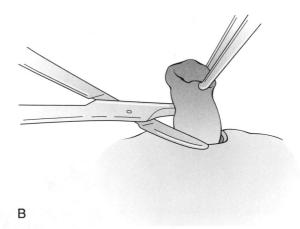

A

B

FIGURE 4-15 **A**, Skin tag. **B**, Scissors removal. (**A** from Habif TP: *Clinical Dermatology: A Color Guide to Diagnosis and Therapy*, ed 4, Philadelphia, 2004, Mosby.)

On the CMS-1500 claim form, report the number of lesions treated in 24G, Days or Units (see Fig. 4–14).

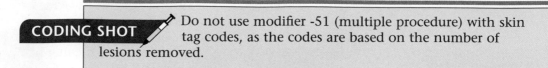

CODING SHOT Do not use modifier -51 (multiple procedure) with skin tag codes, as the codes are based on the number of lesions removed.

Shaving of Epidermal or Dermal Lesions

The shaving of a lesion (11300-11313) can be performed by using a scalpel blade or other sharp instrument. The shaving of a lesion is illustrated in Fig. 4–16.

The blade is held horizontal to the skin and an epidermal or dermal lesion is sliced off. Anesthesia and cauterization (electrocautery or chemical cautery) to control bleeding are included in the lesion-shaving codes.

Electrocautery is sometimes used to finish the edges of the shaving, but if electrocautery is the main method by which the lesion was removed, you would use codes from the Destruction, Benign or Premalignant Lesions category (17000-17250), not from the Shaving category. Electrosurgery used in shaving a superficial lesion will eventually burn (destroy) the lesion, so the destruction code would be reported.

The Shaving codes are further defined according to the **location** of the lesion—trunk, neck, nose—and the size of the lesion. If more than one lesion was removed, you would add modifier -51 (multiple procedures) to any codes after the first code. For example, if one 2.0-cm lesion was removed from the trunk, and a 1.0-cm lesion was removed from the hand, you list the 2.0-cm lesion first with no modifier and the 1.0-cm lesion second, with modifier -51 added. Many third-party payers reimburse 100% for the first lesion and 50% for the second lesion, so by placing the more intensive procedure first, you optimize reimbursement.

Excision of Benign Lesions

The CPT divides the category of excision of lesions on the basis of whether a lesion is benign or malignant. Although at the time of excision it is not known for certain whether the lesion is benign or malignant, the physician makes an assessment of the lesion's status and usually plans the extent of the excision based on that assessment. The codes in the Excision—Benign Lesions category (11400-11471) are used for all benign lesions **except** skin tags, which you learned about earlier.

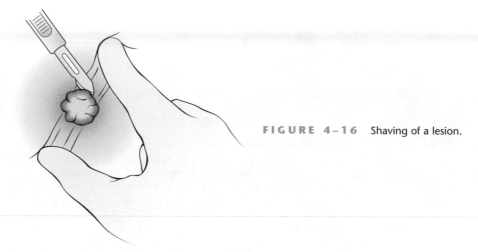

FIGURE 4–16 Shaving of a lesion.

The codes include local anesthesia, so do not code for local anesthesia separately, as that would be unbundling. The excision codes also include simple closure (see Fig. 4–11) of the excision site. If the closure is noted in the medical record as being more than simple (intermediate or complex) you would code the more complicated closure using a separate code from Repair subheading (12031-13160).

You are not to use the shaving codes **if** the shaving had penetrated through the dermis (full thickness). Full-thickness shavings are to be coded using the excision codes found in the Excision—Benign Lesions or Excision—Malignant Lesions categories.

> **CODING SHOT** — For unusual or complicated excisions, you will use a code from the Musculoskeletal section.

The codes in the Excision—Benign Lesions category are based on the **location** of the excision (e.g., trunk, scalp, ears, etc.) and the **size** of the lesion (e.g., 0.6-1.0 cm, 1.1-2.0 cm).

> **CODING SHOT** — In excision of either benign or malignant tissue, focus on the dimension of the normal tissue margin excised with the lesion. This normal tissue margin is the determining factor in selecting the correct CPT code.

Excision of Malignant Lesions

Codes in the Excision—Malignant Lesions subheading (11600-11646) are used for malignant lesions and include local anesthesia and simple closure. As with the benign lesion codes, these codes refer to *each* lesion removed and are divided according to the lesion's **location** and **size.** If you are coding a lesion removal that has been performed by a method other than excision (e.g., electrosurgery), the notes preceding the excision codes direct you to the Destruction codes (17260-17286). If the closure is more than simple you would also use a repair code.

> **CODING SHOT** — If the excision is of a malignant lesion on the eyelid, and if the excision involves more than the skin of the eyelid (lid margin, tarsus, or conjunctiva), do not use malignant lesion excision codes. Instead, you would use a surgery code from the subsection Eye and Ocular Adnexa, Excision category (67800-67850).

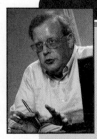

From the Trenches

Would you recommend coding as a profession?

"I would for people who are meticulous and have a mind for detail . . . People who take pride in their work. Someone who will say, 'I can find things out. I can learn things, and I can make it worthwhile for the physician to employ me.' "

CHRIS

NAILS

Within the category Nails (11719-11765) are codes for the trimming of fingernails and toenails, debridement of nails, removal of nails, drainage of hematomas, biopsies of nails, repair of nails, reconstruction of nails, and excision of cysts of the nails. **Podiatrists** are physicians who specialize in the care of the foot; as such, these physicians use this category of codes extensively. However, all physicians can and do use these codes when providing nail care services to both the feet and the hands.

The first code in the Nails category is 11719, used for the trimming of nails that are not defective. This is a minimal service and the code covers trimming one fingernail/toenail or many fingernails/toenails. **Debridement** (11720) is a more complex service—the manual cleaning of up to five nails—and it includes the use of various tools, cleaning materials/solutions, and files. You **would not report** separately for the supplies used for a nail debridement service, as these supplies are included in the codes. The two debridement codes are divided according to the number of nails attended to during the service. If the payer requires HCPCS codes, you would use G0127.

Avulsion is the separation and removal of the nail plate (11730, 11732), leaving the root so the nail will grow back. An anesthetic is administered, the nail is lifted away from the nail bed, and a portion or all of the nail plate is removed.

Place the number of nails treated in the units column (G) of the CMS-1500 form.

> **CODING SHOT**
>
> Do not use modifier -51 (multiple procedures) with nail removal codes, as there are two codes available: one for a single nail and one for each additional nail. For example, if three nails were removed, you would report: 11730 (for the first nail) and 11732 × 2 (for the second and third nails). Often, third-party payers require the use of HCPCS modifiers (F1-FA to indicate the finger and T1-TA to indicate the toe; Fig. 4-17) and the separate reporting of each digit treated.

A subungual hematoma (blood trapped under the nail) is evacuated by puncturing the nail with an electrocautery needle (11740). The trapped blood and fluid are drained by applying pressure to the top of the nail.

Onychocryptosis (ingrown toenail) is the most common condition of the great toe, as illustrated in Fig. 4–18.

The nail grows down and into the soft tissue of the nail fold, causing extreme pain and often infection. Treatment for severe cases is a partial onychectomy (removal of the nail plate and root). The toe is anesthetized and a portion of the nail plate and root is removed (11750-11752). The nail will not grow back where the base has been removed.

> **CODING SHOT**
>
> Use of HCPCS modifiers is very important. For example, nail biopsies (11755) were performed on the left third finger (F2) and the left fourth finger (F3), in addition to the right fourth digit (F8). The reporting would be 11755-F2, 11755-F3, 11755-F8.

Pilonidal Cyst

The codes for the excision of a pilonidal cyst or sinus are 11770-11772. A pilonidal cyst is located in the sacral area and is most often caused by an ingrown hair. The codes are divided according to the complexity of the excision—simple, extensive, or complicated. For a simple cyst, the physician

F1	Left hand, second digit	T1	Left foot, second digit
F2	Left hand, third digit	T2	Left foot, third digit
F3	Left hand, fourth digit	T3	Left foot, fourth digit
F4	Left hand, fifth digit	T4	Left foot, fifth digit
F5	Right hand, thumb	T5	Right foot, great toe
F6	Right hand, second digit	T6	Right foot, second digit
F7	Right hand, third digit	T7	Right foot, third digit
F8	Right hand, fourth digit	T8	Right foot, fourth digit
F9	Right hand, fifth digit	T9	Right foot, fifth digit
FA	Left hand, thumb	TA	Left foot, great toe

FIGURE 4–17 HCPCS modifiers used to indicate digits of hands and feet.

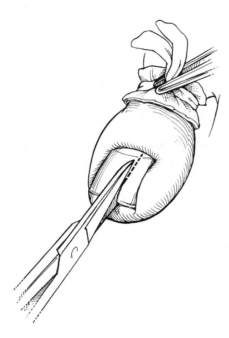

FIGURE 4–18 Removal of ingrown toenail. (From Rakel RE: *Saunders Manual of Medical Practice,* ed 2, Philadelphia, 2000, Saunders.)

would excise the cyst and suture the skin together. A cyst larger than 2 cm is considered complicated and requires more extensive excision and closure. A complicated excision is very extensive and usually requires reconstructive repair.

Introduction

Within the Introduction category of codes (11900-11983) you will find lesion injection, tattooing, tissue expansion, contraceptive capsule insertion/removal, and hormone implantation services. Lesions are injected with medication to treat conditions such as acne, keloids (scar tissue), and psoriasis. Lesion injection codes are divided according to the number of lesions injected (1-7 or 8+).

CODING SHOT Lesion injection code 11901 is not an add-on code! You use 11900 to report lesion injections numbering one through seven, and you use 11901 to report injections eight and above. For example, if seven lesions are injected in one patient, the service is reported using 11900. If eight lesions are injected in another patient, the service is reported using 11901.

Tattooing codes (11920-11922) are also located in the Introduction category. Tattooing is coded on the basis of square centimeters covered. Sometimes physicians use tattooing as a way to disguise birthmarks or scars.

Codes for subcutaneous injection of filling material (11950-11954) are located in the Introduction category and are used for services such as collagen or silicone injections (injectable dermal implants), which are used as a wrinkle treatment. The codes are based on the amount of material injected. The procedure is usually repeated at 2- to 3-week intervals until the results are those desired.

Tissue-expander codes (11960-11971) are also located in the Introduction category. A tissue expander is an elastic material formed into a sac that is then filled with fluid or air so it expands like a balloon. The expander is placed under the skin and then it is filled, stretching the skin. Expanders are most often used to prepare a site for a permanent implant. Expanders are also used to assist in the repair of scars and the removal of tattoos by stretching the skin, removing the expander, removing the scar or tattoo, and suturing the skin edges together. The codes are divided according to whether the service is an insertion, a removal, or an expander removal with replacement of a prosthesis.

CODING SHOT Do not use an expander code from the Introduction category after a mastectomy in which a temporary expander has been inserted. Code 19357 from the reconstruction section of the Integumentary subsection is a combination of mastectomy and the insertion of an expander. If at a later date the expander was replaced with a permanent prosthesis, you would assign 19342, replacement of tissue expander with permanent prosthesis.

You will also find insertion of **implantable contraceptive capsules** in the Introduction category. Implantable contraceptive capsules such as Norplant are inserted under the skin by means of a small incision on the upper arm. A capsule is effective for a number of years; at the end of that time, it must be removed. Read the descriptions in the implantable contraceptive capsule codes (11975-11977) carefully, as there are codes for insertion, removal, and removal with insertion.

CODING SHOT In addition to reporting the service of the introduction of the implantable contraceptive capsule, you report the supply of the contraceptive system using HCPCS code J7307.

Subcutaneous hormone pellet implantation is commonly used for the insertion of a hormone in a time-release capsule into the buttocks of women needing hormone replacement therapy after menopause, and the code for this implantation is in the Introduction category (11980). The implantation area is anesthetized and the pellet is inserted through a tube. The pellet is completely absorbed into the system and so does not need to be removed, as does a contraceptive capsule. However, a new pellet must be inserted every 6 to 9 months (11980), and each reinsertion is reported.

EXERCISE 4–4 *Skin, Subcutaneous, and Accessory Structures*

Apply the information about lesion procedures by coding the following:

1 Paring of three warts

     Code: _____

2 Removal of 15 skin tags

     Code: _____

3 Shaving of 1-cm lesion of face

     Code: _____

REPAIR (CLOSURE)

Repair Factors

When coding wound repair, the following three factors must be considered:

1. Length of the wound in centimeters
2. Complexity of the repair
3. Site of the wound repair

Remember **length**, **complexity**, and **site**. Fig. 4–19 illustrates an example from the CPT manual of these three factors in the wound repair codes.

There are many different types of wounds (Fig. 4–20). Wound repair is classified by the type of repair necessary to repair the wound. There are three types of repair:

- Simple
- Intermediate
- Complex

1. **Simple:** superficial wound repair (12001-12021) that involves epidermis, dermis, and subcutaneous tissue and requires only simple, one-layer suturing. If the simple wound repair is accomplished with tape or adhesive strips, the charge for the closure is included in the E/M service code and would not be coded separately with a repair code. The repair codes are for suture closure.

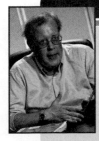

From the Trenches

"[It's my job] to make sure physicians are saying [everything] into their microrecorder, or writing it down. You would be surprised how many physicians [diagnose a patient] mentally, as an automatic thing as part of their evaluation of the patient's condition—then they do the medical decision making on how to treat the patient. Sometimes a third of it doesn't even get put down, and the coder can only count that third of information, until it's in the record . . . I've told doctors 'You dictated this, and this is all you're going to get' so they can see the consequences."

CHRIS

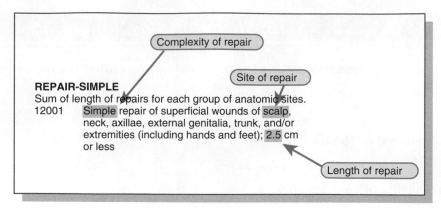

REPAIR-SIMPLE
Sum of length of repairs for each group of anatomic sites.
12001   Simple repair of superficial wounds of scalp,
        neck, axillae, external genitalia, trunk, and/or
        extremities (including hands and feet); 2.5 cm
        or less

Complexity of repair

Site of repair

Length of repair

FIGURE 4–19   Wound repair. Note that metric measure is used throughout the CPT.

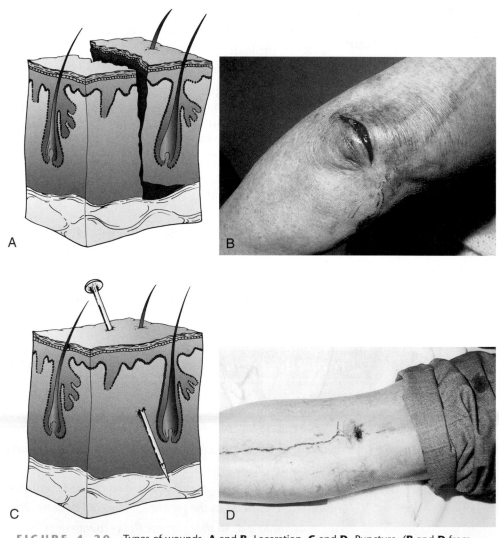

FIGURE 4–20   Types of wounds. **A** and **B,** Laceration. **C** and **D,** Puncture. (**B** and **D** from Henry MC, Stapleton ER: *EMT Prehospital Care,* ed 3, St. Louis, 2004, MosbyJems.)

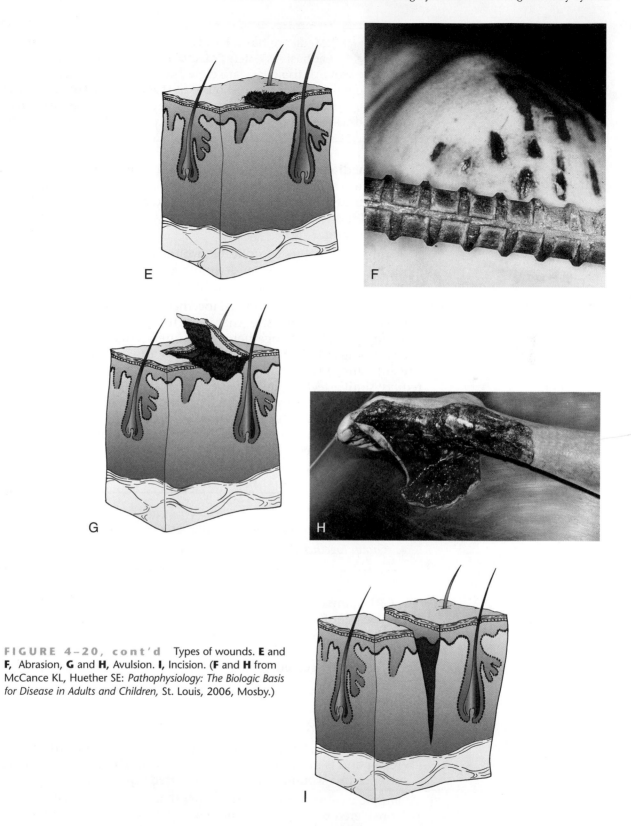

E

F

G

H

I

FIGURE 4–20, cont'd Types of wounds. **E** and **F,** Abrasion. **G** and **H,** Avulsion. **I,** Incision. (**F** and **H** from McCance KL, Huether SE: *Pathophysiology: The Biologic Basis for Disease in Adults and Children,* St. Louis, 2006, Mosby.)

CODING SHOT ✎ Medicare has a HCPCS code to report skin closures using adhesives (such as Dermabond, a special glue that is put into the wound, the edges are closed together, and a bandage is placed over the wound. It is used in place of stitches.): **G0168.** All other third-party payers use the simple repair code to report these skin closures using adhesives.

2. **Intermediate:** requires closure of one or more layers of subcutaneous tissue and superficial (non-muscle) fascia, in addition to the skin closure. You can use the codes for intermediate closure (12031-12057) when the wound has to be extensively cleaned, even if the closure was a single-layer closure.

3. **Complex:** involves complicated wound closure including revision, debridement, extensive undermining, stents or retention sutures, and more than layered closure (13100-13160).

The lengths of wounds are totaled together by complexity (simple, intermediate, complex) and anatomic site (that is, all the simple wounds of the same site grouping are reported together; all the intermediate wounds of the same site grouping are reported together; and all the complex wounds of the same site grouping are reported together). The codes group together sites that require similar techniques to repair. For example, 12001 groups superficial scalp, neck, axillae, external genitalia, trunk, and extremities. When there is more than one repair type, the **most complex** type is listed as the first (primary) procedure. The secondary procedure is then reported using modifier -51 (multiple procedure). Remember that the placement of the -51 indicates a discounted service to the payer.

✋ **CAUTION** *For repairs:*
- *Group together the same anatomic sites, such as face and hand.*
- *Group together the same classification, such as simple or intermediate.*

The CPT manual notes that are found under the subheading Repair include extensive definitions of each of these levels of repair. These notes must be read carefully before you code repairs.

Repair Components

Three things are considered components (parts) of wound repair:
- Ligation
- Exploration
- Debridement

1. Simple **ligation** (tying) of small vessels is considered part of the wound repair and is not listed separately. Simple ligation of medium or major arteries in a wound is, however, reported separately.

2. Simple **exploration** of surrounding tissue, nerves, vessels, and tendons is considered part of the wound repair process and is not listed separately.

3. Normal **debridement** (cleaning and removing skin or tissue from the wound until normal, healthy tissue is exposed) is not listed separately.

If the wound is grossly contaminated and requires extensive debridement, a separate debridement procedure may be coded (11000-11044 for extensive debridement). Fig. 4–21 illustrates a nonsurgical type of debridement.

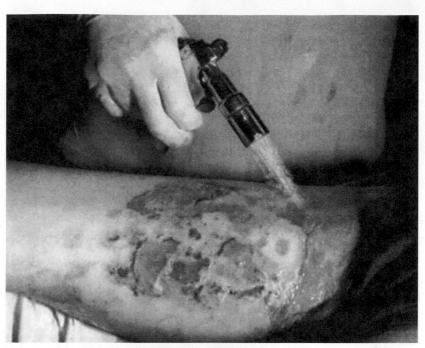

FIGURE 4–21 Burn debridement. (From Converse JM, ed: *Reconstructive Plastic Surgery: Principles and Procedures in Correction, Reconstruction and Transplantation,* vol 1, Philadelphia, 1964, WB Saunders.)

Tissue Transfers, Grafts, and Flaps

There are many types of grafting procedures that can be performed to correct a defect (e.g., adjacent tissue transfers or rearrangements, skin replacement surgery and skin substitutes, flaps). To understand skin grafting, you must know that the **recipient site** is the area of defect that receives the graft, and the **donor site** is the area from which the healthy skin has been taken for grafting. (If a skin graft is required to close the donor site, the closure is coded as an additional procedure.) A brief description of some different types of skin grafting and coding guidelines specific to their use follows.

Adjacent Tissue Transfer or Rearrangement. There are many types of adjacent tissue transfers (14000-14350). Some of them are Z-plasty (Fig. 4–22), W-plasty, V-Y plasty, rotation flaps (Fig. 4–23), and advancement flaps. These procedures are various methods of moving a segment of skin from one area to an adjacent area, while leaving at least one side of the flap (moved skin) intact to retain some measure of blood supply to the graft. Incisions are made, and the skin is undermined and moved over to cover the defective area, leaving the base, or connected portion, intact. The flap is then sutured into place.

Adjacent tissue transfers are coded according to the size of the **recipient site.** The size is measured in square centimeters. Simple repair of the donor site is included in the tissue transfer code and is not coded separately. If there is a complex closure, or grafting of the donor site, this could be coded separately. Adjacent Tissue Transfer or Rearrangement in the CPT manual is divided based on the **location** of the defect (trunk or arm) and the **size** of the defect. In addition, there are codes at the end of the category for coding defects that are extremely complicated. Both the primary defect (results from the excision) and the secondary defect (results from the flap design) are added together to determine code selection.

Any excision of a lesion that is repaired by adjacent tissue transfer is included in the tissue transfer code. If you report the excision in addition to the transfer, it would be considered unbundling.

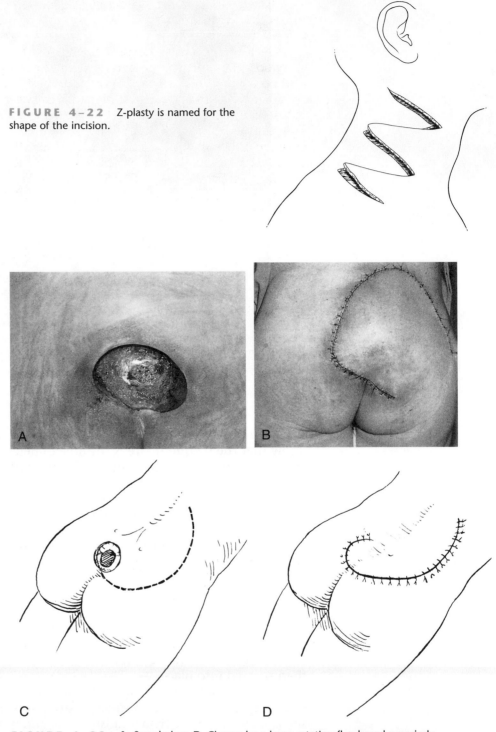

FIGURE 4-22 Z-plasty is named for the shape of the incision.

FIGURE 4-23 **A,** Sacral ulcer. **B,** Closure by a large rotation flap based superiorly. **C** and **D,** Outline of flap and rotation downward and medially. (**A** and **B** from McCarthy, JG., ed: *Plastic Surgery,* vol 6, Philadelphia, 1990, WB Saunders. **C** and **D** from Converse JM, ed: *Reconstructive Plastic Surgery: Principles and Procedures in Correction, Reconstruction and Transplantation,* vol 5, Philadelphia, 1964, WB Saunders.)

Adjacent tissue transfer codes can be located in the CPT manual index under the term Skin.

Skin Replacement Surgery and Skin Substitutes (15002-15431).

These codes report site preparation using a variety of grafting materials and repair methods using skin or skin substitutes. The site of the defect (recipient) site may require surgical preparation before repair, and these repairs are reported with 15002-15005 based on the size of repair and site. Free skin grafts (such as 15100/15101 and 15120/15121) are pieces of skin that are either **split thickness**, which consists of epidermis and part of the dermis, or **full thickness**, which consists of the epidermis and all of the dermis, as illustrated in Fig. 4–24. The grafts are completely freed from the donor site and placed over the recipient site. There is no connection left between the graft and the donor site (Fig. 4–25). Free skin grafts are reported by recipient **site**, **size** of defect, and **type** of repair. The size is measured in square centimeters.

Many of the code definitions in the Skin Replacement Surgery and Skin Substitutes category refer to a measurement in square centimeters and a percentage of body area. The square centimeters measurement is to be applied to adults and children over 10 years of age and the percentage of body area is applied to infants and children under the age of 10.

A **pinch graft** (15050) is a small, split-thickness repair. Often a split-thickness graft is referred to in the patient record as STSG, and a full-thickness skin graft as FTSG.

Autografts are grafts that are taken from the patient's body, whereas allografts are grafts that are taken from a human donor. Epidermal autografts (15110-15116) and dermal autografts (15130-15136) are reported based on

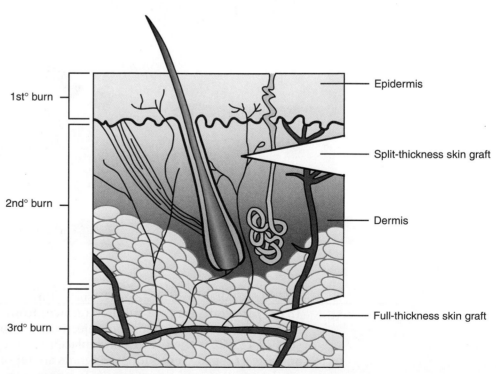

FIGURE 4–24 First, second, and third degree burns, in addition to split-thickness skin graft and full-thickness skin graft.

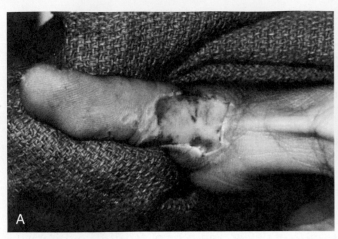

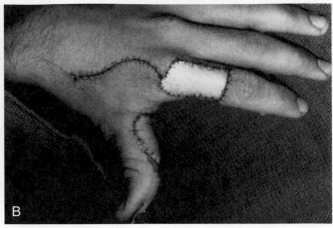

FIGURE 4–25 **A,** Small, localized, full-thickness burn of the first web space. **B,** Immediate postoperative results, after a dorsal metacarpal artery flap was transposed into the defect. (From Achauer BM, et al, eds: *Plastic Surgery: Indications, Operations, and Outcomes* vol 4, St. Louis, 2000, Mosby.)

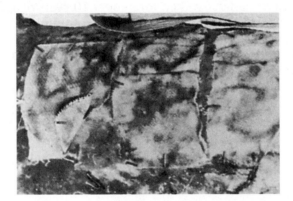

FIGURE 4–26 Three sheets of cultured epithelial autograft are in place on the left anterior thigh, which 3 weeks before was excised to muscle fascia and covered with cadaver allograft. (From Gallico GG, O'Connor NE: Cultured epithelium as a skin substitute. *Clin Plast Surg* 12:155, 1985.)

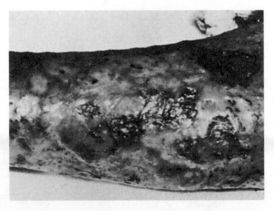

FIGURE 4–27 The same area of left anterior thigh in Fig. 4–26, 1 month after grafting. (From Gallico GG, O'Connor NE: Cultured epithelium as a skin substitute. *Clin Plast Surg* 12:155, 1985.)

graft depth, location, and size. Tissue cultured epidermal autografts (15150-15157) are grafts that are cultured (grown) from the patient's own skin cells, thereby reducing the chances of rejection. Acellular dermal replacement (15170-15176) is the use of skin replacement products based on the location and size of repair. **Temporary** allografts are reported with 15300-15321 based on the location and size of repair. Temporary grafts are used to help protect defect sites while healing is taking place (Figs. 4–26 and 4–27). A **permanent** graft may be placed over the site at a later date to complete the repair process.

autograft

Allograft and Tissue Cultured Allogeneic Skin Substitutes (15300-15366) are grafts from one's own body (allograft), and allogeneic grafts are from a different person of the same species. Xenografts (15400-15431) are grafts taken from a different species (cross species, such as pigskin grafts).

Flaps. A physician may decide to develop a donor site at a location far away from the recipient site. The graft may have to be accomplished in stages. The graft code can be assigned more than once when the surgery is done in stages. Notes specific to this group of codes state that when coding transfer flaps (in several stages), report the **donor site** when a **tube graft** (Fig. 4–28) is formed for later use or when a **delayed flap** is formed before it is transferred (Fig. 4–29). The **recipient site** is reported when the graft is attached to its final site.

In a **delayed graft**, a portion of the skin is lifted and separated from the tissue below, but it stays connected to blood vessels at one end. This keeps the skin viable while it is being moved from one area to another, and at the same time, it lets the graft get used to living on a small supply of blood. It is hoped that living on a small blood supply will help to give the graft a better chance of survival when it is inserted into the recipient site.

There are two categories of codes for flaps. The first category, Flaps (Skin and/or Deep Tissues) (15570-15738), is subdivided based on the type of flap (i.e., pedicle, cross finger, delayed, or muscle flaps) and then by the location of the flap (scalp, trunk, or lips). The codes do not include any extensive immobilization that may be necessary, such as a large plaster cast or other immobilizing device. Extensive immobilization would be coded in addition to the flap procedure. Also not included in the flap procedure codes is the closure of a donor site, which would be reported in addition to the flap procedure.

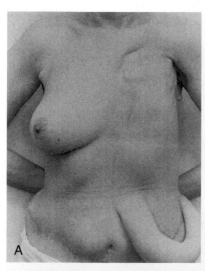
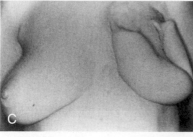
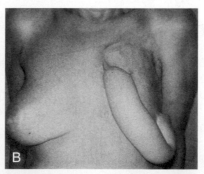
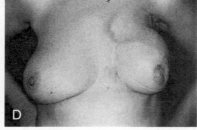

FIGURE 4–28 **A,** Correction of a radical mastectomy defect with a tube flap, created from the abdominal pannus. **B,** Intermediate inset of the tube flap following separation from its abdominal blood supply. This process of "waltzing" a tube-flap from the abdomen to the chest was used by Halsted and Billroth. **C,** Final inset into the sternum before shaping. **D,** The lateral half of the tube flap was then detached laterally and inset into the upper sternum to create the breast shape. This type of reconstruction usually took more than a year to complete, with more than a dozen procedures. (From Bland KI, Copeland EM: *The Breast: Comprehensive Management of Benign and Malignant Disorders,* ed 3, St. Louis, 2004, Saunders.)

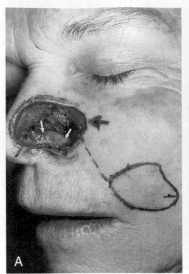
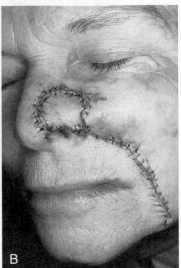

FIGURE 4-29 **A,** A skin and soft tissue defect extends from alar lobule into medial cheek. The cheek advancement flap is designed to repair cheek defect. Separate subcutaneous pedicle transposition flap is designed to resurface the alar lobule after placement of auricular cartilage graft *(arrows)* along the missing alar margin. **B,** Two flaps are in position. (From Cummings CW, Flint PW, Harker LA, Haughey BH, Richardson MA, Robbins KT, Schuller DE, Thomas JR, editors: *Cummings Otolaryngology: Head & Neck Surgery,* ed 4, Philadelphia, 2005, Mosby.)

The second category, Other Flaps and Grafts (15740-15776), is subdivided based on the type of flap (free muscle, free skin, fascial, or hair transplant).

Within the flap codes (15740-15750) the flap (donor site and recipient site remain connected for a period of time) can be an island pedicle or a neurovascular pedicle. The pedicle is the end of the flap that remains connected to the donor area. An **island pedicle flap** contains an artery and vein, and a **neurovascular pedicle flap** contains an artery, vein, and nerve. The term "island" refers to the removal of the fat and subcutaneous tissue prior to implantation into the recipient site. The neurovascular pedicle flap is used when the area of defect requires restoration of sensation in the area; for example, the end of a finger that has sustained damage that destroyed the sensation on the tip of the finger. A neurovascular graft from an adjacent finger could restore sensation to the defective area. A flap from the donor area is freed up and grafted into the recipient area. The connection between the donor and the recipient sites remains in place until the graft has satisfactorily healed, at which time the connection is severed. The donor area may require a separate skin graft and would be reported separately.

QUICK CHECK 4-2

There are three types of measurements utilized in the Integumentary System subsection of CPT. Match the procedure with the type of measurement.

a. length in cm
b. area in square cm
c. diameter in cm

1. Skin Grafts/Flaps _____
2. Lesion Removal _____
3. Wound Repair _____

Other Procedures

The Other Procedures category (15780-15879) contains codes for a wide variety of repair services, such as abrasion, chemical peel, and blepharoplasty. The codes are often divided based on the site or extent of repair.

Dermabrasion is used to treat acne, wrinkles, or general keratoses (horny growth). The skin area is anesthetized by a chemical that freezes the area (a cryogen), and the area is sanded down using a motorized brush. The facial dermabrasion codes (15780-15783) are divided according to the surface area of the face treated (total, segment, region).

A tattoo can be removed by dermabrasion. The process involves the use of a high-speed mechanical wheel to remove the epidermis and part of the papillary dermis. The service is reported with code 15783.

The **abrasion** codes (15786, 15787) are used to report the use of abrasion to remove a lesion, such as scar tissue, a wart, or a callus. This technique is often used to remove areas of sun-damaged skin. The first abraded lesion is reported with 15786, and each additional four or fewer lesions are reported with 15787.

Chemical peels, also known as chemexfoliation, are treatments in which a chemical is applied to the skin and then removed. The skin surface will then shed its outer layer, much as it does after a sunburn. The treatment is used for cosmetic purposes, such as smoothing the wrinkles around the mouth or removing liver spots (lentigines). The chemical peel codes (15788-15793) are divided according to whether the peel is on the face or not on the face, in addition to the depth of the peel (epidermal or dermal).

Cervicoplasty, 15819, is the surgical procedure whereby the physician removes excess skin from the neck, usually for cosmetic reasons. **Blepharoplasty** (15820-15823), also performed predominantly for cosmetic purposes, is the removal of excess skin and the support of the muscles of the upper eyelid. Rhytidectomy is the removal of wrinkles by pulling the skin tight and removing the excess. **Rhytidectomy** codes (15824-15829) are used to report these cosmetic services. Excision of excess skin elsewhere on the body—thigh, leg, hip, buttock, arm, and so forth—is reported by using codes in the range 15830-15839.

Grafts for facial nerve paralysis (15840-15845) are procedures in which the physician harvests a graft from some location on the body and grafts the area damaged by facial paralysis.

There are also codes in the Other Procedures category for the removal of sutures and for dressing changes (15850-15852) performed under anesthesia.

Lipectomy (commonly called liposuction) codes (15876-15879) are divided according to the body area that is being treated—head, trunk, upper extremities, and so forth. Again, if the procedure is done bilaterally, add modifier -50.

Pressure Ulcers

Pressure ulcers are also known as decubitus ulcers or bedsores (Fig. 4-30, *A*). Pressure ulcers are found on areas of the body that have bony projections, such as the hips and the area above the tailbone. Pressure on these areas causes decreased blood flow, and sores form. With continued pressure, the sores ulcerate, and deeper layers of tissue, such as fascia, muscle, and bone, may be affected. As illustrated in Fig. 4-30, *B*, the depth of the ulcer is referred to in stages—I, II, III, IV. Pressure ulcers commonly occur in patients who are unable to change position or have devices that prevent mobility (splints, casts).

Although a pressure ulcer can be seen, the depth to which the ulceration has penetrated cannot be seen. The ulcer may involve only superficial skin or may affect deeper layers. The treatment for a pressure ulcer (15920-15999) is excision of the ulcerated area to the depth of unaffected tissue, fascia, or muscle (see Fig. 4-23).

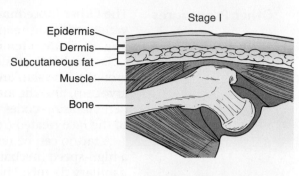

Stage I

Epidermis
Dermis
Subcutaneous fat
Muscle
Bone

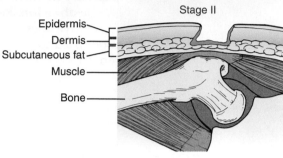

Stage II

Epidermis
Dermis
Subcutaneous fat
Muscle
Bone

FIGURE 4–30 **A,** Decubitus ulcer. **B,** Stage I, II, III, and IV of pressure ulcers. (**A** from Callen J, Greer K, Hood A, et al: *Color Atlas of Dermatology,* Philadelphia, 1993, Saunders.)

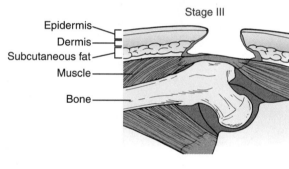

Stage III

Epidermis
Dermis
Subcutaneous fat
Muscle
Bone

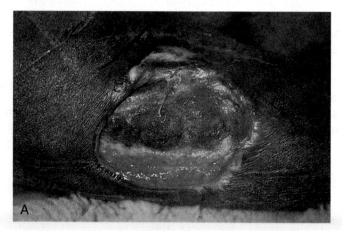

A

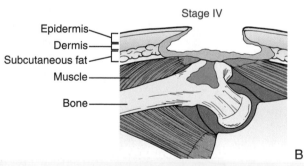

Stage IV

Epidermis
Dermis
Subcutaneous fat
Muscle
Bone

B

CODING SHOT Only an adjacent tissue transfer is included in the pressure ulcer codes. If the medical record indicates a myocutaneous flap closure, or a muscle flap, use codes from both the Pressure Ulcer category (15920-15999) and from the Flaps (Skin and/or Deep Tissue) category (15570-15738). Also, if a free skin graft is used to close the ulcer, that closure would be coded separately too, using a code from the Free Skin Grafts category.

You will note that many of the Pressure Ulcer codes have "with ostectomy" as the indented code. An ostectomy is the removal of the bone that underlies the ulcer area. The bony prominences are chiseled or filed down to alleviate future pressure.

Read the code descriptions carefully when coding from the ulcer repair category, as the codes are divided based on the location, type, and extent of closure needed.

BURNS

Fig. 4-31 illustrates the Rule of Nines, which is used to calculate the percentage of body area in adults. Fig. 4-32 illustrates the Lund-Browder classification of burns, which is often used to calculate the percentage of body area in infants. Although the Lund-Browder approach is similar to the Rule of Nines, adjustments are made in the percentages because an infant's head is larger in proportion to the rest of his or her body. If the donor site for the graft requires repair by grafting, an additional graft code is used. Simple repair (closure) of the donor site is included in the graft code.

Burn treatment is unique in that it is common for a patient to undergo multiple dressing changes or debridements (see Fig. 4–21) during the healing period. Dressing and debridement codes are either initial or subsequent treatments. Burn dressing and/or debridement codes (16020-16030) are divided based on whether the dressing or debridement is of a small, medium, or large area. The definition of small is less than 5% of the total body surface area, medium is the whole face or an extremity equalling 5%-10% of the total body surface area, and large is more than one extremity or greater than 10% of the total body area.

Bundled into codes 16000-16036 is the application of dressing, such as temporary skin replacement. The notes in the Burn, Local Treatment category refer to Biobrane® as one of the bundled materials. Biobrane® is a biosynthetic skin substitute that is constructed of a silicone film with a nylon fabric embedded into the film. Collagen is then embedded into the film and fabric. There are small pores on the skin substitute to make the covering permeable to allow for application of topical antibiotics.

The Burn category contains codes for **escharotomy** (16035, 16036), a procedure in which the physician cuts through the dead skin that covers the surface when there is a full-thickness burn. The crust covers the surface and diminishes blood flow and healing.

CODING SHOT Some third-party payers allow you to submit charges for burn care using the first date of service to the last date of service. This allows you to indicate multiples of the same service (e.g., ×5 or ×3). Other payers require you to list each date of service and to code each service separately. So if the patient received five burn debridements on five separate days, you would report the code five separate times, once for each day of service.

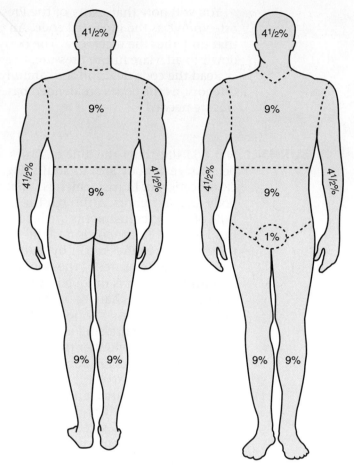

FIGURE 4–31 Rule of nines, adults.

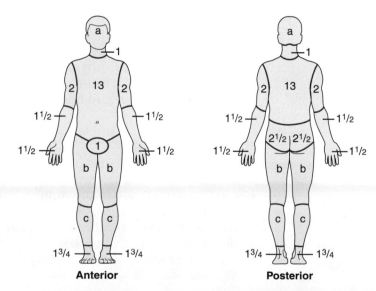

Relative percentage of body surface areas (% BSA) affected by growth

	0 yr	1 yr	5 yr	10 yr	15 yr
a – ½ of head	9½	8½	6½	5½	4½
b – ½ of 1 thigh	2¾	3¼	4	4¼	4½
c – ½ of lower leg	2½	2½	2¾	3	3¼

FIGURE 4–32 Lund-Browder chart for estimating the extent of burns on children.

EXERCISE 4-5 *Repair (Closure) and Burns*

Pay special attention to the following descriptions of main terms. The main term, as introduced in Chapter 1, is the primary word or phrase that identifies the service or procedure, anatomic site, condition, or disease. In this example, the patient record states: **"simple wound repair 12-cm wound, left hand."**

To locate the code for the repair in the CPT manual index using the *condition method*, you first locate the main term, **"Wound,"** and then the subterm, **"Repair."** Wound is the condition and Repair is the procedure. Finally, you identify the type (i.e., complex, simple).

To locate the code using the *service* or *procedure method*, you would first locate the main term, **Repair.** Repair is the service or procedure. The subterm, **Wound,** is located next, and finally the type (i.e., complex, simple). These are just two of the ways to locate this service in the index.

From the main term, Wound, subterm Repair, simple, you are directed to a range of codes, 12001-12021. Locate this range in the CPT manual. The notes under the subheading Repair (Closure) are "must" reading. Also, read the description of the first code in the category (12001). The description specifies that the code includes the term "hands," which is what you are looking for. Now locate the correct length (12 cm), and you will have the correct code—12004.

Now you code the following:

The patient record states: "complex wound repair on leg, 3.1 cm."

1 What is the correct code?

Code: _____

2 After an assault with a knife, a patient requires simple repair of a 3-cm laceration of the neck, simple repair of a 4-cm laceration of the back, simple repair of a 5-cm laceration of the forearm, and complex repair of a 3-cm laceration of the abdomen. (Note: Remember to use modifier -51 with the least intensive repair.)

Code: _____

3 Harry Torgerson, a 42-year-old construction worker, is injured at work when a box containing wood scraps and shingles falls from a second story scaffolding and strikes him on the left forearm, causing multiple lacerations. Forearm repairs: a 5.1-cm repair of the subcutaneous tissues and a 5.6-cm laceration, with particles of shingles and wood materials deeply embedded, both requiring intermediate closure. There is also a superficial wound of the scalp of 3.1 cm that requires simple closure.

Code: _____

4 A patient with multiple healed scars requests that they be removed and repaired for cosmetic reasons. The defects include a 100-cm² scar of the right cheek and a 200-cm² defect of the left upper chest. Several split-thickness skin grafts totaling 300 cm² are harvested from the left and right thighs. The scar tissue is cut away, and the sites are prepared for grafting.

Cheek graft: _____

Upper chest graft: _____ _____

Site prep, cheek, 100 cm²: _____

Site prep, chest, 200 cm²: _____ _____

5 The patient had a 20-cm² defect of the right cheek that was repaired with a rotation flap (adjacent tissue transfer).

Code(s): _____

6 The patient had a 10-cm² malignant neoplasm removed from the forehead. Z-plasty was used to repair this site. How would the excision and repair be coded?

⚕ Code(s): _____

7 A patient has had a portion of his mandible removed due to excision of a malignant tumor. Repair of the site is now performed by use of a myocutaneous flap graft.

⚕ Code(s): _____

8 A patient incurs second- and third-degree burns of the abdomen and thigh (10%) when she pulls a pan of boiling water off the stove. She requires daily debridements or dressing changes for the first week (Monday through Friday, ×5). She is in severe pain and requires anesthesia during these treatments. During the following 2 weeks she will be receiving dressing changes every other day (Monday, Wednesday, Friday, ×6), and it is expected that enough healing will have taken place that anesthesia will not be necessary. What codes would be reported for services during the 3-week treatment period?

Week 1 code: _____

Weeks 2 and 3 code: _____

DESTRUCTION

The next subheading in the subsection of the Integumentary System is Destruction. The codes are for destruction of lesions by means **other than excision.** The codes 17000-17286 are for benign, premalignant, or malignant lesions destroyed by means of electrosurgery (use of various forms of electrical current to destroy the lesion), cryosurgery (use of extreme cold), laser (light amplification by stimulated emission of radiation), or chemicals (acids). Read the notes under the Destruction subsection heading; they contain a list of types of lesions. Destruction codes state "any method" and are divided according to type of lesion (benign or malignant). Further divisions are based on the number of lesions destroyed or the size of the area destroyed. The malignant lesions are divided based on location (nose, ear, and so forth) and size (0.6-1.0 cm, and so forth), regardless of the method used.

Mohs' Micrographic Surgery

One sophisticated procedure is Mohs' micrographic surgery (17311-17315). The **Mohs' microscope** is used by the surgeon during the surgical procedure to view the lesion and assess its pathology. If the lesion is malignant, it is immediately removed. Mohs' micrographic surgery is especially useful in cases of large tumors. The procedure involves mapping the exact contour of the tumor and removing tissue down to the level at which cancerous cells are no longer found. The process involves stages, whereby the surgeon

---

From the Trenches

"Get to know what your doctors are doing—how they do procedures and how they document . . . You can get all the codes correct up front. It sets the stage for anything you have to do with the insurance companies later."

CHRIS

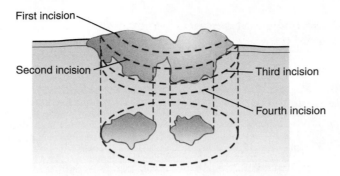

First incision

Second incision

Third incision

Fourth incision

FIGURE 4-33 Mohs' micrographic surgical technique.

removes a layer of skin and examines it under a microscope for cancerous cells, then returns to the lesion to remove another layer of skin, again examining it under a microscope (Fig. 4–33). This process is continued until cancerous cells are no longer identified in the layers being removed. The surgeon acts as both the pathologist and the surgeon.

If a biopsy is performed on the same day as the Mohs' surgery, and there was no previous pathology report to confirm the diagnosis, report the diagnostic biopsy with 11100 or 11101 (-59, distinct procedural service, would be added to the chosen code) and the pathology consultation during surgery with 88331-59.

The codes in the category include the removal of the lesion(s) and pathologic evaluation of the lesion(s). These codes are also divided based on the stage (e.g., first, second) of the surgery and the number of tissue blocks the surgeon takes during the surgery for pathologic examination.

QUICK CHECK 4-3

Review the Mohs' notes before 17311-17315 to determine if repairs are reported:

    a. bundled
    b. reported separately

EXERCISE 4–6 *Destruction*

1 Electrosurgical destruction of a herpetic lesion

    Code(s): _____

2 Cryosurgical destruction of 14 actinic keratoses

    Code: _____ and _____ × _____

3 Mohs' micrographic surgery by a single physician removing and examining three specimens, first stage of the neck

    Code(s): _____

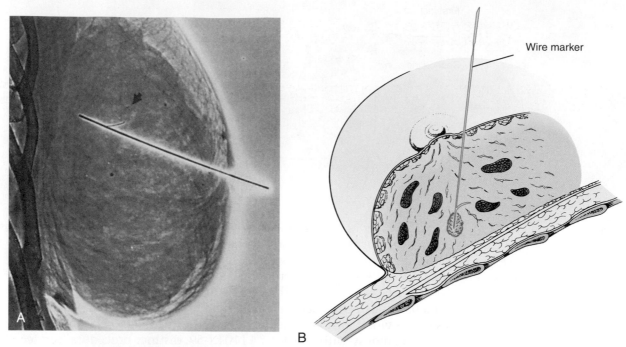

Wire marker

FIGURE 4–34 Wire marker used to mark breast lesion. **A,** Mammography is used to place a preoperative needle used to mark a lesion. **B,** The wire marker serves as a guide for the surgeon to perform the biopsy. (Modified from Bland KI, Copeland EM, eds: *The Breast: Comprehensive Management of Benign and Malignant Disorders,* ed 3, St. Louis, 2004, Saunders.)

BREAST PROCEDURES

Breast procedures (19000-19499) are divided according to category of procedure (e.g., incision, excision, introduction, repair and/or reconstruction). You must read the documentation to identify the procedure used, such as incisional versus excisional biopsies. In an **incisional biopsy,** an incision is made into the lesion and a small portion of the lesion is taken out. In an **excisional biopsy,** the entire lesion is removed for biopsy. In some cases it may be necessary to mark the lesion preoperatively by placing a thin wire (radiologic marker) down to the lesion to identify its exact location (Fig. 4–34). The placement of the wire is coded 19290, and the excision of the lesion identified by the marker is coded separately.

Multiple codes are used to identify mastectomies. You should carefully review the operative report to confirm whether pectoral muscles, axillary lymph nodes, or internal mammary lymph nodes were also removed. This information will be necessary to determine the correct mastectomy code.

CODING SHOT Any breast procedure done on **both** breasts must be coded as a bilateral procedure (modifier -50).

EXERCISE 4–7 *Breast Procedures*

Locate the correct code for the following procedures. Be sure to read all notes in the CPT manual and the description of the code before applying the code.

1 Aspiration of one cyst, breast

   Code(s): _____

2 Simple, complete bilateral mastectomies

   Code(s): _____

3 Right modified radical mastectomy, including axillary lymph nodes without any muscles

   Code(s): _____

4 Preoperative placement of one breast wire, left breast

   Code(s): _____

5 Reconstruction of nipple/areola, right breast

   Code(s): _____

CONGRATULATIONS! You made it through the entire Integumentary System subsection! The subsection is quite complicated and you have done a great job if you understand the basics of these codes. As you use them here and on the job, your knowledge will continue to grow.

CHAPTER REVIEW

CHAPTER 4, PART I, THEORY

Now is an excellent time to put all your newly learned coding skills to work by completing a Chapter Review.

1 What is the largest section of the six CPT manual sections? _____.

2 How many subsections does the Surgery section have? _____

3 Most surgery subsections are defined according to _____.

4 Measurement in the CPT manual is in what system? _____

Wound repair codes are determined by what three criteria?

5 _____

6 _____

7 _____

What are the three classifications of wound repair?

8 _____

9 _____

10 _____

11 What is the bilateral procedures modifier? _____

List the three times when multiple procedures are coded:

12 _____

13 _____

14 _____

15 Modifier -51 indicates what? _____

16 What is the title for the information that precedes each section? _____

17 What is the first subsection in the Surgery section? _____

18 If an unlisted procedure code is used, what must accompany submission of the code?

_____

19 Surgery package and surgical global fee are terms used to describe what?

_____

20 What is the five-digit code number used for documentation purposes to report nonbilled postoperative services provided to the patient under the umbrella of a surgical package?

_____

21 The major distinction in coding destruction of lesions is whether the lesion is

_____ or _____.

22 The division of malignant lesion excision is based on _____ and

_____.

23 What symbol in the CPT manual indicates the beginning and ending of a text change?

_____

24 What kind of package is developed by third-party payers and may go beyond the package described in the CPT manual?

_____

25 What two words following a procedure description alert you to the fact that you can code the procedure only if it is not done as a part of a more extensive procedure?

_____

CHAPTER 4, PART II, PRACTICAL

Code the following cases for the surgical procedures and office visits only. Do not code the radiology services or laboratory work that may be included.

26 Margaret Wilson, a 26-year-old mother of three (new patient), has routine screening mammography of both breasts. (You do not need to code the mammography.) A shadow is visualized in the right breast. The physician performs a biopsy (needle core). The biopsy indicates malignancy. The patient agrees to and has a mastectomy (simple, complete) 1 week later.

There is no global period on this procedure.

Code(s): _____

27 Shirley Peters, age 80, an established patient, presents to the office for removal of 12 skin tags.

Code(s): _____

28 Removal of 180-cm² nevus of left cheek, autograft with split-thickness skin graft of 180 cm²

Code(s): _____

29 Nipple reconstruction

Code(s): _____

30 Destruction of 0.4-cm malignant lesion of the neck

Code(s): _____

31 Simple repair of a superficial wound of the genitalia; 2.4 cm

Code(s): _____

32 Adjacent tissue transfer of chin defect; 9 cm²

Code(s): _____

QUICK CHECK ANSWERS

QUICK CHECK 4-1
False

QUICK CHECK 4-2
1. b
2. c
3. a

QUICK CHECK 4-3
b. reported separately

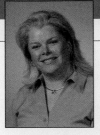

What is the most rewarding part of your job?
"The opportunity to 'serve and protect' physicians and the opportunity to share knowledge."

Judy Breuker, CPC, CCS-P, CHBME, ACS, PCS

President, Medical Reimbursement Services, Inc.

Director, Medical Education Services, LLC

Jenison, Michigan

Musculoskeletal System

Chapter Topics

Format

Coding Highlights

General

Application of Casts and Strapping

Endoscopy/Arthroscopy

Chapter Review

Quick Check Answers

Learning Objectives

After completing this chapter, you should be able to

1. Differentiate among fracture treatment types.

2. Understand types of traction.

3. Identify services/procedures included in the General subheading.

4. Understand elements of arthroscopic procedures.

5. Analyze cast application and strapping procedures.

6. Demonstrate the ability to code musculoskeletal services and procedures.

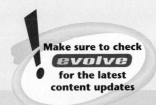

Make sure to check **evolve** for the latest content updates

FORMAT The Musculoskeletal System subsection is formatted by anatomic site. The subheadings in the Musculoskeletal subsection are as follows:

- General
- Head
- Neck (Soft Tissues) and Thorax
- Back and Flank
- Spine (Vertebral Column)
- Abdomen
- Shoulder
- Humerus (Upper Arm) and Elbow
- Forearm and Wrist
- Hand and Fingers
- Pelvis and Hip Joint
- Femur (Thigh Region) and Knee Joint
- Leg (Tibia and Fibula) and Ankle Joint
- Foot and Toes
- Application of Casts and Strapping
- Endoscopy/Arthroscopy

The first subheading in this subsection is General; it contains procedures that are applicable to many different anatomic sites. The other subheadings are further divided by anatomic site, procedure type, condition, and description. They usually include:

- Incision
- Excision
- Introduction or Removal
- Repair, Revision and/or Reconstruction
- Fracture and/or Dislocation
- Arthrodesis
- Amputation

Any or all of these categories of procedures may be found under each subheading.

The codes found in the Musculoskeletal System subsection are used extensively by orthopedic surgeons to describe the services they provide to restore and preserve the function of the skeletal system. There are many codes, however, that are used frequently by a wide variety of primary care and family practice physicians, such as the splinting, casting, and fracture codes. Your study of the Musculoskeletal subsection of the CPT will focus on the format of the subsection, fracture types and repair, application of casts and strapping, the General subheading, and endoscopic procedures.

CODING HIGHLIGHTS Thorough review of the medical record will help you to identify key information necessary for coding. The following tips will help you to choose the most correct code from this subsection:

1. Identify whether the procedure is being performed on soft tissue or bone.
2. Determine whether treatment is for a traumatic injury (acute) or a medical condition (chronic). The ICD-9-CM diagnosis codes indicating acute or chronic must match the treatment codes. E codes from ICD-9-CM should also be used to describe accidents and injuries.

From the Trenches

Why did you choose coding as a profession?
"It chose me; I was fascinated and challenged by the differences in rules and interpretations."
JUDY

3. Identify the most specific anatomic site. For example, when coding vertebral procedures, it is necessary to know whether the procedure was for cervical, thoracic, or lumbar vertebrae.

4. Determine whether the code description includes grafting or fixation. If grafting or fixation is not listed within the major procedure code description, each may be coded as an additional procedure.

5. Read the code carefully to determine whether it describes a procedure done on a single site (e.g., each finger). If the same procedure is performed on multiple sites (e.g., multiple fingers), you must indicate the number of units done (such as, 26060 × 2) or list the code multiple times. HCPCS modifiers are used to identify the digit treated.

6. Check any medical terms you do not understand in a medical dictionary or in the Glossary at the back of the book.

Fractures

Fractures are coded by treatment—open, closed, or percutaneous. **Open treatment** of a fracture is made when a surgery is performed in which the fracture is exposed by an incision made over the fracture and the fractured bone is visualized. **Closed treatment** is performed when the physician repairs the fracture without directly visualizing the fracture. The treatment method used—open or closed—depends on the type and severity of the fracture. A closed fracture (Fig. 5–1) may receive either closed, open, or percutaneous fixation. Whereas, a more complicated compound fracture usually requires an open treatment so as to provide internal fixation (e.g., wires, pins, screws). Fractures are coded to the specific anatomic site and then according to whether manipulation was performed. All fractures and dislocations are coded based on the reason for the treatment. For instance, if a hip replacement (arthroplasty) is done for medical reasons such as osteoarthritis, it is coded 27130, located under the subheading Pelvis and Hip Joint, category Repair, Revision, and/or Reconstruction. The osteoarthritis that caused the breakdown of the bone of the hip requiring repair was the reason for the treatment. If the hip replacement was performed for a fracture, it is coded 27236, located under the subheading Pelvis and Hip Joint, category Fracture and/or Dislocation. The fracture, which is not a progressive, degenerative disease, was the reason for the treatment.

The CPT manual more specifically defines closed, open, and percutaneous treatments as follows:

Closed Treatment: This terminology is used to describe procedures that treat fractures by one of three methods: (1) without manipulation, (2) with manipulation, or (3) with or without traction.

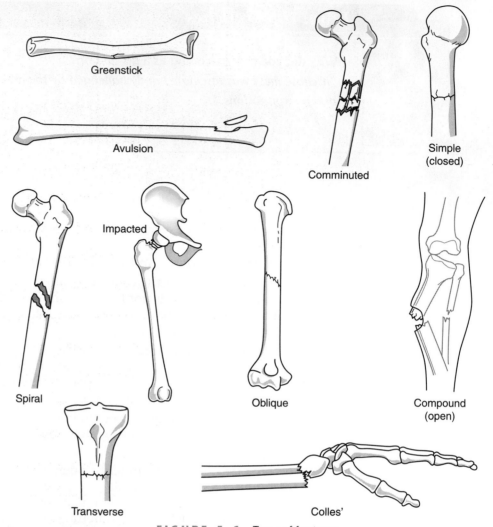

Greenstick

Avulsion

Comminuted

Simple
(closed)

Impacted

Spiral

Oblique

Compound
(open)

Transverse

Colles'

FIGURE 5–1 Types of fractures.

Manipulation is a reduction, which is an attempt to maneuver the bone back into proper alignment. The physician may bend, rotate, pull, or guide the bone back into position.

Closed treatment without manipulation is a procedure in which the physician immobilizes the bone with a splint, cast, or other device but without having to manipulate the fracture into alignment. Code 25500 describes a closed treatment of a radial shaft fracture without manipulation. This code is correctly used when a patient has a broken but stable radial shaft that is not displaced. The physician applies a cast. Initial casting or splinting services are included in the fracture care, but the supplies used are not. Initial splinting or casting of fractures performed by another physician as the only service can be reported by that physician (i.e., an emergency department physician). If the cast needs to be removed and reapplied during the global period, the surgeon that charged the global fee may report the cast/splint application with 29000-29799 and append modifier -58. Only charge for cast removal without reapplication if the physician or physician group is not assuming care for the fracture.

Closed treatment with manipulation is a procedure in which the physician has to reduce (put back in place) a fracture. Code 21320 describes a closed treatment of a nasal bone fracture with stabilization, as illustrated in Fig. 5–2. This code is correctly used when a patient has a displaced broken nose that requires manipulation to return it to the normal position. The physician would then apply external and/or internal splints to immobilize the nose.

Open treatment is used when the fracture is opened (exposed to the external environment). In this instance, the fracture (bone) is open to view and internal fixation (pins, screws, etc.) may be used. For example, 23630, open treatment of greater humeral tuberosity fracture, includes internal fixation when performed. The physician opens the site, reduces the fracture, and applies internal fixation, as needed to maintain anatomic position of the fracture.

Open treatment can also mean that a remote site (not directly over the fracture) is opened to place a nail (intramedullary) across the fracture site.

QUICK CHECK 5-1

Which code would be used to repair a femoral shaft fracture using an intramedullary rod?

a. 27506
b. 27507

Percutaneous skeletal fixation describes fracture treatment that is neither open nor closed. In this procedure, the fracture is not open to view, but fixation (e.g., pins) is placed across the fracture site, usually under x-ray imaging. For example, percutaneous skeletal fixation of a fracture of the great toe, phalanx, or phalanges (28496). This procedure is performed entirely percutaneously.

Areas of bones, as illustrated in Fig. 5–3, the tibia, are important to know when identifying the location of a fracture. For example, there may be an open treatment of a proximal fibula fracture (27784), proximal being closer to the body, or of a distal fibula fracture (27792), distal being farther from the body.

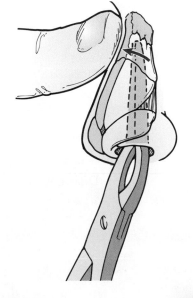

FIGURE 5–2 Realignment and support of nasal fracture.

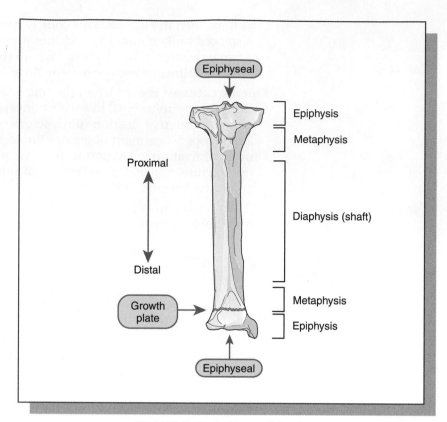

Epiphyseal

Epiphysis

Metaphysis

Proximal

Distal

Diaphysis (shaft)

Growth plate

Metaphysis

Epiphysis

Epiphyseal

FIGURE 5–3 Areas of the tibia.

> **CODING SHOT** 🖋 If the physician attempts a reduction but is unable to correct the fracture successfully, you still report a reduction service. List the attempted reduction service code and then list the more involved fracture care (i.e., open, endoscopic) the physician successfully performed to reduce the fracture with modifier -58 appended.

Traction definitions are as follows:

> **Traction** is the application of pulling force to hold a bone in alignment (Fig. 5–4).
>
> **Skeletal traction** is the use of internal devices, such as pins, screws, or wires, that are inserted into the bone through the skin, with ends of the pins, screws, or wires sticking out through the skin, so traction devices can be attached (Fig. 5–5).
>
> **Skin traction** involves strapping, elastic wrap, or tape that is fastened to the skin or wrapped around the limb; weights attached to them apply force to the fracture (Fig. 5–6).

Dislocations   Dislocation is the displacement of a bone from its normal location in a joint, and the treatment of the dislocation injury is to return the bone to its normal location (anatomic alignment) by a variety of methods. For example, if a finger was dislocated and the bone did not protrude through the skin, the physician would administer a digital block (Fig. 5–7) and apply gentle traction until the finger was realigned. A splint would then be applied to keep the finger immobile for about 3 weeks. If the shoulder was dislocated,

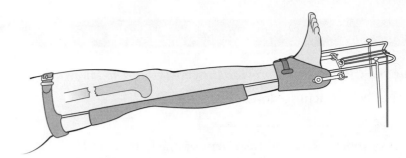

FIGURE 5-4 Traction is the application of a pulling force to hold a bone in alignment.

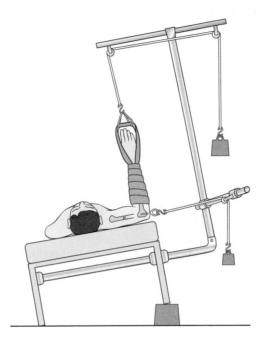

FIGURE 5-5 Skeletal traction uses the patient's bones to secure internal devices to which traction is attached.

FIGURE 5-6 Skin traction utilizes strapping, wraps, or tape to which traction is attached.

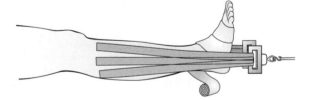

the physician might elevate the arm and rotate the humerus while applying pressure to the head of the humerus. Or the patient might lie facedown on a table with the arm hanging off the edge while a weight is attached to the hand; the weight is sufficient to pull the arm back into place (Fig. 5–8). If external measures such as those just described do not relocate the joint, a surgical reduction might be indicated.

QUICK CHECK 5-2

According to the Musculoskeletal System notes before 20000, does the type of fracture/dislocation (i.e., open, closed) determine the type of treatment (e.g., open, closed)?

Yes or No?

EXERCISE 5-1 *Fractures and Dislocations*

Using the CPT manual, provide the code(s) for the following:

1 Nasal bone fracture, closed treatment

Code: _____

2 Uncomplicated, closed treatment of one fractured rib

Code: _____

3 Interphalangeal joint dislocation of toe, open treatment with internal fixation

Code: _____

4 Open distal fibula fracture repair with internal fixation

Code: _____

5 Femoral shaft fracture repair using closed treatment

Code: _____

6 Percutaneous skeletal fixation of impact fracture of proximal end, femoral neck

Code: _____

7 Open treatment of shoulder dislocation with greater humeral tuberosity fracture

Code: _____

8 Closed treatment of mandibular fracture, including interdental fixation

Code: _____

9 Percutaneous skeletal fixation of distal radius fracture

Code: _____

10 Ankle dislocation, closed treatment

Code: _____

GENERAL The first subheading in the Musculoskeletal subsection is General. As the name implies, this subheading includes miscellaneous procedures that are not specific to an anatomic site.

Incisions The first codes 20000 and 20005 are for the incision of a **soft tissue abscess** that is superficial or deep. There are codes in the Integumentary System for incisions that are for skin only. What makes the 20000/20005 codes different from those in the Integumentary System is that 20000 or 20005 is used when the abscess is associated with the deep tissue and possibly down to the bone that underlies the area of abscess. The physician would make an incision into the abscess, explore and clean the abscess, and debride it (remove dead tissue). This procedure is very different from the procedures you find in the Integumentary System codes for incision of an abscess.

Wound Exploration The Wound Exploration codes (20100-20103) are used for traumatic wounds that result from a penetrating trauma (e.g., gunshot, knife wound). Wound Exploration codes include basic exploration and repair of the area of trauma. These codes are used specifically when the repair requires enlargement of the existing wound for exploration, cleaning, and repair. Included in the

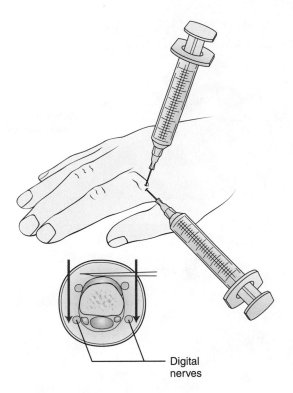

FIGURE 5–7 Digital nerve block.

Digital
nerves

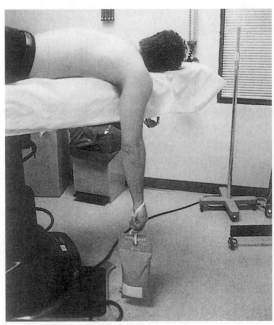

FIGURE 5–8 External technique for relocation of a shoulder. (Stimson technique). (From Rakel RE: *Saunders Manual of Medical Practice,* ed 2, Philadelphia, 2000, Saunders.)

Wound Exploration codes are not only the exploration and enlargement of the wound but also debridement, removal of any foreign body(ies), ligation of minor blood vessels, and repair of subcutaneous tissues, muscle fascia, and muscle, as would be necessary to repair the wound (Fig. 5–9).

If the wound does not need to be enlarged, you would use a code from the Integumentary System, Skin Repair codes. If, however, the wound is more severe than a Wound Exploration code would indicate, the repair code would come from the specific repair by anatomic site codes. For example, for a bullet wound to the chest with suspicion of cardiac injury, the treatment will be thoracotomy of any approach, as illustrated in Fig. 5–10,

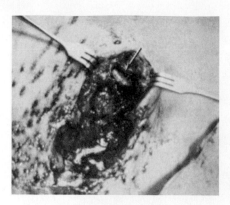

FIGURE 5–9 Gunshot wound requiring exploration. (From Swan KG, Swan RC: Principles of ballistics applicable to the treatment of gunshot wounds. *Surg Clin North Am* 71:221-239, 1991.)

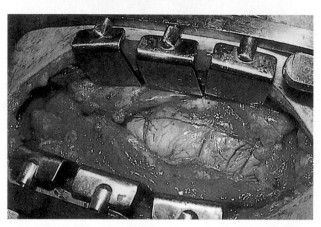

FIGURE 5–10 Median sternotomy was performed because of the position of the entrance wound and the suspicion of cardiac injury. Palpation of the left hemidiaphragm revealed a defect and indicated laparotomy. (From Swan, KG, Swan RC: *Gunshot Wounds: Pathophysiology and Management,* ed 2, Chicago, Year Book Medical Publishers, Inc.)

with control of the hemorrhage and repair of any injured intrathoracic organ. The thoracotomy code would come from the subsection Respiratory System under the subheading Lungs. As you can see from this example, you have to assess the extent of the procedure carefully, reading the medical record to ensure you are in the correct area so you can choose the correct service code. In this case, the wound exploration is included in the thoracotomy, and would not be reported separately.

QUICK CHECK 5-3

Penetrating wound exploration may be coded from the Musculoskeletal System, Integumentary System, or the appropriate _____ site.

Excision

The Excision category (20150-20251) contains codes for the biopsies of muscle and bone. The codes are divided based on the type of biopsy (muscle, bone), the depth of the biopsy (superficial, deep), and, in some codes, the method of obtaining the biopsy (e.g., percutaneous needle).

The procedure for a muscle or bone biopsy typically includes the administration of local anesthetic into the biopsy area, an incision into the area allowing exposure of the muscle or bone, removal of tissue for biopsy, and suturing of the area. A **percutaneous biopsy**, as represented in 20206, differs in that the area is not opened to the physician's view. A trocar (hollow needle) or needle is placed into the muscle or bone by passing the needle through the skin and into the muscle or bone and withdrawing a sample.

When the percutaneous method is used to obtain a biopsy, the area does not require suturing. If the biopsy is extremely complicated, a surgeon may request the assistance of ultrasound to be able to view the biopsy area during the procedure and receive guidance as to the placement of the needle. Notice the guideline in the CPT following 20206 that directs you to the radiology codes if imaging guidance is performed during the procedure.

Biopsy codes in the Excision category of the General subheading are not to be used for the excision of tumors on muscle. If the medical record indicates excision of a muscle tumor, you would have to choose a code from the correct Musculoskeletal subsection. For example, 24076 is used to report the excision of a tumor from the deep (subfascial or intramuscular) tissue of the upper arm or elbow.

Biopsy codes do not include the pathology workup that is done on the sample. You will also learn more about pathology services later in this text.

General Introduction or Removal

Within the Introduction or Removal category you will find a wide variety of injection, aspiration, insertion, application, removal, and adjustment codes. Because the category is within the General subheading of the Musculoskeletal subsection, the codes also have a wide application in coding for services.

Therapeutic **sinus tract injection** procedure codes are within this category. You may initially think of the nasal sinuses, but these are not the sinuses that are being injected here. The term "sinus" refers to a cyst or abscess inside the body with a tract (otherwise known as a fistula) connecting to another surface—internal (to the gut) or external (to the skin). The infection is treated by injecting an antibiotic or other substance into the sinus by way of the sinus tract (passage from the outer surface to the inner cavity). With certain sinus injections, a radiologist provides guidance to ensure the correct placement of the needle and the guidance is reported separately. For example, an interstitial abscess located perirectally that develops a sinus tract opening perianally may be treated by instilling a caustic substance to stimulate healing. Other methods that may be used in treatment of the sinus tract (fistula) are the incision or opening of the tract (fistulotomy) to promote healing or by means of excision (fistulectomy).

Removal codes located in the Introduction or Removal category (20520-20525) are used to report the removal of foreign bodies that are lodged in muscle. Recall that the Integumentary System removal codes were used for foreign bodies lodged in the skin. **Injection** codes in this category are used for injections made into a tendon, ligament, or ganglion cyst (cystic tumor). An example of the use of these injection codes would be a corticosteroid injection as a ganglion cyst treatment.

CODING SHOT You must read the codes carefully. For most injection codes (i.e., 20550, 20551, 20553) the code description states "Injection(s)." This means that one or more injections is/are reported with the same code with no modifier.

Arthrocentesis is aspiration of a joint (Fig. 5–11), and the codes used to report such a service are in the range of 20600-20610. This is a procedure commonly used in the treatment of joint conditions. The area over the involved joint is injected with anesthetic, a needle is inserted into the joint, and fluid is drawn out during the aspiration procedure.

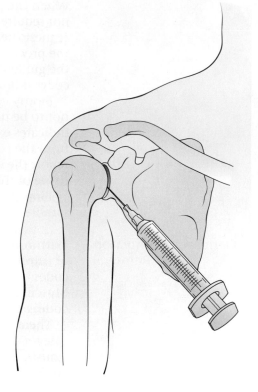

FIGURE 5–11 Arthrocentesis of a joint.

CODING SHOT   The code descriptions for arthrocentesis indicate that the codes can be used for an aspiration, an injection, or both an aspiration and an injection. You would not report the performance of both an aspiration and an injection at the same session by using multiple codes, as that would be unbundling. You would instead report the dual service using a single code.

The arthrocentesis codes are divided according to whether the joint is small (finger, toe), intermediate (ankle, elbow), or major (shoulder, hip). Note that while the shoulder is a major joint, the acromioclavicular joint, which is a part of the shoulder, is only an intermediate joint. This often leads to incorrectly coding the acromioclavicular joint as a major joint rather than as an intermediate joint.

Lidocaine, Marcaine, and so forth, when used as anesthetics, are not reported separately. Any injected therapeutic drug such as a steroid is reported separately using a J code (drug code) from the HCPCS (CMS's Healthcare Common Procedural Coding System).

Insertion of wires or pins to repair bone (20650) is a procedure often used by orthopedic physicians. The procedure is performed using a local or general anesthetic. The bone is drilled through with a power drill and pins and/or wires are placed through the holes in the bone and allowed to emerge through the skin on each side of the bone. A traction device is then attached to the pins or wires to hold the bone immobile while healing takes place. This may sound painful, but actually, the procedure is used to allow well-aligned healing, as well as alleviate pain.

CODING SHOT The removal of the external wires or pins is included in the reimbursement for skeletal fixation; but for internal fixation removal, report separately using 20670, 20680.

The codes to report the **application** of many of the devices used for fixation of the bones of the body during the healing process—cranial tong, cranial halo, pelvic halo, femoral halo, caliper, stereotactic frame—are located in this category. Each of the applications includes the removal of the device, unless the device is removed by another physician (20665). When the application of these devices is performed through an open surgical procedure, the procedure is referred to as an open reduction with internal fixation (**ORIF**) and uses pins, wires, and screws to stabilize a fracture.

Implant removal codes (20670, 20680) are available for reporting the services of removal of buried wires, pins, rods, and so forth previously implanted by another physician or implanted by the same physician at a much earlier date. If, for example, there is a complication, such as pain, the hardware may need to be removed. Diagnosis coding must support the necessity of removal of the deep hardware as a complication. If removed during the global period, report the service with modifier -58 appended to the procedure code for a staged procedure. The implant removal codes are divided according to whether the implants are superficial or deep.

External fixation is the application of a device that holds a bone in place, but rather than internal fixation, the device is placed on the outside of the body and pins or wires are placed into the bone from the outside (Fig. 5–12). These wires and pins, when fastened to the bone, hold the device or system immobile. This type of fixation is commonly used with comminuted fractures that are difficult to hold in place. External fixation is used primarily in cases of limb fracture, major pelvic disruption, osteotomy, arthrodesis, bone infection, and bone lengthening.

The codes (20690, 20692) are divided according to whether the device or system is placed on one surface (uniplane) or several surfaces (multiplane). With the uniplane device, two or more pins are inserted above the fracture

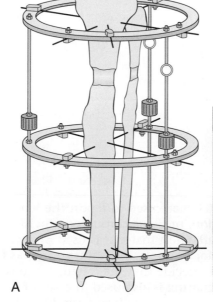

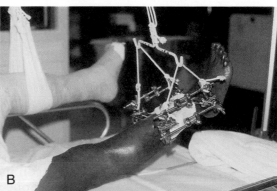

FIGURE 5–12 **A,** External fixation (Ilizarov multiplane). **B,** Example of an external fixation device on the right leg. The left leg is in a splint. (**B** from McCance KL, Huether SE: *Pathophysiology: The Biologic Basis for Disease in Adults and Children,* St. Louis, 2006, Mosby.)

A

B

site and two or more pins are inserted below the fracture site. Multiplane devices are more complicated and are usually reserved for highly complex fractures.

> **CODING SHOT** The **fixation** devices codes are used in addition to the code for the **treatment** of the fracture, unless the application code specifically states that fracture repair is included. For example, see code 25545: "Open treatment of ulnar shaft fracture includes internal fixation, when performed." This code specifies both the **treatment** of the fracture and the **fixation**. External fixation, if performed, would be reported separately.

Note also that the codes in the Introduction or Removal categories are for **unilateral** services, so if a procedure is bilateral you would add modifier -50.

If the device is **adjusted**, the service is reported separately (20693). **Removal** of external fixation devices or systems is usually accomplished under anesthesia and is reported separately from the application (20694). However, if the removal does not require return to the operating room, you would not report the service separately but would consider the removal as being bundled into the application code. If the removal was done outside the global period, some payers may reimburse it as an E/M service.

EXERCISE 5–2 *General*

Using the CPT manual, provide the codes for the following:

1 Exploration of a penetrating wound of the left leg

Code: _____

2 Replantation of right foot after a complete, traumatic amputation

Code: _____

3 Radical resection of malignant neoplasm of cheek

Code: _____

4 Nonoperative, electrical stimulation of nonhealing femur fracture

Code: _____

5 Percutaneous needle biopsy of muscle of upper arm

Code: _____

6 Intra-articular aspiration and injection of finger joint

Code: _____

Grafts (or Implants) Codes 20900-20938 are used to report the harvesting of bone, cartilage, fascia lata, tendon, or tissue through an incision separate from that used to implant the graft. Graft material is used in a wide variety of repair procedures. If, for example, a tibial fracture has failed to heal in 20 weeks, the surgeon may decide that the fracture requires bone grafting to achieve healing. Bone grafting is also used in cases of large defects (>6 cm). Some types of fractures commonly heal with difficulty, so after debridement and a

5- to 7-day healing period, the bone grafting procedure is performed. The grafts are obtained from the patient or a donor. Donors can be either living or deceased (a cadaver). The pieces of bone are shaped into bars or pegs and then used to repair the defect.

Fascia lata grafts are taken from the lower thigh area because the fascia is thickest in this area. Fascia is the fibrous tissue that serves as connective tissue; it may be shaved off with an instrument called a stripper or it may be incised (cut) away. The fascia lata is then used in the repair procedure. Codes for obtaining the fascia lata graft are based on whether a stripper (20920) was used to remove the fascia or whether a more complex removal procedure (20922) was required for removal of the graft material.

Tissue grafts include the obtaining of fat, dermis, paratenon (fatty tissue from the tendon compartment), and other tissue types. **Spine surgery** codes 20930-20938 are used to report the obtaining and shaping of the tissue, whether from the patient (autograft) or from a donor (allograft). The obtaining and shaping of the spine graft material is reported in addition to reporting the implantation procedure, which is the main procedure (the definitive procedure), unless the description of the major procedure includes a graft.

Other Procedures

Other procedure codes (20950-20999) for monitoring muscles, bone grafting with microvascular technique, free osteocutaneous flaps with microvascular technique, electronic/ultrasound stimulation, and computer-assisted navigation procedures are found under Other Procedures. **Monitoring of interstitial fluid pressure** (20950) is a procedure in which the physician inserts a device into the muscle to measure the pressure within the muscle. Increased pressure in the muscle indicates that the tissue is not receiving a sufficient supply of blood due to accumulation of fluid.

Bone grafts in this category (20955-20962) are identified by the site from which the graft is taken. When the bone grafts are taken, the small blood vessels remain attached to the graft. The graft is then inserted and the blood vessels are attached to vessels in the area of implant, using an operating microscope. The bone grafts described by these codes are extremely complicated.

Free osteocutaneous flaps (20969-20973) are bone grafts that include the skin and tissue that overlie the bone. The flap has an arterial pedicle that is attached (anastomosed) to an artery on the recipient site. The surgeon then uses both the skin and tissue and the bone to reconstruct the defect, using an operating microscope. The flap procedures described by these codes are very complicated. The codes are divided based on which part of the body the flap is taken from. The grafts in the Other Procedures category differ from the grafts in the Grafts (or Implants) category; the codes in the Other Procedures category are used for grafts that include skin, blood vessels, and muscle as part of the graft. The use of the operating microscope, 69990, is not reported separately because these procedures already include its use.

Electrical or ultrasound stimulation (20974-20979) is used to promote healing. Low-voltage electricity or ultrasound is applied to the skin, and both are often used in the treatment of fractures.

Computer-assisted surgical navigation (20985) is used to report the use of navigational assistance in musculoskeletal procedures. The code is listed in addition to the primary procedure.

The anatomic subheadings that follow the General subheading (e.g., head, neck, back, spine) contain codes divided based on the procedure; for example, incision, excision, or fracture. There are extensive notes throughout the Musculoskeletal System subsection that provide the specifics for reporting services using the codes. Many of the notes even tell you what specific anatomic areas the codes cover. For example, notes under the subheading

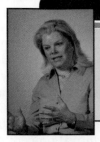

From the Trenches

"Have anatomy and medical terminology reference tools available. Look up every word you do not understand."

JUDY

Shoulder indicate that the areas covered are clavicle, scapula, humerus head/neck, sternoclavicular joint, acromioclavicular joint, and shoulder joint. So be certain to read any notes carefully before using the codes.

CAUTION *As you use the codes, you will begin to know this background information, and the coding process will become faster for you. But at the beginning, reading the notes is the way to gain the knowledge that you are seeking. Now is not the time to take shortcuts.*

Spinal Instrumentation and Fixation

Within the subheading Spine (Vertebral Column) (22010-22899), services are often based on the cervical (C1-C7), lumbar (L1-L5), and thoracic (T1-T12) spinal areas. For example, codes in the range 22210-22216 identify osteotomy of the cervical, lumbar, or thoracic spinal area. Codes are often further divided based on the exact spinal location. For example, codes in the range 22590-22600 identify arthrodesis of three different cervical areas: occiput-C2, C1-C2, or cervical below the C2 segment. Of special note in the CPT manual is that the C1 is often referred to as the **atlas** and C2 is referred to as the axis.

Arthrodesis can be performed with another surgical procedure, such as fracture care or a laminectomy. If arthrodesis is performed with a more major procedure, use modifier -51 on the arthrodesis code to indicate that multiple procedures were performed. An exception to this rule applies when the code is an add-on code, which is exempt from use with modifier -51. For example, 22614 is used to report an arthrodesis of multiple vertebral segments; therefore, the multiple modifier -51 is not needed. A code from 22600-22612 is reported for the first vertebral segment, and 22614 is reported for each additional vertebral segment.

CODING SHOT When choosing procedure codes for spine procedures, verify whether the code is describing a vertebral segment, the actual bony segment, versus an interspace (the space between two vertebral segments). If coding a procedure performed at L4-L5, and the correct code description indicated vertebral segment, you would choose the primary code to report L4, and the add-on code to report L5. If the procedure code description was by interspace, only one code would be chosen.

Spinal instrumentation is used to stabilize the spinal column in some repair procedures. **Segmental instrumentation** is the attachment of a fixative device at each end of the area being repaired and at least one other attachment in the spinal area being fixed. For example, if the repair was at

T10 and T11 (thoracic vertebral bodies 10 and 11) and a rod was attached to T7 and T13, the repair rod may also be attached at T8, T9, T10, T11, and T12.

Nonsegmental instrumentation is the application of the fixative device at each end of the area being repaired, as illustrated in Fig. 5–13. For example, if the repair was of T10, the rod may be attached at T7 and T12. Many of the instrumentation codes are usually add-on codes. Instrumentation procedure add-on codes 22840-22848 and 22851 are reported in addition to the major procedure.

Foot and Toe Repairs

A common procedure performed on the toe is a hallux valgus correction, or bunion surgery. Hallux is the great toe and valgus is the angulation of the toe away from the midline, as illustrated in Fig. 5–14.

A variety of procedures are used to correct the defect, as represented by codes in the range 28290-28299. For example, the Keller type of procedure is reported with 28292, which describes a procedure in which a wire is inserted through the bones of a toe to hold the bones in correct alignment. Each code description indicates the procedure type that is included, many of which include specific eponyms (names of individuals for whom the procedures are named), so careful reading is necessary to choose the correct bunion repair code.

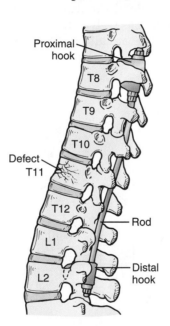

FIGURE 5-13 Fixation at each end of the area to be repaired (nonsegmental spinal instrumentation).

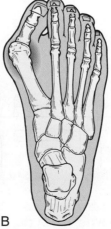

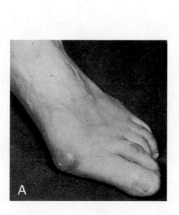

FIGURE 5-14 **A** and **B**, Hallux valgus, or bunion, is a bursa usually found along the medial aspect of the big toe. Most commonly, it is attributed to heredity or to poorly fitting shoes. (**A** from Seidel HM, et al: *Mosby's Guide to Physical Examination,* ed 6, St. Louis, 2006, Mosby)

APPLICATION OF CASTS AND STRAPPING

Application of Casts and Strapping codes (29000-29799) are used for subsequent treatment of fractures of the extremities, ligament sprains or tears, and overuse injuries. They may also be reported for the initial stabilization of an injury until definitive restorative treatment can be provided. Because each injury is unique, each cast is unique in terms of size and position. The cast immobilizes the fracture. Materials used to make casts are usually plaster, fiberglass, or thermoplastics. Each physician has a preference for the types of cast materials he or she uses.

Strapping is the taping of a body part, as illustrated in Fig. 5–15. Strapping is used to exert pressure on a body part to give it more stability; it is used in the treatment of sprains, strains, and dislocations. **Splints** are made of wood, cloth, metal, or plastic, as illustrated in Fig. 5–16, and are used to immobilize, support, or protect a body part, thereby allowing rest and healing. The **removal** of the cast, strapping, or splint is included in each of the Application of Casts and Strapping codes.

CODING SHOT If a cast, strapping, or splint is applied as a part of a **surgical procedure**, you do not use the codes from the Application of Casts and Strapping subheading to code for the service because the musculoskeletal surgical procedure codes include the **first** cast, strapping, or splint as well as its later removal. The surgery, application, and removal are all bundled into the surgical code.

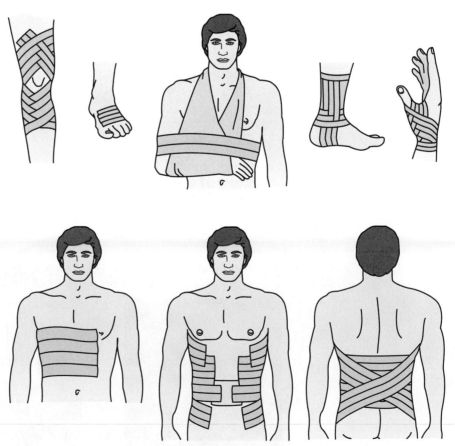

FIGURE 5–15 Types of strapping.

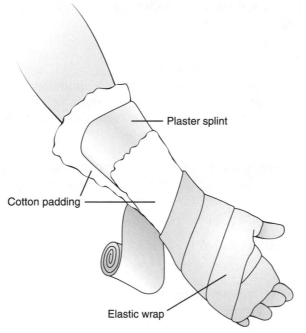

Plaster splint

Cotton padding

Elastic wrap

FIGURE 5-16 Splint used to immobilize a joint or bone.

If the cast, strapping, or splint is applied as a part of a **fracture repair,** you also do not code for the application service separately. The application service is bundled into all fracture repair codes, as is the removal. If a subsequent cast, strapping, or splint is applied within the follow-up period for either the surgical procedure or the fracture repair, you can bill for the application by coding the application and appending a -58 modifier, and the materials (A4580-A4590). You can bill for a separate office visit during which a second cast, strapping, or splint is applied only if the patient is provided some other, separate and significant service in addition to the application if you are not in the global period of a previous procedure. In these situations, modifier -25 would be appended to the E/M code.

QUICK CHECK 5-4

A replacement cast during the global period of fracture care may require which modifier? _____

You can use the Application of Casts and Strapping codes only when the physician:

- applies an initial cast, strapping, or splint for stabilization prior to definitive treatment by another provider
- applies a subsequent cast, strapping, or splint
- treats a sprain and does not expect to provide any other type of restorative treatment

The subheading Application of Casts and Strapping is divided into three major categories:

- Body and Upper Extremity
- Lower Extremity
- Removal or Repair (Note: These are for removal or repair by another physician.)

The subcategories of Body/Upper Extremity and Lower Extremity are:

- Casts
- Splints
- Strapping—Any Age

The codes in all subcategories are divided primarily according to the **location** of the cast, splint, or strapping on the body—head, hand, leg—and often on the **type**—Minerva, Velpeau, static (nonmovable), dynamic (movable).

EXERCISE 5–3 *Application of Casts and Strapping*

Using the CPT manual, provide the codes for the following:

1 Replacement of fiberglass shoulder-to-hand (long-arm) cast for a 54-year-old patient

   Code: _____

2 Initial application of a walking-type short leg cast for a sprain

   Code: _____

3 Removal of a full leg cast by a physician who did not apply the cast

   Code: _____

4 Strapping of a 46-year-old patient's knee

   Code: _____

5 Replacement of a thigh-to-toes cast on the right leg of a 35-year-old female patient

   Code: _____

ENDOSCOPY/ ARTHROSCOPY

Arthroscopy is fast becoming the treatment of choice for many orthopedic surgical procedures. The incisions are smaller, which decreases the risk of infection and speeds recovery time. Several small incisions are made through which lights, mirrors, and instruments are inserted, as illustrated in Fig. 5–17.

The arthroscopy codes are located separately at the end of the Musculoskeletal subsection. If multiple procedures are performed through a scope, they are reported with modifier -51. Bundled into all surgical arthroscopic procedure codes is the diagnostic arthroscopy. You must not unbundle and code a diagnostic arthroscopy and a surgical arthroscopy if both were performed during the same encounter. You also do not want to code separately for things done during a procedure that are considered a part of the procedure, such as shaving, removing, evacuating, casting, splinting, or strapping.

A note preceding the Endoscopy/Arthroscopy codes (29800-29999) states, "When arthroscopy is performed in conjunction with arthrotomy, add modifier -51." This note indicates that if a surgeon performs an arthroscopy and during the procedure extends the procedure to an arthrotomy, you can report both services. For example, a physician performs an arthroscopic shaving of the articular cartilage and also does an open capsulotomy (posterior capsular release) of the knee. Both the arthroscopic shaving (29877) and the capsulotomy (27435) would be reported, and to the least expensive procedure you would add modifier -51 (multiple procedures).

In arthroscopic procedures, it is also applicable to code multiple procedures in different compartments in the joint area. In the knee, there are three

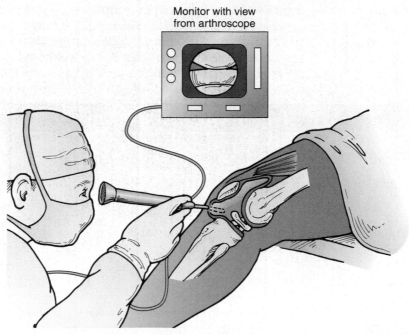

Monitor with view
from arthroscope

FIGURE 5–17 Arthroscopy of knee.

compartments, the medial, lateral, and patellofemoral. If a menisectomy (29881) is performed in the medial compartment, and a shaving (29877) is performed in the patellofemoral compartment, these procedures can both be reported.

CODING SHOT When coding arthroscopic procedures of the knee, note the use of **basket forceps**, which indicates a meniscectomy (meniscus removal) rather than a shaving and debridement.

The codes in this subheading are divided according to body area—elbow, shoulder, knee—and then according to the type and extent of procedure performed. An example of type of service is as follows: code 29805 is for an arthroscopy of the shoulder for **diagnostic** purposes (diagnosis of disease), whereas code 29806 is an arthroscopy of the shoulder for a **surgical** procedure (repair). Not only are there two different codes for surgical and diagnostic arthroscopic procedures, but also the surgical procedure is significantly more expensive than the diagnostic procedure. So great care must be taken to select the code that correctly describes the services supported in the medical record.

CODING SHOT A diagnostic arthroscopy is always included in a surgical arthroscopy.

Note the description for code 29805: "Arthroscopy, shoulder, diagnostic, with or without synovial biopsy (separate procedure)." You will find the statement "separate procedure" several times in the Endoscopy/Arthroscopy subheading because oftentimes a minor arthroscopic procedure is part of a more extensive procedure. You cannot report the service of the minor procedure unless it has been performed as an independent service, addressing a distinctly separate problem. Also note that the parenthetical information indicates the codes "(23065-23066, 23100-23101)" are to be used if the procedure was done as an open (incisional) procedure rather than as an endoscopic procedure.

EXERCISE 5-4 *Endoscopy/Arthroscopy*

Using the CPT manual, provide the codes for the following:

1 Surgical arthroscopy of ankle, which included extensive debridement

Code: _____

2 Diagnostic knee arthroscopy with a synovial biopsy

Code: _____

3 Diagnostic shoulder arthroscopy

Code: _____

4 Arthroscopic repair of tuberosity fracture of knee with manipulation

Code: _____

5 Surgical arthroscopy of ankle, including drilling and excision of tibial defect

Code: _____

CHAPTER REVIEW

CHAPTER 5, PART I, THEORY

Without the use of reference material, complete the following:

1 The Musculoskeletal System subsection is formatted according to what type of sites?

_____

2 Which physician subspecialty can use the codes from the Musculoskeletal System subsection?

_____

3 List the three types of fracture treatments and briefly describe each: _____

_____

_____

_____

4 It is the _____ of the fracture that determines the type of treatment.

5 _____ is the application of pulling force to hold a bone in place.

6 What is the term that describes the physician's actions of bending, rotating, pulling, or guiding the bone back into place?

_____

7 What term is used to mean "put the bone back in place"? _____

8 What term describes a bone that is not in its normal location? _____

9 What term describes the cleaning of a wound?

_____

10 This is a hollow needle that is often used to withdraw samples of fluid from a joint:

_____

11 Would a biopsy code usually include the administration of any necessary local anesthesia?

_____

CHAPTER 5, PART II, PRACTICAL

With the use of the CPT manual, complete the following:

12 Incision of a superficial soft tissue abscess, secondary to osteomyelitis

Code(s): _____

13 Radical resection of a malignant neoplasm of the soft tissue of the upper back

Code(s): _____

14 Closed treatment of three vertebral process fractures

Code(s): _____

15 Under general anesthesia, manipulation of a right shoulder joint with external fixation

Code(s): _____

16 Lengthening of four tendons of elbow

Code(s): _____

17 Incision and drainage of bursa of elbow

Code(s): _____

18 Open treatment of a carpal scaphoid fracture with internal fixation applied

Code(s): _____

19 Arthroplasty of two metacarpophalangeal joints

Code(s): _____

20 Tenotomy of two flexor tendons of a finger using an open procedure

Code(s): _____

21 Amputation, lower arm, using Krukenberg procedure

Code(s): _____

22 Open treatment of radial and ulnar shaft fractures with internal fixation of both radius and ulna

Code(s): _____

23 Osteoplasty for shortening of both of radius and ulna

Code(s): _____

24 Percutaneous lateral tenotomy for tennis elbow

Code(s): _____

25 Replantation of right arm, including the neck of the humerus through the elbow joint, following a complete traumatic amputation

Code(s): _____

QUICK CHECK ANSWERS

QUICK CHECK 5-1
a. 27506

QUICK CHECK 5-2
No

QUICK CHECK 5-3
anatomic

QUICK CHECK 5-4
Modifier -58

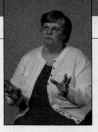

"This is not a profession that one can learn overnight. A person has to be willing to invest their time in continuing education...No matter how old you are, the key to advancement is education."

Christine A. Patterson
Coder and Biller
Reinhart Family Healthcare
Monticello, Arkansas

Respiratory System

Chapter Topics

Format

Coding Highlights

Nose

Accessory Sinuses

Larynx

Trachea and Bronchi

Lungs and Pleura

Chapter Review

Quick Check Answers

Learning Objectives

After completing this chapter you should be able to

1 Understand terms that apply to coding respiratory services.

2 Identify highlights of nasal procedure coding.

3 Differentiate among codes based on the surgical approach.

4 Review the specifics of coding for the sinuses and larynx.

5 Explain the structure of the trachea/bronchi codes.

6 Demonstrate the ability to code respiratory services and procedures.

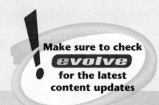

Make sure to check **evolve** for the latest content updates

FORMAT

The Respiratory System subsection is arranged by anatomic site (e.g., nose, accessory sinus, larynx) and then by procedure (e.g., incision, excision, introduction). Your knowledge of respiratory terminology is important (Fig. 6–1), as the coding you will learn about in the Respiratory System subsection covers a wide variety of services. In the Musculoskeletal System section, the arthroscopy codes were placed at the end of the subsection, but in the Respiratory System subsection, the endoscopy codes are listed throughout, according to anatomic site. Fracture repair, such as that of the nose or sternum, is listed in the Musculoskeletal System subsection, not in the Respiratory System subsection. Procedures that are performed on the throat or mouth are not located in the Respiratory System subsection, but instead are located in the Digestive System subsection.

The Respiratory System subsection contains some codes that may be considered cosmetic. It is important to note the extent of the cosmetic repair indicated in a patient's medical record. The extent is important so that you do not report the same service more than once and unbundle a code. For example, under the subheading Nose and the category Repair, there is code 30400 for rhinoplasty. The rhinoplasty can be performed either through external skin incisions (open) or through intranasal incisions (closed), and both approaches can be coded to 30400. The extent of the procedure varies based on the desired outcome, but a rhinoplasty can include fracturing a deformed septum, repositioning the septum, reshaping and/or augmenting the nasal cartilage, removing fat from the area and performing a layered closure, and applying a splint or cast. If all of these components of a rhinoplasty were performed, they would all be bundled into code 30420. You have to read all of the notes and the code information carefully to ensure that you do not code components of the procedure separately if there is one code that includes all the components. Also, be sure to report the service with the code that describes the furthest extent of the service provided.

QUICK CHECK 6-1

Rhinoplasty can be performed either _____, through external skin incisions, or closed, through _____ incisions.

CODING HIGHLIGHTS

Endoscopy

In endoscopic procedures, a scope is placed through an existing body orifice (opening), or a small incision is made into a cavity for scope placement.

When sinus endoscopies are performed, a scope is placed through the nose into the nasal cavity. Codes (31231-31294) for sinuses are used to report unilateral (on one side) procedures except in the case of a diagnostic nasal endoscopy, which is unilateral or bilateral. Multiple procedures may be performed within different sinuses (frontal, maxillary, and ethmoid sinuses) during the same operative session. The CPT manual has combined into a single code some multiple sinus procedures commonly performed at the same operative session.

Example

31276   Nasal/sinus endoscopy, surgical with frontal sinus exploration, with or without removal of tissue from frontal sinus

---

 CAUTION *Code to the full extent of the procedure.*

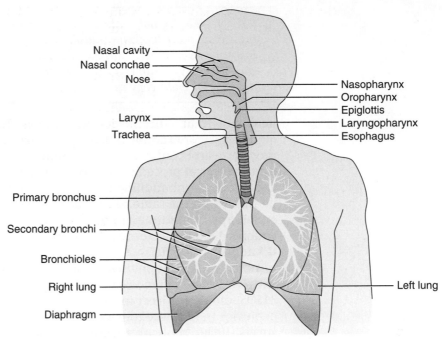

FIGURE 6-1 Respiratory system.

Endoscopic procedures may start at one site (such as the nose) and follow through to another site (such as the larynx or bronchial tubes). It is important to choose the code that most appropriately reflects the farthest extent of the procedure. For example, if a direct laryngoscopy (31515) is performed, the scope is progressed past the larynx and can include examination of the trachea. The 31515 code description states either with or without tracheoscopy. However, if it is necessary to continue the procedure to the bronchial tubes, the only code used would be 31622 (bronchoscopy). The larynx and trachea must be passed to get to the bronchial tubes and can be visualized while progressing to the farthest point (bronchial tubes).

🤚 **CAUTION** *Code the **correct approach** for the procedure.*

The same surgical procedure may be performed using different approaches. For example, code 32141 describes a **thoracotomy** with "excision-plication (removal/shortening) of bullae (blisters); with or without any pleural procedure." Code 32655 describes a surgical **thoracoscopy** with excision-plication of bullae, including any pleural procedures. Code 32655 describes the same procedure as 32141, except that 32655 is a procedure done through very minute incisions utilizing a thoracoscope, whereas code 32141 describes an open incision through the thorax, opening the full operative site to the surgeon.

Multiple endoscopic procedures may be performed through the scope during the same operative session. When this occurs, each procedure should be coded with modifier -51 (multiple procedures) placed on subsequent procedure(s). Suppose, for example, a bronchoscopy with biopsy is performed as well as a bronchoscopy with removal of a foreign body. Not only would you code a bronchoscopy with biopsy, but you would also code the removal of a foreign body. The multiple procedure modifier -51 would have to be placed after the lower priced (least resource-intensive) procedure.

The exception to this occurs when the CPT manual offers a code for which the description includes all the separate elements of the procedure bundled into one code.

CAUTION *Do not confuse the nasal/sinus endoscopic procedures with the intranasal procedures. Intranasal procedures may require that surgical instruments be placed into the nose but do not require the use of an endoscope. When an endoscope is used in a nasal/sinus procedure, use a nasal/sinus endoscopy code.*

Remember that a diagnostic endoscopy is always bundled into a surgical endoscopy. For example, if a physician began a diagnostic endoscopic nasal procedure and continued on to complete a surgical procedure, you code only for the surgical procedure. To code for both a diagnostic *and* a surgical nasal endoscopy is unbundling if the diagnostic and surgical procedures are performed on the same nasal space. For example, if a diagnostic sinus endoscopy is performed to the right maxillary sinus and a surgical endoscopic maxillectomy on the left, both are reportable with appropriate -LT and -RT modifiers.

When coding laryngoscopic procedures, note that the terms "indirect" and "direct" are often used. For example, see codes 31505, indirect, and 31515, direct. **Indirect** in 31505 means that the physician uses a tongue depressor to hold the tongue down and view the epiglottis (the lid that covers the larynx) with a mirror. The patient vocalizes (says "ah") and the physician can then view the vocal cords. **Direct** in 31515 means that the endoscope is passed into the larynx and the physician can look directly at the larynx through the endoscope. The patient's operative note will indicate whether the procedure was indirect or direct.

Locating Endoscopy Codes. Endoscopy codes can be located in the CPT manual index under Endoscopy and then under the anatomic subterm of the site. You can also locate an endoscopic procedure by the anatomic endoscopy title. For example, a bronchial biopsy using endoscopy would be listed under Bronchoscopy and then under the subterm Biopsy.

EXERCISE 6–1 *Endoscopy*

Using the CPT manual, complete the following:

1 Endoscopic maxillary antrostomy

Code: _____

2 Direct laryngoscopy for removal of fish bone

Code: _____

3 After the airway is sufficiently anesthetized, a flexible bronchoscope is inserted through the mouth and advanced to the bronchus, where a transbronchial biopsy of one lobe is obtained.

Code: _____

4 Diagnostic thoracoscopy of the mediastinal space is accomplished with the use of a flexible endoscope that is inserted through a small incision on the chest.

Code: _____

5 Segmental resection of the right lung using a flexible endoscope (surgical thoracoscopy)

Code: _____

NOSE   Many of the codes in the Nose subheading are used by physicians who specialize in treating conditions of the nose (otorhinolaryngologist; ear, nose, and throat specialists), but there are also many codes in the subheading that are more widely used. For example, it is in the Nose subheading that you will find the codes for the following services: control of nosebleeds, incision of abscesses, removal of foreign objects from the nose (think children!), and removal of nasal cysts and lesions, all of which are commonly performed as office procedures.

Incision   Codes for incision of a nasal abscess (30000, 30020) are divided on the basis of whether the abscess is on the nasal mucosa or the septal mucosa. If a nasal abscess is approached from the outside of the nose (**external approach**), you would use a code from the Integumentary System subsection; but if the approach is from the inside of the nose (**internal approach**), you would use a code from the Respiratory System subsection. The medical record will describe the approach procedure used and the approach procedure will direct you to the correct subsection.

After the abscess has been penetrated, the physician may place a tube in the incision to ensure that the pus continues to drain from the abscess area. After the drain is removed, the abscess may be packed with gauze, with one end of the packing material left outside the surface to act as a wick, as illustrated in Fig. 6–2, *A* to *C*.

The incision may also be closed immediately if it is felt that further drainage is not necessary. The insertion and removal of the tube and/or gauze and any required sutures and/or anesthesia are bundled into the code, so you should not report these services separately. You should report any additional supplies over and above those usually used for the procedure by using the Medicine section code for supplies, 99070, or a HCPCS code, as directed by the payer.

Excision   Within the Nose subheading, the Excision category (30100-30160) contains a wide range of procedures that describe removal of tissue from the nose—for example, biopsy, polyp excision, and cyst excision—as well as resection of the turbinate bone.

CODING SHOT   When two procedures are completed during the same surgical session, the most complex procedure is sequenced first.

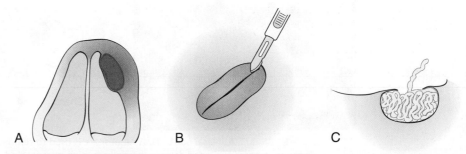

FIGURE 6–2 **A,** Nasal mucosal abscess. **B,** Incision of abscess. **C,** Gauze packed into abscess with end extended outside the abscess, acting as a wick.

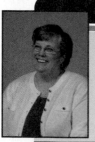
The **biopsy** code (30100) is used for a biopsy that is done intranasally; but for a biopsy of the skin outside of the nose, you would use the biopsy code (11100) from the Integumentary System.

Nasal polyps develop and mature, causing nasal obstruction (Fig. 6–3, *A*). The physician removes the polyps, usually with a snare, as illustrated in Fig. 6–3, *B*.

The excision of **nasal polyps** has two codes (30110 and 30115), with the difference between the codes being the extent of the excision. Code 30110 is used for a simple polyp excision that would usually be performed in the physician's office, whereas 30115 is used for a more extensive polyp excision that would usually be performed in a hospital setting.

CODING SHOT Use modifier -50 (bilateral) if the polyps are removed from both the left and right sides of the nose.

The codes for excision or destruction of **lesions** inside the nose are divided based on the approach—internal or external.

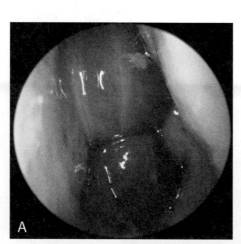
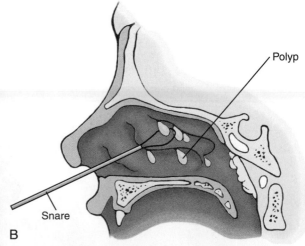

FIGURE 6–3 **A,** Nasal polyp. **B,** A nasal snare is used to remove nasal polyps. The nose is anesthetized, a snare is slipped around the polyp, which is transected, and a forceps is used to remove the polyp. (**A** from Zitelli BJ, Davis HW: *Atlas of Pediatric Physical Diagnosis,* ed 5, Philadelphia, 2007, Mosby. **B** from Monahan FD, et al: *Phipps' Medical-Surgical Nursing: Health and Illness Perspectives,* ed 8, St. Louis, 2007, Mosby.)

CAUTION *Usually, if the approach to the procedure has been external, you are referred to the Integumentary System subsection to locate the correct code; but the nasal lesion excision/destruction codes can be used for either an external or an internal approach to a lesion.*

You have to read the code descriptions carefully to ensure that you understand all of the circumstances that surround using the code, and you have to identify codes such as the lesion excision/destruction codes that are exceptions to the usual rules.

All methods of lesion destruction, including laser, are included in the Excision codes. Usually, if laser was used in the destruction of a lesion, you would be referred to a separate set of codes just for laser destruction; but with the lesion destruction codes in the Nose category, laser is included as one of the destruction methods.

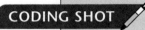 **CODING SHOT** If the lesion destruction or excision is bilateral, remember to use modifier -50.

Turbinates are the bones on the inside of the nose; they are divided into three sections—inferior, middle, and superior (Fig. 6–4). Portions of or all of a turbinate bone may be removed for cosmetic reasons or because of neoplastic growth. Because third-party payers usually do not pay for cosmetic surgical procedures, you must document the medical necessity for noncosmetic procedures carefully to ensure appropriate reimbursement. Watch for and read the extensive notes inside the parentheses throughout this category.

Introduction

Introduction codes (30200-30220) include injection, displacement therapy, and insertion. **Injections** into the turbinates are therapeutic injections usually used to shrink the nasal tissue so as to improve breathing. For example, if a patient has inflamed nasal passages due to an allergic reaction or a deviated septum, he or she may benefit from a steroid injection into

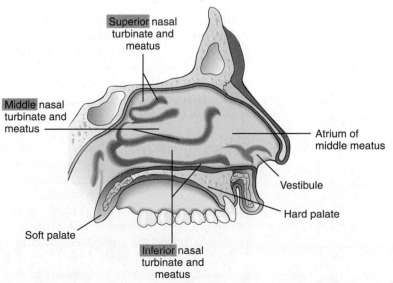

FIGURE 6–4 Superior, inferior, and middle nasal turbinates.

the turbinates. **Displacement therapy** is a procedure in which the physician flushes saline solution into the sinuses to remove mucus or pus. The insertion of a **nasal button** is a technique used for a patient who has a hole in the septum. The physician places the button into the hole and fastens the button in place with sutures. The button is usually made of silicone or rubber. This technique is used as a method of repairing the septum without surgical grafting.

Removal of a Foreign Body

A variety of objects are inserted into the various orifices (openings) of the body, and the nose is a common place into which these foreign objects are placed. The code to report an office procedure for the removal of a foreign body from the nose is 30300. Codes for more extensive procedures are also available for removal of foreign objects from the nose, such as those requiring general anesthesia and a more invasive surgical procedure.

Repair

Within the Repair category (30400-30630) you will find the plastic procedures—rhinoplasty, septoplasty, and septal dermatoplasty. **Rhinoplasty** is a procedure used to reshape the nose internally, externally, or both. The codes are divided based on the extent (minor, intermediate, major), on whether the septum was also repaired (septoplasty), and on whether the procedure was an initial or secondary procedure. **Secondary** procedures are those that are done after an initial procedure. For example, if a rhinoplasty was performed and the results were not as successful as the patient desired, the surgeon could perform a second procedure (secondary) to improve the result.

Septoplasty is rearrangement of the nasal septum. This procedure is commonly performed in a patient with a deviated septum.

 CAUTION *Do not use a septoplasty code if the operative report indicates that only a resection of the inferior turbinate(s) was performed. The resection of the inferior turbinate(s) is reported with 30140 and is not a procedure done on the septum. The septoplasty code, 30520, is used when the nasal septum is resected. There is a note enclosed in parentheses following both codes— 30140 and 30520—that cautions you to use the correct code, which is determined by whether the turbinate or the septum was resected.*

Destruction

Destruction can be accomplished by using either cauterization or ablation. **Ablation** is removal, usually by cutting. Ablation or cauterization is used to remove excess nasal mucosa or to reduce inflammation. The destruction codes are divided according to the extent of the procedure—superficial or intramural. **Intramural** is ablation or cauterization of the deeper mucosa, as compared to **superficial** ablation or cauterization, which involves only the outer layer of mucosa.

Other Procedures

The codes (30901-30999) for the control of nasal hemorrhage are located in the Other Procedures category and are used often. The physician may use anterior or posterior pressure to control the hemorrhage. Anterior nasal packing (Fig. 6–5) is the application of pressure using packing to the anterior aspect of the nasal cavity and posterior nasal packing is the application of pressure to the posterior aspect of the nasal cavity. The nasal pack is inserted via the nasal opening. A balloon may be inserted and inflated to further control bleeding (Fig. 6–6). The codes are divided according to the type and extent of control required.

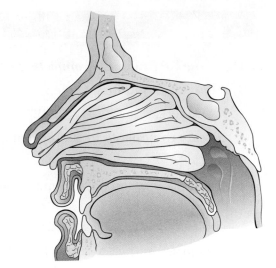

FIGURE 6-5 Anterior nasal packing.

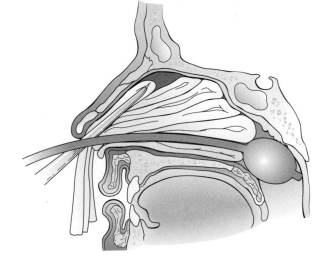

FIGURE 6-6 Posterior nasal packing.

CODING SHOT The key to correctly coding nasal hemorrhage is to know the type of control used by the physician.

There are times when neither cauterization nor packing will control a nasal hemorrhage, and ligation of the bleeding artery may be necessary. Ligation of ethmoidal arteries involves opening the upper side of the nose and locating and tying the ethmoid artery. Ligation of the internal maxillary artery is performed to gain control of nasal hemorrhage by locating and ligating the maxillary artery.

A **therapeutic fracture** of the nasal turbinate is a procedure in which the physician fractures the turbinate bone and then repositions it. The patient receives a local anesthetic. Repositioning the turbinate(s) often alleviates obstructed airflow caused by a previous fracture that has healed out of alignment and resulted in a deviation of the nose.

EXERCISE 6–2 *Nose*

Using the CPT manual, complete the following:

1 Biopsy of an intranasal lesion

Code: _____

2 Primary rhinoplasty including major septal repair

Code: _____

3 Anterior control of nasal hemorrhage by means of limited chemical cauterization and simple packing

Code: _____

4 Septoplasty with contouring and grafting

Code: _____

5 Removal of crayon from nose of 5-year-old boy, conducted as an office procedure

Code: _____

ACCESSORY SINUSES

Incision

Within the Incision category are codes for services that you would not think of as being incisional. For example, the nasal sinuses can be washed (lavage) with a saline solution introduced through a canula (hollow tube) to remove infection. The Incision category code 31000 describes lavage of the maxillary

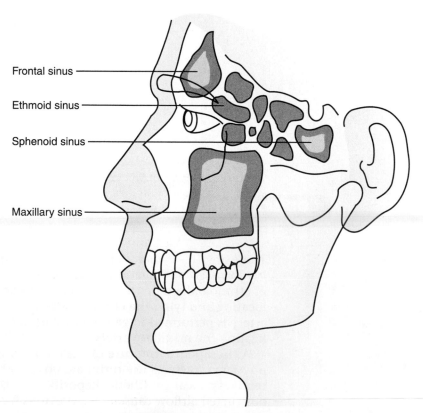

Frontal sinus

Ethmoid sinus

Sphenoid sinus

Maxillary sinus

FIGURE 6–7 Paranasal sinuses.

sinus. Lavage can be done to both the maxillary and the sphenoid sinuses (Fig. 6–7). If the lavage is of the sphenoid sinus, you use 31002 to describe the service.

CODING SHOT 🖊 Use modifier -50 (bilateral) if the lavage is for both the left and right maxillary sinuses.

Many of the codes in the Incision category are for sinusotomies. A **sinusotomy** is a procedure in which the physician enlarges the passage or creates a new passage from the nasal cavity into a sinus. This procedure is performed when a patient has a chronic sinus infection; the procedure enables improved sinus drainage. The codes are divided according to the extent of the procedure.

EXERCISE 6–3 *Accessory Sinuses*

Using the CPT manual, complete the following:

1 Lavage of the maxillary sinus, bilateral

   Code(s): _____ _____

2 Simple frontal sinusotomy using an external approach

   Code: _____

3 Unilateral sinusotomy of frontal, ethmoid, and sphenoid

   Code: _____

4 Radical sinusotomy

   ◉ Code(s): _____

5 Pterygomaxillary fossa surgery, transfacial approach

   Code: _____

LARYNX   The procedures covered by the Larynx subheading (31300-31599) include a wide range of surgical procedures, such as laryngectomy, plastic repair, and nerve destruction. Make certain that you understand the terminology used in the Excision category before you code in the category.

Excision   **Laryngotomy** is an incision that is made over the larynx (thyrotomy) to expose the larynx to view. With the larynx exposed, the physician can remove a tumor, a laryngocele (air-filled space), or a vocal cord (cordectomy). A laryngotomy can also be performed for diagnostic purposes, without a surgical procedure's being performed.

   Be careful not to get the codes from the Laryngotomy category confused with the tracheostomy codes located in the Trachea and Bronchi subheading, Incision category, which you will learn more about later in this chapter. The codes from the two categories differ, depending on the **purpose of the procedure**. The Laryngotomy category codes describe procedures in which the surgeon performs a thyrotomy for the purpose of exposing the larynx. The codes in the Trachea and Bronchi subheading, Incision category

---

describe a procedure in which the surgeon performs only the tracheostomy, usually to establish airflow, and no procedure or exposure of the larynx is planned or is involved.

Radical neck dissection, as referred to in the codes for laryngectomy, is the removal not only of the larynx but also of lymph glands and/or other surrounding tissue. Many of the codes in the Larynx subheading, Excision category are divided according to whether radical neck dissection was or was not performed. The operative report would indicate the extent of the dissection by referring to excision of lymph nodes in a radical procedure.

Introduction

Intubation is the establishment of an airway in a patient. The intubation represented in 31500 is provided on an emergency basis at such time as the patient experiences respiratory failure or the occurrence of an inadequate airway. Fig. 6–8 illustrates endotracheal intubation. The other Introduction code is for the replacement of a previously inserted tracheostomy tube.

Repair

Within the Repair category are several plastic procedures. A laryngoplasty for a **laryngeal web** is a surgical procedure, usually done in two stages, for the repair of congenital webbing between the vocal cords. The surgeon removes the webbing and places a spacer between the vocal cords. At a later time, the surgeon will again expose the vocal cords, using the same tracheostomy incision made on the initial procedure, and remove the spacer.

Closed laryngeal fracture repair used to be reported with Repair codes 31585-31586; however, in 2006 these codes were deleted and a note in the CPT manual directs the coder to report laryngeal fracture repair with appropriate E/M code.

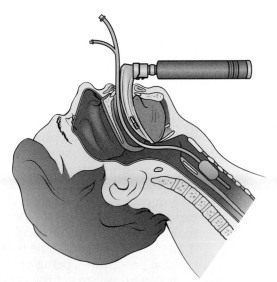

FIGURE 6–8 Endotracheal intubation.

EXERCISE 6–4 *Larynx*

Using the CPT manual, complete the following:

1 Diagnostic laryngotomy

Code: _____

2 Laryngoplasty, two stages, for repair of congenital laryngeal web, removal of spacer

Code: _____

3 Emergency establishment of positive airway by means of endotracheal intubation

Code: _____

4 Subtotal supraglottic laryngectomy with removal of adjacent lymph nodes and tissue

Code: _____

5 Pharyngolaryngectomy with radical neck dissection

Code: _____

TRACHEA AND BRONCHI

Procedures in the Trachea and Bronchi subheading (31600-31899) include incisions, introductions, and repairs, in addition to the endoscopic procedures.

Incision

Tracheostomy is the most common procedure in the Incision category. A tracheostomy can be planned or can be performed as an emergency procedure. A planned tracheostomy is usually done when there is a need for prolonged ventilation support, beyond the level of support that can be provided by endotracheal intubation, or when a patient cannot tolerate an endotracheal tube. Note that code 31603 is used for an emergency **transtracheal** tracheostomy, and code 31605 is used for an emergency **cricothyroid** tracheostomy. These codes represent two different approaches to establishing an airway. Fig. 6–9 illustrates the transverse (across) incision used in a transtracheal approach; it is made between the cricoid cartilage and the sternal notch. Fig. 6–10 illustrates entry into the trachea using the transtracheal approach. Fig. 6–11 illustrates the vertical incision made for a cricothyroid tracheostomy. Fig. 6–12 shows the entry into the trachea using the cricothyroid approach.

Introduction

Codes in the Introduction category are for the catheterization, instillation, injection, and aspiration of the trachea and the placement of tubes into the trachea.

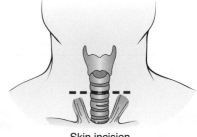

FIGURE 6–9 Transverse incision used in a transtracheal approach.

Skin incision

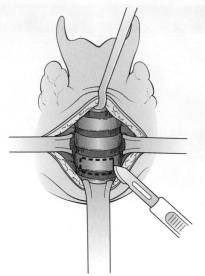

FIGURE 6–10 Transtracheal entry into the trachea using the transtracheal approach.

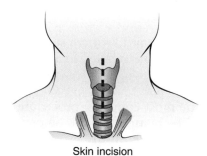

Skin incision

FIGURE 6–11 Vertical incision made for a cricothyroid tracheostomy.

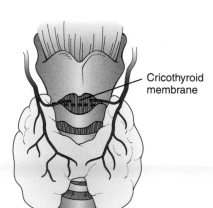

Cricothyroid membrane

FIGURE 6–12 Cricothyroid entry into the trachea.

A transglottic catheterization is one in which the physician punctures the glottis (vocal apparatus) with a needle and inserts a catheter to establish a passage. The catheter is held in place by a suture affixed to the skin and then tied to the catheter.

Some of the Introduction codes represent the instillation of contrast material into the larynx to improve viewing during bronchographic procedures. The contrast material is suspended in a gas that the patient inhales. The gas contains radiant energy that appears darker on the x-ray if there is an obstruction in the area, such as a tumor. Codes from the Radiology section are used in conjunction with injection of contrast material. For example, if a physician provided the service of a bronchography with contrast material injection, you would use code 31715 for the service of injecting the contrast material into the trachea, and 71040 for the supervision and interpretation of the unilateral bronchography. The injection of contrast material is not bundled into the radiology service for a bronchography, so you would have to code each part (component) of the service separately.

Repair Repair procedures in the Trachea and Bronchi subheading include the plastic repairs, such as tracheoplasty and bronchoplasty, in addition to the excision of stenosis or of tumors, the suturing of tracheal wounds, and scar revision.

Tracheoplasty involves the surgical repair of a damaged trachea. The repair may involve reconstruction of the trachea by the use of grafts or splints formed from cartilage taken from other areas of the body or by the use of prostheses. The codes are divided according to the approach used (cervical or thoracic) and the extent and type of repair.

Bronchoplasty is the repair of the bronchus; it often involves the use of grafting repair or stents. A chest tube may be left in the area as a drain after the procedure and is not reported separately. The grafting procedure is part of the bronchoplasty code 31770.

EXERCISE 6–5 *Trachea and Bronchi*

Using the CPT manual, complete the following:

1 Emergency tracheostomy, cricothyroid approach

 Code(s): _____

2 Excision of a tumor of the trachea, cervical

 Code(s): _____

3 Transtracheal injection for bronchography (code only the injection procedure)

 Code(s): _____

4 Planned tracheostomy in 47-year-old patient

 Code(s): _____

5 Catheterization with bronchial brush biopsy

 Code(s): _____

LUNGS AND PLEURA The Lungs and Pleura subheading (32035-32999) includes a wide range of codes that cover such procedures as thoracentesis, thoracotomy, and pneumonostomy, in addition to lung transplants and plastic procedures.

Incision **Thoracotomy** is the procedure of making a surgical incision into the chest wall and opening the area to the view of the surgeon. This is a major surgical procedure in which the patient is under general anesthesia. The codes are divided according to the reason for the procedure, such as biopsy, control of bleeding, cyst removal, foreign body removal, and cardiac massage.

> **CODING SHOT** As a part of a thoracotomy, the surgeon may insert a chest tube to allow for continued drainage of the surgical area. The placement of this tube is bundled into the surgical procedure, so you would not code separately for the placement of the tube.

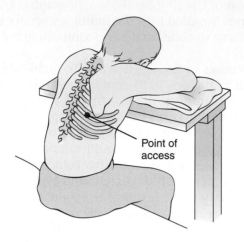

FIGURE 6–13 Patient position for a thoracentesis.

Point of access

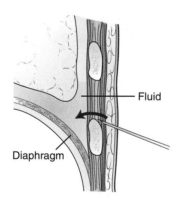

Fluid

Diaphragm

FIGURE 6–14 After administration of local anesthesia, a needle is inserted between the ribs, and fluid is withdrawn (thoracentesis).

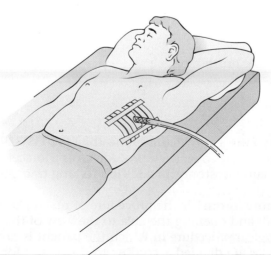

FIGURE 6–15 A chest tube may be inserted after thoracentesis to allow for further fluid draining.

Excision   The Excision category contains codes for pleurectomy, biopsy, pneumonocentesis, removal, and reconstructive lung procedures.

The preferred method of accomplishing a **thoracentesis** is by having the patient sit with arms supported, as illustrated in Fig. 6–13; local anesthesia is administered, a needle is inserted (Fig. 6–14) between the ribs, and fluid is withdrawn. Thoracentesis is performed to withdraw from the pleural space fluid that has accumulated as a result of a variety of conditions, such as congestive heart failure, pneumonia, tuberculosis, or carcinoma.

Thoracentesis may also be performed to insert a **chest tube** as an indwelling method of draining the accumulated fluid in the pleural space (pleural effusion), as illustrated in Fig. 6–15. Local anesthesia is administered, and a small incision is made through the skin, fat, and muscle. The hole is then enlarged by using an instrument, and the tube is inserted into the pleural space. A suture is placed through the skin and tied to the tube. The tube is then secured with tape. The fluid is withdrawn by means of a suction device called a multichamber water-seal suction tube. This therapeutic procedure may be performed when the patient's pleural space contains air or gas (pneumothorax), blood (hemothorax), or a large amount of fluid (pleural effusion). These conditions can be caused by trauma, can be secondary to another disease process, or can occur spontaneously.

Pleurectomy is a procedure in which the physician opens the chest cavity to full view. With the chest open and the ribs spread apart by a rib spreader, the parietal pleura is removed. If a pleurectomy is done as part of another, more major procedure such as the removal of a lung (pneumonectomy), you would not report the pleurectomy separately. Note that after code 32310, pleurectomy, parietal "separate procedure" warns you not to report a separate pleurectomy if the pleurectomy was performed as a part of a more major procedure.

Percutaneous needle lung or mediastinum **biopsy** is often performed under radiologic guidance so that correct placement of the needle can be ensured. As with the bronchography procedure described earlier, in the discussion of the Trachea and Bronchi subheading, if radiologic guidance was used, you also use a code from the Radiology section to describe the guidance service. There is a note following code 32405 (biopsy) that directs you to the Surgery section, General subsection, code 10022, when a fine-needle aspiration is performed.

Pneumonocentesis is the withdrawal of fluid from the lung by means of an aspirating needle. Air or gas in the pleural cavity is known as pneumothorax and is caused when the lung is traumatically ruptured or an emphysematous bulla ruptures. Pneumothorax is the thoracic cavity. When the thoracic cavity (intrathoracic) air pressure increases, the pressure on the lung can result in collapse of the lung. The surgeon withdraws the fluid to allow the lung to reinflate.

From the Trenches

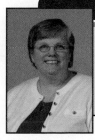

"The benefit to working in medical coding is job security, because the field is constantly expanding."

CHRISTINE

The codes for the removal of the lung are based on how much of the lung is removed—segmentectomy for one segment, lobectomy for one lobe, bilobectomy for two lobes, total pneumonectomy for an entire lung—as well as on the extent of the procedure and the approach.

CODING SHOT

If a part of the bronchus was removed or repaired at the same time as the lobectomy or segmentectomy, you would indicate the service with the use of the add-on code 32501.

Surgical Collapse Therapy; Thoracoplasty

Thoracoplasty is a procedure in which a portion of the internal skeletal support is removed to treat a condition in which pus chronically collects in the chest cavity (chronic thoracic empyema). The procedure is major and requires extensive resecting of the membrane that lines the chest cavity. Gauze is left in the cavity and after several days it is removed. Note that code 32905, thoracoplasty, refers to "all stages." The subsequent stages are for the removal of the packing. Thoracoplasty procedures may also require the use of muscle grafting to close a bronchopleural fistula.

Pneumonolysis is a procedure that is performed to separate the inside of the chest cavity from the lung to permit collapse of the lung.

Pneumothorax injection is a therapeutic procedure in which the surgeon inserts a needle into the pleural cavity and injects air into the pleural cavity. The pressure in the thoracic cavity is increased and the lung partially collapses. This procedure is sometimes performed to treat tuberculosis. A chest tube may be inserted into the space for further injections of air. You would not report the insertion of the chest tube separately, as the insertion is bundled into the procedure code.

EXERCISE 6-6 *Lungs and Pleura*

Using the CPT manual, complete the following:

1 A limited thoracotomy for lung biopsy

    Code(s): _____

2 Percutaneous needle lung biopsy

    Code(s): _____

3 Lobectomy and bronchoplasty performed at same surgical session

    Code(s): _____

4 Resection of an apical lung tumor

    Code(s): _____

5 Pneumonostomy with open drainage of abscess

    Code(s): _____

CHAPTER REVIEW

CHAPTER 6, PART I, THEORY

Without the use of reference material, complete the following:

1 The Respiratory System subsection is arranged by _____ site.

2 The procedure in which a scope is placed through a small incision and into a body cavity is called a(n) _____.

3 When coding endoscopic procedures you must be certain to code to the fullest _____ of the procedure and to code the correct approach for the procedure.

4 If more than one distinct procedure was performed during an endoscopic procedure, what modifier would you add to the lesser-priced service? _____

5 What type of endoscopy is always bundled into a surgical endoscopy?

_____

6 A(n) _____ laryngoscopy is performed when a physician uses a tongue depressor to hold the tongue down and view the epiglottis with a mirror.

7 A(n) _____ laryngoscopy is performed when the endoscope is passed into the larynx and the physician can look at the larynx through a scope.

8 An otorhinolaryngologist is a physician who specializes in treating conditions of the

_____, _____,

and _____.

9 When coding a nasal abscess or a nasal biopsy of the skin using the external approach, you use codes from the _____ System subsection.

10 When coding a nasal abscess or a nasal biopsy using the internal approach, you use codes from the _____ System subsection.

11 What are the three sections of turbinates?

_____, _____,

and _____.

12 What is the name of the therapy in which the physician flushes saline solution into the sinuses to remove mucus or pus?

_____

CHAPTER 6, PART II, PRACTICAL

With the use of the CPT manual, code the following procedures. Code only the physician services in this exercise; do not code the laboratory or radiology services.

13 A unilateral, total lung lavage

Code: _____

14 Performed as a separate procedure, a parietal pleurectomy

Code: _____

15 Resection of apical lung tumor with chest wall resection and reconstruction

Code: _____

16 Removal of a crayon lodged inside nasal passage, office procedure

Code: _____

17 Surgical nasal endoscopy with polypectomy

Code: _____

18 Direct, operative laryngoscopy for removal of button lodged in 2-year-old child's larynx

Code: _____

19 Indirect laryngoscopy with biopsy

Code(s): _____

20 Internal approach used to drain nasal hematoma

Code(s): _____

21 External, simple, frontal sinusotomy

Code(s): _____

22 Surgical sinus endoscopy with sphenoidotomy

Code(s): _____

23 Submucous resection of nose with scoring of cartilage and contouring

Code(s): _____

24 Jack Rogers developed chest pain and difficulty breathing. He has also been coughing up thick, blood-tinged sputum. A chest radiograph shows an ill-defined mass. A diagnostic bronchoscopy of one lung is performed and a specimen of the mass is taken. The pathology report comes back positive for cancer. One week later, a lobectomy is performed.

Code(s): _____

25 James Wilson has been having difficulty breathing and has had continual sinusitis. Dr. Adams takes James to the operating room to perform a sinus endoscopy with anterior and posterior ethmoidectomy and removal of polyps.

Code(s): _____

26 Mary Bronson has a nosebleed that won't stop. She goes to the emergency department, where anterior packing is done to control the nasal hemorrhage.

Code(s): _____

QUICK CHECK ANSWERS

QUICK CHECK 6-1
open, intranasal

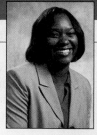
"The world of coding is wide open; coders should explore all available opportunities and find what most interests them."

Letitia Patterson, MPA, CPC, CCS-P
Consultant
A Coder's Resource
Chicago, Illinois

Cardiovascular System

Chapter Topics

Coding Highlights

Cardiovascular Coding in the Surgery Section

Cardiovascular Coding in the Medicine Section

Cardiovascular Coding in the Radiology Section

Chapter Review

Quick Check Answers

Learning Objectives

After completing this chapter you should be able to

1. Understand cardiovascular services across three sections—Surgery, Medicine, and Radiology.

2. Review cardiovascular coding terminology.

3. Recognize the major differences in the subheadings of the Cardiovascular subsection.

4. State the coding rules for arteries and veins.

5. Define rules of coding cardiovascular services when using codes from the Medicine section.

6. Identify the major rules of coding cardiovascular services using the Radiology section codes.

7. Demonstrate ability to code Cardiovascular services.

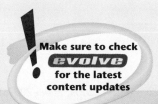
Make sure to check **evolve** for the latest content updates

CODING HIGHLIGHTS

Cardiology is one of the fastest growing subspecialties in medicine, and numerous modern techniques are used to diagnose and treat cardiac conditions. A **cardiologist** is an internal medicine physician who has chosen to specialize in the diagnosis and treatment of conditions of the heart. A cardiologist can further specialize in cardiovascular surgical procedures or other treatment and diagnostic specialties. In a smaller practice a cardiologist may do many of these procedures himself/herself, whereas in a larger practice a cardiologist may be more specialized and provide a more limited variety of services.

Coding from Three Sections

When you are reporting cardiology services you will often be using codes from three sections: Surgery, Medicine, and Radiology.

- The Surgery section contains the codes for cardiovascular surgical procedures.
- The Medicine section contains codes for nonsurgical cardiovascular services.
- The Radiology section contains diagnostic study or radiologic visualization codes.

Fig. 7–1 is a list of the section information that is most often used when reporting cardiovascular services. The confusion in coding cardiology often comes from not understanding the components (parts) of coding cardiovascular services, the various locations of these service codes in the CPT manual, and the terminology associated with cardiovascular services. To clarify cardiology coding, let's begin by reviewing the definitions of invasive, noninvasive, electrophysiology, and angiography as they relate to cardiovascular coding.

Invasive

Invasive cardiology is entering the body—breaking the skin—to make a correction or for examination. An example of an invasive cardiac procedure is the removal of a tumor from the heart. The chest is opened, the ribs

---

From the Trenches

What qualities best describe a medical coder?

"Detail oriented, investigative and research oriented, patient, and excellent analytical skills."

LETITIA

SURGERY SECTION	MEDICINE SECTION	RADIOLOGY SECTION

Cardiovascular System (33010-37799)
  Heart and Pericardium
  Endoscopy
  Arteries and Veins
  Adjuvant Techniques
	Cardiovascular System (92950-93799)
	  Therapeutic Services
	  Cardiography
	  Echocardiography
	  Cardiac Catheterization
	  Intracardiac Electrophysiological Procedures
	  Peripheral Arterial Disease Rehabilitation
	  Other Vascular Studies
	  Other Procedures
		Diagnostic Radiology (75557-75790)
		  Heart
		  Aorta and Arteries
		Diagnostic Ultrasound (various)
		  Ultrasonic Guidance Procedures
		Radiologic Guidance (77001-77032)
		Nuclear Medicine (78414-78499)
		  Cardiovascular System

FIGURE 7-1 A list of the section information that is most often used when reporting cardiovascular services.

spread apart, the heart fully exposed to the view of the surgeon, and the tumor removed. Another example is the removal of a clot from a vessel. The surgeon usually enters the body percutaneously (through the skin) by means of a catheter that is threaded through the vessel to the location of the clot. The clot can then be pulled out of the vessel through the catheter or can be injected with a substance that dissolves it. Although an open surgical procedure was not used, the body was entered—an invasive surgical procedure. Invasive cardiology procedures are also called **interventional** procedures; some codes are located in the Surgery section for the surgical technique, and others are located in the Radiology section for the radiologic supervision and guidance.

Noninvasive

Noninvasive services and procedures—not breaking the skin—are usually performed for diagnostic purposes—for example, electrocardiograms, echocardiography, and vascular studies. Usually, performing these procedures does not require entering the body; rather, they are diagnostic tests that can be done from outside the body, for example, echocardiography (93303-93350) or cardiography (93000-93278) from the Medicine section.

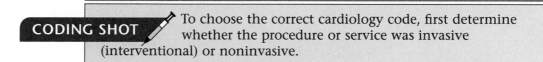

CODING SHOT
To choose the correct cardiology code, first determine whether the procedure or service was invasive (interventional) or noninvasive.

Electrophysiology

Electrophysiology (EP) is the study of the electrical system of the heart and includes the study of arrhythmias. Diagnostic procedures include procedures such as recording from inside the heart by placing an electrical catheter into the heart percutaneously and taking an electrogram of the electrical activity within the heart. The codes for these invasive diagnostic procedures are located in the Medicine section (93600-93662).

As a treatment for abnormal electrical activity in the heart, more invasive treatments can be performed, such as the placement of a pacemaker, cardioverter-defibrillator, or other devices to regulate the rhythm of the heart. These invasive treatments are surgical procedures and the codes are located in the Surgery section, Cardiology subsection, Pacemaker or Pacing Cardioverter-Defibrillator (33202-33249). There are also Surgery codes for operative procedures to correct electrophysiologic problems of the heart (33250-33266) when the electrical problems are corrected surgically by incision, excision, or destruction.

Angiography

Nuclear cardiology is a diagnostic specialty that plays a very important role in modern cardiology. A physician who specializes in nuclear cardiology uses radioactive radiologic procedures to aid in the diagnosis of cardiologic conditions. For example, during angiography of peripheral vessels, a nuclear cardiologist may inject a radioactive dye into the bloodstream to improve the detail of the study. The code for the angiography comes from the Radiology section (Heart, 75557-75564; Aorta and Arteries, 75600-75790; Veins and Lymphatics, 75801-75893), and the code for the injection procedure comes from the Medicine section. For example, 75600 reports the radiological portion of an aortography and 93544 reports the injection portion of the procedure.

EXERCISE 7–1 *Coding Highlights*

Complete the following:

1 This term means entering the body. _____

2 A cardiologist is a(n) _____ medicine physician who has chosen to specialize in the diagnosis and treatment of conditions of the heart.

3 What three sections of the CPT will you often use to code cardiology services?

_____, _____, and _____

4 What type of cardiology enters the body—breaks the skin—to make a correction or for

examination? _____

5 What is the term that describes the study of the electrical system of the heart and includes the

study of arrhythmias? _____

6 A(n) _____ is an x-ray examination that enables the study of the patient's blood vessels and organs by injecting contrast media into the blood vessels and viewing the results on x-ray film.

Now that you are familiar with the terms "invasive," "noninvasive," "electrophysiology," and "nuclear," let's look at the three sections where you will find the components (parts) of cardiovascular coding: Surgery, Medicine, and Radiology.

CARDIOVASCULAR CODING IN THE SURGERY SECTION

The Cardiovascular System subsection (33010-37799) of the Surgery section contains diagnostic and therapeutic procedure codes that are divided on the basis of whether the procedure was done on the heart/pericardium or on arteries/veins. It is in the Heart and Pericardium subheading (33010-33999) that you will find codes for procedures that involve the repair of the heart and coronary vessels, such as placement of pacemakers, repair of valve disorders, and graft/bypass procedures. In the Arteries and Veins subheading (34001-37799) you will find many of the same types of procedures, but for noncoronary (nonheart) vessels. For example, a thromboendarterectomy is the removal of a thrombus (stationary obstruction) and a portion of the lining of an artery. When a thromboendarterectomy is performed on a coronary artery, you would use a code from the Heart and Pericardium subheading; but if the procedure was done on a noncoronary artery, you would use a code from the Arteries and Veins subheading.

CODING SHOT The location of the procedure—coronary or noncoronary— is the first step in selecting the correct cardiovascular surgical code, because the CPT codes are divided on the basis of whether a procedure involved coronary or noncoronary vessels.

Heart and Pericardium

The Surgery section, Cardiovascular System subsection, Heart and Pericardium subheading (33010-33999) contains procedures that are performed both percutaneously and through open surgical sites. There are always many revisions and additions in this subheading each year to reflect the many advances in this important health care area. Numerous notes are located throughout the subheading, and they must be read prior to coding in the subheading. Codes in the Heart and Pericardium subheading are for services provided to repair the heart (Fig. 7–2), pericardium, or coronary vessels (Fig. 7–3). Pericardium codes 33010 and 33011 are divided based on initial or subsequent service.

QUICK CHECK 7-1

Using Fig. 7–3, name the coronary arteries:

_____

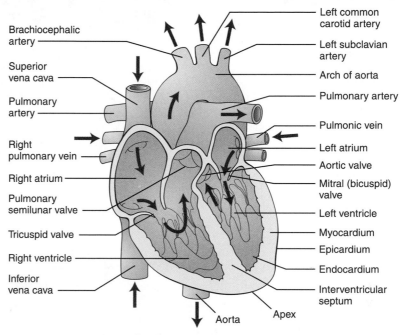

FIGURE 7–2 Internal view of heart.

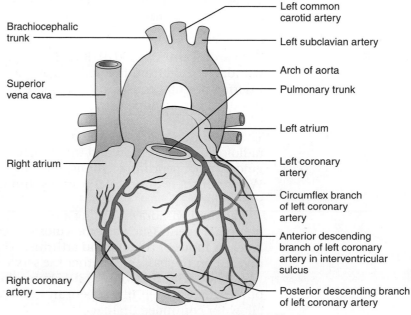

FIGURE 7–3 External view of heart.

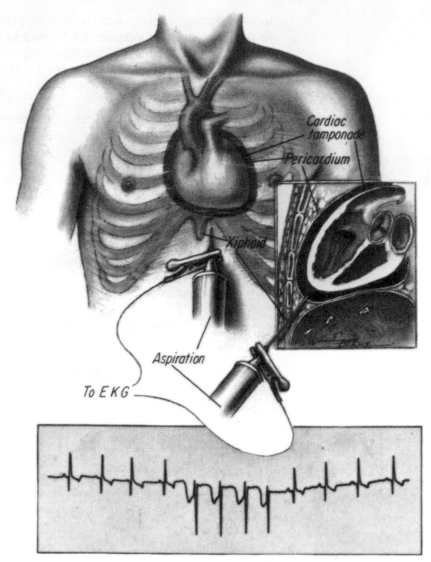

FIGURE 7–4 Pericardiocentesis is the withdrawal of fluid from the pericardium by means of aspiration. (From Sellke FW, editor: *Sabiston & Spencer Surgery of the Chest, Volume II,* ed 7, Philadelphia, 2005, Saunders.)

Pericardium

Pericardiocentesis (33010, 33011) is a procedure in which the surgeon withdraws fluid from the pericardial space by means of a needle that is inserted percutaneously into the space as illustrated in Fig. 7–4. The insertion can be done using radiologic (ultrasound) guidance—the use of which would be reported with a separate code from the Radiology section. There is a note following the pericardiocentesis codes that states: "(For radiological supervision and interpretation, use 76930)"; that is, ultrasonic guidance for pericardiocentesis, imaging supervision, and interpretation. Watch for these directional features throughout the Cardiovascular System subsection.

The fluid withdrawn during a pericardiocentesis is then examined for microbial agents (such as tuberculosis), neoplasia, or autoimmune diseases (such as lupus or rheumatoid arthritis). The pericardiocentesis codes are divided on the basis of whether the service was initial or subsequent.

A tube pericardiostomy (33015) uses the same procedure described earlier, but a catheter is left in the pericardium leading to the outside of the body to allow for continued drainage.

The remaining procedures in the Pericardium category (33020-33050) are open surgical procedures for the removal of clots, foreign bodies, tumors, cysts, or a portion of the pericardium or to create a window for pericardial fluid drainage into the pleural space.

Cardiac Tumor

A procedure performed to remove a tumor of the pericardium is reported using a code from the Pericardium category (33010-33050), but if a tumor is removed from the heart, you would select a code from the category Cardiac Tumor (33120, 33130). There are only two tumor-removal codes in the Cardiac Tumor category, one for a tumor that is removed from inside the heart (intracardiac) and one for a tumor that is removed from outside the heart (external). Both procedures are open surgical procedures that involve opening the chest, spreading the ribs, and excising the tumor.

Transmyocardial Revascularization

Laser transmyocardial revascularization describes a procedure in which areas of cardiac ischemia (reversible muscle damage) are exposed to a laser beam to create holes in the surface of the heart. This procedure encourages new capillary growth, thereby revitalizing the damaged area by increasing the blood flow in the area. This procedure can be performed as the only surgical procedure (33140) or at the time of another cardiac procedure (add-on code 33141).

Pacemaker or Pacing Cardioverter-Defibrillator

A pacemaker and a cardioverter-defibrillator (33202-33249) are devices that are inserted into the body to electrically shock the heart into regular rhythm. When a pacemaker is inserted, a pocket is made and a generator and lead(s) are placed inside the chest (Fig. 7–5). Sometimes, only components of the pacemaker are reinserted, repaired, or replaced. You need to know three things about the service provided to correctly code the pacemaker:

1. Where the electrode (lead) is placed: atrium, ventricle, or both ventricle and atrium

2. Whether the procedure involves initial placement, replacement, or repair of all components or separate components of the pacemaker

3. The approach used to place the pacemaker (epicardial or transvenous)

CODING SHOT A single pacemaker has one lead (atrium or ventricle), a dual pacemaker has two leads (one lead in the right atrium and one in the right ventricle), and a biventricular pacemaker has three leads (one in the right atrium, one in the right ventricle, and one in the left ventricle via the coronary sinus vein).

Approaches. The two approaches that can be used when inserting a pacemaker are epicardial (on the heart) and transvenous (through a vein), and the codes are divided according to the surgical approach used.

1. The **epicardial** approach involves opening the chest cavity and placing a lead on the epicardial sac of the heart. A pocket is formed in either the upper abdomen or just under the clavicle, and the pacemaker generator is placed into the pocket. The wires are then connected to the pacemaker generator and the chest area is closed. Codes for the epicardial process are further divided based on the approach to the chest wall that was used— thoracotomy or upper abdominal (xiphoid region).

2. The **transvenous** approach involves accessing a vein (subclavian or jugular) and inserting an electrode (lead) into the vein. The pacemaker is

affixed by creating a pocket into which the pacemaker generator is placed. The fluoroscopic portion of the procedure is coded separately using a radiology code (71090) because it is not bundled into the pacemaker codes. Transvenous codes are further divided based on the area of the heart into which the pacemaker is inserted. For example, 33207 (single-chamber pacemaker) is reported for transvenous placement of a pacemaker into the ventricle of the heart. If the pacemaker components were placed in both the atrium and the ventricle, 33208 (dual-chamber pacemaker) is reported.

The documentation in the medical record will indicate whether a pacemaker or cardioverter-defibrillator was inserted or replaced.

The same set of criteria applies to choosing the correct cardioverter-defibrillator codes:

1. Revision or replacement of lead(s)

2. Replacement, repair, removal of components

3. Approach used for insertion or repair

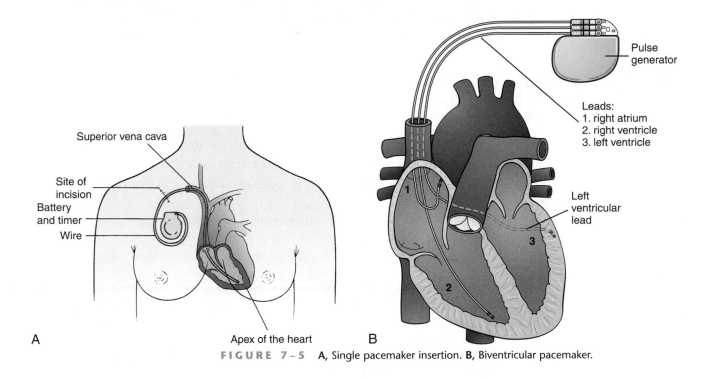

FIGURE 7-5 **A,** Single pacemaker insertion. **B,** Biventricular pacemaker.

CODING SHOT A change of batteries in a pacemaker or cardioverter-defibrillator is a **removal** of the implanted generator and the **reimplantation** (insertion) of a new generator. Both the removal and the reimplantation are coded separately.

Electrophysiology (EP) that was used in the diagnosis of a condition and that resulted in the insertion of a pacemaker or cardioverter-defibrillator is not included in the surgery code. If EP diagnostic services of the pacemaker system are provided, you would report services using the Medicine section codes 93279-93292.

Radiology supervision and interpretation are not included in the pacemaker implantation codes. If radiology supervision and interpretation are provided, you would report the service using the Radiology section code 71090, Insertion of pacemaker, fluoroscopy, radiography, radiological supervision and interpretation.

Remember to use modifier -26 on a radiology service when only the professional portion of the service was provided and -TC when only the technical portion was provided.

CODING SHOT If a patient with a pacemaker or other implantable device is seen by the physician within the 90-day follow-up (global) period for implantation but for a problem not related to the implantation, the service for the new problem can be billed. Documentation in the medical record must support the statement that the service is unrelated to the implantation. Append the unrelated E/M service code with modifier -24. If the patient is returned to the operating room for repositioning or replacement of the pacemaker or cardio-defibrillator during the global period, modifier -78 would be appended to the code.

EXERCISE 7–2 *Pericardium, Cardiac Tumors, and Pacemakers*

Using the CPT manual, code the following:

1 Allen Jackson gets very tired walking up and down stairs. He has a hard time catching his breath and experiences instances when his heart feels as if it is beating fast. His physician has told him that he will require a pacemaker implantation. Allen goes to surgery and has a single-chamber pacemaker implanted with a ventricular lead.

    Code: _____

2 Five days after the pacemaker is implanted, Allen (from Question 1) feels very dizzy and his electrocardiogram is showing some abnormalities. His physician takes him back to the operating room and discovers that the pacemaker lead is malfunctioning. The pacemaker lead is replaced, and Allen recovers nicely.

    Code: _____

3 Five years later, the battery in Allen's pacemaker is found to have become depleted. He is also having some other symptoms that his physician believes necessitate not only a replacement pacemaker but also an upgrade to a dual-chamber device.

    Code: _____

4 A new patient with a chief complaint of sharp, intermittent retrosternal pain that is reduced by sitting up or leaning forward is evaluated by a cardiologist. Chest films reveal pulmonary edema with pericardial effusion. The physician performs a pericardiocentesis. (Code only the procedure.)

Code: _____

5 Resection of an intracardiac tumor in which cardiopulmonary bypass is required

Code: _____

Electrophysiologic Operative Procedures

Electrophysiology, as you learned earlier in this chapter, is the study of the electrical system of the heart, and most of the codes for the EP tests are in the Medicine section (93600-93662). The codes in the Surgery section (33250-33266) apply to the surgical repair of a defect that causes an abnormal rhythm. Cardiopulmonary bypass is usually required during these major operative procedures in which the chest is opened to expose the heart to the full view of the surgeon. New codes in 2007 (33265, 33266) are used to report endoscopic approach for EP procedures. The surgeon maps the locations of the electrodes of the heart and notes the source of the arrhythmia. The source of the arrhythmia is then ablated (separated). The codes are divided on the basis of the need for cardiopulmonary bypass, the reason for the procedure (atrial fibrillation, atrial flutter, etc.), and the approach. Percutaneous electrophysiology is discussed later in this chapter under the heading Intracardiac Electrophysiologic Procedures.

Patient-Activated Event Recorder

A patient-activated event recorder is also known as a cardiac event recorder or a loop recorder. Codes 33282, 33284 involve surgical implantation into the subcutaneous tissue in the upper left quadrant, with leads running to the outside of the body. The recorder senses the heart's rhythms, and when the patient presses a button, the device records the electrical activity of the heart. The recording can assist the physician in making a diagnosis of a hard-to-detect rhythm problem. Codes are divided on the basis of whether the device was implanted or removed.

Cardiac Valves

The category Cardiac Valves (33400-33496) has subcategory codes of aortic, mitral, tricuspid, and pulmonary valves. The procedures are about the same for each valve; some are a little more extensive than others. Code descriptions vary depending on whether a cardiopulmonary bypass (heart-lung) machine is used during the procedure. The cardiopulmonary bypass is a resource-intensive procedure that requires a heart-lung machine to assume the patient's heart and lung functions during surgery.

The cardiac valve procedures are located in the CPT manual index under the valve type or under what was done, such as a repair or a replacement. For example, the replacement of an aortic valve is located in the CPT index under "Aorta," subterm "Valve," subterm "Replacement."

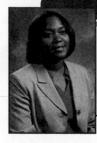

From the Trenches

"It is important to be a multi-tasker in the work environment. Also, be as flexible as possible. Learn the basics of the entire practice if the opportunity presents itself."

LETITIA

EXERCISE 7–3   *EP, Event Recorder, and Valves*

Using the CPT manual, code the following:

1 Mary Black's echocardiogram and cardiac catheterization show severe mitral stenosis with regurgitation. Her physician believes that because she is symptomatic, she should have her mitral valve replaced. The mitral valve replacement includes cardiopulmonary bypass.

   Code: _____

2 Andrew Nelson has a loud heart murmur and, after study, is found to have severe aortic stenosis. He elects to have an aortic valve replacement. He is taken to the operating room and placed on a heart-lung machine. He then has his aortic valve replaced with a prosthetic valve.

   Code: _____

3 With the heart exposed through the sternum and the patient's functions supported by a cardiopulmonary bypass, the right atrium is opened and the arrhythmia focuses are ablated by using electrical current. Bypass is discontinued and the atrium and sternum are closed in the usual fashion.

   Code: _____

4 Implantation of a patient-activated cardiac loop device with programming

   Code: _____

Coronary Artery Anomalies

The Coronary Artery Anomalies category (33500-33507) contains codes to report the services of repair of the coronary artery by various methods, such as graft, ligation (tying off), and reconstruction. The codes include endarterectomy (removal of the inner lining of an artery) and angioplasty (blood vessel repair). Do not unbundle the codes and report the endarterectomy or angioplasty separately. Also, the procedures often require the use of cardiopulmonary bypass to allow the surgeon to repair the defect while the heart is without bloodflow, which makes a difference in the choice of codes.

Coronary Artery Bypass

Arteries deliver oxygenated blood to all areas of the body, and veins return to the heart blood that is full of waste products. The pulmonary vessels, however, are not included in this cycle. The pulmonary vein carries oxygenated blood and the pulmonary artery carries waste products. The heart muscle is fed by coronary arteries that encircle the heart. When these arteries clog with plaque (known as arteriosclerotic coronary artery disease) (Fig. 7–6), the flow of blood lessens. Sometimes the arteries clog to the point that the heart muscle begins to perform at low levels due to lack of blood **(reversible ischemia)** or to actually die **(irreversible ischemia).** Reversible ischemia means that if the bloodflow is increased to the heart muscle, the heart muscle may again begin to function at normal or near-normal levels. **Coronary artery bypass grafting** is one way to increase the flow of blood. The diseased portion of the artery is "bypassed" by attaching a healthy vessel above and below the diseased area and allowing the healthy vessel to then become the conduit of the blood, thus bypassing the blockage (Fig. 7–7). Blockage can also be pushed to the sides of the coronary arterial walls by a procedure in which a balloon is expanded inside the artery. This procedure is known as a **percutaneous transluminal coronary angioplasty (PTCA)** (Fig. 7–8).

QUICK CHECK 7-2

What is the acronym commonly used for "coronary artery bypass graft"? (Hint: It is in the index of the CPT.) _____

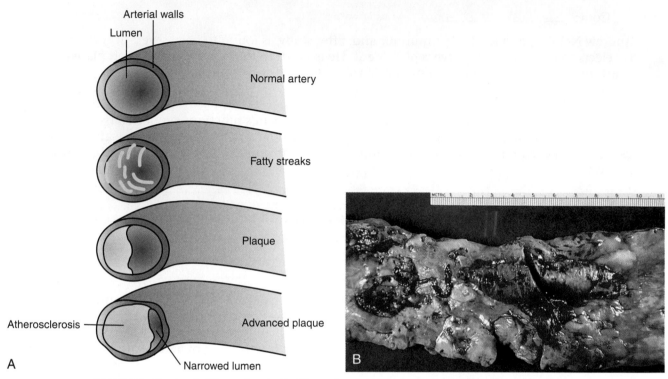

FIGURE 7–6 **A,** Atherosclerosis. **B,** Atherosclerotic vessel. (**B** from Damjanov I: *Pathology for the Health-Related Professions,* ed 3, St. Louis, 2006, Saunders.)

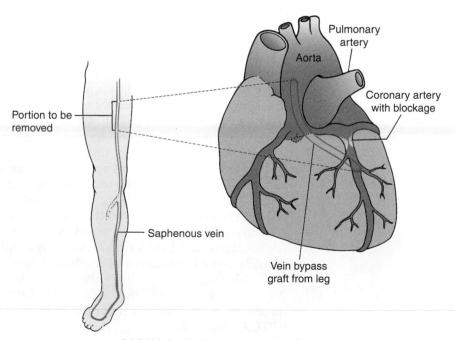

FIGURE 7–7 Coronary artery bypass.

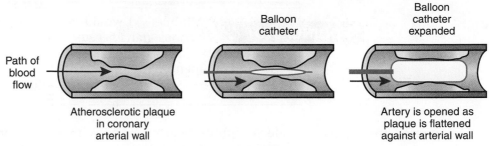

Path of blood flow

Atherosclerotic plaque in coronary arterial wall

Balloon catheter

Balloon catheter expanded

Artery is opened as plaque is flattened against arterial wall

FIGURE 7–8   Percutaneous transluminal coronary angioplasty.

To correctly code coronary bypass grafts, you must know whether an artery (33533-33536), a vein (33510-33516), or both (33517-33523) are being used as the bypass graft. You must also know how many bypass grafts are being performed. There may be more than one blockage to be bypassed and, therefore, more than one graft. If only a vein is used for the graft (most often the saphenous vein from the leg is harvested and used for this purpose; see Fig. 7–7), the code reflecting the number of grafts would be chosen from the category Venous Grafting Only for Coronary Artery Bypass (33510-33516).

The following exercise will help you learn the differences in coding for bypass grafts using arteries, veins, or both, and for coding anomalies.

EXERCISE 7–4   *Coronary Artery Bypass and Anomalies*

Using the CPT manual, code the following:

1   Two coronary bypass grafts using veins only

  Code: _____

The code for Question 1 came from the category Venous Grafting Only for Coronary Artery Bypass because the bypass was accomplished using a venous graft. If the bypass had been accomplished using an arterial graft, the codes in the category Arterial Grafting for Coronary Artery Bypass would be used to report the service. If both veins and arteries were used to accomplish the bypass, you would report the service by using an artery bypass code and a code from the category Combined Arterial-Venous Grafting for Coronary Bypass. Because the title of the category contains the words "arterial-venous," you might think that the codes in the category report both the artery and the vein; but this is not the case. The category codes under "arterial-venous" are used only when a venous graft has been used in addition to an arterial graft and these arterial-venous codes are used only in combination with the arterial graft codes (33533-33536).

For example, a patient has had a **five-vessel** coronary artery bypass graft, for which two bypasses were accomplished using internal mammary arteries and three bypasses were accomplished using veins (reported with 2A and 2B):

2A   Coronary artery bypass using two arterial grafts

  Code: _____

2B   Coronary artery bypass using three venous grafts in addition to the arterial grafts

  Code: _____

3   Coronary artery bypass using one internal mammary artery graft and three venous grafts

  Code(s): _____ and _____

CODING SHOT Modifier -51 would not be used with the code for the venous grafts because codes 33517-33523 are add-on codes. Parenthetical notations with each code indicate the code is to be used in conjunction with 33533-33536. This means that the venous code is never used alone, but always follows an arterial code.

Arteries and Veins

Code groupings for arteries and veins vary according to procedures such as thrombectomies, aneurysm repairs, bypass grafting, repairs, angioplasties, and all other procedures. A good book about vascular procedures will be an invaluable tool for you when coding cardiovascular services as you begin your career as a coder. Codes in the subheading Arteries and Veins (34001-37799) refer to all arteries and veins except the coronary arteries and veins (Figs. 7–9 and 7–10).

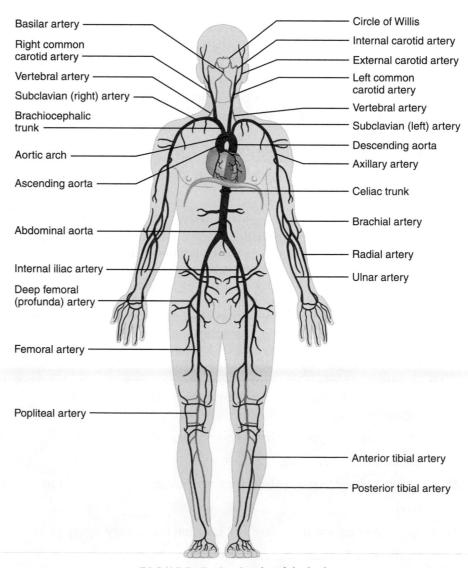

Basilar artery
Right common carotid artery
Vertebral artery
Subclavian (right) artery
Brachiocephalic trunk
Aortic arch
Ascending aorta
Abdominal aorta
Internal iliac artery
Deep femoral (profunda) artery
Femoral artery
Popliteal artery

Circle of Willis
Internal carotid artery
External carotid artery
Left common carotid artery
Vertebral artery
Subclavian (left) artery
Descending aorta
Axillary artery
Celiac trunk
Brachial artery
Radial artery
Ulnar artery
Anterior tibial artery
Posterior tibial artery

FIGURE 7–9 Arteries of the body.

**Vascular Families—
Selective or
Nonselective
Placement**

A vascular family can be compared to a tree with branches. The tree has a main trunk from which large branches and then smaller branches grow. The same is true with vascular families. A main vessel is present, and other vessels branch off from the main vessel. Vessels that are connected in this manner are considered families.

Catheters may have to be placed in vessels for monitoring, removal of blood, injection of contrast materials, or infusion. When coding the placement of a catheter it is necessary to know where the catheter starts and where it ends up.

Catheter placement is nonselective or selective. **Nonselective catheter placement** means the catheter or needle is placed directly into an artery or vein (and not manipulated farther along) or is placed only into the aorta from any approach. **Selective catheter placement** means the catheter must be moved, manipulated, or guided into a part of the arterial system other than the aorta or the vessel punctured (that is, into the branches), generally under fluoroscopic guidance. The following codes illustrate nonselective and selective placement:

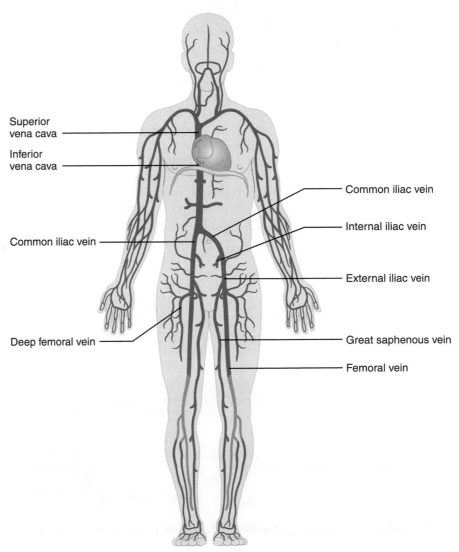

Superior
vena cava

Inferior
vena cava

Common iliac vein

Internal iliac vein

Common iliac vein

External iliac vein

Deep femoral vein

Great saphenous vein

Femoral vein

FIGURE 7-10   Veins of the body.

Example

| Nonselective: | 36000 Introduction of needle or intracatheter, vein |
| Selective: | 36012 Selective catheter placement, venous system; second order, or more selective, branch |

Code 36000 describes the placement of a needle or catheter into a vein with no further manipulation or movement. Code 36012 describes the placement of a catheter into a vein and its manipulation or moving to a second-order vein or farther.

The first note in the Cardiovascular System subsection in the CPT manual refers to selective placement. The note appears at the beginning of the section because it is very important and applies to the entire Cardiovascular System subsection. When coding selective placement for any procedure, you report the fullest extension into one vascular family, just as you would when coding a gastrointestinal endoscopic procedure, when you code to the farthest extent of the procedure. The same is true of selective placement into a vascular family: code to the farthest extent of the placement within the vascular family.

The **first order** is the main artery in a vascular family, the **second order** is the branch off the main artery, the **third order** is the next branch off the second order, and so on. A vascular family can have more than one second-order, third-order, and so on, vessel, as illustrated in Fig. 7–11. If the farthest extent of the placement was to the third order, only the third-order code would be reported. For example, if a catheter was placed into the first-order brachiocephalic artery and from there manipulated through the second-order artery, and finally into the third-order artery, you would report only the third-order artery, with code 36217, which describes an initial third-order placement within the brachiocephalic family.

If the catheter placement continued from one branch of the brachiocephalic artery into another branch of the artery, you would report the additional second order, third order, and beyond using an add-on code—36218. Oftentimes, a physician will investigate not only one branch of an

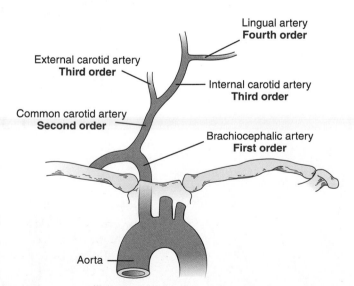

FIGURE 7–11 Brachiocephalic vascular family with first-, second-, third-, and fourth-order vessels.

artery but several others. Report all subsequent catheter placement to the farthest extent of each placement.

> **CODING SHOT** Code to the farthest extent of the vascular family using an initial code; then code any additional services of the second order, the third order, or beyond by using an add-on code.

Catheter placement codes may vary according to the vascular family into which the catheter is placed. Look at the following two codes and note the difference in vascular families:

Example

36215   Selective catheter placement, arterial system; each first order **thoracic or brachiocephalic** branch, within a vascular family

36245   Selective catheter placement, arterial system; each first order **abdominal, pelvic, or lower extremity** artery branch, within a vascular family

QUICK CHECK 7-3

Which CPT Appendix would be a resource for selective vascular coding?

_____

Embolectomy/Thrombectomy. An **embolus** is a mass of undissolved matter that is present in blood and is transported by the blood. A **thrombus** is a blood clot that occludes, or shuts off, a vessel. When a thrombus is dislodged, it becomes an embolus. Thrombectomies or embolectomies are performed to remove the unwanted debris, or clot, from the vessel and allow unrestricted bloodflow. A thrombus or embolus may be removed by opening the vessel and scraping out the debris or by percutaneously placing a balloon within the vessel to push the material to the sides and out of the vessel (see Fig. 7–8). A catheter may also be used to draw a thrombus or embolus out of the vessel, as illustrated in Fig. 7–12. Embolectomy/Thrombectomy codes (34001-34490) are divided based on the artery or vein in which the clot or thrombus is located (e.g., radial artery, femoropopliteal vein), with the site of incision for the catheter specified in the code description (e.g., by arm, by leg, by abdominal incision). You can locate these codes in the CPT manual index under embolectomy or thrombectomy, subdivided by arteries and veins (e.g., carotid artery, axillary vein).

When more involved procedures such as grafts are performed, inflow and outflow establishment is included in the major procedure codes. This means that if a thrombus is present and a bypass graft is performed, the removal of the thrombus is bundled into the grafting procedure if done on the same vessel. Also bundled into the aortic procedures is any sympathectomy (interruption of the sympathetic nervous system) or angiogram (radiographic view of the blood vessels).

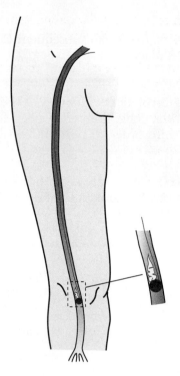

FIGURE 7–12   Embolectomy.

EXERCISE 7–5   *Embolectomy/Thrombectomy*

Using the CPT manual, code the following:

1 Thrombectomy of the femoropopliteal aortoiliac artery, by leg incision

    Code: _____

2 Embolectomy, carotid artery, by neck incision

    Code: _____

3 Thrombectomy of venous bypass graft

    Code: _____

Cardiovascular Repairs

The category Venous Reconstruction (34501-34530) contains codes for the various repairs made to the valves of the vena cava, saphenous vein, and femoral vein. The repair to heart valves is made by opening the site and clamping off the vessels that lead to the heart. The surgeon then tacks down excess material of the valve with sutures (plication). If there is a defect in the valve, the surgeon repairs the defect with a graft, usually harvested from elsewhere in the body. **Vein repairs** are done by locating the defective vessel, clamping the vessel off, and bypassing or grafting the defect.

The category Direct Repair of Aneurysm or Excision (Partial or Total) and Graft Insertion for Aneurysm, Pseudoaneurysm, Ruptured Aneurysm, and Associated Occlusive Disease (35001-35152) contains **aneurysm repair** codes that are divided according to the type of aneurysm (e.g., pseudoaneurysm [false], ruptured) and the vessel the aneurysm is located in (subclavian artery, popliteal artery). The aneurysm is formed by the dilation of the wall of an artery, a vein, or the heart; it is filled with fluid or clotted blood. During repair, the aneurysm is located, and clamps are placed above and below it. The section containing the aneurysm is then removed or bypassed. The aneurysm codes often refer to a pseudoaneurysm, which is an aneurysm in which the vessel is injured and the aneurysm is being contained by the tissue that surrounded the vessel.

Endovascular aneurysm repair (EVAR) is an emerging technology that involves placing a stent graft, a fabric tube, inside the affected area of the blood vessel by access through an artery. For example, abdominal aortic aneurysm repair by endovascular technique is reported with codes 34800-34834 and an iliac aneurysm endovascular repair is reported with 34900.

Repair, Arteriovenous Fistula category codes (35180-35190) are used for **fistula repair** and are divided on the basis of whether the fistula (abnormal passage) is congenital, has been acquired, or is traumatic. An arteriovenous fistula occurs when blood flows between an artery and a vein. An example of an acquired arteriovenous fistula is the creation of an arteriovenous connection that is used for a hemodialysis site (Fig. 7–13). In repairing a fistula, the surgeon separates the artery and vein and then patches the area of separation with sutures or a graft.

If an **angioscopy** of the vessel or graft area is performed during a therapeutic procedure, code 35400, Angioscopy (noncoronary vessels or grafts) during therapeutic intervention, is listed in addition to the procedure code. For example, suppose the surgeon performed the repair of an acquired arteriovenous fistula (of the neck, 35188) and then placed a scope into the artery to determine visually whether the repair was complete. Code 35188 would describe the primary therapeutic procedure of repair of the acquired arteriovenous fistula, and code 35400 would describe the use of the angioscopy to accomplish the repair. Note that 35400 is an add-on code and cannot be used alone, but only in conjunction with a therapeutic procedure code.

A **transluminal angioplasty** is a procedure in which a vessel is punctured and a catheter is passed into the vessel for the purposes of stretching the vessel. The category codes (35450-35476) are divided on the basis of whether the catheter was passed into the vessel by incising the skin to expose the vessel (open) or by passing the catheter through the skin (percutaneous) into the vessel. Further divisions of the codes are based on the vessel into which the catheter is placed (e.g., iliac, aortic).

A **transluminal atherectomy** (35480-35495) is a procedure in which a vessel is punctured and a guide wire is threaded into the vessel. The surgeon then inserts a device called an atherectomy catheter into the vessel; this catheter contains a device that can destroy the materials clogging the vessel. This procedure can be done by an open or a percutaneous method, and the codes are divided on the basis of the method used and the vessel into which the catheter is passed.

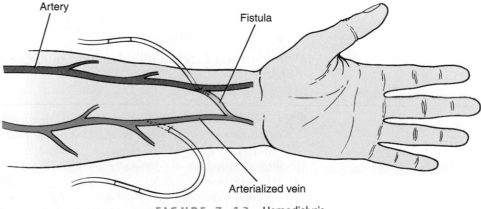

FIGURE 7–13 Hemodialysis.

Bypass Grafts, Veins

As with coronary artery bypass grafting, you must know the type of grafting material being used for vascular bypass grafts (Bypass Grafts 35500-35671). Grafts can be vessels harvested from other areas of the body or they may be made of artificial materials. Codes are chosen on the basis of the type of graft and the specific vessel(s) that the graft is being bypassed from and to. For example, code 35506 describes a graft that is placed to bypass a portion of the subclavian artery. During this procedure the surgeon would sew a harvested vein to the side of the carotid artery and attach the other end of the vein to the subclavian artery below the damaged area, creating a bypass around the defect.

One way to locate the graft codes in the CPT manual index is to look under "Bypass Graft" and then under the subterm type (e.g., carotid, subclavian, vertebral).

QUICK CHECK 7-4

According to the CPT notes for bypass grafts, which of the following procurements is bundled in the bypass?

a. Upper extremity graft
b. Composite graft(s)
c. Saphenous vein graft
d. Femoropopliteal vein graft

Vascular Access

Some treatments are given through the blood by means of vascular access. For instance, in patients receiving hemodialysis, arteriovenous fistulas may be created for dialysis treatments (see Fig. 7–13). This means that an artificial connection is made between a vein and an artery, allowing blood to flow from the vein through the graft for dialysis (cleansing of waste products) and then be returned to the artery.

Vascular Injection Procedures

Bundled into the vascular injections (36000-37216) are the following items:

■ Local anesthesia

■ Introduction of needle or catheter

■ Injection of contrast media

■ Pre-injection care related to procedure

■ Post-injection care related to procedure

Vascular injections bundles do not include the following items:

■ Catheter

■ Drugs

■ Contrast media

For items not bundled into the injection procedure, code each item separately.

 CAUTION *Just for a moment, think about what a difference a seemingly small fact—such as what is included in the vascular injection procedures—makes in the amount received for the procedure over the course of a year! It is your responsibility as the coder to know the rules of coding to ensure appropriate reimbursement for services provided by physicians. Details are important in the business of coding!*

You will use code 99070, supplies and materials, from the Medicine section to code items such as catheters, drugs, and contrast media if the procedure is performed in the clinic facility. If the procedure is performed in the hospital catheterization laboratory, the hospital-based coder would report the supply. There are also specific HCPCS Level II codes for many of these supply items that the third-party payer may require.

As previously discussed, knowledge of the vascular families is critical in coding vascular injection procedures because the initial placement and the extent of placement are usually the characteristics that determine the codes. You now know that the initial placement of the catheter is reported first and that add-on codes report any additional services. For example, review the following initial and additional third-order placement code descriptions in this example:

Example

36217	Selective catheter placement into the brachiocephalic branch, **initial** third order placement
36218	Selective catheter placement into an **additional** third order brachiocephalic branch

---

In the service described in 36217, the physician inserts a needle through the skin and into an artery. The needle has a guide wire attached to it, as illustrated in Fig. 7–14, and when the needle is withdrawn, the guide wire is left inside the artery. The guide wire can then be manipulated into the particular artery. Once the guide wire is in the correct artery, a catheter is threaded into place over the guide wire and into the first-order brachiocephalic artery. The catheter is manipulated through the second-order artery and arrives at the third-order artery, where contrast material is injected into the artery through the catheter and an arteriography is completed.

After the completion of the service described in 36217, the physician pulls the catheter back into the artery and then manipulates the catheter into another third-order artery (36218), where contrast material is again injected into the artery through the catheter and another arteriography is completed.

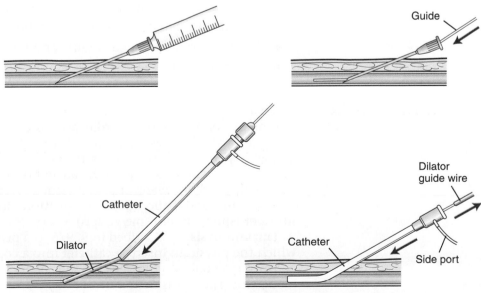

FIGURE 7-14 Catheter insertion.

EXERCISE 7–6 *Repairs, Grafts, and Vascular Access*

Using the CPT manual, code the following:

1 Bypass graft, with vein; carotid-subclavian

   Code: _____

2 Bypass graft, with vein; femoral-popliteal

   Code: _____

3 Bypass graft, using Gore-Tex; axillary-axillary

   Code: _____

4 Excision, with application of a patch graft, for an aneurysm, common femoral artery

   Code: _____

5 From a right femoral artery approach, the catheter is placed in the abdominal aorta and is then threaded into the left internal iliac artery where contrast material is injected and angiography is done. The surgeon then pulls back the catheter into the right internal iliac where contrast is injected and angiography is completed. The catheter is withdrawn. *Note: Report only the catheterization as radiographic guidance services (75600-75790) would be reported separately.*

   Code(s): _____ -RT and _____ -59-LT

CARDIOVASCULAR CODING IN THE MEDICINE SECTION

Services in the Cardiovascular subsection of the Medicine section (92950-93799) can be either invasive/noninvasive or diagnostic/therapeutic. The invasive treatments are not a matter of cutting open the body so the surgeon can view it, as was the case in the Cardiovascular subsection of the Surgery section, but are invasive in that there is an incision into or a puncture of the skin. The subheadings in the Cardiovascular subsection in Medicine are

- Therapeutic Services and Procedures
- Cardiography
- Echocardiography
- Cardiac Catheterization
- Intracardiac Electrophysiological Procedures/Studies
- Peripheral Arterial Disease Rehabilitation
- Noninvasive Physiologic Studies and Procedures
- Other Procedures

Therapeutic Services

It is within the Therapeutic Services and Procedures subheading that you find many commonly used cardiovascular codes, such as cardioversion, infusions, thrombolysis, placement of catheters and stents, atherectomy, and angioplasty. Many of these services used to be performed as open operative procedures, but with the advent of modern techniques, many are now performed by means of percutaneous access. Division of the codes is based on **method** (balloon, blade), **location** (aorta or mitral valve), and **number** (single or multiple vessels).

Thrombolysis, as described in 92975, is a percutaneous procedure in which the physician inserts a catheter into a coronary vessel and injects contrast material into the vessel to further enhance the visualization of a blood clot. The clot is then destroyed by a drug. The Medicine section code 92975 represents the total procedure when the thrombolysis is performed in a coronary vessel. If vessels other than the coronary vessels are treated, a code from the Surgery section, Cardiovascular subsection, would be used to indicate an infusion of a thrombus (37201).

Intravascular ultrasound of the coronary vessels can be reported using the two codes 92978 and 92979, depending on the number of vessels diagnosed. A needle is inserted percutaneously into the vessel and a guide wire introduced, followed by an ultrasound probe. The probe allows a two-dimensional image of the inside of the vessel to be viewed on the ultrasound monitor. The physician can assess the vessel before and after treatment. The physician may reposition the probe to assess additional vessels, and code 92979 is used to indicate this subsequent placement. Note that both 92978 and 92979 are add-on codes and are intended to be used only in conjunction with the primary procedure. For example, intravascular ultrasound with coronary stent placement would be coded as 92980 (placement of stent) and 92978 (intravascular ultrasound).

Intracoronary stent placement (92980, 92981) using a catheter is a procedure that is performed to reinforce a coronary vessel that has collapsed or is blocked. The placement of the stent is usually accomplished with radiographic guidance. The surgeon usually reports the stent placement, and the radiologist who provides the ultrasonic guidance reports the guidance.

The codes are divided on the basis of whether more than one coronary vessel was cleared of obstruction and had a stent placed within it.

Fig. 7–15 illustrates an angioplasty/stent report in which the coronary artery is repaired by placement of a stent. Percutaneous transluminal coronary angioplasty (PTCA), as illustrated in Fig. 7–8, is described in codes 92982 and 92984. The codes are divided on the basis of whether a single vessel or multiple vessels are treated during the procedure. Add-on code 92984 (PTCA for each additional vessel) is of interest because it can be used not only with 92982 but also with other codes in the category. For example, 92984 can be used with code 92980, placement of a stent, when a stent is placed in one vessel and the PTCA is done in a different vessel. If a patient had an intracoronary stent placed in one coronary vessel, you report 92980,

---

Angioplasty/Stent

Patient: Marlene Castello   **Number:** 45900   **Room:** Cardiac Cath Lab 5F

DOB: 02/13/43   **Attending Physician:** Dr. Helen Palmer

DATE OF STUDY: 04/06/0X

PROCEDURE: Angioplasty/stent of 80 to 90 percent proximal/mid-right coronary artery stenosis.

INDICATIONS: Chest pain and abnormal Cardiolite stress test.

COMPLICATIONS: None

RESULTS: Successful angioplasty/stent of 80 to 90 percent proximal/mid-right coronary artery stenosis with no residual stenosis at the end of the procedure.

David H. Robinson, MD

David H. Robinson, MD

Cardiology Department

DHR/jkl

FIGURE 7–15 Angioplasty/stent report.

and if the physician also performed a PTCA on another coronary vessel, you report 92984. This is the first time that you have used an add-on code with a code other than the one(s) that appears directly above it in the same group of codes, so be certain to read the code descriptions for each of the codes used in the example above and pay special attention to the notes that follow 92984.

CODING SHOT There are HCPCS modifiers to identify the specific coronary arteries that are treated, such as **RC**, right coronary; **LC**, left circumflex; and **LD**, left anterior descending.

Valvuloplasty can also be performed by inserting a catheter percutaneously. The procedure opens a blocked valve by using a balloon, which is inflated to clear the blockage. The codes (92986-92990) are divided based on the valve being repaired.

The balloon technique is also used to treat congenital heart defects such as vessels that are too narrow. A blade can also be used inside the coronary vessels. A special catheter that has a retractable blade is guided into the vessel and the surgeon manipulates the blade to enlarge the area, using ultrasound or fluoroscopic guidance.

Cardiography

This category (93000-93278) of the Cardiovascular System subsection contains frequently used codes, such as those for electrocardiograms and heart monitoring, which are certain to be used in most office practices, even if the practice does not include a cardiologist.

The Cardiography subheading is used to report diagnostic electrocardiographic procedures such as stress tests. **Stress tests** are performed to test the adequacy of the amount of oxygen getting to the heart muscle (at rest and during exercise) and thus indicate the presence or absence of heart disease. The top number on a blood pressure reading is systole (heart muscle is contracting); the bottom number is diastole (heart muscle is relaxing). The heart muscle is fed by three coronary arteries and their branches. If these arteries are clear, the amount of blood going to the muscle is adequate during rest and exercise. The heart muscle is fed only during diastole. Normal blood pressure is about 120/80 mm Hg, and the normal heart rate is about 60-100 beats per minute. During low blood pressure, little blood and oxygen get to the heart.

As the heart beats faster, such as during exercise, the heart rate increases and diastolic pressure time decreases, meaning that there is less time to supply blood to the heart muscle. As the heart beats faster, more oxygen is also required. With narrowing of coronary arteries and branches, too little blood may circulate to the heart muscle, supplying even less oxygen than during rest, and chest pain may result as an indication that heart muscle tissue is dying. Indications of heart disease during a stress test are chest pain and a depressed or elevated ST wave segment on the ECG, as illustrated in Fig. 7-16.

The **Holter monitor** is similar to an **electrocardiogram (ECG)**, as illustrated in Fig. 7-17, in that leads are attached to the patient. It is portable and records the patient's ECG readings for 24 hours. Leads are attached to the chest and to a cassette machine. The monitor converts the ECG readings to sound, and the sound is converted back to an ECG reading when completed. The reading is then sped up to hundreds of times faster than normal by computers. Any reading that varies from a normal reading will be identified. The Q, R, and S waves are related to the contraction of the

ST dip indicates abnormal stress test

P QRS T

ST

A. Normal Stress Test

P QRS

ST

B. Abnormal Stress Test

FIGURE 7–16 Normal and abnormal ECG test results. **A,** Normal ECG reading. **B,** Abnormal ECG reading. The ST segment dips. QRS complex and T waves are related to the contraction of the ventricles. Indications of heart disease during a stress test are chest pain and lengthened ST segments.

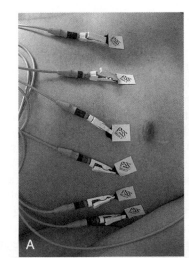

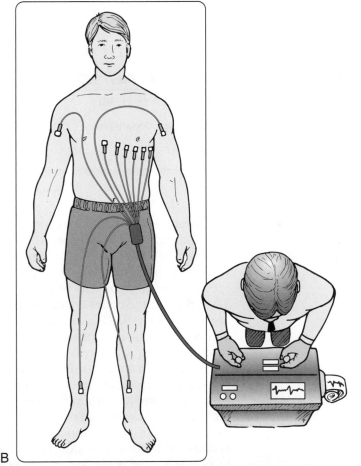

A B

FIGURE 7–17 **A** and **B,** Placement of the electrodes for a standard ECG. The ECG is a visual record of the electrical activity of the heart. (**A** from Young AP, Proctor DB: *Kinn's The Medical Assistant: An Applied Learning Approach,* ed 10, St. Louis, 2007, Saunders.)

ventricles of the heart. The QRS waves and heartbeats can be monitored by Holter monitors. Cardiac arrhythmias can be identified using the Holter monitor process. An example of a Holter report is presented in Fig. 7–18.

An ECG is typically conducted by attaching 10 electrodes (leads) to the patient's chest to monitor 12 areas. The ECG provides a reading of the electrical currents of the heart and is a standard test conducted to detect suspected cardiac abnormalities, such as arrhythmias and conduction

Holter Report

INDICATIONS: Patient with atrial fibrillation on Lanoxin. Patient with known cardiomyopathy.

BASELINE DATA: 84-year-old gentleman with congestive heart failure on Elavil, Vasotec, Lanoxin, and Lasix.

The patient was monitored for 24 hours.

INTERPRETATION:
1. The predominant rhythm is atrial fibrillation. The average ventricular rate is 74 beats per minute, minimal 49 beats per minute, and maximum 114 beats per minute.
2. A total of 4948 ventricular ectopic beats were detected. There were 4 forms. There were 146 couplets with 1 triplet and 5 runs of bigeminy. There were 2 runs of ventricular tachycardia, the longest for 5 beats at a rate of 150 beats per minute. There was no ventricular fibrillation.
3. There were no prolonged pauses.

CONCLUSION:
1. Predominant rhythm is atrial fibrillation with well-controlled ventricular rate.
2. There are no prolonged pauses.
3. Asymptomatic, nonsustained ventricular tachycardia.

Raymond P. Price, MD

Raymond P. Price, MD

Cardiology Department

RPP/lpm

FIGURE 7-18 Holter report.

abnormalities. Some codes are to be used for the tracing only (the technical component), for the interpretation and report only (the professional component), or for the entire procedure of tracing and interpretation (the technical and professional components). The patient's medical record will indicate the components provided. Codes 93000-93010 are for the standard 12-lead ECG; the codes are divided on the basis of the component(s) provided.

Codes 93040-93278 are used for other various ECGs and are divided according to the type of recording and the component(s) provided. Only careful reading will reveal the often slight differences between codes.

Of special note is **signal-averaged electrocardiography (SAECG)**, as represented in 93278. SAECG is a type of electrocardiography that can help physicians predict certain tendencies to abnormalities such as ventricular tachycardia. The signal is recorded during nine periods, each lasting 10 to 20 minutes, and the computer manipulates the data produced and predicts certain tendencies. The SAECG is a more sophisticated ECG than the standard ECG and is used when a standard ECG is unable to demonstrate the suspected conductive abnormalities.

CODING SHOT If only the interpretation and report are done with an SAECG, report 93278-26 to indicate that only the professional component was provided.

Telephonic transmission of an electrocardiogram is made possible by a device the patient wears that records irregular rhythms. The readings from the ECG can then be sent to the physician by using a telephone to transmit the information, which is subsequently printed for the physician's review. Third-party payers usually restrict the payment of telephonic transmissions to one every 30 days. The codes 93012, 93014 are divided on the basis of the component(s) the physician provides.

A **cardiovascular stress test** is a test that is used to evaluate and diagnose chest pain, to screen for heart disease, to evaluate irregular heart rhythms, and to investigate many other cardiovascular abnormalities. The patient is placed on a treadmill or a stationary bicycle and ECG leads are attached. The patient then exercises until he or she reaches maximal (220 minus age) or submaximal (85% of maximal) heart rate. During certain intervals, the physician or technician records the ECG, heart rate, and blood pressure of the patient.

The codes for stress tests (93015-93018) are divided on the basis of the components provided with 93015, which is used to report the global outpatient service, and 93016-93018, which are used to report components (parts) of the service. The ECG is bundled into the stress test, so do not unbundle and report an ECG or any reading separately. Medication can be administered to mimic the stressing of the heart; it is used when factors are present that limit a patient's ability to exercise, such as arthritis, morbid obesity, or stroke. Stress test codes are used for both stress-induced (exercise) and pharmacologically induced (drug) studies. Medications and radiology services may be reported separately.

Echocardiography

Echocardiography is a noninvasive diagnostic method that uses ultrasonographic images to detect the presence of heart disease or valvular disease. A sliced image is used to detail the various walls of the heart. A **transducer** is placed on the outside of the chest wall, and it sends sound waves through the chest (Fig. 7–19).

As the sound reflects back from each organ wall, dots are recorded, indicating the point of reflection. When the heart is in systole, it is contracting, and the dots on the recording appear farther apart. When the heart is in diastole, it is relaxing, and the dots on the recording appear closer together.

Bundled into the complete echocardiography procedures (93303-93350) are the obtaining of the signal from the heart and great arteries by means of two-dimensional imaging and/or Doppler ultrasound, the interpretation,

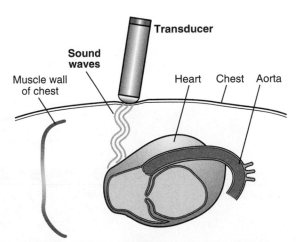

FIGURE 7–19 Echocardiography. A transducer is placed on the outside of the chest wall, and it sends sound waves through the chest. When the heart is in systole, the heart is contracting and the dots on the echocardiogram appear farther apart. When the heart is in diastole, it is relaxing and the dots on the echocardiogram appear closer together.

and the report. Modifiers -26, professional service only, and -TC, technical component, may be applied to these codes if only one component is provided. The codes are divided on the basis of whether it was a complete echocardiogram or a follow-up/limited study, the type of echocardiogram, and the approach used.

EXERCISE 7-7 *Therapeutic Services, Cardiography, and Echocardiography*

Using the CPT manual, code the following:

1 A physician provides CPR to a patient in cardiac arrest.

Code: _____

2 Cardiovascular stress test using submaximal bicycle exercise with continuous ECG; physician was in attendance for supervision and provided the interpretation and report

Code: _____

3 Percutaneous transluminal coronary balloon angioplasty of three vessels

Code(s): _____ and _____

4 SAECG with ECG, interpretation and report only

Code: _____

Cardiac Catheterization

Catheterization (93501-93572) is an invasive diagnostic medical procedure in which the physician percutaneously inserts a catheter and manipulates the catheter into coronary vessels and/or the heart. Fig. 7–20 illustrates a percutaneous method of catheterization called the Seldinger technique, after the inventor of the method. This catheterization is at the right subclavian artery. Following insertion of the fine-gauge needle, a guide wire and then a catheter are inserted. The cardiac catheter is used to measure pressure, oxygen, and blood gases, take blood samples, and measure the output of the heart. A cardiac catheterization is a study of both the circulation and the movement of the blood of the heart; the physician may inject a dye into

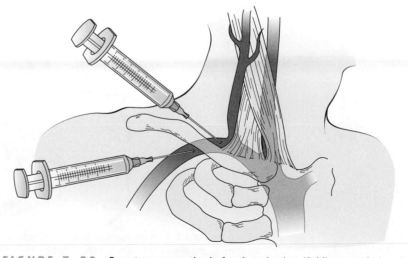

FIGURE 7-20 Percutaneous method of catheterization (Seldinger technique).

the vessel or heart and observe the movement of the dye by means of angiography. When injection of contrast material is used to improve visualization, additional injection procedure codes (such as 93540 or 93544) must be used to specify the site of the injection.

Example

During a cardiac catheterization procedure, contrast medium is injected into a bypass graft and into the coronary arteries. CPT codes would be used to identify each of the areas of injection as follows:

93540   injection into the bypass graft

93545   injection into selective coronary arteries

Each of these two codes would be reported in addition to the code reflecting the type of cardiac catheterization (e.g., left and right heart catheterization, 93526). But you wouldn't be finished coding this one yet. If the cardiologist also supervises, interprets, and reports on the x-ray imaging of the angiography, codes 93555 and 93556 would be used to report the imaging services. This is a good example of component coding. Component coding requires you to examine services that were provided to the patient, identify each component, or part, of that service, identify who performed each component, and code each service provided.

If the private physician (such as the clinic physician) performs the catheterization procedure in the catheterization laboratory at the hospital, you would add modifier -26 to each code. The hospital would submit charges for the technical component of the procedure.

Access for cardiac catheterization can be made in several locations, depending on the patient's condition and the physician's preference—for example, under sterile preparation (prep) and drape, the right femoral artery (access site) was accessed.

Cardiac catheterization can indicate valve disorders, abnormal flow of blood, and a variety of cardiac output abnormalities. Often, a cardiac catheterization leads to a more definite treatment, such as a valvoplasty, stent placement, or angioplasty.

Bundled into the cardiac catheterization codes are the introduction, positioning, and repositioning of the catheter(s); the recording of pressures inside the heart or vessels; the taking of blood samples; rest/exercise studies; final evaluation; and final report.

There are three components in the coding of cardiac catheterization:

1. **Placement** of the catheter, using codes 93501-93533
2. **Injection** procedure, using codes 93539-93545
3. **Imaging** supervision, interpretation, and report on the injection procedure, using codes 93555, 93556

From the Trenches

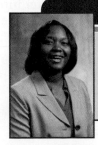

"Teamwork is important in this environment . . . As a profession, we must be a resource to each other and the health care community as a whole."

LETITIA

CODING SHOT Some cardiac catheterizations codes (93544-93556) are modifier -51 exempt. The remainder of the codes (93501-93543) are subject to multiple procedure rules and reporting of modifier -51.

In the case of a complete cardiac catheterization, which is the usual procedure, you will find all the codes you need to fully report the service in the Medicine section, Cardiac Catheterization category. It is a good idea to make a notation of the code ranges for the three components of cardiac catheterization so you remember to look for the components when coding.

CAUTION *The Cardiac Catheterization injection codes (93539-93545) are not to be used unless the injection procedure is a part of a cardiac catheterization.*

There are several codes (93561-93572) in the category that are not a part of the usual three components of the cardiac catheterization. These codes are for the **indicator dilution studies**, which are already bundled into the cardiac catheterization codes and are to be coded only when the complete cardiac catheterization procedure was not done. For example, if only the dye or thermal dilution study was done, without a cardiac catheterization, an indicator dilution study code would be used to report the service.

Intracoronary Brachytherapy

Intracoronary brachytherapy is the use of radioactive substances as a therapy for in-stent restenosis of a coronary vessel. For example, a patient has a coronary artery stent placed to open a vessel that is blocked with plaque (stenosis). The stent reopens the vessel so blood can once again flow without obstruction. However, the stent can also become occluded with plaque and when this happens, the physician can use intracoronary brachytherapy in which a radioactive strip of material is inserted by means of a catheter to the area of blockage, where it is left for up to 45 minutes and then removed.

The procedure would usually be performed by an interventional cardiologist and a radiation oncologist. The interventional cardiologist would place the radioactive-element guide wire and report that service with 92974, which is the catheter placement code. The radiation oncologist would then place the radioactive elements and report the services with whichever codes applied to the service, such as planning (77261, 77263), simulation (77280, 77295), dosimetry (77300-77370), and/or clinical brachytherapy codes (77785-77787).

EXERCISE 7–8 *Cardiac Catheterization*

Answer the following:

1 Right heart catheterization was performed by means of the introduction of a cardiac catheter into the venous system, with further manipulation into the right atrium, including injection into the right atrium of contrast material, multiple measurements, and sampling; image supervision was provided by the physician.

Code(s):

_____ Catheterization procedure

_____ Injection procedure

_____ Supervision, interpretation, and report for injection procedure

2 Retrograde left heart catheterization of left ventricle was performed, with cutdown entry into the brachiocephalic artery, and contrast medium was injected for left ventricular angiography, including supervision, interpretation, and report.

🔵 Code(s): _____

3 Indicator dilution studies when done with a cardiac catheterization are to be billed separately.

True   False

4 Bundled into the cardiac catheterization codes are the positioning and repositioning of the catheter(s).

True   False

5 Modifier -51 can be added to all codes in the Cardiac Catheterization subheading.

True   False

Intracardiac Electrophysiologic Procedures/Studies

As you learned earlier in this chapter, surgical electrophysiologic procedures (33250-33261) are those that repair the electrical system of the heart using invasive surgical procedures. In the Medicine section, the Intracardiac Electro-physiological Procedures/Studies category (93600-93662) contains codes that are used to describe services that diagnose and treat the electrical system of the heart using less invasive procedures. Although the Medicine section procedures are invasive, they are percutaneous procedures.

Fig. 7–21 illustrates the electrical conduction system of the heart, which begins with the sinoatrial node (SA), known as the heart's pacemaker. The sinoatrial node sends impulses to the atrioventricular (AV) node, which in turn passes the impulses to the bundle of His, and finally on to the Purkinje fibers to stimulate the ventricles of the heart. Lesions or diseases involving these structures along the electrical conduction pathway underlie many of the disturbances of cardiac rhythm.

To diagnose the origin of an electrophysiologic abnormality, the physician takes recordings at various sites along the pathway. The physician may also stimulate the heart to induce arrhythmia by means of a catheter attached to a pacing device that sends electrical impulses to various sites within the heart. A protocol (a set order) for the placement of the catheter is a **programmed stimulation.**

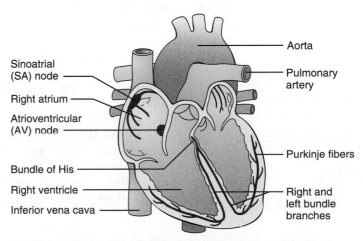

FIGURE 7–21   Electrical conduction system of the heart.

Pacing is the regulation of the heart rate. A cardiac pacemaker is a permanent pacer; but the pacing referred to in the EP codes is a temporary pacing done in an attempt to stabilize the beating of the heart. **Recording** is a record of the electrical activity of the heart taken by means of an ECG. Recording services are reported using codes in the range of 93600-93603, and pacing services are reported using the codes 93610 and 93612. Combination codes that indicate both recording and pacing begin with 93619. These codes are not used as much as they used to be when EP was a new technique and readings were commonly taken at just one site. Today, more complex EP studies are usually done, including multiple pacings and recordings in combinations based on established protocols using three or more catheters. These complex services are reported with codes in the 93619-93622 range. Carefully read the notes in parentheses following several of the combination codes, as the notes indicate when the use of the combination code is appropriate and even indicate the codes that are bundled into the one combination code.

 CAUTION *Most of the EP codes have many items bundled into them, so read the description of each code completely so as to avoid unbundling the services.*

A **bundle of His recording** is a reading taken inside the heart (intracardiac) at the tip of the bundle of His. The physician percutaneously inserts into a vessel a special catheter that can sense electrical impulses. The catheter is advanced to the right heart. The femoral vein is the usual site of entry and fluoroscopic guidance is usually used for placement of the catheter into the heart.

Codes 93602 and 93603 describe a **single recording** based on the location—intra-arterial, right ventricle, or left ventricle. Codes 93610 and 93612 describe **single pacing** in an atrial or a ventricular location.

Code 93631 is used to report pacing and mapping done during an open surgical procedure in which the surgeon opens the chest and exposes the heart. The EP physician performs the **mapping** (locating the origin of the arrhythmia and defining the pathway), and the surgeon then destroys the source of the arrhythmia. When reporting the services of both physicians for this procedure, use 93631 to report the mapping service and a surgery code from the range 33250-33261 to report the arrhythmia ablation. Make a notation next to the mapping code 93631 to report any surgical ablation (33250-33261) to remind yourself to code both procedures if required. If the mapping is not done intraoperatively (during surgery), report the service with 93609 or 93613.

Ablation can also be performed by using a catheter with a tip that emits electric current. When the tip is placed on tissue and activated, the tissue is destroyed. Sometimes physicians destroy certain sites along the conduction pathway as a treatment for slow (bradycardia) or fast (tachycardia) heart rhythms. Ablation procedures are reported with codes 93651 and 93652, according to whether they were performed above the ventricles (supraventricular) or in the ventricles.

There are two ways ablation can be performed. The first way does not require surgery. An area of the patient's upper thigh is numbed, but the patient is awake. Then the physician inserts a thin tube through a blood vessel (usually in the upper thigh) and all the way up to the heart. At the tip of the tube is a small wire that can deliver **radiofrequency** energy to burn away the abnormal areas of the heart. Then the heart can beat normally again.

The second way ablation can be performed is by means of surgery. In the Maze procedure, the surgeon makes small **cuts** in the heart to direct healthy electrical rhythms. In **cryoablation**, a very cold substance is used to freeze the cells that are creating problems so they cannot cause more damage. In **endocardial resection**, the surgeon removes a section of the thin layer of the heart where the abnormal rhythms originate.

CODING SHOT There are no codes that specifically indicate the technical component only or the professional component only of EP, so if only the professional component was performed, use modifier -26. If only the technical component was performed, add the HCPCS modifier -TC.

Peripheral Arterial Disease Rehabilitation

Peripheral arterial disease (PAD) rehabilitation sessions (93668) last 45 to 60 minutes; these are rehabilitative physical exercises done either on a motorized treadmill or on a track to build the patient's cardiovascular endurance. An exercise physiologist or nurse supervises the sessions. If a session produces symptoms of angina or other negative symptoms, the physician reviews the information and may determine to reevaluate the patient. The physician services are reported with an additional Evaluation and Management (E/M) code.

Noninvasive Physiologic Studies and Procedures

If a patient has a pacemaker or defibrillator in place, periodic monitoring must occur to ensure that the device is functioning properly. Codes from the Noninvasive Physiologic Studies and Procedures (93701-93790) category reflect these services. Codes are chosen according to the type of pacemaker (single- or dual-chamber) and whether reprogramming of an existing pacemaker or defibrillator was done.

Plethysmography (93720-93722) is a recording of the change in the size of a body part when blood passes through it and is used to determine vascular abnormalities. Respiratory function especially is assessed using total body plethysmography. There are two components in a plethysmography process—the professional component and the technical component. There are codes for the total procedure, for only the technical component of tracing, and for only the professional component of interpretation and report.

Electronic analysis is an analysis of the electronic function of devices such as pacemakers and cardioverter-defibrillators after they have been implanted into a patient. The physician analyzes the devices by means of an electrocardiogram and other analyses of the device. The majority of codes in the range 93279-93299 describe a variety of electronic analytic procedures used in a variety of devices. The codes describe analysis and reprogramming of single- or dual-chamber pacemakers and cardioverter-defibrillators. Some of the pacemaker analysis codes are specifically for **remote analysis**, which is the analysis of a pacemaker using the telephone to transmit the information about the function of the device.

Ambulatory blood pressure monitoring (93784-93790) is an outpatient procedure that is done over a 24-hour period by means of a portable device worn by the patient. There is a code for the total procedure—including recording, analysis, and interpretation/report—and there are codes for each of the individual components—recording only, analysis only, and interpretation/report only.

Other Procedures   The Other Procedures codes (93797-93799) are used for physician services that are provided for cardiac rehabilitation of outpatients, either with or without electrocardiographic monitoring.

EXERCISE 7–9   *EP and Vascular Studies*

Using the CPT manual, code the following:

1 Bundle of His recording

  Code(s): _____

2 Comprehensive electrophysiologic evaluation was performed, including recording and pacing of the right atrium and right ventricle. Three electrodes were repositioned. Left ventricular recordings were also made, with pacing and induction of arrhythmia.

  Code(s): _____

3 Total body plethysmography, including tracing, interpretation, and report

  Code(s): _____

CARDIOVASCULAR CODING IN THE RADIOLOGY SECTION

Before 1992, the Radiology section of the CPT manual contained combination codes that included both the **professional** and **technical components** in one code. For example, 75659 existed to report the services of both the angiography (technical component) and the injection procedure (professional component) in a brachial angiography procedure. When the complete procedure code, 75659, was deleted, the injection procedure (professional component) was moved to the Surgery section and a code to report the technical component (angiography) remained in the Radiology section. Now, to report both the injection procedure and the angiography services (the complete procedure), the coder uses a Surgery code to report the professional component and a Radiology code to report the technical component. The division of the technical and professional components makes it possible to specify the various parts of a procedure, which is important because some cardiologists perform both components of these cardiovascular procedures, and some cardiologists perform only the injection procedure and have a radiologist do the angiography portion of the procedure. Component coding allows for the flexibility necessary to code these various situations. Component coding also makes it easier to identify the various diagnostic tests that are used in cardiovascular conditions. For example, one cardiologist may prefer to use an ultrasonic procedure in the diagnosis of arterial stenosis and another may prefer angiography. Both procedures require the insertion of a catheter and, as such, the insertion code remains the same, but the diagnostic tools may change.

Radiology codes often contain the statement "supervision and interpretation." **Supervision** is the radiologist's overseeing of the technician who is performing the procedure or indicates that the radiologist is performing the procedure himself/herself. **Interpretation** is the summary of the findings, also known as the final report, and only the radiologist does this portion of the service. There are actually two components (parts) in a code with supervision and interpretation in the description—the professional and technical components. The technical component is the equipment and the technician who actually provides the service. The professional component is the interpretation of the results and the writing of a report about the results, as illustrated in Fig. 7–22. Both components are not necessarily done by the same organization. Let's take an x-ray as an example of a service and see how you report the components.

If a clinic owns its own x-ray equipment and employs a radiologist to interpret the x-rays and write the reports, and also employs the technician who, under the supervision of the radiologist, takes the x-rays, the clinic could report the x-ray service using the appropriate radiology code, with supervision and interpretation in the description and *no modifier.* The clinic provides the total service, also known as the **global service.**

Another clinic owns the equipment and employs the technician who takes the x-ray, but then the clinic sends the x-ray out to a radiologist at another clinic who reads the x-ray and writes the report. The radiologist would report the service with the appropriate radiology code and *modifier -26* to indicate that he or she provided only the professional component of the service. The clinic that employs the technician and owns the equipment would report the same radiology code but would attach the HCPCS *modifier -TC* (technical component) to indicate that only the technical component of the service was provided by it.

 CAUTION *The **professional component** (interpreting results and writing the report) is reported using modifier -26. The **technical component** (technician and equipment) is reported using modifier -TC.*

Examination:	Chest
Clinical symptoms:	Aortic stenosis, abnormal cardiac stress test
Date ordered:	Today's date
Date Completed:	Today's date
Ordering Dr.:	Dr. Timothy Swenson
Attending Dr.:	Dr. Timothy Swenson
Date of Birth:	04/13/65 Record #: 456980
PA & Lateral chest:	Radiographic examination reveals no abnormality of the lungs, heart, mediastinum, or visualized bony structures.
Impression:	Radiographically normal chest.

Ronald A. Potts, MD

Ronald A. Potts, MD

Radiologist

RAP/rnf

FIGURE 7–22 The final radiology report contains the radiologist's interpretation of findings.

A third clinic has no x-ray equipment, so the physicians in the clinic send patients to an outside radiologist who hires the technician who takes x-rays on equipment owned by the radiologist, the radiologist interprets the results, and writes the report. The outside radiologist would report the service using the global radiology code with *no modifier,* because both the professional component and the technical component were provided.

Contrast material is commonly used with radiology procedures to enhance the image. If the Radiology section code states "with contrast" or "with or without contrast," you will know that the injection of contrast material and the contrast material itself (the substance used for contrasting) are bundled into the code; therefore, you would not code for the contrast material or injection separately. If, however, there is no indication of contrast in the code description, and the physician used contrast, you would code both for the injection of the contrast material and for the contrast material itself. Injection of contrast is usually included in the radiology code. If guidelines state that you should code injections separately, they are coded with the appropriate code from the surgery section—for example, 47500, Injection procedure for percutaneous transhepatic cholangiography, and 74320 for the radiology portion of the service. The contrast material is reported separately using code 99070 from the Medicine section, Special Services, Procedures, and Reports subsection or with a HCPCS code.

CODING SHOT Not all contrast material can be coded separately! Oral or rectal contrast is considered a part of the procedure and is not coded separately. Intravenous, intra-arterial, or intrathecal injection of contrast material can be coded separately if the code description does not refer to inclusion of contrast material.

STOP *Now, don't be getting discouraged with all of these codes from all of these sections! Remember that only with repeated use of these codes can you master them. At first, it sounds so confusing that you might wonder if you can ever absorb all of this information and the variations. You can. But you must be patient with the process. To be a coder is to be able to concentrate on details and commit yourself to the process of learning the details through repeated use. Everyone starts at the same place.*

Now, let's get back to learning about component coding. Two physicians, a cardiologist and a radiologist from the same facility, perform an angiography of the brachiocephalic artery (third order) using contrast material. The coding is as follows:

- Cardiologist placing the catheter: 36217, Surgery section
- Radiologist performing the angiography: 75658, Radiology section
- Supply of the contrast material: 99070, Medicine section, or with a HCPCS Level II code

Two physicians, a cardiologist and a radiologist from different facilities, perform an angiography of the brachiocephalic artery (first order) using contrast material. The coding for the cardiologist is as follows:

- Cardiologist placing the catheter: 36215, Surgery section

The coding for the radiologist is as follows:

- Radiologist performing the angiography: 75658, Radiology section
- Supply of the contrast material: 99070, Medicine section, or a HCPCS Level II code

CODING SHOT If the radiologist is at the same facility as the equipment, you use code 75658 (angiography). If the radiologist is hospital-based, you use code 75658-26 on the CMS-1500 (hospital outpatient) and 75658 on the UB-04 (hospital inpatient).

Heart

The Heart subsection (75557-75564) of the Radiology section contains codes that are used to report cardiac magnetic resonance imaging (MRI) of the heart.

The remaining codes in the Heart subsection of the Radiology section are used to report cardiac magnetic resonance imaging (MRI). An **MRI**, as illustrated in Fig. 7–23, *A* and *B*, is the use of radiation to show the body in a cross-sectional view. MRI may include the use of injectable dyes (radiographic contrast) to aid in imaging. Other MRI codes are located throughout the Radiology section according to body part being imaged, but the codes in the Heart subsection are just for cardiac MRIs.

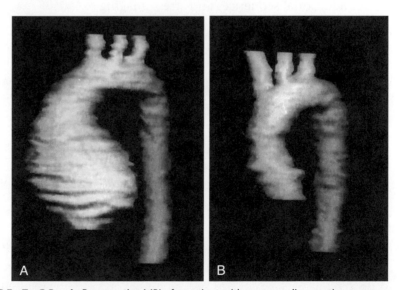

FIGURE 7–23 **A,** Preoperative MRI of a patient with an ascending aortic aneurysm. **B,** Post-operative MRI of the same ascending aortic area. (From Bennett JC, Plum F: *Cecil Textbook of Medicine,* ed 20, Philadelphia, 1996, WB Saunders.)

Aorta and Arteries   In Radiology, the Aorta and Arteries subsection (75600-75790) includes codes for aortography excluding the heart—thoracic, abdominal, cervicocerebral, brachial, external carotid, carotid, vertebral, spinal, extremity, renal, visceral, adrenal pelvic, pulmonary, and internal mammary.

The codes found in the Aorta and Arteries subsection are often used in coding components of cardiovascular services.

EXERCISE 7–10   *Heart, Aorta, and Arteries*

Using the CPT manual, code the following:

1 Code a selective catheter placement in the first-order brachiocephalic artery, with angiography, including contrast done at the clinic catheterization laboratory.

   Code(s): _____, _____, and _____

2 A cardiologist performs a selective catheter placement into the left external carotid artery (first-order branch) via a direct puncture to the left common carotid artery. A radiologist performs an angiographic procedure without contrast.

   Code(s): _____ and _____

3 A cardiologist performs selective catheter placement via the femoral artery. The catheter is advanced into the aorta and then into the left common carotid artery, terminating in the left external carotid artery. The radiologist performs an angiographic procedure without contrast.

   Code(s): _____ and _____

4 Complete cardiac MRI for morphology and function without contrast followed by contrast along with four additional sequences and stress imaging

   Code: _____

CHAPTER REVIEW

CHAPTER 7, PART I, THEORY

Without the use of reference material, complete the following:

1 What are the two subheadings within the Cardiovascular System subsection?

_____ and _____,

_____ and _____

2 The subspecialty of internal medicine that is concerned with the diagnosis and treatment of the heart is _____.

3 In Chapter 7 you learned about coding from which three sections of the CPT?

_____, _____, and

_____

4 Procedures that break the skin for correction or examination are known as

_____ procedures.

5 Procedures that do not break the skin

are known as _____
procedures.

6 The study of the heart's electrical system is

known as _____.

7 The use of radioactive radiologic procedures to aid in the diagnosis of cardiologic conditions

is termed _____

_____ cardiology.

8 A catheter that is inserted into an artery and manipulated to a further order is termed

_____ placement.

9 A catheter that is inserted into an artery and not manipulated to a further order is termed

_____ placement.

10 Surgical procedures in the Heart and Pericardium subheading contain procedures that are performed through both open surgical

sites and _____.

CHAPTER 7, PART II, PRACTICAL

Code the following cases for the surgical procedures, the office visits, and the cardiology-related Radiology and Medicine section codes. Do not code the laboratory work.

11 Dennis Smith, a 42-year-old railroad employee (established patient), has a history of severe mitral stenosis with regurgitation. He is now symptomatic and his physician recommends a mitral valve replacement, to be done in 2 weeks. Dennis agrees to the surgery, and the physician does a comprehensive history and physical in preparation for surgery. The physician orders a general health panel blood workup and a urinalysis (automated). Two weeks later, the physician performs a mitral valve replacement. Dennis recovers uneventfully and is discharged from the hospital 5 days later.

   Code(s): _____

12 Thrombectomy of arterial graft

   Code(s): _____

13 Direct repair of aneurysm and graft insertion for occlusive disease of the common femoral artery

   Code(s): _____

14 A surgical assistant performs five venous grafts in a coronary artery bypass.

   Code(s): _____

15 Open-heart repair of mitral valve with use of cardiopulmonary bypass

   Code(s): _____

16 Removal of a single-chamber pacing cardioverter-defibrillator pulse generator, subcutaneous

   Code(s): _____

17 Pericardiotomy for removal of clot

   Code(s): _____

18 Complete repair of tetralogy of Fallot is made with closure of a ventricular septal defect, and a conduit from the pulmonary artery to the right ventricle is constructed. A pulmonary graft valve is then secured. Cardiopulmonary bypass is required.

   Code(s): _____

19 Shunting from subclavian to pulmonary artery using the Blalock-Taussig operation

   Code(s): _____

20 Pulmonary endarterectomy with embolectomy requiring cardiopulmonary bypass

   Code(s): _____

21 Direct repair of aneurysm associated with occlusion of the vertebral artery

   Code(s): _____

22 Thromboendarterectomy with patch graft of iliac artery

   Code(s): _____

QUICK CHECK ANSWERS

QUICK CHECK 7-1
Left and right coronary arteries. The rest are branches, e.g., circumflex branch of the left coronary artery.

QUICK CHECK 7-2
CABG

QUICK CHECK 7-3
Appendix L

QUICK CHECK 7-4
c. Saphenous vein graft

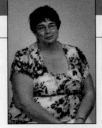
"Teamwork is so important! You have to be able to work with other people, and keep your mind open at all times...Coding can be subjective; there is no one who knows everything."

Stephanie A. Lewis, CPC, ACS-EM, CCP
Compliance Analyst
University of Missouri Health Care
Columbia, Missouri

Female Genital System and Maternity Care and Delivery

Chapter Topics

PART I: *Female Genital System*

Format

Coding Highlights

PART II: *Maternity Care and Delivery*

Format

Coding Highlights

Chapter Review

Quick Check Answers

Learning Objectives

After completing this chapter you should be able to

1 Understand the format of the Female Genital System subsection.

2 Explain the use of incision and destruction codes in the vulva, perineum, and introitus.

3 Define the extent and size of vulvectomy procedures.

4 Differentiate between colpotomy and colpocentesis.

5 Demonstrate an understanding of LEEP procedures.

6 Differentiate between biopsy and conization.

7 Define laparoscopic, hysteroscopic, and abdominal procedures.

8 Identify elements of component coding with Female Genital System codes.

9 Define the critical terms in maternity and delivery services.

10 Define services in the global maternity and delivery package.

11 Analyze abortion procedures.

12 Understand the format of the Maternity Care and Delivery subsection services.

13 Demonstrate the ability to code the Female Genital and Maternity Care and Delivery subsection.

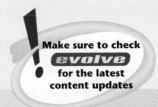
Make sure to check **evolve** for the latest content updates

PART I ▪ *Female Genital System*

FORMAT

The Female Genital System subsection (56405-58999) is divided according to anatomic site, from the vulva up to the ovaries (Fig. 8–1). The anatomic sites are then divided on the basis of category of procedure (i.e., incision, excision, destruction). Codes for in vitro fertilization are found at the end of the subsection.

The subsection has a wide variety of codes for minor procedures that are performed in a physician's office as well as for major procedures that are performed in a hospital. It is important to read the descriptions of the codes as well as the notes to avoid unbundling in this subsection. For example, if a total abdominal hysterectomy was performed as well as a bilateral oophorectomy (removal of ovaries), only CPT code 58150 would be used. CPT code 58150 includes in the description the statement "with or without removal of ovary(s)." Bundled into the code are both the abdominal hysterectomy and the bilateral oophorectomy.

CODING HIGHLIGHTS

Vulva, Perineum, and Introitus

You will see a repeated note in the Vulva, Perineum, and Introitus subheading (56405-56821) indicating procedures performed on the Skene's glands are not coded using codes in the Female Genital System subsection but instead are coded using Surgery section, Urinary System subsection codes. That is because Skene's glands, also known as the **para-urethral ducts**,

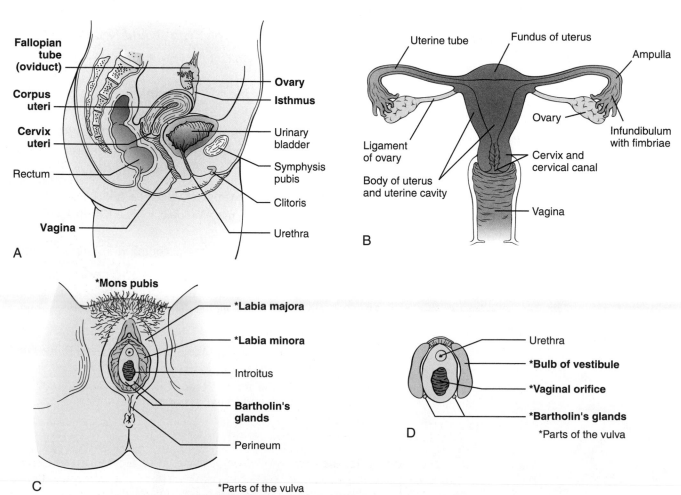

FIGURE 8–1 **A,** Female genital system. **B,** Anterior view, female genital system. **C,** External female genital system. **D,** Parts of vulva.

is a group of small mucous glands located near the lower end of the urethra and is part of the urinary system. Procedures involving Skene's glands are, therefore, always coded using Urinary System codes (53060 or 53270).

Incision. The vulva includes the following parts: mons pubis, labia majora, labia minora, bulb of vestibule, vaginal orifice or vestibule of the vagina, and the greater (Bartholin's gland) and lesser vestibule glands (see Fig. 8–1, *C* and *D*). When the code description indicates the incision and drainage of an abscess of the vulva, the code covers an abscess of any of the anatomic areas just listed. For example, if a medical record indicates "an incision and drainage of an abscess of Bartholin's gland," you must know that Bartholin's gland is considered a part of the vulva, so the code will be located in that subheading.

Destruction. Destruction of lesions of the vulva, perineum, or introitus can be accomplished using a variety of methods—laser surgery, cryosurgery, electrosurgery, or chemical destruction. Destruction codes are divided on the basis of whether the destruction is simple or complex, although the code description does not define simple or complex. Complexity is based on the physician's judgment of complexity, and the complexity should be stated in the medical record.

 CAUTION *Destruction is not excision. Destruction is obliteration or eradication. Excision is removal. With destruction no tissue is removed, as the tissue is destroyed. There is no pathology report after a lesion has been destroyed because there is nothing for the pathologist to analyze.*

Excision. The first two codes (56605 and 56606) in the Excision category are for biopsies in which the physician takes a tissue sample by removing a piece of tissue with a scalpel or punch. The area to be biopsied is anesthetized with local anesthetic before the biopsy is performed. The physician may suture the area or use clips for closure. The anesthesia and closure are included in the package of an excision code, so be careful not to unbundle. The codes are also divided on the basis of number of lesions, one and each additional lesion. Be certain to specify the number of lesions biopsied by listing the number of units on the CMS-1500 form in Block 24-G (refer to Fig. 4–14).

Vulvectomy is the surgical removal of a portion of the vulva. Usually a vulvectomy is performed to treat a malignant or premalignant lesion. The following definitions apply to the vulvectomy codes (56620-56640) and describe the extent and size of the vulvar area removed during the procedure.

EXTENT

- Simple   skin and superficial subcutaneous tissue
- Radical   skin and deep subcutaneous tissue

SIZE

- Partial   less than 80%
- Complete   greater than 80%

The vulvectomy codes are divided on the basis of these definitions of extent and size. The extent and size are stated in combination. For example, the term "simple partial vulvectomy" describes a *superficial subcutaneous tissue* (extent) removal of 78% (size) of the vulvar area. Bundled into the codes is usual closure, but if plastic repair is required, you would report the repair in addition to the procedure. The operative report will indicate the extent of the procedure and the closure.

CODING SHOT There are two labia: labia minora and labia majora. A partial vulvectomy (less than 80%) pertains to leaving at least 20% of the vulvar area.

The more radical procedures involving the vulva are usually performed because of a demonstrated malignancy, and more extensive removal takes place. This radical removal can include the removal of deep lymph nodes, saphenous veins, ligaments, or large amounts of tissue from the lower abdomen or even from the thigh. The procedure may also be done bilaterally, so don't forget modifier -50, bilateral procedure.

Repair. The procedure codes in the Repair category (56800-56810) describe plastic repair of the vulva, perineum, or introitus. Plastic repair of the **introitus** is surgical repair of the opening of the vagina. The extent and nature of the procedure are determined by the defect being repaired and hence vary greatly from patient to patient. **Clitoroplasty** is surgical reduction of a clitoris that has become enlarged due to an adrenal gland imbalance. **Perineoplasty** is plastic repair of the perineum, usually to provide additional support to the perineal area.

Vagina

The Vagina codes are 57000-57425. **Colpotomy** (57000-57010) is cutting into the vagina to gain access to the pelvic cavity. The procedure is performed to explore the pelvic cavity or to drain a pelvic abscess. **Colpocentesis** is insertion of a long needle (puncture) attached to a syringe through the back wall of the vagina to gain access to the peritoneal cul-de-sac—the area between the uterus and the rectum—to drain fluid. If the colpocentesis is a part of a more major procedure, you do not code it separately, as it is considered to be bundled into the more major procedure. Note that the code 57020 (colpocentesis) has a "(separate procedure)" after it to designate colpocentesis as a minor procedure; it is reported only if it is the only procedure of the area performed.

Destruction. As with the destruction codes for the vulva, the destruction codes for the Vagina subsection are divided on the basis of whether the destruction was simple or extensive, in the judgment of the physician. Any method of destruction is acceptable for assignment of these codes.

Excision. The Excision category of the Vagina subsection contains codes for reporting the services of biopsy, vaginectomy (removal of part or all of the vagina), colpocleisis (closure of the vaginal canal), and cyst/lesion

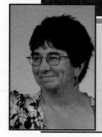

From the Trenches

"I often tell the coders and auditors I work with that they are detectives and should think and act like a detective, never giving up until they have dug up all the information that they can to back up what they are telling a physician or non-physician practitioner."

STEPHANIE

removal. The vaginectomy codes are divided according to the extent of the procedure—partial or total—and the extent to which tissue and adjacent structure(s) are removed.

Introduction. The Introduction category contains codes for vaginal irrigation. Also included is the insertion of a tandem/ovoid for brachytherapy. The tandem and ovoid are internal implants that contain a radioactive substance and are often used in the treatment of cervical cancer. A tandem is a small, hollow metal tube that is inserted through the vagina into the uterus (intrauterine tandem). An ovoid is a small metal cylinder that is placed into the vagina and up against the cervix (intravaginal ovoid). The implants then deliver a concentrated dose of radiation to the site of the tumor. Other codes in the Introduction category report the insertion of a support device (pessary), diaphragm, or cervical cap (to prevent pregnancy); and packing of the vagina (for vaginal hemorrhage). The pessary and diaphragm/cervical cap are not included in these Introduction codes. The supply of these devices would be billed using code 99070, supplies, or a HCPCS code (e.g., A4561).

Repair. The Repair category is rather extensive, as the possible forms of repair of the vagina are many. A note in parentheses, "(nonobstetrical)," sometimes follows the code description in the Female Genital System subsection because if the procedure was performed as a part of an obstetric procedure, you would use a code from the Maternity Care and Delivery subsection.

A surgeon performs a **colporrhaphy** to strengthen an area of the wall of the vagina that is weak by pulling together the weakened vaginal area with sutures. The vaginal wall can also be reinforced with sutures placed in weakened areas. Also, excess tissue can be removed to tighten the area. The reinforcement might be performed for several reasons, but it is commonly done to prevent the bladder from protruding into the weakened vaginal wall (cystocele) or when the rectum protrudes into the vagina (rectocele).

In this Repair category, the codes are often divided on the basis of the approach used. For example, an abdominal approach (open, 57270) to the repair of an enterocele (herniation of intestines through intact vaginal mucosa) has a different code than does a vaginal approach (57268) to the same repair; and an anterior colporrhaphy (vaginal repair) (57240) differs from a posterior colporrhaphy (57250). So, you must pay particular attention to the **approach** used. You will find that the approach used is noted in the operative report.

One method of vaginal repair that is *not* in the Repair category is the laparoscopic repair. Codes for repair of the vagina using a colposcope (microscope) are located in the Vagina subheading, Endoscopy category. The colposcope enables the physician to directly view changes in the vagina and cervix. For example, Fig. 8–2 illustrates an endocervical polyp protruding through the external os (mouth of the cervix) as seen by the physician using a colposcope.

 CAUTION *Coders need to pay close attention to the method as well as to the approach. For example, a surgeon might perform an open procedure as opposed to a laparoscopic procedure.*

Notes throughout the Repair category will often direct you to the correct code or code range in the Urinary System subsection. Often, the only difference between surgical procedures coded with Female Genital System

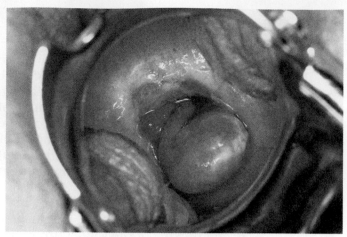

FIGURE 8-2 Endocervical polyp protruding through the mouth of the cervix as seen through a colposcope. (From Baggish MS: *Colposcopy of the Cervix, Vagina, and Vulva: A Comprehensive Textbook,* Philadelphia, 2003, Mosby.)

codes and those coded with the Urinary System codes is the approach. For example, Female Genital System code 57330 describes the closure of a vesicovaginal fistula (abnormal channel between bladder and vagina) using a vaginal approach, whereas Urinary System code 51900 describes the same procedure using an abdominal approach. The approach method would be described in the operative report.

Manipulation. **Manipulation** of the vagina includes dilation (stretching), pelvic examination, and removal of foreign material. What these three different procedures have in common is that they are all performed under **general anesthesia** because a patient cannot tolerate the procedure while awake. If a local anesthetic or no anesthetic was used, which is the usual case, you would not use a Manipulation code; instead, the service would be included in the Evaluation and Management (E/M) service. For example, if a physician removed an impacted tampon from the vagina and used no anesthetic during the procedure, only the office visit at which the removal took place would be coded.

Endoscopy. As discussed earlier in this chapter, the endoscopic procedure codes in the Endoscopy category of the Vagina subheading are for colposcopic procedures. The colposcopic procedures are often bundled into other, more major procedures. Only when a colposcopic procedure is performed as the only procedure or is unrelated to another procedure(s) being done is the colposcopy coded.

If a biopsy of the vagina or cervix is performed with colposcopy, the code to report the service is 57421. The codes specifies "biopsy(s)," so whether one or multiple biopsies were taken, 57421 represents the total number.

Cervix Uteri

The Cervix Uteri subheading contains codes (57452-57800) for endoscopy, excision, repair, and manipulation.

Endoscopy. Similar to the vaginal endoscopic codes, the colposcopy codes are used in procedures of the cervix uteri (57452-57461). A loop electrode excision procedure is referred to as LEEP, LETZ, or cervical loop diathermy and is an office procedure that uses heated wire (Fig. 8–3) to remove cervical tissue. The device is attached to an electric generator that heats the wire. The procedure has a lower risk level and is less expensive than other

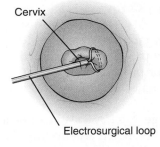

Cervix

Electrosurgical loop

FIGURE 8-3 The loop used in the electrosurgical excision procedure.

methods. A LEEP would usually be done after an abnormal Pap smear result or an abnormal examination. The cervix is moistened, and the loop is positioned over the cervix and drawn across the area. The resulting slice is examined by a pathologist. The device is also used to cauterize the area at the end of the procedure by means of a different attachment.

Excision. The codes in the Excision category often specify "(separate procedure)" because many times, the procedures are bundled into a more major procedure. For example, the excision procedure of a biopsy is often incidental to a more major surgical procedure, such as a hysterectomy, and the biopsy would not be coded separately.

Codes for **conization** of the cervix are divided on the basis of the method used to obtain the tissue. In conization, a cone of tissue is removed from the cervix for a biopsy or treatment of a lesion by means of excision of the lesion. Although a laser is an often used method of conization, LEEP technology is also widely used. The LEEP device can be used for various procedures. The code for a LEEP procedure with **cervical biopsy** in the Cervix Uteri subheading, Endoscopy category, is 57460, and the code for a LEEP procedure with **cervical conization** is 57461. The difference between the codes is that the cervical biopsy procedure only removes a certain sample with return in the future if the lesion is to be completely removed. The conization procedure removes a cone-shaped tissue of the cervix when it encompasses the identified abnormal tissue highlighted by iodine. Also, the cervical biopsy is performed with the use of a colposcope (endoscopy), and the conization is performed using a speculum (an instrument inserted into a cavity to stretch the opening). Be certain, when coding cervical biopsy and conization, that the information in the medical record provides sufficient detail to allow you to distinguish between a biopsy and a conization. If the record is not complete enough to make the determination, obtain the information from the physician before choosing a code.

Repair. Nonobstetric **cerclage** (repair of the cervix) involves extensive suturing of the cervix to decrease the size of the opening into the vagina. **Trachelorrhaphy** is a complex cervical repair in which plastic methods are used to repair a laceration of the cervix. Both Repair codes use a vaginal approach to the procedure.

Manipulation. Dilation of the cervix is coded separately only if it is the only procedure performed. Dilation of the cervix, like dilation of the vagina, is often bundled into a more major procedure.

Corpus Uteri   The corpus uteri (58100-58579) is the anatomic area above the isthmus and below the opening for the fallopian tubes. The subheading contains the categories of excision, introduction, repair, and laparoscopy/hysteroscopy procedures. Many of the procedures in the category are very complex, and some of them have several variations.

Excision. Endometrial **sampling** is a biopsy of the mucous lining of the uterus. The physician inserts a curet (spoon-shaped instrument) into the endocervical canal to extract tissue samples for pathologic examination. If the sampling is the only procedure performed, it is reported, but if it is done as a part of a more major procedure involving the cervix, it is considered incidental to the more major procedure and is bundled into the surgical package.

Dilation and curettage (D&C; 58120) can be a diagnostic or therapeutic procedure that is performed when an endometrial biopsy has failed or was inconclusive, to determine the cause of abnormal bleeding or to locate a neoplasm. Clamps are used to manipulate the cervix, a curet is inserted into the uterus, and fragments are removed from the endometrium. The tissue is sent to pathology for analysis. The D&C in the Corpus Uteri subheading is for nonobstetric patients only. If a D&C is performed because of postpartum hemorrhage, a code from the subsection Maternity Care and Delivery would be used to report the service (59160).

CODING SHOT Many third-party payers will not reimburse for a dilation and curettage if it is performed with any other pelvic surgery because it is thought to be integral to or a part of the procedure. The CPT manual does not list a D&C as a "(separate procedure)"; therefore, you need to be familiar with reimbursement policies in your area.

Hysterectomy codes (58150-58294) represent the majority of the codes in the Corpus Uteri subheading. A **hysterectomy** is the removal of the uterus, but in the CPT manual there are many variations of the procedure. The divisions of the hysterectomy codes are based first on the **approach** (abdominal or vaginal), then on the **secondary procedures** that were performed (removal of tubes, biopsy, bladder, etc.). You have to read the code descriptions carefully to determine what is bundled into the code. Because so many procedures are bundled into several of the codes, you also have to be careful not to unbundle and code for items already covered in the main procedure. For example, a total abdominal hysterectomy can include the removal of the ovaries and/or the fallopian tubes; therefore, billing separately for the removal of the ovaries or tubes would be unbundling.

Within the Excision category there are codes for abdominal approaches for hysterectomies. An **abdominal approach** is one in which the surgeon opens the abdomen to view by means of an incision. Review the codes in the

QUICK CHECK 8-1

1. What is the difference between codes 58260 and 58290?

_____

2. Look up the term "myomectomy" in the CPT Index. Look at the codes listed. What are the determining factors in selecting a code?

a. Approach, location, number

b. Approach, number, weight

c. Location, weight, pathological outcome

d. Weight, number, age of patient

range 58150-58240 and underline "abdominal" in each of the codes as a reminder of the approach used in these codes. The other type of surgical approach for hysterectomies listed in the Excision category is the vaginal approach. Using the **vaginal approach**, the surgeon makes an incision in the vagina around the cervix and removes the uterus and/or ovaries/fallopian tubes (salpingo-oophorectomy) through the incision. The cuff of the vagina is then closed with sutures. Review the codes in the range 58260-58294 and underline "vaginal" as a reminder of the approach used in these codes. The uterus and/or ovaries/fallopian tubes can also be removed during a **surgical laparoscopy**.

Introduction. It is in the Introduction category that you will find the codes for some very common procedures such as the insertion and removal of an **intrauterine device (IUD)** for birth control and for some not-so-common procedures such as artificial insemination. There are also several codes that have radiology components—your component coding skills will again be used.

Because intrauterine device (IUD) insertion is coded using Introduction category codes, you might think IUD removal would be in a removal category, but it is in the Introduction category.

CODING SHOT

The cost of the IUD is not included in the code for the insertion of the IUD. You report the cost of the device separately, using 99070 or a HCPCS code.

Don't confuse the insertion of an IUD with the placement of an implantable contraceptive such as Norplant, as described in the Integumentary subsection.

The specialized fertility procedure of **artificial insemination** and the preparation of the sperm for insemination are coded using Introduction category codes. During the insemination procedure, sperm is injected into the cervix and often a cervical cap is inserted to keep the sperm in the cervical area. **In vitro fertilization** is a different procedure in which an egg from the female is withdrawn and fertilized with sperm in a laboratory for 2 to 3 days, then implanted into the uterus. There is an In Vitro Fertilization subheading containing codes to report these services, located at the end of the Female Genital System subsection (58970-58976).

Catheterization and introduction (58340) of saline or contrast material through the cervix and uterus and into the fallopian tubes (hysterosalpingography) is used by a physician to identify blockage or abnormalities of the fallopian tubes. Ultrasound can also be used for the same procedure (hysterosonography). You need to remember your component coding and code the radiology or ultrasound portion of the procedure with a code from the Radiology section. A note following 58340 in the CPT manual directs you to the correct component code. For the radiographic supervision and interpretation, the component code is 74740; for the ultrasound, the code is 76831.

The other procedure in the Introduction category that may have a radiology component is the introduction of a catheter into the fallopian tubes (58345). The catheter is passed through the fallopian tube, and an x-ray will show where the catheter encounters an obstruction or a narrowing of the tube. A code from the Radiology section, Gynecological and Obstetrical subsection, would be used to report the radiology portion of the service (74742).

Hysterosalpingraphy is a diagnostic procedure to test for patency of the tubes. **Chromotubation** (58350) is a surgical procedure to open obstructed tubes.

Laparoscopy/Hysteroscopy. An increasing number of procedures are being performed by using an endoscope instead of opening the area to complete view. With an endoscopic procedure, usually two or three small incisions are made through which lights, cameras, and instruments may be passed. The surgeon first inserts an instrument into the vagina, and it is used to grasp the cervix. Another scope is inserted into the abdomen, and the uterus and/or ovaries/fallopian tubes may be excised. An incision is made in the vagina and the surgically excised material is removed. The vagina is then repaired by means of sutures. Review the codes in the range 58541-58579 and underline "Laparoscopy" or "Hysteroscopy" as a reminder of the approach used in these codes. It is very important to read the full code description to identify the approach. Because endoscopic procedures are less invasive, patients are more accepting of the procedures, and recovery times and risks are reduced. Fig. 8–4 illustrates a laparoscopy procedure and Fig. 8–5 illustrates a laparoscopy/hysteroscopy procedure.

The first rule of a laparoscopy or hysteroscopy is that all surgical procedures include a diagnostic procedure. You never unbundle a surgical laparoscopic procedure and also report a diagnostic procedure. If a procedure started out as a diagnostic laparoscopic procedure and ended up being a surgical laparoscopic procedure, still being performed through a laparoscope, you code only for the surgical laparoscopy.

✋ **CAUTION** *If the laparoscopy is of the peritoneum, you use a code (49320) from the laparoscopy category of the Digestive System, Abdomen, Peritoneum, and Omentum subheading.*

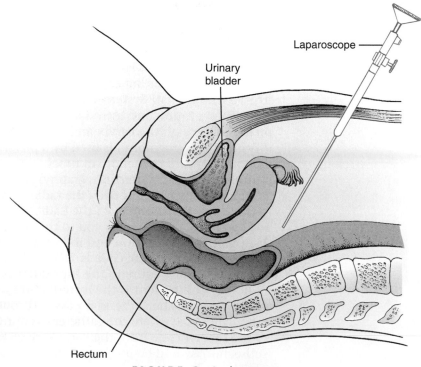

Laparoscope

Urinary bladder

Rectum

FIGURE 8–4   Laparoscopy.

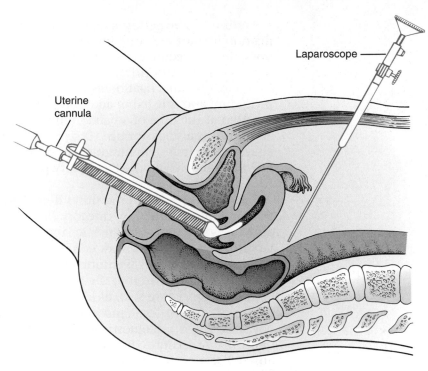

FIGURE 8–5 Hysteroscopy/laparoscopy.

The codes in the Laparoscopy/Hysteroscopy category are divided on the basis of approach—laparoscopy or hysteroscopy—and further divided by other procedures that might have been performed. For example, a hysteroscopy with removal of a foreign body and a hysteroscopy with ablation have different codes.

Oviduct/Ovary

The Oviduct/Ovary subheading (58600-58770) is divided into incision, laparoscopy, excision, and repair. Fallopian tube procedures are located in this subheading.

Incision. The Incision category is where you will locate the codes for tubal ligation. **Tubal ligation** is a permanent, highly effective method of birth control. The codes are divided according to the type of ligation performed and the circumstances at the time of the ligation. The types of ligation are as follows: **tying** off the tube with suture material (ligation), **removing** a portion of the tube (transection), and **blocking** the tube with a clip, ring, or band (occlusion). The circumstances under which the procedure is done affect the choice of codes. For example, a procedure can be done either on one side (unilateral) or on both sides (bilateral). The procedure can be done at different times, such as during the same hospitalization period as the period of delivery, during the postpartum period, or during another surgical procedure.

CODING SHOT Do not use a bilateral procedure modifier (-50) with codes in the Incision category because the code descriptions indicate "tube(s)" or "unilateral or bilateral." Also, do not code tubal ligations performed by means of a laparoscopic procedure using the Incision category codes. There are codes for laparoscopic tubal ligation procedures in the Laparoscopy category of subheading Oviduct/Ovary (58660-58679).

A ligation can be performed by an abdominal or a vaginal approach. If a ligation or transection of the fallopian tube(s) is done during the same operative procedure as a cesarean delivery or other intra-abdominal surgery, you code the ligation/transection using code 58611. Code 58611 is used only to report the tubal ligation as a component of the more major surgical procedure and is listed in addition to the primary code.

Often at the time of an abdominal tubal ligation, lysis (loosening) of adhesions is also performed. Lysis is not bundled into the ligation code. You code for the lysis of adhesions separately, using the Repair category code 58740, if allowed by the third-party payer.

Laparoscopy. The procedures described in the Oviduct/Ovary subheading, Laparoscopy category (58660-58679) are surgical laparoscopy and always include a diagnostic laparoscopy. If only a diagnostic laparoscopy was performed, you use code 49320 from the Digestive System subsection, Abdomen, Peritoneum, and Omentum category, because the scope is being passed into the abdomen for examination only. Once a definitive procedure such as a tubal ligation has begun, the examination/diagnostic laparoscopic procedure is bundled into the surgical procedure. For example, if a diagnostic laparoscopy was done and did not lead to a definitive procedure, the diagnostic laparoscopic code 49320 from the Surgery section would be submitted to describe the procedure of examining the abdomen using an endoscope. But if a diagnostic laparoscopy was done and did lead to a fulguration of the oviducts, code 58670 from the Female Genital System subsection would be used. The terminal (end or final) procedure dictates the code choice.

The laparoscopy codes are divided on the basis of the procedure performed—for example, lysis of adhesions, oophorectomy, and lesion excision.

Excision. The Excision category codes are for salpingectomy (removal of uterine tube) or salpingo-oophorectomy (removal of uterine tube and ovary). Both codes describe unilateral or bilateral procedures that are either complete or partial. An unbundling issue presents itself with the use of these codes. If either procedure is done with a more major procedure such as a hysterectomy, each is considered bundled into the more major procedure and is not reported separately.

Repair. Within the Repair category are codes for lysis of adhesions and various repairs to the fallopian tubes. All of the repairs are performed for the purpose of restoring fertility. Often the repairs are made through small incisions above the pubic hairline, but they can also be made through a laparoscope, so pay special attention to the approach used for repairs to the fallopian tubes.

Lysis of adhesions performed on the fallopian tubes (**salpingolysis**) or the ovaries (ovariolysis) uses a small incision to insert instrumentation to complete the repairs. Lysis is a procedure that is often performed at the time

From the Trenches

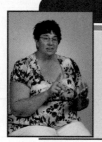

"Coding is an evolving science; in order to be successful a coder needs to be willing to use everyday to the fullest by continuing their education and learning something new and useful."

STEPHANIE

of another, more major procedure and it is usually bundled into the more major procedure. If the lysis takes an extensive amount of time, you can report the service separately.

Ovary   The subheading Ovary (58800-58960) contains two categories of codes: Incision and Excision. The Incision codes are used to report ovarian incision and drainage. The Excision codes are used to report ovarian biopsy, cystectomy, and oophorectomy procedures.

QUICK CHECK 8-2

Review code range 58950-58956. Which of the codes include "total abdominal hysterectomy?"

_____

In Vitro Fertilization   In vitro fertilization means to fertilize an egg outside the body, and the codes in the In Vitro Fertilization category describe several methods that are used in modern fertility practice. Third-party payers often do not pay for the fertility treatments, and you will have to be certain that you know the policy of the payer regarding fertility treatments.

Code 58970, aspiration of the ova, is often performed with ultrasonic guidance and when it is, you use the Radiology section, Ultrasonic Guidance Procedures category code 76948 to report the radiology service.

EXERCISE 8–1 *Female Genital System*

Using the CPT manual, code the following:

1 Simple destruction of one lesion of the vaginal vestibule

Code: _____

2 Biopsy of three lesions of the vulva

Code(s): _____

3 Closure of rectovaginal fistula, abdominal approach

Code: _____

4 Cone biopsy (laser) of cervix with dilation and curettage

Code(s): _____

5 Unilateral, laparoscopic, ovarian cystectomy

Code(s): _____

Using the vulvectomy notes in the CPT manual, match each of the following procedures with its correct definition:

PROCEDURE	THE REMOVAL OF:
6 simple _____	a. greater than 80% of the vulvar area
7 radical _____	b. skin and deep subcutaneous tissues
8 partial _____	c. skin and superficial subcutaneous tissues
9 complete _____	d. less than 80% of the vulvar area

PART II ■ *Maternity Care and Delivery*

FORMAT

The Maternity Care and Delivery subsection (59000-59899) is divided according to type of procedure. As a general rule, the subsection progresses from antepartum procedures through delivery procedures. The guidelines are very detailed as to the services included in antepartum and delivery care, not only to facilitate coding but also to help guard against unbundling. Notes found at the beginning of this subsection describe, in depth, the services listed in obstetric care. Be certain to read these notes.

Abortion codes, whether for spontaneous abortion, missed abortion, or induction of abortion, are found at the end of the subsection. Abortion codes indicate treatment of a spontaneous abortion or missed abortion, including additional division on the basis of trimester and induction of abortion by method. You must be aware of the gestational age of the fetus to determine the correct code.

Treatment for ectopic pregnancies is based on the site of the pregnancy, the extent of the surgery, and whether the approach was by means of laparoscopy or laparotomy.

CODING HIGHLIGHTS

Maternity and Delivery

The gestation of a fetus takes approximately 266 days; but when the **estimated date of delivery (EDD)** is calculated, 280 days are often used, counting the time from the **last menstrual period (LMP)**. The gestation is divided into three time periods, called trimesters. The trimesters are as follows:

First   LMP to week 12
Second   Weeks 13-27
Third   Weeks 28-EDD

When a maternity case is uncomplicated, the service codes normally include the antepartum care, delivery, and postpartum care in the global package. **Antepartum care** is considered to include both the initial and subsequent history and physical examinations, blood pressures, patient's weight, routine urinalysis, fetal heart tones, and monthly visits to 28 weeks of gestation, biweekly visits from gestation weeks 29 through 36, and weekly visits from week 37 to delivery when these services are provided by the same physician. If the patient is seen by the same physician for a service other than those identified as part of antepartum care, you would report that service separately. For example, if a patient in week 32 came to the office because of cold symptoms, an E/M service code would be billed.

Delivery includes admission to the hospital, which includes the admitting history and examination, management of an uncomplicated labor, and delivery that is either vaginal or by cesarean section (including any episiotomy and use of forceps).

Included in **postpartum care** are the hospital visits and/or office visits for 6 weeks after a delivery. If the postpartum care is complicated or if services are provided to the patient during the postpartum period, but the services are not generally part of the postpartum care, you would report those services separately.

Routine Obstetric Care

There are four codes that describe the global routine obstetric care that includes the antepartum care, delivery, and postpartum care, based on the delivery:

59400   Vaginal delivery
59510   Cesarean delivery
59610   Vaginal delivery after a previous cesarean delivery
59618   Cesarean delivery following attempted vaginal delivery after previous cesarean delivery

Two abbreviations commonly found on the delivery record are VBAC (vaginal birth after cesarean) and VBACS (vaginal birth after cesarean section), which help to direct the choice of the correct code.

CODING SHOT ✎ Bundled into the vaginal delivery codes are an episiotomy (cutting of the perineum) and/or the use of forceps during delivery and, therefore, neither is reported separately.

If the physician provided only a portion of the global routine obstetric care, the service is reported with codes that describe that portion of the service as delivery only or postpartum care only, based on the delivery method. For example, if a physician provided only the delivery portion of the service, you would report the service with:

59409   Vaginal delivery only
59514   Cesarean delivery only
59612   Vaginal delivery only, after previous cesarean delivery
59620   Cesarean delivery only, following attempted vaginal delivery after previous cesarean delivery

If the global obstetric care is provided and twins are delivered, the same codes are still used but, depending on the third-party payer, modifier -22 (Increased Procedural Services) or -51 (Multiple Procedures) is added. Usually, if both twins are delivered vaginally, report 59400 for Twin A and 59409-51 for Twin B. If one is delivered vaginally and one is delivered cesarean, report 59510 for Twin B and 59409-51 for Twin A. If both are delivered via cesarean, report only 59510 (because only one cesarean was performed).

Antepartum Services

Amniocentesis (59000-59001) is a procedure in which the physician inserts a needle into the pregnant uterus to withdraw amniotic fluid. The procedure cannot be done in the first 14 weeks of pregnancy. In this procedure, ultrasound is used to guide the needle, and the supervision and interpretation (S&I) service is reported using a code from the Radiology section, Ultrasonic Guidance Procedures subsection, code 76946.

Several of the antepartum services require component coding in order to fully report the services provided. Attention to the code descriptions and parenthetic statements is necessary to ensure that all services are reported.

Cordocentesis (59012) is a procedure in which fetal blood is drawn. This procedure is done under ultrasonic guidance to assess the status of the fetus. Cordocentesis is not included in normal antepartum care and should be reported separately. The ultrasonic guidance (76941) would also be reported separately.

Excision. Abdominal **hysterotomy** is performed to remove a hydatidiform mole (cystlike structure) (Fig. 8–6) or an embryo. If a tubal ligation is performed at the same time as a hysterotomy, be certain to use an additional code (58611) to indicate the ligation.

An **ectopic pregnancy** is one in which the fertilized ovum has become implanted outside of the uterus, as illustrated in Fig. 8–7. The surgical treatment for this condition can use either an abdominal or a vaginal approach; most often, the abdominal approach is used. If the area has not ruptured, the pregnancy is removed. If a rupture has occurred, a more extensive procedure is required. You have to know the location of the ectopic pregnancy, the extent of the necessary repair, and the approach to the repair—vaginal, abdominal, or laparoscopic to correctly code the procedure.

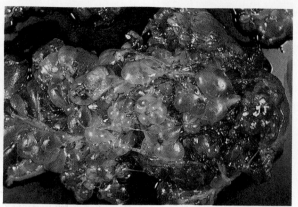

FIGURE 8-6 Hydatidiform. (From Damajnov I, Linder J: *Pathology: A Color Atlas,* St. Louis, 1999, Mosby.)

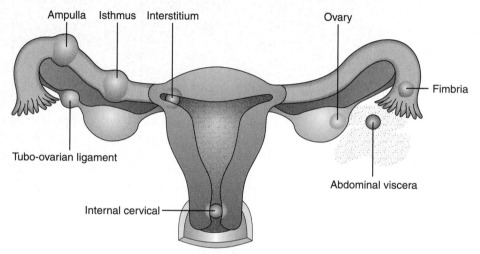

FIGURE 8-7 Implantation sites of ectopic pregnancy.

Score	Dilation (cm)	Effacement (%)	Station	Consistency	Cervical Position
0	Closed	0-30	−3	Firm	Posterior
1	1-2	40-50	−2	Medium	Midposition
2	3-4	60-70	−1, 0	Soft	Anterior
3	>4	>70	+1, +2	—	—

FIGURE 8-8 The Bishop Scoring System of cervical ripening.

Postpartum curettage is performed within the first 6 weeks after delivery to remove remaining pieces of the placenta or clotted blood. Code 59160 is only for use with postpartum curettage. If the curettage is nonobstetric, you would use 58120.

Introduction. A cervical dilator may be inserted prior to a procedure in which the cervix is to be dilated; it prepares the cervix for an abortive procedure or a delivery. The dilator initiates uterine contractions, which in turn cause cervical dilatation. Induction can be elective—at the convenience of the patient or the physician—or required, based on a medical risk factor to the mother or fetus. Physicians use a scoring system to measure the stage of cervical ripening, as illustrated in Fig. 8-8.

To induce cervical ripening, a preparation such as Prepidil gel is introduced intracervically using a catheter. The cervical ripening takes place in the delivery ward.

CODING SHOT You can report 59200 (cervical ripening) with an induced abortion (59840 or 59841), but not with an abortion induced by means of vaginal suppositories (59855-59857). Also, do not report an induction procedure using a code that describes a manual dilation as a part of the procedure, such as D&C.

Many third-party payers will not pay separately for an induction procedure, as it is considered to be part of the package for obstetric care. You will have to check with your payers to determine their policies regarding the induction procedure.

Repair. The obstetric repairs can be to the vulva, vagina, cervix, and uterus. All of these repairs are also located in the Female Genital subsection, but here in the Maternity Care and Delivery subsection, the codes are used only for repairs made during pregnancy. Repairs made during delivery or after pregnancy are reported using the postpartum codes, 59400-59622.

CODING SHOT Vaginal repairs can be reported separately only by a physician other than the attending physician. When the attending physician performs a procedure such as an episiotomy, it is considered part of the package for obstetric care. Each third-party payer determines what is included in its own obstetric package.

Abortion Services. The abortion codes (59812-59857) include services for treatment for several types of procedures. A **spontaneous** abortion (miscarriage) is one that happens naturally. If the uterus is completely emptied during the miscarriage and the physician manages the postmiscarriage, the services are reported with E/M codes. Sometimes the abortion is **incomplete** and requires intervention to remove the remaining fetal material (59812-59830). A **missed** abortion is one in which the fetus has died naturally sometime during the first half of the pregnancy but remains in the uterus. The physician removes the fetal material from the uterus and reports the service based on the trimester in which the service was provided. A **septic** abortion is similar to a missed abortion but has the added complication of infection. The physician removes the fetal material from the uterus and vigorously treats the infection.

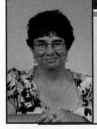

From the Trenches

"Having good working relationships with physicians is the #1 priority. You need to be confident that what you are telling them is correct, and when they realize that you know what you are talking about, they will respect you."

STEPHANIE

The induced abortions are those in which the death of the fetus is brought about by medical intervention (59840-59857). One of three methods is used: **dilation** with either curettage (scraping) or evacuation (removal by means of suction), intra-amniotic **injections**, or vaginal **suppositories**. The selection of the code depends on which of the three methods was used to accomplish the abortion. Dilation and **curettage** is a procedure in which the cervix is dilated and the fetal material is scraped out by means of a curet. When the dilation and **evacuation** method is used, the cervix is dilated and the contents are suctioned out by means of a vacuum aspirator. The intra-amniotic **injections** are of urea or saline, which induces an abortion. Vaginal **suppositories** (such as prostaglandin) can be inserted into the uterus, with or without cervical dilation, and that induces an abortion. A **hysterotomy** (cutting into the uterus) may be performed if the medical intervention by injection or vaginal suppositories fails.

EXERCISE 8–2 *Maternity Care and Delivery*

Using the CPT manual, code the following:

1 Laparoscopic salpingectomy for tubal ectopic pregnancy

Code: _____

2 Version or breech presentation, successfully converted to cephalic presentation, with normal spontaneous delivery

Code(s): _____

3 Thirty-year-old woman, 20 weeks' gestation, with cervical cerclage by vaginal approach

Code(s): _____

CHAPTER REVIEW

CHAPTER 8, PART I, THEORY

Without the use of reference material, complete the following:

1 The Female Genital System subsection is divided by _____ site from the vulva to the ovaries.

2 Skene's glands procedures are reported using codes from which subsection?

_____

3 The vulva includes the following:

mons _____,

labia _____,

labia _____,

bulb of _____,
vaginal orifice or vestibule, greater and

lesser _____ glands.

4 Who is responsible for determining the complexity of destruction procedures?

_____

5 Destruction of a lesion is also known as excision.

True   False

6 Would you expect a pathology report to be available for a lesion that was obliterated?

Yes   No

7 The term that describes the removal of a portion of the vulva is

_____.

8 The removal of the vulvar area is reported with which two measures?

_____ and _____

9 Vulvar area tissue removal that involves the skin and superficial subcutaneous tissues is

termed _____.

10 Vulvar area tissue removal that involves the skin and deep subcutaneous tissues is termed

_____.

11 This vulvectomy involves less than 80% of the vulva: _____; and
this one involves more than 80%:

_____.

CHAPTER 8, PART II, PRACTICAL

Using the CPT manual, code the following:

12 Sue Lind, age 29, has a Pap test. The pathology report comes back positive for malignancy. Her physician recommends and performs a diagnostic colposcopy. Evidence of further malignancy of the uterus is seen and the physician does a laparoscopically assisted vaginal hysterectomy 20 days later of a 236-gram uterus. Report only the hysterectomy.

Code(s): _____

13 Laparoscopy with fulguration of oviducts

Code(s): _____

14 Oocyte retrieval by means of a follicle puncture with radiologic assistance

Code(s): _____

15 The attending physician, who has provided Sally Fisher's obstetric care, performed a cesarean delivery and ligation of the fallopian tubes and routinely followed up with Sally in the postpartum period.

Code(s): _____

16 Colpopexy using an abdominal approach

Code(s): _____

17 Biopsy of three lesions of the vulva

Code(s): _____

18 Fitting and supply of a diaphragm with instructions for use

Code(s): _____

19 Extensive biopsy of mucosa of vagina, requiring closure

Code(s): _____

20 Using instrumentation, the cervical canal was dilated and examination was completed.

Code(s): _____

21 Simple incision and drainage of an abscess of the vulva

Code(s): _____

22 Colpocentesis

Code(s): _____

QUICK CHECK ANSWERS

QUICK CHECK 8-1
1. The weight of the uterus.
2. b. Approach, number, weight

QUICK CHECK 8-2
Codes 58951, 58953, 58954, 58956

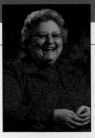

"My motto for my billing and coding students is, 'Persist until you succeed.'"

Patricia Sommerfeld, CPC
Senior Client Manager
HealthMed Inc.
Adjunct Instructor
Mercy College of Health Sciences
Des Moines, Iowa

General Surgery I

Chapter Topics

Male Genital System

Intersex Surgery

Urinary System

Digestive System

Mediastinum and Diaphragm

Chapter Review

Quick Check Answers

Learning Objectives

After completing this chapter you should be able to

1 Understand the format and codes of the Male Genital System subsection.

2 Review the subheadings and categories of the Male Genital System subsection.

3 Understand the format and codes of the Urinary System subsection.

4 Review the subheadings and categories of the Urinary System subsection.

5 Understand the format and codes of the Digestive System subsection.

6 Review the specialty terminology of the Digestive System subsection.

7 Understand the format of the Mediastinum/Diaphragm subsection codes.

8 Demonstrate the ability to code male genital, urinary, digestive, and mediastinum/diaphragm services.

Make sure to check **evolve** for the latest content updates

MALE GENITAL SYSTEM

Format

The Male Genital System subsection (54000-55899) of the CPT manual is divided into anatomic subheadings (penis, testis, epididymis, tunica vaginalis, scrotum, vas deferens, spermatic cord, seminal vesicles, and prostate) (Fig. 9–1). The category codes are divided according to procedure. The greatest number of category codes fall under the subheading Penis because there are many repair codes in this subheading. The other subheadings are mainly for incision and excision, with only a few repair codes for the remaining subheadings.

Penis

Incisions and Destruction. Under the Incision category (54000-54015) of the subheading Penis, there is an incision and drainage code (54015). Recall that under the Integumentary System section there are incision and drainage codes. The code from the Penis subheading is for a deep incision, not just an abscess of the skin. For the deep abscess described in 54015, the area is anesthetized, the abscess is opened and cleaned, and often a drain is placed to maintain adequate drainage.

QUICK CHECK 9-1

For a superficial incision and drainage of the penis, you would select a code from the _____ subsection of CPT.

Destruction. Under the Destruction category (54050-54065) of the subheading Penis there are also destruction codes for lesions of the penis. These lesion destruction codes are divided on the basis of whether the destruction is simple or extensive. Simple destruction is further divided

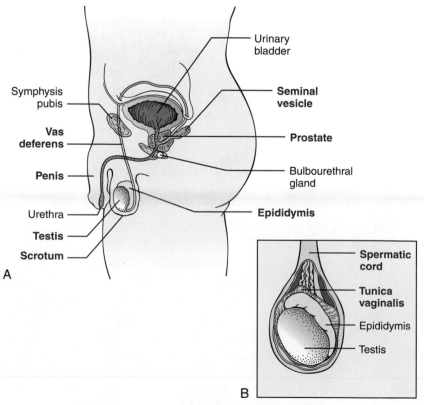

FIGURE 9–1 **A,** Male genital system. **B,** Testis.

according to the method of destruction (e.g., chemical, cryosurgery, laser). The code for extensive lesion destruction can be used no matter which method was employed.

Excision. Excision codes (54100-54164) include codes to report biopsy of the penis (54100, 54105). Note that the procedure code 54100 has a designation of separate procedure, which means that it is reported when it is the *only* procedure performed during the operative session. The physician removes a portion of a lesion by excision of a small section of the lesion (scalpel or scissors) or by a punch biopsy. A punch biopsy is commonly used with skin lesions. A punch biopsy instrument is a pencil-shaped instrument (Fig. 9-2) that removes a round disk of tissue. The opening left by the punch may require simple closure (suture) depending on the size of the skin defect. A more complex biopsy (54105) of the penis involves the deeper layers of the penis and may require layered closure.

Peyronie disease is a curvature of the penis that results from plaque formation on the cavernous sheaths of the penis as illustrated in Fig. 9-3. The plaque develops on the lower and upper side of the penis where the erectile tissue is located. Inflammation results and leads to the formation of scar tissue. Over time, this fibrous plaque bends the penis. In severe cases, the penis arches during erection causing pain. Surgical correction involves removal of the penile plaque (54110-54112). Grafting of the defect may be necessary, depending on the extent of the removal. CPT code 54110 reports the excision of penile plaque when no grafting is required and 54111, 54112 report excision when grafting is required.

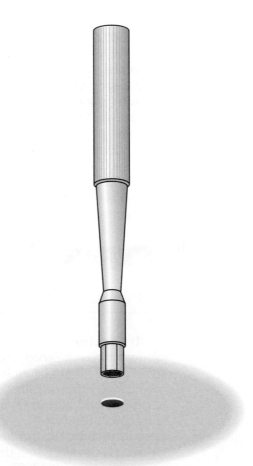

FIGURE 9-2 A punch biopsy is used for deeper lesions and the area may require closure.

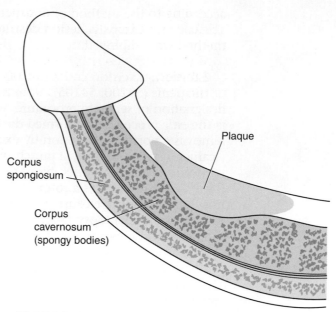

FIGURE 9–3 Curvature of penis due to Peyronie disease.

Penile amputation can occur as a result of trauma or as a surgical procedure for penile cancer. If the procedure is the removal of only the penis (partial or complete) report the service with 54120 or 54125. If the procedure includes removal of the inguinofemoral lymph nodes, report the service based on the extent of the removal (54130, 54135). A lymphadenectomy performed as a separate procedure is reported with a code from the range 38760-38765.

Circumcision codes 54150-54161 are divided based on whether the circumcision was accomplished by means of a clamp/other device or surgical excision and whether the procedure was performed on a neonate or non-neonate. A clamp is a device that is used to restrain the foreskin of the penis while the skin is trimmed. Report newborn circumcisions that utilize a clamp or other device with code 54150. A surgical excision of the foreskin is a procedure in which a clamp or other device is not used, and the surgeon excises the skin from the penis. Once the skin has been removed, the incision is closed with sutures. Report the surgical excision without the use of a clamp or other device with 54160 (neonate) or 54161 (except neonate).

QUICK CHECK 9-2

Circumcision code 54160 is used for infants aged _____ days or less.

Introduction. Introduction codes (54200-54250) are used to report various injection procedures, irrigations, plethysmography, and other tests. An example would be an injection procedure for Peyronie disease in which steroids are injected into the fibrous tissue of the penis to decrease pain, deformity, and fibrous tissue size. There are two ways the fibrous tissue can be injected: the first way is to inject steroids directly into the area of the lump formed by the fibrous tissue (54200), and the second way is to first expose the fibrous tissue through an incision and then inject steroids into the fibrous tissue (54205).

Priapism is a state of prolonged erection that can last from hours to days because of the inability of the blood to flow from the penis, which returns the penis to a flaccid state. The condition may be caused by medications used to treat impotence, such as sildenafil citrate (Viagra) or medical conditions, such as leukemia, multiple myeloma, or tumor infiltrate. If medical intervention is necessary, the surgeon introduces a large needle into the corpus cavernosum and aspirates blood. (This is what is keeping the penis erect.) The corpus cavernosum is then irrigated with a saline solution. The entire procedure is reported with 54220.

Repair. Repair category (54300-54440) contains codes for various repairs made to the penis. The Repair procedure code descriptions often state the condition for which the procedure is being performed. For example, 54304 is plastic repair for correction of chordee or a first-stage hypospadias (defined in next paragraph) repair, and 54380 is plastic repair for epispadias. Also many other codes in the Repair category indicate the stage of the procedure.

Many of the Repair codes refer to repair of chordee and hypospadias. **Chordee** is a condition in which the penis has a ventral (downward) curve and is a congenital deformity. **Hypospadias** is a congenital abnormality in which the urethral meatus (opening) is abnormally placed, usually along the ventral aspect (underside) of the shaft. Degrees of hypospadias are classified according to location: anterior, middle, or posterior. Hypospadias may lead to chordee. The farther from the glans penis the opening is, the more chordee. Read the code descriptions for Repair codes carefully as many of the descriptions have only slight differences.

Codes in the range 54400-54417 are used to report insertion, repair, or removal of various types of penile prostheses. The codes are divided based on the type of service and often on the circumstances of the service. Erectile dysfunction (impotence) is a condition in which the penis does not become erect. Impotence may be caused by a variety of conditions, such as obesity, chronic illness, or as a result of medication. One surgical solution to impotence is insertion of a **penile implant**. There are various types of penile implants, but mainly there are two broad categories: non-inflatable (malleable or flexible, 54400) and inflatable (54401). These implants are inserted deep within the penile tissue. When the implant is subsequently removed, the removal procedure is reported with 54406 (inflatable) or 54115 (non-inflatable).

On occasion, removal and replacement are accomplished during the same operative session. Removal of a previously placed prosthesis with insertion of a new prosthesis during the same operative session is reported with 54410, 54411 (inflatable) or 54416, 54417 (non-inflatable).

QUICK CHECK 9-3

When coding for penile prostheses the code selection is determined by the type of implant, which may be _____ or _____, and the type of service insertion, repair, removal, and/or replacement.

Testis

Excision. The Excision category (54500-54535) of codes is used to report services such as biopsy, excision, orchiectomy, and exploration of the testis. Biopsies may be percutaneous (54500) or incisional (54505). If incisional biopsies of the testis are performed bilaterally, report modifier -50 with 54505.

Extraparenchymal is defined as unrelated to the essential elements of an organ. Removal of an extraparenchymal lesion of the testis is reported with 54512. An incision is made on the scrotum, and the testicle is pulled out through the incision where the tunica vaginalis is opened and the lesion removed. The testicle is retuned to the scrotum and the area is sutured closed.

An **orchiectomy** is the removal of a testis. CPT codes 54520-54535 report orchiectomies if the procedure was simple/radical, unilateral/bilateral, with/ without testicular prosthesis insertion, and the approach used to gain access to the site. Watch for codes that specify unilateral or bilateral. For example, a simple orchiectomy with or without testicular prosthesis insertion (54520) reports a unilateral procedure. When the procedure is bilateral, modifier -50 must be added to correctly report the procedure. However, a radical orchiectomy as reported with 54530 reports the removal of both testes and does not require modifier -50.

Repair and Laparoscopy. **Undescended testis** (cryptorchidism) is a congenital condition in which the testis(es) did not descend into the scrotal sac. The condition may be unilateral or bilateral. The testis(es) may remain in the abdominal, inguinal, or prescrotal areas or may move back and forth between areas. Often, undescended testis is associated with a hernia. During the hernia repair procedure, the undescended testis is brought down into the scrotum where it is anchored with sutures (orchiopexy). An exploration may be necessary to locate the undescended testis(es) and the choice of CPT codes (54550, 54560) is determined based on the approach used (inguinal/scrotal or abdominal) to gain access to the area. The exploration codes report a unilateral procedure, so if a bilateral procedure was performed, add modifier -50. During an exploration, when no more definitive procedure is performed, it is only coded as an exploration. If the testis was located during the exploration and the surgeon moved the testis into the scrotal sac, the procedure is no longer an exploration, but it has become a corrective procedure (orchiopexy). An orchiopexy is reported with codes from the Repair category or the Laparoscopy category, depending on the technique used. An orchiopexy in which the operative site is opened to the surgeon's view is reported with 54640 or 54650 depending on whether the approach was inguinal or abdominal. If the orchiopexy is performed laparoscopically, report the procedure with 54692.

QUICK CHECK 9-4

If during an exploratory procedure the testis is located and moved to the scrotal sac, the procedure becomes the corrective procedure an

_____.

Epididymis

The **epididymis** is a narrow, coiled tube that connects the efferent ducts at the back of each testicle to the vas deferens. The epididymis is divided into the caput (head), corpus (body), and cauda (tail). The epididymis can become infected, inflamed, or obstructed. When an abscess or hematoma forms in the epididymis, the surgeon may incise and drain the area (54700). At times, the testis, scrotal space, and epididymis are the site of abscess or hematoma. When any or all of these areas are incised and drained, the service is reported with 54700. For example, if the surgeon incised and drained the scrotal space, the service is reported with 54700. Or, if the surgeon incised and drained the testis, scrotal space, and epididymis, the service is reported with 54700. The one code reports incision and drainage of *each* or *all* of the areas.

QUICK CHECK 9-5

Code _____ is used to report incision and drainage of abscess or hematoma of the testis, scrotal space, and/or epididymis.

Excision. The Excision category (54800-54861) of the Epididymis codes reports biopsy, exploration (with/without biopsy), lesion or spermatocele excision, and unilateral or bilateral removal. A spermatocele is a cyst that contains sperm, and during the excision of the cyst the epididymis may or may not be removed depending on the damage to the area caused by the presence of the cyst. Code 54840 reports the excision of a spermatocele with or without an epididymectomy.

Repair. Repair to the epididymis is an **epididymovasostomy**, also known as vasectomy reversal. During epididymovasostomy, the epididymis is connected to the vas deferens. The surgical procedure is reported with 54900 or 54901 depending if the procedure was unilateral or bilateral. An operating microscope is often used during this procedure and is reported separately with 69990.

Tunica Vaginalis

Incision. The **tunica vaginalis** is a serous sheath of the testis, which can be the site of hydrocele (fluid collection). The physician may aspirate the fluid or inject a substance such as a sclerosing agent (55000) to help prevent further accumulation of fluid. Another method of management of a hydrocele is excision (unilateral, 55040 or bilateral, 55041), which may be accompanied by a hernia repair that is reported separately (49495-49501).

Repair. A **Bottle type** repair (55060) is a surgical procedure performed to remedy a hydrocele of the tunica vaginalis. An incision is made in the inguinal or scrotal area, and the hydrocele is drained and repositioned. A catheter may be left in place to ensure continued drainage of the area and to prevent further fluid accumulation.

Scrotum

Incision. The **scrotum** is the sac that contains the testes. If a lesion of the skin of the scrotum is removed, use codes from the Integumentary System to report the service. However, if the abscess is in the scrotal wall and requires drainage report the procedure with 55100. If the abscess is of the epididymis, testis, and/or scrotal space, report the service with 54700.

Repair. Scrotoplasty, also known as oscheoplasty, is repair of a congential abnormality or traumatic defect of the scrotum. Skin flaps may be utilized during a simple repair (55175) and in the more complex repair (55180) rotational pedicle grafts and/or free skin grafts may be used. Simple skin flaps are included in the scrotoplasty and are not reported separately, but the more complex grafts are reported in addition to the scrotoplasty.

Vas Deferens

Incision. The **vas deferens** is the tube that conducts the sperm from the testes to the urethra. A vasotomy is cutting into the vas deferens. Usually the procedure is performed to obtain a semen sample or to determine if the tube is obstructed. Code 55200 also includes cannulization of the vas deferens. The code describes a unilateral *or* bilateral procedure, so there is no need for modifier -50 with this code.

Excision. A **vasectomy** is a procedure in which a section of the vas deferens is removed for purposes of sterilization. A small incision is made on the scrotum, and the vas deferens is identified and brought out through the incision. A section of the cord is removed, and the vas deferens is returned to its natural position. The procedure is reported with 55250 and includes a unilateral or bilateral procedure and postoperative semen examination(s).

Introduction. A **vasotomy** may also be performed for a **vasogram**, vesiculogram, or epididymogram in which colored dye is traced through the vas deferens to visualize any obstruction. The vasotomy is reported with 55300, and the radiological supervision/interpretation is reported separately with 74440.

Repair. A **vasovasostomy** or **vasovasorrhaphy** is a procedure performed to remove obstruction from the vas deferens. Injection of dye is often used during the procedure to identify the area of blockage. Once the area is identified, it is removed, and the ends of the vas deferens are anastomosed (reconnected end to end). Semen sampling may be conducted to ensure the removal of the blockage. A unilateral procedure is reported with 55400, so modifier -50 should be added to indicate a bilateral procedure. An operating microscope is often used during the procedure and is reported separately with 69990.

Spermatic Cord

Excision and Laparoscopy. The **spermatic cord** is a collection of structures that suspends the testes in the scrotum as illustrated in Fig. 9–4. The spermatic cord may be the site of formation of a hydrocele, lesion, or varicocele. Unilateral excision of a spermatic cord hydrocele is reported with 55500 with modifier -50 added to report a bilateral procedure. A **varicocele** is a mass of enlarged vessels that occurs when the valves that control blood flow in and out of the vessel become defective, and the blood is not able to circulate out of the vessel. The trapped blood causes the vessel to swell. Excision of a varicocele by means of a scrotal approach is reported with 55530, and an abdominal approach with 55535. A hernia repair may be performed during the same operative session, and with other procedures in this section has been reported separately. However, there is a single code (55540) to report both the varicocele excision and a hernia repair. If the varicocele is repaired using surgical laparoscopy, report the procedure with 55550.

Seminal Vesicles

The **seminal vesicles** are a pair of glands that are located posterior to (behind) the bladder. The glands provide the majority of the fluid that becomes semen and empties into the urethra.

Incision. A **vesiculotomy** is surgical cutting into the seminal vesicles. The approach can be by an incision into the lower abdomen or the perineum (between the anus and scrotum). Frequently, the procedure is performed to relieve pressure due to inflammation. There are two codes to report a vesiculotomy based on the extent of the dissection required to accomplish the procedure. If the procedure required simple dissection, report 55600, and if complicated dissection was required, report 55605. The codes are unilateral, so a bilateral procedure requires modifier -50.

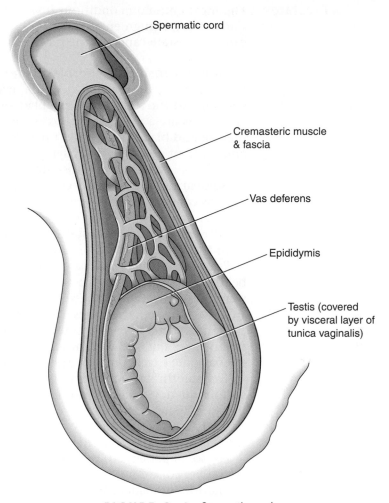

Spermatic cord

Cremasteric muscle & fascia

Vas deferens

Epididymis

Testis (covered by visceral layer of tunica vaginalis)

FIGURE 9–4   Spermatic cord.

QUICK CHECK 9-6

A vesiculotomy may be performed by incision either in the lower _____ area or the _____ (between the anus and scrotum).

Excision. A **vesiculectomy** is the removal of one of the seminal vesicles. The procedure is performed to remove a tumor, calculus (stone), or other obstruction. The approach may be through the lower abdomen or perineum, but the choice of codes is the same (55650) because the code description indicates "vesiculectomy, any approach." The code reports a unilateral procedure, so modifier -50 is required for a bilateral procedure.

The **Mullerian ducts** develop prenatally in females, and the Wolffian ducts degenerate. In males it is the opposite, the Wolffian ducts develop, and the Mullerian ducts degenerate. The Mullerian system develops into oviduct, uterus, and upper vagina. The Wolffian ducts develop into epididymis, vas deferens, and seminal vesicles. In some males a remnant of the Mullerian duct remains, and a cyst may form at that site. The cyst may be excised using a lower abdominal or perineal approach and reported with 55680.

Prostate

The most common conditions involving the prostate are inflammation (prostatitis), benign enlargement (BPH, benign prostatic hypertrophy), and cancer. Prostate cancer is the most common type of cancer in men.

Benign Prostatic Hyperplasia and Prostatectomy. The symptoms of BPH are urinary frequency, nocturia, urgency, decreased force of urine stream, and the feeling that the bladder has not completely emptied. These symptoms are a result of the excess prostate tissue pressing against the urethra and bladder. Treatment for BPH is based on the degree of prostate enlargement and severity of symptoms. Minimally invasive treatments include balloon dilation, prostatic stents, and thermal based therapies. If these treatments are not successful, surgical intervention may be necessary, such as coagulation, transurethral resection, laser vaporization, or open surgical procedure.

BPH treatment and prostatectomies procedures are reported with codes from the Urinary System and/or the Male Genital System:

Prostatic **stents** (52282) are flexible metal mesh tubes that are designed to be inserted into the urethra at the level of the prostate and expanded. The stent keeps the urethra open. Over time, the urothelial tissue grows over the stent and the stent becomes incorporated into the urethral wall.

Transurethral microwave heat treatment (**TUMT**, 53850) is the use of microwaves that are sent through a catheter and introduced into the urethra to coagulate excess prostate tissue and allow the urethra to be less constricted.

Transurethral needle ablation (**TUNA**, 53852) is a procedure that utilizes radiofrequency to create heat that is applied to the prostate to destroy excess prostate tissue. During this procedure the urethra is punctured to allow the needles to be placed directly into the prostate. The needles are insulated, so the urethra is not damaged when pierced.

For some patients these less radical treatments are not effective or advisable. For example, for patients with renal insufficiency, recurrent gross hematuria, or bladder stones because of BPH, a surgical procedure is the recommended treatment option. Surgical therapies include transurethral prostate incision, electrovaporization, and laser ablation/coagulation. Let's do a closer review of each of these surgical options:

Transurethral resection of the prostate (**TURP**, 52601, 52630) is the gold-standard of surgical procedures for removal of tumor or prostatic tissue. A special type of cystoscope is inserted through the urethra. The scope has lights, valves for controlling irrigation fluids, and an electrical loop to remove obstructions and cauterize blood vessels. For the first stage of a **TURP,** report 52601; for partial **TURP,** report 52601 with modifier -58 (reduced service); and for resection of residual or regrown tissue, report 52630.

Transurethral incision of the prostate (**TUIP**, 52450) is used when the prostate is slightly enlarged. Two incisions are made in the prostate to relieve the pressure on the urethra without removing tissue.

When a laser is used to accomplish the prostatectomy, the choice of codes is first based on whether the procedure was a *coagulation* (52647) or *vaporization* (52648). Code 52648 includes vaporization with or without transurethral resection of the prostate.

LASER *COAGULATION* (52647)

- Transurethral ultrasound-guided laser induced prostatectomy (TULIP, non-contact) is a procedure in which a laser is used to *coagulate* prostate tissue. There is no direct visualization of the prostate using this method, and the penetration is not as deep as with other more commonly performed methods.

▪ Visual laser of the prostate (VLAP, non-contact) is under the direct vision of the surgeon, but the laser fiber does not come in direct contact with the prostate. This method *coagulates* the tissue rather than vaporizing it. Once coagulated, the tissue dies and is sloughed off, which relieves the pressure.

▪ Interstitial laser coagulation of prostate (ILCP, contact) uses several laser fibers that are placed directly into the prostate to coagulate the tissue. There is no direct visualization with the ILCP.

QUICK CHECK 9-7

Code 52647, laser coagulation of the prostate, may be accomplished by one of three techniques: TULIP (non-contact, no direct visualization), _____ (non-contact, direct visualization), or _____ (contact, no direct visualization).

LASER *VAPORIZATION* (52648)

▪ Transurethral vaporization of the prostate (TUVP or TVP, contact) uses electrical current to *vaporize* tissue of the prostate by means of a ball that is rolled over the tissue. The ball contains a current that vaporizes the tissue. This procedure is a modification of a TURP.

LASER *VAPORIZATION WITH/WITHOUT RESECTION* (52648)

▪ Holmium laser enucleation of the prostate (HoLEP, contact), also known as transurethral holmium laser resection (THLR), is a procedure used to resect prostate tissue by means of a holmium laser fiber. There is less intraoperative bleeding with this procedure than with a TURP.

There are many different techniques used to remove the prostate (prostatectomy). Codes in the Excision category (55801-55845) represent open surgical procedures. Determination of the correct code to report a prostatectomy (removal of the prostate) is based first on the approach (perineal, suprapubic, or retropubic).

▪ Perineal approach is through the space between the rectum and the base of the scrotum, and it is used to gain access to a prostate that is located closer to the perineal area.

▪ Suprapubic approach is through the lower abdominal region, and it is used to gain access to the front (anterior) surface of the bladder. The access to the prostate is gained by an opening in the bladder neck.

▪ Retropubic approach is also through the lower abdominal region and is used to gain access to the front (anterior) of the prostate.

Once the correct approach has been identified, the extent of the procedure will determine code selection. The term subtotal used in many of the code descriptions means anything less than the total prostate is removed, and the term radical means total removal of the prostate.

QUICK CHECK 9-8

There are different approaches to an open prostatectomy. Match the approach with the definition.
1. Perineal _____
2. Suprapubic _____
3. Retropubic _____

a. Through the lower abdominal region to gain access to the anterior prostate
b. Through the space between the rectum and the base of the scrotum
c. Through the lower abdominal region to gain access to the anterior surface of the bladder, opening the bladder neck to access the prostate

Codes 55812-55815 and 55842-55845 include code selection based on the lymph node biopsy/removal performed. If lymph node biopsy (single or multiple) and limited removal of pelvic lymph node(s) was performed, report 55812 (perineal approach) or 55842 (retropubic approach). If lymph nodes were removed bilaterally and include the external iliac, hypogastric and obturator nodes, report 55815 (perineal approach) or 55845 (retropubic approach).

A laparoscopic retropubic prostatectomy (**LRP**, 55866) is a minimally invasive procedure that may be utilized instead of an open procedure. Robotic assisted prostatectomy (**RAP**) is a new development used with LRP and is designed to assist in the performance of some surgical tasks. Several small incisions are made through which robotic instrumentation is inserted. The surgeon operates the instrumentation from a console. The use of RAP necessitates an assistant during surgery. Surgeons who use a RAP system are trained by the manufacturer of the system before using the system during surgery. The training is extensive, but the new robotic systems enhance the precision with which the procedure can be performed. One such robotic system is the da Vinci® prostatectomy system and a video about the procedure can be viewed at *http://www.davinciprostatectomy.com/video.html*.

Now that you have reviewed BPH treatment and prostatectomies, let's review the remaining codes in the Prostate category.

Biopsy. Biopsy of the prostate may be performed with a needle, punch, or by incision. Report a prostate biopsy with 55700 (needle, punch), 55705 (incisional), or 55706 (transperineal, stereotactic). Do not report these codes during the same procedure. For example, if, during the same operative session, a needle or punch biopsy of the prostate (55700) is undertaken, and it is followed by an incisional biopsy (55705) either to supplement or to obtain adequate tissue, the appropriate CPT code to report is 55705, not both codes. Do not confuse a prostate biopsy with a fine needle aspiration (**FNA**). During a FNA, fluid is withdrawn for analysis and is reported with 10021 or 10022.

QUICK CHECK 9-9

Biopsy of the prostate may be accomplished by one of three methods: incision, _____, or _____ stereotactic.

A **prostatotomy** is an incision into the prostate. Codes 55720 and 55725 describe prostatotomies performed to drain an abscess. The surgeon inserts a needle into the prostate via the perineum or through the rectum. Reporting of the procedure is based on if the procedure was simple or complicated. A complicated prostatotomy would document excess bleeding or other factors that increase time and effort necessary to complete the service.

Brachytherapy. Brachytherapy (55860-55865) is a type of radiation treatment for prostate cancer and utilizes high dose rate (HDR, temporary method) or low dose (permanent seeds) and may be used in combination with biopsy/removal of lymph nodes. The placement of the brachytherapy element(s) can be accomplished by transperineal placement or with open exposure of the prostate. The transperineal (through the area between scrotum and anus) placement involves the fastening of a template to the perineal area. The template contains a pattern of holes that indicate where the catheters or needles are to be placed to correctly access the area around the prostate. Approximately 100 permanent seeds are placed for the low dose method.

For the high dose method of temporary delivery, small catheters are placed into the prostate, and a series of radiation treatments are delivered. For example, a patient would present to an outpatient department of the hospital where a template would be fastened to the perineal area. The catheters would be inserted through the holes in the template into the prostate. The treatment plan is established by the physician, and the computer that is attached to the catheters is set to deliver the prescribed dose of radiation. If the prescribed dose cannot be administered in one session, the catheters remain in place, and the patient remains in the hospital overnight. The next day, the patient would receive another radiation treatment. The catheters would be removed, and the patient would be discharged from the hospital. An advantage of the HDR is that the physician can regulate the radiation dosage more precisely than with the low dose method.

The transperineal placement is reported with 55875 and includes the use of a cystoscope if applicable. The placement of the radioelements is reported separately with 77776-77787. If ultrasound guidance is used during the placement, the guidance is reported separately with 76965, ultrasonic guidance for interstitial radioelement application.

Another approach for placement of radioactive substances is the open approach in which the prostate is viewed by the surgeon. The exposure procedure is reported with 55860, and the application of the radioelements is reported with 77776-77778, based on the number of sources placed: simple (1-4), intermediate (5-10), complex (>10). During the same operative session in which the radioelements are placed, the surgeon may biopsy lymph nodes and/or may perform a lymphadenectomy (55862). If a bilateral pelvic lymphadenectomy is performed and includes the external iliac, hypogastric, and obturator nodes, the procedure is reported with 55865.

Transrectal ultrasound (**TRU**, 76872, 76873) is guidance that is often used when reporting biopsy, evaluation and staging for prostate cancer, delivery of brachytherapy, evaluation or aspiration of prostate abscess, evaluation of infertility, diagnosis of prostate abnormalities, and monitoring of treatment response.

EXERCISE 9–1 *Male Genital System*

Using the CPT manual, code the following:

1 Simple orchiectomy with insertion of prosthesis using scrotal approach

Code: _____

2 Epididymis exploration without biopsy

Code: _____

3 Aspiration of fluid sac on the testicular covering

Code: _____

4 Extensive electrodesiccation of a condyloma on the penis

Code: _____

5 Reversal of previously completed vasectomy, bilateral

Code: _____

6 A 75-year-old male patient presents with a PSA of 8.1. He has a 100-gram prostate, and 1 out of 10 cores were positive for adenocarcinoma. The patient was placed in the supine position and a number 20 French Foley catheter was inserted into the bladder. A lower abdominal midline incision was made and the retropubic space was entered. Bilateral pelvic lymphadenectomy was performed in the usual manner and included the external iliac, obturator, and hypogastric nodes. Lymph nodes were small and were sent for permanent section to pathology. The prostate was extremely large. The prostate was mobilized using blunt dissection technique. The area was closed in the usual manner. Pathology report later indicated primary malignant neoplasm of the prostate.

Code: _____

7 The diagnosis is azoospermia and the procedure bilateral testicular biopsies. The patient was given a general mask anesthetic, prepped and draped in supine position. Bilateral testicular cord blocks were performed. Beginning on the right side, a scrotal incision was made. The tunica vaginalis was identified, opened, and a stay stitch placed in the testis. A small incision was made, tubules delivered, resected and sent for permanent section. The testis, vaginalis, and skin were closed with 3-0 chromic. The procedure was repeated in identical fashion on the contralateral side.

Code: _____

8 The 68-year-old male patient presents with BPH. Two 18-gauge needles were affixed to the catheter, and by means of a rigid cystoscope, the needles were transurethrally inserted into the prostate. Radiofrequency waves were set at 490 kHz and 99° C was obtained. Ablation of the area was completed and the cystoscope withdrawn.

Code: _____

9 Patient presents for removal of a previously implanted semi-rigid penile implant.

Code: _____

INTERSEX SURGERY The Intersex Surgery subsection (55970-55980) is located after the Male Genital Surgery subsection and contains only two codes: one for a surgical procedure to change the sex organs of a male into those of a female and one for changing the sex organs of a female into those of a male. These procedures are very specialized and are performed by physicians who have special skills and training in the procedures.

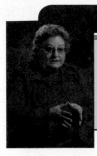

From the Trenches

"Be willing to learn everything there is to know. Medical terminology and anatomy/physiology are a must for the successful coder."

PATRICIA

Intersex surgeries include a series of procedures that take place over an extended period of time. The procedure for changing the male genitalia into female genitalia involves removing the penis but keeping the nerves and vessels intact. These tissues are used to form a clitoris and a vagina. The urethral opening is shifted to be in the position of that of a female.

The surgical procedure for changing the female genitalia into male genitalia involves a series of procedures that use the genitalia and surrounding skin to form a penis and testicle structures into which prostheses are inserted.

URINARY SYSTEM

Format

The Urinary System subsection (50010-53899) of the CPT manual is arranged anatomically by the subheadings of kidney, ureter, bladder, and urethra, with category codes arranged by procedure (i.e., incision, excision, introduction, repair). A wide range of terminology is used in the subsection because the four major subheadings have their own terminology (Fig. 9–5). The Glossary at the back of the book includes many of the terms that you will encounter

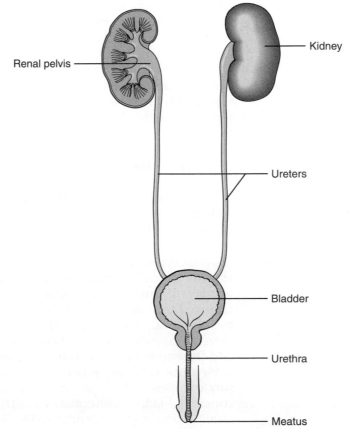

FIGURE 9–5 The four subheadings of the Urinary System subsection in the CPT manual are: Kidney, Ureter, Bladder, and Urethra.

in the CPT manual. Always be certain you know the meaning of all the words in the code description before you assign a code.

Kidney

The first subheading in the Urinary subsection is Kidney (50010-50593).

Incision. The Incision codes (50010-50135) are assigned to exploration, nephrostomy, drainage, nephrolithotomy, and pyelotomy services.

Renal exploration is a procedure that is utilized if the cause of a patient condition is unknown. An example of this is surgical exploration of an injured kidney when a patient is clinically unstable and appears to be losing blood from the kidney. Access for the exploration is from the side (flank). Note that a parenthetical statement preceding 50010 indicates "For retroperitoneal exploration, abscess, tumor, or cyst, see 49010, 49060, 49203, 49205." Code 49010 reports an exploration of the retroperitoneum. The term **retroperitoneal** refers to that area located behind (retro) the abdominal cavity. The retroperitoneal space may also be accessed by means of a flank incision or abdominal incision. When coding an exploration, you have to be careful to determine the exact anatomical location(s) explored to report the correct code(s). The kidney is located in the retroperitoneal space. If only the kidney was explored, report the service with 50010; if the retroperitoneal area was explored, report the service with 49010.

If the exploratory procedure becomes a definitive or corrective procedure, such as repair of a lacerated kidney, only the definitive procedure is reported. The exploration is considered a diagnostic procedure that is normally included in the definitive procedure when both are performed during the same operative session.

Open drainage of a perirenal or renal abscess (50020) specifically reports the drainage of a kidney abscess or the surrounding kidney tissue. If an abscess of the retroperitoneum was drained, the service would be reported with 49060. Again, the exact location of the abscess is the critical factor when assigning an abscess drainage code. The renal abscess can also be accessed percutaneously, which is then reported with 50021. When performing a percutaneous access of the kidney, fluoroscopy, ultrasound, or computer tomography may be used for guidance of needle placement and is reported separately with 75989. Also note that 50021 has the symbol next to it to indicate that conscious (moderate) sedation is included with the procedure and therefore is not reported separately.

A **nephrostomy** is a procedure that is used to decompress the renal system by means of inserting a catheter into the kidney while leaving the other end of the catheter outside the body to temporarily drain the kidney. The renal collecting system may be obstructed by a calculus or defect of the renal pelvis or ureter. Code 50040 reports an incisional placement of the drainage tube.

A **nephrotomy** is the exploration of the inside of the kidney. During this exploration, no definitive procedure is performed. For example, if the surgeon began the procedure as an exploration to determine the cause of urinary obstruction and identified a renal calculus (kidney stone) and removed the calculus, the procedure no longer would be an exploration but removal procedure 50060, kidney stone removal (nephrolithotomy). The surgeon may also do a renal endoscopy at the same time as the nephrotomy, and the endoscopy is reported separately with 50570-50580.

Nephrolithotomy procedures are removal of calculus (50060), secondary surgical operation for calculus (50065), a procedure complicated by congenital kidney abnormality (50070), and removal of a staghorn calculus (50075). The staghorn calculus (Fig. 9–6) is shaped like a deer antler and can become large and create extensive obstruction. If the calculus involves the renal pelvis and at least two calyces, it is classified as a staghorn calculi.

These types of stones account for about 30% of stones reported in the world and are usually associated with urinary infections. With a staghorn, a nephrolithotomy may be performed after extracorporeal shock wave lithotripsy (ESWL), which fragments the stones without incision (52352).

ESWL used to be performed with a machine in which the patient was submersed in a fluid. Newer machines do not require submersion, rather the patient is placed on an x-ray table, and a water-filled cushion is placed under the patient's back (Fig. 9–7). The procedure is performed in an operating room with a built-in ESWL machine. The procedure is performed under

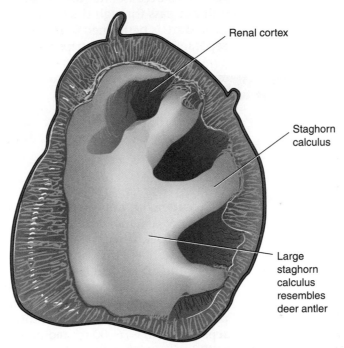

Renal cortex

Staghorn calculus

Large staghorn calculus resembles deer antler

FIGURE 9–6   Large staghorn calculus inside the kidney filling the pelvis and calyceal system.

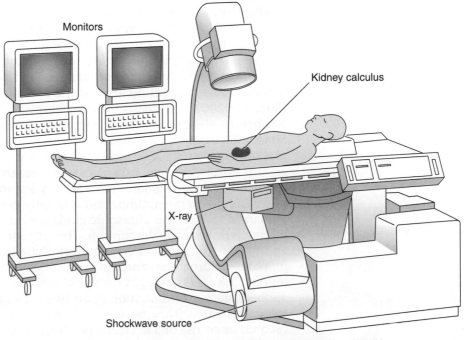

Monitors

Kidney calculus

X-ray

Shockwave source

FIGURE 9–7   Extracorporeal shockwave lithotripsy (ESWL).

general anesthesia. The shock waves are targeted to the stones by means of x-ray and pulverize the stones with repeated shocks. Usually, the particles subsequently pass through the urinary tract.

Percutaneous nephrolithotomy (nephrolithotripsy) is a method of treating kidney stones that is invasive and usually uses ultrasound. An incision is made over the kidney, and a probe is inserted. The shock waves then pulverize the stone. Electrohydraulic or mechanical lithotripsy may be used instead of shock waves, but the use of shock waves is the most often used method. A basket may also be attached to the probe, and the stones removed. Because the stone fragments of a staghorn are so large, they often will not pass through the urinary system, and an open or percutaneous procedure is performed to remove the fragments. The lithotripsy is reported separately (50590 lithotripsy or 52353 cystourethroscope with lithotripsy).

QUICK CHECK 9-10

When lithotripsy is performed to fragment kidney stones, the particles always pass out of the body through the urinary system.

True or False?

Percutaneous **nephrostolithotomy** (PCNL) or a **pyelostolithotomy** is a procedure to remove kidney stones. In this procedure, entry is through the patient's back. The procedure is reported based on the size of the stone removed (50080, to 2 cm; 50081, >2 cm). Internal lithotripsy is included in 50080 and 50081 and is not reported separately. External lithotripsy is not included in the codes and can therefore be reported in addition to the 50080 and 50081; but remember to attach modifier -51 to the lesser procedure. The procedure is performed with fluoroscopic guidance that is reported separately with 76000 for radiological physician time or 76001 for a radiological physician assisting a nonradiological physician.

Excision. There are Excision codes in the Kidney subheading for biopsy, nephrectomy (removal of the kidney), and removal of a cyst. The biopsy codes (50200, 50205) are based on the approach, either percutaneous (through the skin) or by surgical exposure of the kidney.

A **nephrectomy** is the removal of a kidney, either partial or radical (total). A radical nephrectomy includes removal of the fascia and surrounding fatty tissue, regional lymph nodes, and the adrenal gland. The nephrectomy codes (50220-50240) are all based on the complexity and extent of the procedure. Nephrectomies can also be performed by means of a laparoscope (50543, 50545-50548), based on whether the procedure was partial, radical, donor, and included a partial or total ureterectomy.

Ablation is, as previously discussed, the cutting away or erosion of tissue. Code 50250 reports ablation of a kidney lesion by means of cryosurgery (use of subfreezing temperatures) and is usually performed with ultrasonic guidance. If used, the ultrasonic guidance is not reported separately as it is included in the code description. The surgeon accesses the kidney through an incision and inserts a cryosurgical probe into the lesion. The cryosurgical machine is turned on, and subfreezing temperatures are delivered to the lesion. The area is brought back to above freezing, and the treatment is applied again. At times, more than two cycles are applied to ensure the lesion is ablated. This procedure can also be performed percutaneously (50593) or by use of a laparoscope (50542).

Renal Transplantation. Allotransplantation is the transfer of tissue or an organ between two people who are not related (genetically different). Autotransplantation is transfer of tissue from one part of a person's body to another part of that person's body. This is also known as autograft or autotransplant. A surgeon would perform a renal autotransplant to reposition the kidney, which may be necessary when the kidney has been severely damaged from trauma or disease. A renal autotransplantation is reported with 50380. If backbench procedures were performed, those services would be reported in addition to the transplantation service with modifier -51 added to indicate multiple procedures. Backbench work is the work involved in preparation for the transplant surgery and includes:

1. Open organ **retrieval** from a deceased (50300) or living (50320) donor; laparoscopic organ retrieval from a living (50547) donor.
2. Standard **preparation** based on deceased (50323) or living (50325) donor. As a part of this preparation the surgeon may perform additional surgery on the organ, such as venous, arterial, or ureteral anastomosis (50327-50329).
3. **Transplant** service reported with 50360 (without nephrectomy) or 50365 (with nephrectomy) with modifier -50 added for a bilateral procedure.

If the recipient requires a nephrectomy, the procedure is reported separately with 50340 with modifier -50 for a bilateral procedure.

Introduction. Introduction category codes in the Kidney subheading are for aspiration, catheters, injections for radiography, guides, and tube changes. There are extensive notes within the category, so you must be certain to read all notes when coding in this area.

Codes in the range 50382-50389 are percutaneous, transurethral, or externally accessible procedures that report removal and/or replacement of renal stents and tubes. These stents are not renal artery stents but are ureteral stents placed through the renal pelvis. The codes only report a unilateral procedure, so if a bilateral procedure was performed, add modifier -50. Imaging guidance is used for the codes in this range and is included in the code description, so be careful not to report the guidance separately. If imaging guidance was *not* used for removal and/or replacement of externally accessible stents, you would report the removal with an E/M code.

QUICK CHECK 9-11

An Evaluation and Management (E/M) code is used to report removal of an _____ accessible stent when imaging guidance is not used.

Approximately half of the population over age 50 has renal cysts that are asymptomatic and are often discovered as an incidental finding on ultrasound or computed tomography. When these cysts are symptomatic, percutaneous aspiration or injection may be performed. The procedure is performed by use of local anesthetic on an outpatient basis. A sclerosing agent (such as alcohol) may be injected into the cyst. The code description indicates "and/or," which means if both an aspiration and injection are performed at the same operative session, the code is reported only one time (50390). Image guidance is not included in the code description and is reported separately.

Repair. Repair category codes include plastic surgery (pyeloplasty), suturing (nephrorrhaphy), and closure of fistula.

Pyeloplasty is a surgical procedure for an obstruction of the ureteropelvic junction (UPJ), which connects the renal pelvis to the ureter. Usually, this is a congential condition, but it may also be an acquired condition. If an obstruction occurs the urine will not drain, which results in dilatation of the collecting system and enlargement of the renal pelvis (hydronephrosis). The goal of a pyeloplasty is to remove the obstruction and repair the renal pelvis (Fig. 9–8). As a part of the repair, a nephropexy (surgical fixation of mobile kidney), nephrostomy (a passageway from the kidney to exterior of the body), pyelostomy (a passageway between the renal pelvis and the exterior of the body), and ureteral splinting are included in the codes for a **simple** pyeloplasty (50400). A **complicated** pyeloplasty (50405) includes all of the procedures in the simple pyeloplasty, as indicated by the placement of the semicolon in 50400. Note that the semicolon is after the term splinting, which means that all the terms that precede the semicolon are included in the code description for the indented code 50405. In addition to all the procedures in the simple pyeloplasty, the **complicated** pyeloplasty is more difficult, because the procedure may be repair of a congenital kidney abnormality (which can be extensive), further plastic repair of the pelvis of the kidney, repair of a solitary kidney (patient only has one kidney), or a calycoplasty. A calycoplasty is repair of the calyx (the cup-shaped structure) of the kidney.

Closures of nephrocutaneous, pyelocutaneous, or nephrovisceral fistulas (abnormal opening) are reported with codes from the 50520-50526 range. Code 50520 reports the closure of a fistula between the renal pelvis and the exterior of the body or of the kidney and the exterior. Codes 50525 and 50526 report closure of a fistula between the kidney and another organ, such as the kidney and the bladder. The codes report the abdominal approach (50525) to close the fistula or a thoracic approach (50526).

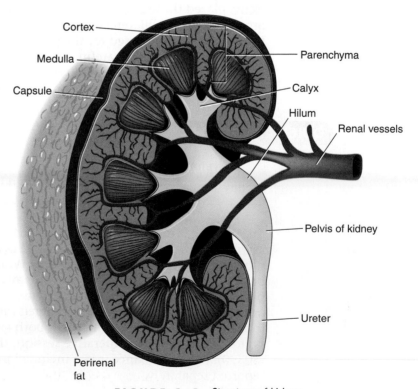

FIGURE 9–8 Structure of kidney.

Laparoscopy. The Laparoscopy codes report ablation of renal cysts (50541) or lesions (50542). Cryosurgical ablation is reported with 50250, and percutaneous ablation of renal tumors is reported with 50593. The code reports a unilateral procedure.

Laparoscopic nephrectomies and pyeloplasty are also reported with codes from in the Laparoscopy category and are based on the extent of the procedure.

Endoscopy. Endoscopy codes are frequently reported for various kidney procedures, because they are less invasive than the open procedures and are often performed on an outpatient basis. Renal endoscopies may be performed through an established connection between the kidney and the exterior of the body. The codes in the Endoscopy category are divided into those procedures performed through an established nephrostomy or pyelostomy and those that are not. The codes are then further divided based on the reason the procedure is being performed: ureteral catheterization, biopsy, fulguration, or foreign body/calculus removal. There is a code for renal endoscopy through an established access for resection of a tumor (50562) that does not have a counterpart in the range of codes for without established access.

The code descriptions in the Endoscopy category (50551-50580) indicate that these codes are "exclusive of radiologic service," which means that the radiologic services are reported *in addition to* the endoscopic procedures. If, for example, a ureteropyelogram was performed, you would report the service in addition to the endoscopy code.

QUICK CHECK 9-12

Renal Endoscopy codes 50551-50562 are used when the scope is inserted through an established _____ or _____ opening.

Kidney Index Locations. You will locate the kidney codes in the CPT manual index under "Kidney"; they are subtermed primarily by category (e.g., insertion, excision, or repair). Another method of locating kidney codes in the CPT manual index is to look under the medical term for the procedure (e.g., nephrostomy or nephrotomy). Again, there are other index location methods; these are just a couple to help you get started locating the codes.

Ureter

The next subheading (50600-50980) in the Urinary System subsection is Ureter. The category codes are based on procedure (i.e., incision, excision, introduction, repair, laparoscopy, or endoscopy). The ureter is the tube that leads from the kidney to the bladder and may be the site of an assortment of conditions, such as obstruction by calculus, cysts, or lesions in addition to reflux, congenital abnormalities, and fistulas.

Incision. The Incision codes are used to report open procedures to explore or drain (50600), insert indwelling stent (50605), and removal of calculus (ureterolithotomy) based on the location of the calculus as upper third, middle third, or lower third of the ureter (50610-50630). The incisional procedures also have laparoscopic, endoscopic, and/or transvesical counterparts. For example, to report a laparoscopic ureterolithotomy of the upper third of the ureter report 50945 and for an incisional ureterolithotomy report 50610.

Excision. The codes in the Excision category (50650, 50660) report ureterectomy either with bladder cuff or a total excision. The bladder cuff is the tissue that connects the ureter to the bladder, and the excision of the bladder cuff is only reported if it is the only procedure performed during the surgical session. A total ureterectomy may be performed by means of an abdominal, vaginal, or perineal approach or a combination of the three approaches.

Introduction. The Introduction codes include injection procedures, manometric studies, and change of tubes and/or stents. Code 50684 reports an **injection** procedure that is performed through an indwelling catheter to determine the status of the renal collecting system. The physician injects a contrast agent through the catheter and an x-ray is taken, which is reported separately with 74425.

Manometric studies (50686) are tests to measure kidney and ureter flow and pressure. The study is conducted by means of a machine (manometer) through an established access (ureterostomy or catheter). A tube carrying sterile fluid is inserted through the access site and into the kidney or bladder and the area flooded. Pressures are then measured.

Repair. Repair procedures include plastic repair of the ureter (**ureteroplasty**), **ureterolysis** (freeing fibrous tissue), revisions of surgical opening, **ureteropyelostomy** (connection of upper ureter to renal pelvis), ureterocalicostomy (connection of upper ureter to renal calyx), and uretero-ureterostomy (bypass of obstructed ureter), in addition to numerous other procedures to repair the ureter.

 CAUTION *Watch the Repair codes for use of modifier -50! Unless specifically stated the procedure is unilateral and requires modifier -50 for bilateral procedures.*

Laparoscopy. Laparoscopy procedures of the ureter are performed for placement of a ureteral stent (50947, 50948), which may be performed in conjunction with or without cystoscopic placement. The stent is placed because of an obstruction of the UVJ. The surgeon laparoscopically repositions the ureter on the bladder and then by means of the cystoscope places the ureteral stent.

Endoscopy. The Endoscopy codes (50951-50961) in this subheading are used for procedures that are performed through an established stoma (ureterostomy) or through an incision (50970-50980) into the ureter (ureterotomy). The procedures conducted through a ureterostomy are similar to the types of procedures conducted through a nephrostomy (e.g., 50551-50562, biopsy, catheterization, irrigation, and instillation). Excellent medical terminology skills are essential for working within this subheading, because the words can be intimidating. Keep your medical dictionary close by to look up any words you are not absolutely sure about. You can also refer to the Glossary at the back of the book. The time you spend now increasing the depth and breadth of your medical terminology vocabulary is an excellent investment and will greatly increase your coding accuracy.

The endoscopy procedures are for irrigation, instillation, catheterization, biopsy, fulguration, and foreign body or calculus removal. The procedures often utilize radiological services, but these services are reported separately. Note that the stand-alone code descriptions in the category (50951, 50970) indicate that the service is "exclusive of radiologic service" meaning that you report those services in addition to the procedure.

Bladder

The Bladder subheading (51020-52700) is next and contains category codes not only for the usual services, such as incision and excision but also for some unique services such as urodynamics and procedures performed on the prostate. Review the anatomy of the bladder in Fig. 9–9.

Incision/Removal. Aspiration of urine from the bladder may be accomplished by means of needle, trocar (a sharply pointed surgical instrument), or intracatheter (plastic tube with a needle on the end). A suprapubic (above the pubic bone) catheter may also be inserted during the aspiration service (51010). Aspirations are often performed by means of imaging guidance, which is reported separately.

Cystotomy (51020-51050) is often performed to fulgurate (use of electric current), insert radioactive material, or cryosurgically to destroy a lesion. In addition, the procedure is used for drainage, placement of catheter/stent, or a **cystolithotomy** (removal of calculus).

A **transvesical ureterolithotomy** (51060) is one that is performed through the bladder for the removal of calculus. The procedure is an open procedure that utilizes a midline incision of the abdomen. The calculus of the ureter is identified, and the surgeon makes an incision in the bladder and removes the calculus through the incision. Ureter calculus is also removed transvesically in 51065, but in this procedure the calculus is first fragmented by ultrasound or electrohydraulic means. Electrohydraulic fragmentation is the use of a probe containing two electrodes that are applied, one on each side, of the calculus. Electrical current is then directed through the electrodes, which fragments the calculus. Ultrasound is also used in a similar manner to fragment ureter calculus.

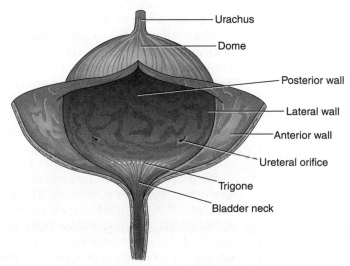

Urachus

Dome

Posterior wall

Lateral wall

Anterior wall

Ureteral orifice

Trigone

Bladder neck

FIGURE 9–9 Bladder anatomy.

Excision. A **urachal cyst** is between the umbilicus and bladder dome and is often diagnosed in young children when the cyst becomes infected. Because of the proximity to the abdominal cavity and potential to rupture, a urachal cyst is a condition that warrants prompt medical attention. A **urachal sinus** is a congenital abnormality in which prenatal tissue remains, causes drainage to the umbilicus, and results in infection and umbilicus drainage. The excision of a urachal cyst or sinus is assigned 51500 and may or may not include umbilical hernia repair.

Cystotomies and cystectomies (51520-51596) are performed for a variety of reasons, such as excision of a portion or all of the bladder, repair of a ureterocele, or to replant a ureter into the bladder. The codes are divided based on the extent of the procedure. If the procedure is performed transurethrally, such as a bladder resection, codes from the Transurethral Surgery category (52204-52318) should be assigned.

Pelvic exenteration (51597) is also known as total pelvic exenteration (TPE) and is the removal of the pelvic organs and adjacent structures due to malignancy. If the TPE is performed due to gynecologic malignancy, report the service with 58240. A hysterectomy may be performed with 51597, but the initial and primary reason the procedure is being performed is for other than a gynecological malignancy.

QUICK CHECK 9-14

Pelvic exenteration is reported with 51597, unless the diagnosis is a gynecologic malignancy, then code _____ should be reported.

Introduction. The **injection procedures** reported with codes 51600-51610 are for urethrocystography. The radiological supervision and interpretation are reported in addition to the injection procedure. Note that the parenthetical statements after each of the injection codes direct the coder to the correct code(s).

Insertion of bladder catheters may be non-indwelling (51701) or temporary indwelling (51702, 51703). The non-indwelling catheter is the type that is inserted into the urethra and manipulated into the bladder to drain residual urine. The temporary indwelling can be a simple catheterization (such as with a Foley) or a complicated catheterization (anatomical anomaly or catheter fracture). Catheter fracturing may occur when, for example, a patient pulls the catheter out.

Instillation is a procedure that is performed for bladder cancer where the anticarcinogenic agent is introduced into the bladder by means of a catheter. For example, immunotherapy is the instillation of a non-active tuberculosis agent into the bladder. The agent is retained in the bladder for a period of time with the patient in a lying position. The agent is then drained and the treatment is concluded. A series of these instillations is in a course of treatment. Code 51720 reports the instillation and the retention time.

Urodynamics. Urodynamics pertains to the motion and flow of urine. Urinary tract flow can be obstructed by renal calculi, narrowing (stricture) of the ureter, cysts, and so forth. The procedures in the subheading are to be conducted by or under the direct supervision of a physician, and all the instruments, equipment, supplies, and technical assistance necessary to conduct the procedure are bundled into the codes. If the physician performs only the professional service (e.g., interpretation of the results), modifier -26 (professional component) is used with the code to indicate that the technical portion of the service (performance of test or tests) was provided elsewhere. For example, if a physician provides only the interpretation (-26) of a urethral pressure profile (UPP) (51772), you would report the professional component of the service as 51772-26.

Repair and Laparoscopy. Repair procedures (51800-51980) include procedures such as cystoplasty (bladder repair), cystourethroplasty (bladder and urethra), vesicourethropexy/urethropexy (repair for urinary incontinence), and closure of fistulas.

Stress incontinence is surgically repaired by a colposuspension procedure in which a urethral sling is placed to support and elevate the UVJ (ureterovesical junction, where ureter joins with bladder). There are several types of these sling procedures, such as the Marshall-Marchetti-Krantz (MMK), Burch, paravaginal repair, anterior vesicourethropexy, or urethropexy. These procedures are reported with 51840 for a simple procedure and 51841 for a complicated repair, which would include a secondary repair of the bladder. The urethral suspension and sling operation are also performed by means of laparoscopy (51990, 51992). A sling operation for stress incontinence is also reported with 57288 when vaginal and abdominal incisions are used. A Pereyra procedure (57289) is also known as a needle bladder neck suspension in which sutures are used to support and anchor the bladder. The codes (57287-57289) are in the Female Genital System subsection, Vagina subheading because the procedure includes repair of the vagina. There are also codes in the Urethra subsection (53431-53442) that also refer to the creation, removal, or revision of a sling operation for male urinary incontinence and plastic repair of the bladder for incontinence.

Endoscopy. There are codes for bundled endoscopy procedures (i.e., cystoscopy, urethroscopy, and cystourethroscopy). The codes contain the primary procedure of a cystourethroscopy (endoscopic procedure to view the bladder and urethra) and minor related procedures or functions performed at the same time. For example, if a cystourethroscopy is done for biopsy of the ureter with radiography, bundled into the code for the procedure (52007) are catheterization, endoscopic procedure, and biopsy or biopsies. To unbundle individual components of the procedure would not be correct. If the secondary procedure(s) required significant additional time or effort, the procedure can be identified using modifier -22 (increased procedure). There are combination codes that include many components of a procedure. For example, 52005 reports a cystourethroscopy with ureteral *catheterization*, with/without *irrigation, instillation,* or *ureteropyelography* with the one code. Be careful to read the details of each description in this category before assigning the code to be certain you have identified each component included in the code before assigning the code or reporting additional services. For example, you cannot report a cystourethroscopy (52005) with a catheterization (51701) because a catheterization is included in the code description. Many third-party payers, such as CMS, have lists of codes (also known as edits) that cannot be reported with other codes. For example, 52000 (cystourethroscopy) cannot be reported with 51701 (catheterization), even though the catheterization is not stated in the code description. So, you need to know not only the limitations set by the notes and codes in the CPT manual but also the limitations set by the third-party payer. If the additional service(s) required a significant amount of additional time and effort, the service can be reported with modifier -22.

QUICK CHECK 9-15

To locate endoscopy codes in the CPT index, use the main terms
_____, _____, or cystourethroscopy.

CODING SHOT For a complete list of the CMS Correct Coding Initiative (CCI) edits, check out *http://www.cms.hhs.gov/National CorrectCodInitEd/.*

A cystourethroscopy is a diagnostic procedure to assess lower urinary tract symptoms (LUTS), such as incontinence or BPH. The procedure is reported only if it is performed as the only procedure during the operative session, because it is designated a separate procedure.

CODING SHOT Usually, third-party payers will not reimburse for more than two cystourethroscopic procedures per episode of illness unless bladder or urethral malignancies are being treated.

Transurethral Surgery. Transurethral Surgery (52204-52355) codes are for the urethra/bladder (52204-52318) and ureter/pelvis (52320-52355).

Code 52204 reports a cystourethroscopy with biopsy and, as you recall, 52000 is also a cystourethroscopy. The difference is that 52000 is a diagnostic procedure only. No additional procedure was performed when reporting 52000. When reporting 52204 a biopsy was performed, so the procedure was not diagnostic. The procedure may have begun as a diagnostic procedure, but it progressed to a biopsy on identification of a lesion. The diagnostic procedure is then bundled into the surgical procedure and not reported separately.

CODING SHOT Many third-party payers will bundle the code 52204 (diagnostic cystourethroscopy) into the more major procedure. For example, Medicare bundles the cystourethroscopy into the transurethral resection of a bladder tumor (52234-52240).

A **transurethral resection of a bladder tumor** (TURBT) is a procedure in which a bladder tumor is removed by fulguration (electric current) or excision. Note that the code descriptions 52234-52240 contain multiple methods of removal of the bladder tumor, i.e., "with fulguration (including cryosurgery or laser surgery) and/or resection." If any, or a combination of, these methods has been used to eradicate the tumor, you can assign a code based on the size of the bladder tumor. The code description indicates the size as minor (<0.5 cm), small (0.5-2.0 cm), medium (2.0-5.0 cm), and large (>5 cm). Code 52224 is a cystourethroscopy with fulguration or treatment of a minor (<0.5 cm) lesion(s). The lesion(s) are treated with cryosurgery or a laser. This procedure may or may not include a biopsy.

Many of the code descriptions require the coder to be familiar with the anatomy of the bladder and surrounding structures. For example, 52214 (cystourethroscopy) with fulguration (including cryosurgery or laser surgery) of trigone, bladder neck, prostatic fossa, urethra, or periurethral glands. Refer to Fig. 9–9 for bladder anatomy and location of the trigone and bladder neck. To code correctly the coder also needs to know the anatomy surrounding the bladder, such as the prostatic fossa, which is the depression or cavity (the bed) in which the prostate is located, also known as the prostatic bed.

The codes in the Ureter and Pelvis subsection (52320-52355) all include insertion and removal of *temporary* stents during the procedure, even though the code descriptions may not all state that fact. You know this only when you read the notes preceding code 52320. That does not mean that insertion and/or removal of *temporary* stents cannot be reported with other procedures, such as ESWL (50590), only that *temporary* stents are not reported separately with the codes in the 52320-52355 range. Make a note in your CPT manual next to this range of codes stating "includes insertion/removal of *temporary* stents" as a reminder of this important point. Insertion of indwelling stents is reported separately with 52332-51 in addition to the primary procedure. Code 52332 reports insertion of unilateral stents, so modifiers to indicate bilateral procedures were performed would also be needed; for example, 52332-51-50. To report removal of indwelling stents, use 52310 (simple removal) or 52315 (complicated removal) with modifier -58, staged or related procedure or service by same physician during the postoperative period. It is a good idea to place a bracket next to codes 52310 and 52315 and write "-58" as a reminder of how to report these codes, considering the direction for the use of this modifier with these codes is located in notes before code 52320.

Vesical Neck and Prostate. The Vesical Neck and Prostate codes 52400-52700 contain codes to report cystourethroscopy and transurethral procedures. Many of these codes were reviewed in the Male Genital System information because many of these procedures are of the prostate with access through the urethra, such as 52450, transurethral incision of the prostate.

When the procedure is a transurethral *resection* of the bladder neck, report 52500. If a transurethral *incision* of the bladder neck is performed, report 52276.

Urethra The subheading Urethra contains codes (53000-53899) for the usual procedures of incision, excision, and repair. For endoscopic procedures of the urethra, refer to codes 52000-52700, which contain cystoscopy, urethroscopy, and cystourethroscopy procedures.

If the physician performs the injection procedure for radiology studies for examination of the *urethra*, report 51600-51610 based on the type of study being performed. The radiological supervision and interpretation is reported separately with 74430 (cystography), 74450 (retrograde urethrocystography), or 74455 (voiding urethrocystography).

Incision. A meatotomy is surgical incision of the meatus, which is the opening of the urethra to the outside of the body (urethral meatus) and is often bundled into other more major procedures. Codes 53020 (except infant) and 53025 (infant) report a meatotomy if it is done as a separate procedure. Because 53025 is specifically for infants, do not append modifier -63, Procedure performed on infants less than 4 kg.

The **Skene's glands** are also known as the paraurethral or the lesser vestibular glands and are located on either side of the urethra. These glands drain into the urethra near the meatus (urethral opening). When infected, the gland will become enlarged and tender and may require drainage or excision. Drainage of an abscess or cyst of the Skene's glands is reported with 53060. Excision of the Skene's glands is reported with code 53270.

Excision. The Excision category of codes includes services such as biopsy, urethrectomy, lesion excision, fulguration, and marsupialization (creating a pouch).

When the urethra is totally surgically removed (urethrectomy), the service is reported with 53210 for a female and 53215 for a male. The procedure involves removal of the urethra and creation of an opening from the bladder to the skin that is then used to drain urine. The procedure would include removal of any tumors of the urethra. If the urethra was not removed and only the tumor was, report 53220.

The bulbourethral gland is also known as the Cowper's gland and is a pair of glands about the size of a pea that is located beneath the prostate. These glands produce some of the fluid for semen and drain directly into the urethra. Excision of the bulbourethral gland is reported with 53250.

Repair. A urethroplasty may be completed in one stage or two stages (53400-53431). The choice of codes to report a urethroplasty is based on the number of stages, type of repair, and for some codes, gender of the patient (53410, male; 53430, female).

Codes 53420 (first stage) and 53425 (second stage) report the two stages of an urethroplasty, and 53415 reports a one-stage urethroplasty.

A tandem cuff or dual cuff is an artifical urinary sphincter (AUS) that is placed due to atrophy, disease, or defect of the urinary sphincter and reported with 53444. An artificial sphincter that is inflatable and includes a pump, reservoir, and cuff, is inserted through a subpubic incision and is illustrated in Fig. 9–10. The small switch in the scrotum can be manipulated to activate the pump and control urinary continence. Codes 53446-53448 report the removal and/or replacement of AUS system, and 53449 reports repair of the system.

Urethromeatoplasty is repair of the meatus and the urethra (53450, 53460) and is performed to open and/or reconstruct the urethra.

Manipulation. The Manipulation category (53600-53665) has codes that are a bit different from those you have encountered previously. Manipulation is performed on the urethra (e.g., dilation or catheterization). Dilation stretches, or dilates, a passage that has narrowed. The Dilation

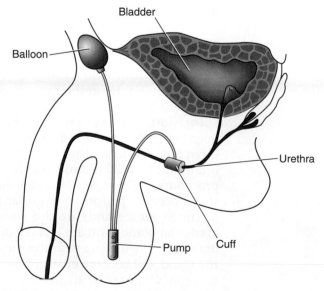

FIGURE 9-10 The cuff on the urethra squeezes the urethra closed.

codes are based on initial or subsequent dilation of a male or female patient. The catheterization codes in the Manipulation category are for either a simple or a complicated procedure.

EXERCISE 9–2 *Urinary System*

Using the CPT manual, code the following:

1 Needle aspiration of bladder

Code: _____

2 Endoscopy for establishment of a Gibbons ureteral stent

Code: _____

3 Repeat nephrolithotomy

Code: _____

4 Closure of a urethrostomy in a 54-year-old man

Code: _____

5 Second stage, surgical reconstruction of the urethra, with urinary diversion

Code: _____

6 The patient presents for a nephrostomy tube exchange. The patient was placed prone on the angiographic table and has preexisting left nephrostomy tube. The patient did not receive conscious sedation. The back was prepped and draped in the usual sterile fashion. A guide wire was advanced through the nephrostomy tube. The tube was exchanged, and the tube was secured to the skin with suture.

Code: _____

7 The patient presents with right renal calculus with stent for a right ESWL, cystoscopy, and stent removal. The patient was placed on the lithotripsy table and administered a general anesthetic. The stone was targeted, shock head engaged. Total of 2400 shocks at maximum kV of 24 were administered to the stone. Good fragmentation was noted. The patient was then prepped and draped in the supine position. The urethra was anesthetized with 2% Xylocaine jelly. The patient was cystoscoped with the flexible instrument; stent was visualized, grasped, and removed intact.

Codes: _____ and _____

8 The patient has been diagnosed with incontinence and presents for an urethropexy. The patient was brought to the operating room and placed on the operating table in the supine position, prepped, and draped. A small horizontal incision is made in the abdomen just above the symphysis pubis. The bladder was then suspended by placing sutures bilaterally at the mid-portion of the urethra 1 cm lateral and at the bladder neck 2 cm lateral. The sutures were then suspended to the Cooper's ligament bilaterally. The urethra was then elevated to the horizontal position.

Code: _____

9 The 33-year-old patient has postoperative diagnosis of left ureteral calculus and presents for a cystoscopy, bilateral retrograde pyelograms, left ureteroscopy, and stone extraction. The patient was cystoscoped using a 21-French instrument. There was no evidence of urethral or bladder abnormality. *Bilateral retrograde pyelograms* were performed that showed normal collecting system of the right-hand side. There was only a minimal suggestion of a filling defect in the distal ureter on the left. A guide wire was advanced up the ureter under fluoroscopic control and then a rigid short ureteroscope followed this. A stone was visualized and was entrapped in a basket and withdrawn under visual guidance.

Codes: _____ and _____

10 Cystoscopy, left retrograde pyelogram using contrast, under fluoroscopic control, insertion of left ureteral stent

Code: _____

DIGESTIVE SYSTEM

Format

The format of the Digestive System subsection (40490-49999) is divided according to anatomic site (Fig. 9–11) and procedure. Included in this subsection are codes for sites beginning with the mouth and ending with the anus.

Note that also included are those internal organs that aid in the digestive process, including the pancreas, liver, and gallbladder. This subsection includes codes for procedures of the abdomen, peritoneum, omentum, and all types of hernia repairs. Endoscopic codes can be found throughout the subsection on the basis of the anatomic site where the particular procedure is performed.

Lips. Codes in the Lips subheading (40490-40799) include the three categories of Excision, Repair (Cheiloplasty), and Other Procedures.

A **vermilionectomy** (40500) is shaving of the lip. The vermilion zone is the red part of the lips. The surgeon removes an area of tissue and repairs the defect by moving the mucosal surface to reconnect the lip, thereby forming a new vermillion border. If the area of defect is larger, a more extensive

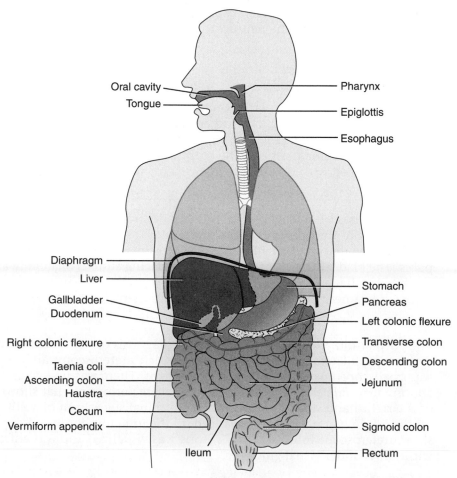

FIGURE 9–11 Digestive system.

excisional procedure may be necessary (40510-40527). For example, a **transverse wedge excision** (40510) is when a wedge of lip tissue is removed, and tissue flaps are used to repair the defect. The **Abbe-Estlander** (40527) is a reconstruction procedure in which a graft is taken from a portion of the lip and above the lip that is non-defective and is used to repair the area of defect that remains after an excision. For example, a patient has cancer of the lower lip caused by smoking, as illustrated in Fig. 9–12, *A*, for which the surgeon removes the area of defect from the lower lip and identifies a superior flap. In Fig. 9–12, *B*, the superior flap is moved to cover the area of defect. Fig. 9–12, *C*, illustrates the results of the reconstruction. If more than one-fourth of the lip surface is removed, the procedure is considered a resection and is reported with 40530. If **reconstruction** of the lip is required to repair the defect that remains after the resection, the procedure is reported with 13131-13153, complex repair of lip and face. The proper reconstruction code is selected based on location and size of the defect.

QUICK CHECK 9-16

Reconstruction of a lip defect may be accomplished with a local flap (same lip) or _____ flap (flap from upper lip to defect in lower lip).

The codes for **cheiloplasty** (lip repair) are located in the Repair category. There are two types of Repair codes: those that report full thickness repair of the lip (40650-40654) and those that report cleft lip repair (40700-40761). The full thickness repairs are based on the extent of the repair, for example, vermilion only, up to half of the vertical height of the lip, and over one-half of the vertical height of the lip, also known as complex repair. A cleft lip is a congenital defect in which the muscle and tissue of the lip did not close properly. Fig. 9–13, *A*, illustrates a unilateral defect and Fig. 9–13, *B*, illustrates a bilateral defect. Some of the cleft lip Repair codes report bilateral procedures (40701, 40702) and other codes report unilateral procedures (40700, 40720). If a bilateral procedure was performed and the code

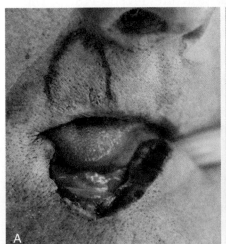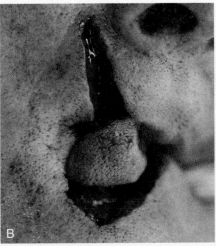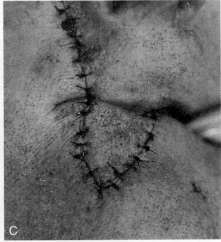

FIGURE 9–12 **A,** Abbe-Estlander flap for lip reconstruction with defective area excised and flap area outlined. **B,** Abbe-Estlander flap for lip reconstruction with flap moved down and positioned in defect area. **C,** Completed Abbe-Estlander flap. (From Kavanagh KT: Abbe-Estlander Flap for Lip Reconstruction in a Patient With Skin Cancer of the Lower Lip, *Ear Nose & Throat - U.S.A.* (website): http://www.entusa.com/abbe_estlander.htm. Accessed January 25, 2008.)

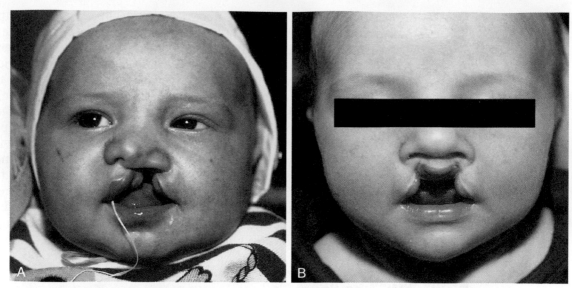

FIGURE 9–13 **A,** Unilateral cleft lip. Note the nasal deformity in which the nose is out of normal position. **B,** Bilateral cleft lip. (**A** and **B** from Zitelli BJ, Davis HW: *Atlas of Pediatric Physical Diagnosis,* ed 5, Philadelphia, 2007, Mosby.)

description does not indicate a bilateral procedure, add modifier -50. A **rhinoplasty** may be required if a nasal deformity has occurred with the cleft lip defect. This happens when the muscle, rather than encircling the mouth, attaches to the nose and pulls the nose out of normal position. If a rhinoplasty is performed with a cleft lip repair, the rhinoplasty is reported separately with 30460 or 30462. A **cleft palate** may also be present with a cleft lip, and if repair of the palate is performed at the time of the lip repair, the palate repair is reported separately with codes from the 42200 series. For example, 42205 is used to report a palatoplasty for a cleft palate with closure of alveolar ridge.

Vestibule of Mouth. The vestibule of the mouth is also known as the buccal cavity and is part of the oral cavity. Codes for the Vestibule of Mouth (40800-40899) do not include codes for services of the tongue and floor of mouth (41000-41599) or for dentoalveolar structures (41800-41899). The categories included within the Vestibule of the Mouth subheading are incisions (e.g., abscess, cyst, or hematoma), excision/destruction (e.g., biopsy, lesion excision), and repair (e.g., closure or vestibuloplasty). The procedures are based on the complexity of the procedure (e.g., simple or complex), and whether the procedure is bilateral or unilateral.

Tongue and Floor of Mouth. The Tongue and Floor of Mouth subheading (41000-41599) includes codes to report the incision and drainage of abscess, cyst, or hematoma of the tongue or floor of the mouth. These incision and drainage codes (41000-41009) are based on the location of the abscess, cyst, or hematoma, such as under the tongue **(sublingual)**, under the mandible **(submandibular)**, or within the space from the floor of the mouth to the hyoid bone **(masticator space)**. The sublingual is further based on whether the abscess, cyst, or hematoma is superficial or deep.

The **lingual frenum** is the flap of skin under the tongue. The procedure in which an incision is made in this flap is termed a frenotomy. The incision procedure (41010) would be performed to free the tongue to allow greater motion. During a frenotomy, the lingual frenum is only incised, not excised. If a frenectomy (excision of the lingual frenum) is performed, the service is reported with 41115 from the Excision category. If the lingual frenum is surgically repaired, the procedure is reported with 41520 from the Other Procedures category.

Extraoral incision and drainage (I&D) is performed on an abscess, cyst, or hematoma that is located outside the mouth or on the floor of the mouth. The codes in the 41015-41018 range report extraoral I&D based on the location of sublingual, **submental** (under the chin), submandibular, or masticator space.

Excision category (41100-41155) is for oral biopsies, excision of oral lesions, and removal of all or part of the tongue (glossectomy). Note that the biopsy codes (41100-41108) are reported based on the location from which the biopsy is obtained. The codes for excision of a lesion are also based on the location such as floor of mouth, tongue, or lingual frenum. If a local tongue flap is required to repair the excisional defect, report the repair with 41114 in addition to the excision.

Repair (41250-41252) of the tongue is reported based on the size of the repair (2.5 or less and over 2.6) and the location: anterior two thirds, posterior one third, or floor of mouth.

Dentoalveolar Structures. The dentoalveolar structures are the bone (osseous) and soft structures of the mouth that anchor the teeth. Codes 41800-41899 report incision, excision/destruction, and other types of procedures performed on the dentoalveolar structures. Examples of these procedures include drainage of an abscess, cyst, or hematoma (41800) or excision of a lesion with simple repair (41826). Some of the codes are based on the quadrant in which the procedure is performed, such as a gingivectomy (excision of the gingiva, 41820), each quadrant, or excision of the alveolar mucosa, 41828, each quadrant. Fig. 9–14 illustrates the alveolar mucosa.

Palate and Uvula. Services to the palate (roof of mouth) and uvula (pendulous structure at the back of the throat) are reported with codes 42000-42299. This subheading contains the usual codes for incision, excision, and repair. If grafting is required to repair the area of defect after excision of a lesion, the grafting service is reported *in addition to* the excision code. The choice of grafting codes is based on whether a skin graft (14040-14300) or an oral mucosal graft (40818) is used. Within the Repair codes you will also locate the codes to report the repair procedures for cleft palate (42200-42225), as discussed previously.

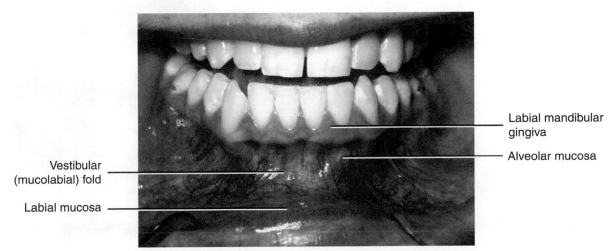

FIGURE 9–14 Alveolar mucosa. (From Liebgott, B: *The Anatomical Basis of Dentistry*, ed 2, St. Louis, 2001, Mosby, Inc.)

Salivary Gland and Ducts. There are three salivary glands as illustrated in Fig. 9–15 (parotid, submandibular, and sublingual). The codes in the Salivary Gland and Ducts subheading (42300-42699) are often divided based on the gland. For example, excision of a tumor of the parotid gland is reported with 42410; of the submandibular gland, 42440; and of the sublingual gland, 42450. Other services are reported on the number of glands involved. Examples are diversion of the parotid duct with excision of one submandibular gland (42508) or both submandibular glands (42509).

Imaging guidance may be used for salivary gland biopsy (42400) and is reported in addition to the biopsy service with 77002 (fluoroscopic), 77012 (CT), 77021 (MRI), or 76942 (ultrasound).

Pharynx, Adenoids, and Tonsils. It is within this range of codes (42700-42999) that you will locate the often reported codes for tonsillectomy and adenoidectomy, in addition to codes for biopsy, excision of brachial cleft cysts, pharyngoplasty, and pharyngostomy.

The Incision category (42700-42725) reports the drainage of an abscess and codes are assigned based on the **location** (peritonsillar, retropharyngeal/parapharyngeal) and **approach** (intraoral or external). Careful reading of the operative report is necessary to identify the location and approach to ensure correct code assignment.

The **biopsy** codes 42800-42806 include obtaining the biopsy sample but do not include the use of a scope. If a laryngoscopic biopsy is performed, the service is reported with 31510 (indirect laryngoscopy, that is viewing the larynx through reflection) or 31535, 31536 (direct laryngoscopy, that is viewing the larynx directly).

A **branchial cleft cyst** is a congenital defect that appears as a gill and is located on the neck. Branchia is Greek for gills, which the cyst resembles. Reporting an excision of the branchial cleft cyst is based on the extent of the procedure—the defect was confined to the skin and subcutaneous tissue (42810) or extended beneath the subcutaneous tissue and perhaps into the pharynx (42815).

Tonsillectomy and **adenoidectomy** are commonly reported surgical procedures (42820-42836). The tonsils are two glands located at the back of the throat (Fig. 9–16A), and the adenoids (Fig. 9–16B) are located behind the

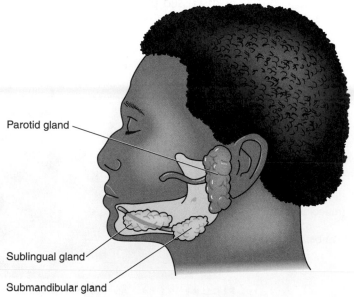

Parotid gland

Sublingual gland

Submandibular gland

FIGURE 9–15 Salivary glands.

nose and above the soft palate (roof of mouth) and cannot be visualized without a mirror or scope. The selection of the correct code is based on if only the tonsils are removed, only the adenoids are removed, or both the tonsils and adenoids are removed, and if the patient is over or under 12 years of age. Note that the code descriptions for some of the tonsillectomy and adenoidectomy procedures include the definition of "primary" or "secondary."

- **Primary** procedure—Tonsils/adenoids are removed for the first time.
- **Seconday** procedure—Tonsils/adenoid tissue has grown back and needs to be removed.

A **pharyngoplasty** (42950) is the surgical repair of the pharynx and includes the use of flaps fashioned from the skin, tongue, and/or tissue located near the area of defect (regional cutaneous flaps). If a pharyngeal flap is used, report the service with 42225.

A **pharyngostomy** (42955) is a procedure to create an opening for insertion of a long-term feeding tube. An incision is made below the jaw line on the skin and the incision is carried down to the pharynx. The opening is reinforced with sutures, and a long-term feeding tube is inserted through the opening into the pharynx. A nasogastric feeding tube is a more well-known method, but in some patients (i.e., severe facial trauma), pharyngostomy is the necessary approach.

Codes to report the control of oropharyngeal or nasopharyngeal hemorrhage are located in the Other Procedures subheading. The codes in the range 42960-42972 are reported based on if the procedure is a primary or secondary procedure and the level of complexity.

Esophagus. Procedures of the esophagus are reported with codes in the 43020-43499 range. The Incision codes include both a cervical approach (43020) and a thoracic approach (43045) for removal of a foreign body. It is important to confirm the approach used when coding removal of a foreign body from the esophagus. Some of the Excision codes also include various approaches in the code description, such as cervical, thoracic, and abdominal.

If a lesion is removed from the esophagus, report the service with 43100 (cervical) or 43101 (thoracic or abdominal) depending on the approach used. If a partial, near total, or total removal (wide excision) of the esophagus with

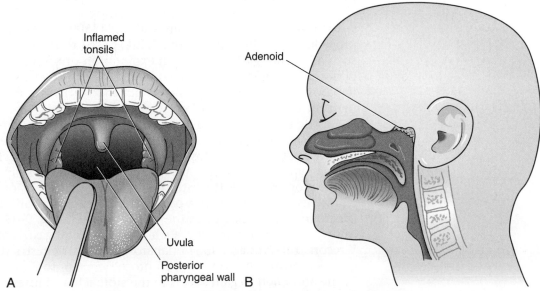

Inflamed tonsils

Adenoid

Uvula

Posterior pharyngeal wall

A   B

FIGURE 9-16 **A**, Tonsils. **B**, Adenoid.

the total removal of the larynx (may or may not include extensive [radical] neck dissection) is performed, the service is reported with 43107, 43116 (with graft), 43124, or 31360 (total laryngectomy). Note that some of these codes also specify the approach. For example, 43116 indicates a cervical approach.

The **Endoscopy** subheading (43200-43273) contains many codes to describe procedures that are conducted to diagnose or treat conditions of the esophagus and the hepatobiliary system.

The types of **esophagus** procedures are diagnostic endoscopy, injection, biopsy, removal of foreign body, insertion of plastic tube/stent, dilation, and hemorrhage control. Some codes, such as 43220 (balloon dilation), do not include imaging guidance (74360), whereas other codes include the guidance, such as 43231 (diagnostic esophagoscopy with endoscopic ultrasound examination). Note that many codes include conscious sedation as a part of the service as indicated by the bullseye symbol to the left of the code.

An endoscopic gastrostomy tube placement (43246) is a procedure in which an endoscope is passed through the patient's mouth into the esophagus and may progress to the stomach, duodenum, or jejunum. The endoscope is used to assist in the guidance of a percutaneous gastrostomy tube that is passed through the skin. Percutaneous gastrostomy tube placement (43750) is accomplished by a small incision made in the skin and a needle with a suture attached being passed through the incision into the stomach. The needle is snared and the needle and the suture are removed through the patient's mouth. The tube is then connected to the suture and then passed back through the mouth into the stomach and out the abdominal wall where the tube is then sutured to the skin.

An **endoscopic retrograde cholangiopancreatography** (ERCP, 43260-43272) is an endoscopic procedure of the pancreatic ducts, hepatic ducts, common bile ducts, duodenal papilla, and/or gallbladder (hepatobiliary system). The scope is advanced through the esophagus, into the stomach, to the duodenal papilla (papilla of Vater) and contrast is injected to visualize the bile ducts and biliary tract, including the gallbladder. Assignment of these codes is based on if the procedure was diagnostic or included a therapeutic procedure, such as dilation. The codes do not include the radiological supervision and interpretation, so if used, assign 74328 (biliary ductal system), 74329 (pancreatic ductal system), or 74330 (biliary and pancreatic ductal systems).

Stomach. The Stomach subheading (43500-43999) includes incisional procedures in which the stomach is exposed to the view of the surgeon, such as 43500 (gastrotomy with exploration or foreign body removal). Other procedures are performed by means of a scope, such as 43653 (laparoscopic gastrostomy). Be certain to identify the method used to perform the procedure before assigning a code.

Gastric bypass surgery is performed on patients who are morbidly obese with the outcome of decreasing the size of the stomach and/or intestines to aid with patient weight loss. There are many different techniques used for gastric bypass procedures. A **Roux-en-Y** (RNY) is a Y-shaped surgical connection in which the intestine is detached from its original origin and reattached so as to bypass a part of the stomach and all of the duodenum (first part of the small intestine) as illustrated in Fig. 9–17. This term is used in several code descriptions, such as 43621 (total gastrectomy with Roux-en-Y reconstruction) and 43644 (laparoscopic gastric restriction with Roux-en-Y gastroenterostomy). For an open procedure, a 6- to 9-inch incision is made in the abdomen to gain access to the stomach and intestines, whereas with a laparoscopic procedure about six access ports are established measuring

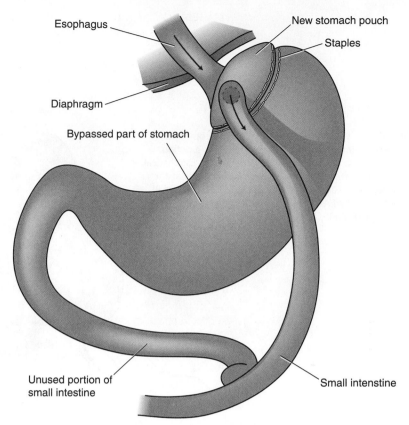

Esophagus

New stomach pouch

Staples

Diaphragm

Bypassed part of stomach

Unused portion of
small intestine

Small intenstine

FIGURE 9-17 Roux-en-Y (RNY) gastric bypass.

about ¼ to ½ inch each in diameter through which the surgical instruments are inserted. The laparoscopic procedures are much less invasive and decrease the time the patient spends in the hospital, recovery time, and complications.

Bariatric Surgery codes 43770-43774 are also procedures performed for morbidly obese patients and are gastric restrictive procedures that are accomplished by placing a restrictive device around the stomach to decrease its functional size. Code 43770 reports "placement of adjustable gastric restrictive device (e.g., gastric band and subcutaneous port components)." The band is adjustable because the band is hollow and contains a tube that can be inflated with fluid. After surgery, fluid is gradually inserted into the tube through a subcutaneous port (just beneath the skin) with a syringe. The physician can adjust the amount of fluid in the tube and thereby adjust the amount of food that can pass through the banded area. The procedure can be performed on an outpatient basis and can be reversed by removal of the banding apparatus.

Intestines (Except Rectum). Separate procedures are common in this subheading. Colostomies are always bundled into the major procedure unless the code specifically states to code it separately. For example, code 44141 is a partial colectomy with cecostomy or colostomy (creation of an artificial opening). Included in the description for 44141 is the establishment of the colostomy; thus, it would not be correct to report a separate code (44320) for the establishment of a colostomy.

Many procedures are performed through endoscopes (such as the gastroscopy in Fig. 9-18). Endoscope codes are available for procedures throughout the digestive system depending on how far down (through the mouth) or up (through the anus) the scope is passed. The code selection

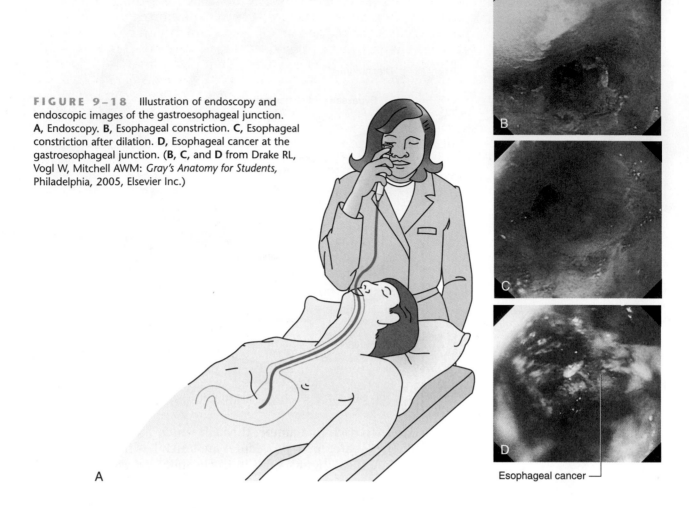

FIGURE 9–18 Illustration of endoscopy and endoscopic images of the gastroesophageal junction. **A,** Endoscopy. **B,** Esophageal constriction. **C,** Esophageal constriction after dilation. **D,** Esophageal cancer at the gastroesophageal junction. (**B, C,** and **D** from Drake RL, Vogl W, Mitchell AWM: *Gray's Anatomy for Students,* Philadelphia, 2005, Elsevier Inc.)

Esophageal cancer

varies according to the procedure(s) performed and includes the sites the scope passed through to accomplish the procedure. To choose the proper code, the **extent** of the procedure must be determined. For example, if a scope is passed to the esophagus only, the code would be chosen from the endoscopy codes 43200-43232. If the scoping is continued through the esophagus to the stomach, duodenum, and/or jejunum, the code selection would be from the endoscopy codes 43234-43259. Once the anatomic site of the endoscope procedure is correctly identified, the surgical procedure(s) performed guides the selection of the code. A surgical endoscopy always includes a diagnostic endoscopy, so do not code for both. Remember to use modifier -51 if more than one procedure is performed.

CODING SHOT To choose the correct endoscopy code from the Digestive System subsection, choose the farthest extent to which the scope was passed and then the procedure performed.

Resection of the intestine means taking out a diseased portion of the intestine and either joining the remaining ends (anastomosis) directly or developing an artificial opening (exteriorizing) through the abdominal wall.

Fig. 9–19 illustrates three types of anastomoses. The artificial opening (stoma) allows for the removal of body waste products (Fig. 9–20), as with the colostomy. The type of anastomosis or exteriorization depends on the medical condition of the patient and on the amount of intestine (large or small) that has to be removed. Some patients have temporary exteriorization for the length of time it takes the remaining small or large intestine to heal itself so it can perform the necessary functions. Other patients have permanent exteriorization because too much of the intestine has been removed to allow for adequate functioning. Openings to the outside of the body are named for the part of the intestine from which they are formed—colostomy is an artificial opening from the colon, ileostomy from the ileum, gastrostomy from the stomach, and so forth (Fig. 9–21). Therefore, to choose the correct code it is critical that you identify the correct anatomic site from which the ostomy originated, as well as the procedure used to establish the ostomy.

QUICK CHECK 9-17

The suffix for resection is _____.

Sometimes, a laparotomy is used as the approach in digestive system surgeries. When it is used as a surgical approach, a laparotomy is never coded separately. An exploratory laparotomy may be done to investigate the cause of a patient's illness. If only the exploratory laparotomy is performed, it is appropriate to report the service with an exploratory laparotomy code, such as 49000. However, if the exploratory procedure progressed to a more definitive surgical treatment (such as an appendectomy), only the definitive treatment (appendectomy) is reported.

Anastomoses

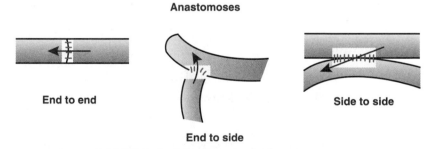

End to end

End to side

Side to side

FIGURE 9–19   Three types of anastomoses.

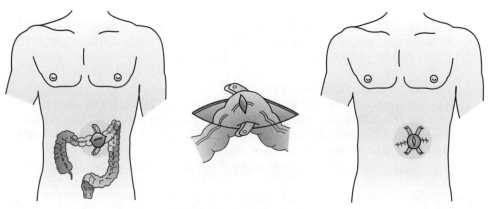

FIGURE 9–20   Stoma.

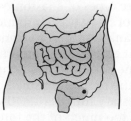
Sigmoid colostomy

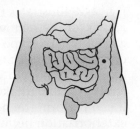
Descending colostomy

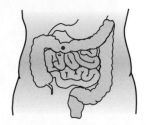
Transverse (single B) colostomy

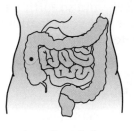
Ascending colostomy

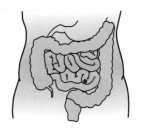
Ileostomy

FIGURE 9–21 Various ostomies.

EXERCISE 9–3 *Resections*

Using your knowledge of medical terminology, identify what the following procedures surgically accomplish:

1 Coloproctostomy _____

2 Ileostomy _____

3 Colostomy _____

4 Enteroenterostomy _____

Using the CPT manual, code the following:

5 Partial bowel resection with colostomy

Code: _____

6 Resection of small intestine, single resection, with anastomosis

Code: _____

7 A sphincterotomy and one quadrant hemorrhoidectomy for an anal fissure is performed. During the procedure an enlarged hemorrhoid/sentinel tag was noted at the 10 o'clock position and a fissure right at the base of this. Anoscope and a Kelly clamp were placed, and a sentinel tag excised. The defect was closed with sutures.

Code: _____

8 The patient presents for removal of sigmoid and rectal polyps. The Pentax video sigmoidoscope was inserted and four polyps were seen scattered between the rectum and proximal sigmoid colon. The largest measured about 1.5 cm in diameter. The others were diminutive, about 4 or 5 mm in diameter. Biopsies were taken of two of these polyps.

The pathology report indicated benign polyps.

Code: _____

Meckel's Diverticulum and the Mesentery. A Meckel's diverticulum is a fairly common congenital pouch on the wall of the small bowel and may contain pancreatic or stomach tissue and may be surgically removed (44800). The omphalomesenteric duct is included in the code description of 44800 and refers to the embryonic passage that connects an egg sac to the intestine of an embryo.

Appendix. Surgical procedures of the appendix may be accomplished by means of open procedures, such as 44900 (open I&D of abscess) or 44950 (open appendectomy); percutaneous procedures, such as 44901 (percutaneous I&D of abscess); or laparoscopic procedures, such as 44970 (laparoscopic appendectomy). If an appendectomy is performed incidentally during another intra-abdominal surgical procedure, do not report the appendectomy separately (44955), unless the procedure was significantly complex or significantly extended the procedure. If the appendectomy is reported separately, append modifier -52, Reduced Service. If you only appended modifier -51, the third-party payer would remove the service assuming an unbundling error had occurred. See the parenthetical note that follows 44950 for example, which directs the coder to add -52 to identify separate identification of the appendectomy.

Add-on code **44955** is appended to indicate that the appendectomy was done at the same time as another major procedure and is listed in addition to the code for the primary procedure.

Rectum. Rectal endoscopic procedures are:

- **Proctosigmoidoscopy:** Endoscopic examination of the rectum (procto = rectum) and the sigmoid colon (45300-45327)
- **Sigmoidoscopy:** Endoscopic examination of the sigmoid colon and may include the descending colon (45330-45345)
- **Colonoscopy:** Endoscopic examination of the colon (from rectum to cecum, which is the uppermost portion of the large intestine and may include the lower portion of the small intestine, ileum) (45355-45392)

The codes are divided based on the extent and the purpose of the procedure. Note that the stand-alone codes 45300, 45330, and 45378 each have a list of indented codes based on the purpose (such as biopsy, foreign body removal, ablation, control of bleeding, etc.).

If the patient is fully prepared for the endoscopic procedure, and the procedure has begun but is not completed because of extenuating circumstances, use modifier -53 (Discontinued Procedure), with the endoscopic code. Some payers, such as Medicare, require the coder to report -53 for a procedure that could not be completed. These extenuating circumstances could be that the patient has become unstable, the bowel preparation for the surgery was not sufficient to continue the procedure, or an equipment failure has occurred. Use either -52 or -53 and provide documentation.

EXERCISE 9–4 *Endoscopic Procedures*

Using the CPT manual, code the following:

1 Esophagogastroduodenoscopy with control of bleeding

    ❀ Code(s): _____

2 Flexible sigmoidoscopy with three biopsies

  ❧ Code(s): _____

3 Colonoscopy with removal of polyp by a snare

  ❧ Code(s): _____

Anus. Abscess is a common anal condition that is usually treated with I&D; however, when this fails to satisfactorily treat the abscess, other methods may be used.

Several of the codes in the Anus subheading refer to a seton, such as 46020 (seton placement) or 46030 (seton removal). A **seton** is a treatment for anal fistula (abnormal passage between anus and skin), which is usually the result of a previous abscess that has drained but not completely healed. A non-absorbable suture is threaded through the fistula, out through the anus, and the two ends of the suture are tied together. The seton is left in place until healing has occurred. Scar tissue forms around the suture, and the ends of the seton are eventually cut away. Usually the seton can be placed during an office procedure that does not require anesthesia. If the fistula is more complex and requires opening of the fistula track, report the service with 46270-46285.

Hemorrhoids are another frequent condition of the anus. A hemorrhoid (piles) arises from an inflammation of the venous plexuses around the anus and may be inside or outside of the anal canal. Hemorrhoids are classified into four degrees depending on severity:

- First degree may bleed but does not protrude outside of the anal canal.
- Second degree protrudes outside of the anal canal occasionally but then retracts spontaneously.
- Third degree protrudes outside the anal canal more often and must be manually placed back into the anal canal.
- Fourth degree protrudes outside the anal canal but cannot be manually placed back into the anal canal. Often, the fourth degree hemorrhoid will be strangulated or thrombosed.

The type of surgical treatment of the hemorrhoid is determined by the severity of the hemorrhoid. For example, 46250 reports a complete external hemorrhoidectomy, and 46260 reports a complex hemorrhoidectomy of both internal and external hemorrhoids. Sometimes hemorrhoids are treated by injection of a sclerosing (caustic) solution, which causes irritation of the tissue that results in increased healing.

An anoscope is an instrument that is inserted a short distance into the anal canal. Once inserted, various procedures are performed, such as dilation, biopsy, removal of a foreign body, lesion removal, and control of hemorrhage. Procedures that utilize the anoscope are reported with codes in the Endoscopy subheading (46600-46615).

Liver. Biopsy of the liver may be performed percutaneously (47000) and usually uses imaging guidance that is reported separately. If the biopsy is performed at the time of a more major procedure, report the biopsy with 47001, which is an add-on code. A liver biopsy may also be performed as a wedge biopsy (47100) that involves removal, through an incision, of a small fan-shaped section of tissue for examination.

A liver transplant is a complex procedure that usually involves the surgical expertise of several physicians and a trained surgical team. The transplant procedure involves obtaining the graft to be transplanted (from a cadaver or living donor), backbench work (special preparation of the graft before transplantation), and transplantation into the recipient, and each component should be coded separately. There are extensive notes preceding the transplant codes 47133-47147 that must be carefully read before assigning codes to these complex procedures.

Biliary Tract. The gallbladder is connected to the liver and the small intestine by the biliary tract. The tract can be the site of conditions such as calculus and tumor that may obstruct the flow of bile. An incisional procedure to explore the tract may be performed to determine the cause of obstruction (47400) and may include removal of calculus or drainage of bile from the tract. A **choledochotomy** is an incision into the biliary tract, and a **cholecystostomy** is the formation of a stoma between the abdominal wall and the gallbladder. You can locate the codes for these procedures in the Incision category of the Biliary Tract codes 47400-47490.

An **injection** procedure may be necessary to determine if the biliary tract is obstructed. The choice of code is based on if the injection is performed percutaneously (47500) or through an existing catheter (47505). **Stents** may be placed in the biliary tract (47511), changed (47525), or revised/reinserted (47530).

Laparoscopic cholecystectomy involves the placement of ports through the abdominal wall into which the laparoscope and instrumentation are inserted to remove the gallbladder. You can locate these codes in the Laparoscopy category (47560-47579). The operative report indicates the method used for the removal of the gallbladder, which determines the assignment of the code. For example, 47562 reports a laparoscopic removal of the gallbladder, and 47600 reports the removal of the gallbladder through an incision.

Pancreas. The pancreas is located behind (posterior to) the stomach and produces enzymes and hormones. The pancreas may become inflamed (pancreatitis). Drains may be placed into the pancreas to drain excess fluid. If the procedure is performed by means of an incision, report the drain placement with 48000, and if the procedure also included cholecystostomy, gastrostomy, and jejunostomy report the service with 48001. The pancreas can also be the site of a calculus that may be removed through an incision (48020).

Biopsies can also be performed by means of an open procedure (48100) or percutaneously (48102). The guidance is not included in the percutaneous biopsy code, so guidance must be reported separately and depends on the type of guidance used. The injection portion of the intraoperative pancreatogram is reported separately with add-on code 48400 (injection procedure, intraoperative pancreatography).

The pancreas can be totally or partially removed and codes for the pancreatectomies (48140-48160) are divided based on the extent of removal and other procedures that may be performed during the same operative session.

The pancreas may be transplanted (48550-48554) and includes harvesting the pancreas graft from a cadaver, backbench work in preparation for transplantation, and transplantation of the graft into the recipient.

Abdomen, Peritoneum, and Omentum. The laparoscopy code 49320 is used to report a diagnostic laparoscopic procedure. If the procedure was a surgical procedure, the diagnostic laparoscopy is included in the surgical procedure and not reported separately. For example, if the procedure began as a diagnostic laparoscopy but then a lymphocele of the peritoneal cavity

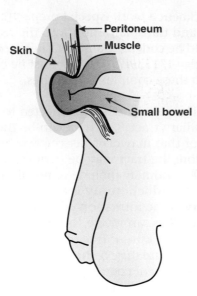

FIGURE 9–22 Hernia.

was identified and drained, the diagnostic laparoscopy becomes a surgical laparoscopy and would be reported with 49323.

Hernia codes are listed according to type of hernia (see Repair 49491-49611 and Laparoscopy 49650-49659). Fig. 9–22 is an illustration of an inguinal hernia that would be surgically repaired by a herniorrhaphy. The defect would be closed with sutures. Other factors in coding hernias are whether the hernia is **strangulated** (the blood supply is cut off) or **incarcerated** (cannot be returned to the abdominal cavity); whether the repair is an initial or subsequent repair; whether the hernia is reducible (can be returned to the abdominal cavity); and the age of the patient.

Hernia repairs using an abdominal approach are located in the Abdomen, Peritoneum, and Omentum subsection, Repair subheading (49491-49611). Laparoscopic hernia repairs are in the Laparoscopy subheading (49650-49659).

QUICK CHECK 9-18

Name two hernia types (locations) that affect code selection for hernia repair.

_____ and _____

EXERCISE 9–5 *Miscellaneous Digestive System Coding*

Using the CPT manual, code the following:

1 Exploratory laparotomy with a laparoscopic cholecystectomy

🔗 Code(s): _____

2 Cholecystotomy with exploration and removal of calculus

🔗 Code(s): _____

3 Repair of recurrent reducible incisional hernia, with implantation of a mesh graft, abdominal approach

🔗 Code(s): _____

4 Repair of an initial incarcerated inguinal hernia in a $5\frac{1}{2}$-year-old

  Code(s): _____

5 Biopsy of lip

  Code: _____

From the Trenches

"Teamwork with other coders gives you support with the 'problem' codes. It is extremely important with the physicians because services must be presented accurately and correctly to the insurance companies."

PATRICIA

MEDIASTINUM AND DIAPHRAGM

Format

The mediastinum is the area between the lungs (Fig. 9–23). The Mediastinum subheading of the Mediastinum and Diaphragm subsection (39000-39599) of the CPT manual is divided by procedures and includes the categories of Incision, Excision, and Endoscopy. The difference between the mediastinum incision codes is the surgical approach. The approach can be either cervical (neck area) or across the thoracic area (transthoracic) or sternum. The excision codes vary based on whether a cyst or tumor was excised. Codes for the mediastinum procedures are usually located in the CPT manual index under "Mediastinum."

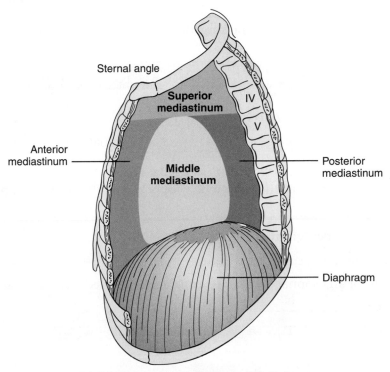

FIGURE 9–23 Mediastinum and diaphragm.

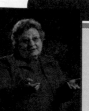

From the Trenches

"Certification means that the coder has been exposed to a lot more knowledge about coding than simply what is used in a particular workplace. It also means more money for the coder."

PATRICIA

The diaphragm is the wall of muscle that separates the thoracic and abdominal cavities. The codes in the Diaphragm subheading are repair codes. Repairs are usually to a hernia or laceration. Diaphragm codes are usually located in the CPT manual index under "Diaphragm."

Coding Highlights

Mediastinum. The mediastinum category of codes (39000-39499) are based on the surgical approach taken to perform the mediastinotomy. A cervical or anterior mediastinotomy is a surgical procedure in which an incision is made in the lower portion of the front of the neck for exploration, drainage, biopsy, or removal of a foreign body. Exploration, drainage, removal of foreign body, or biopsy is done with a mediastinotomy (39000-39010). The codes for Excision use a surgical approach in which the surgeon makes the operative incision just below the nipple line, pulls back the rib cage, retracts the muscles, and has exposure of the thoracic cavity. The cyst or tumor is removed and the incision closed.

Diaphragm. Other than one code for unlisted diaphragm procedures, all diaphragm codes (39501-39599) are for repair of the diaphragm. The repairs are for lacerations or hernias, with one code for imbrication of the diaphragm. An imbrication of the diaphragm may be performed for eventration, which is when the diaphragm moves up, usually because of the paralysis of the diaphragmatic nerve (phrenic nerve). In this case the surgeon sutures the diaphragm back into place.

EXERCISE 9–6 *Mediastinum and Diaphragm*

Using the CPT manual, code the following:

1 Repair of paraesophageal hiatus hernia, abdominal approach, with limited fundoplasty

Code: _____

2 Exploratory mediastinotomy with biopsy accomplished with approach through the neck

Code: _____

3 Excision of benign tumor of the mediastinum

Code: _____

4 Repair of an esophageal hiatal hernia accomplished with approach across the thoracic area

Code: _____

CHAPTER REVIEW

CHAPTER 9, PART I, THEORY

Complete the following:

1 The greatest number of category codes in the Male Genital System fall under the

_____ subheading because of the numerous repairs made to this anatomic area.

2 In what section of the CPT manual would you find a code for a superficial abscess of the skin

of the penis? _____

3 How many codes are there in the Intersex

Surgery subsection? _____

4 What is the term that pertains to the motion and flow of urine? _____

5 What is the modifier that indicates that only the professional portion of the service was

performed? _____

6 The codes in the Digestive System subsection begin with this anatomic part,

_____, and end with this

anatomic part, _____.

7 In the Digestive System, many of the procedures performed to view the esophagus and stomach are done with this instrument.

_____

8 What type of endoscopy is always included in a surgical endoscopy and would therefore never be reported separately?

_____

9 What is the term that describes a surgical opening into the abdomen?

_____

10 When a hernia can be returned to the abdominal

cavity, it is said to be _____.

11 The difference between the mediastinum incision

codes is the surgical _____.

CHAPTER 9, PART II, PRACTICAL

Code the following cases:

12 Mary Carter, age 72, has an exploratory laparotomy with cholecystectomy through an incision.

Code(s): _____

13 Incision and drainage of deep penis abscess

Code(s): _____

14 Repair of recurrent, reducible incisional hernia

Code(s): _____

15 Extensive destruction of penile herpetic vesicle lesions using cryosurgery

Code(s): _____

16 Repair of an esophageal hiatal hernia using a transthoracic approach

Code(s): _____

17 Excision of full thickness of lip lesion with Abbe-Estlander flap reconstruction

Code(s): _____

18 Thoracic approach used in a diverticulectomy of hypopharynx

Code(s): _____

19 Endoscopic retrograde cholangiopancreatography (ERCP) with multiple biopsies

Code(s): _____

20 Total open abdominal colectomy with ileostomy

Code(s): _____

21 Multiple biopsies of the small intestine by means of endoscopy with progression past the second portion of the duodenum

Code(s): _____

22 Proctosigmoidoscopy using rigid endoscope with collection of multiple specimens by brushing

Code(s): _____

23 Biopsy of kidney with percutaneous incision by trocar

Code(s): _____

24 Physician providing the technical and professional component of a cystography with contrast and four views

Code(s): _____

25 Drainage of abscess of Skene's glands

Code(s): _____

QUICK CHECK ANSWERS

QUICK CHECK 9-1
Integumentary

QUICK CHECK 9-2
28

QUICK CHECK 9-3
non-inflatable, inflatable

QUICK CHECK 9-4
orchiopexy

QUICK CHECK 9-5
54700

QUICK CHECK 9-6
abdomen, perineum

QUICK CHECK 9-7
VLAP, ILCP

QUICK CHECK ANSWERS

QUICK CHECK 9-8
1. b
2. c
3. a

QUICK CHECK 9-9
needle (or punch), transperineal

QUICK CHECK 9-10
False

QUICK CHECK 9-11
externally

QUICK CHECK 9-12
nephrostomy, pyelostomy

QUICK CHECK 9-13
50945

QUICK CHECK 9-14
58240

QUICK CHECK 9-15
cystoscopy, urethroscopy

QUICK CHECK 9-16
cross

QUICK CHECK 9-17
-ectomy

QUICK CHECK 9-18
Any two of the following: inguinal, lumbar, incisional (ventral), epigastric, umbilical, spigelian, diaphragmatic (hiatal)

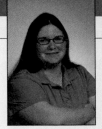

"Reading operative notes is a key to surgery coding. Try to read as many operative reports as possible; the more you can practice, the more comfortable the work will be."

Ellen Dooley, BA, CPC-A
Compliance Analyst
University of Missouri Health
  Care
Columbia, Missouri

General Surgery II

Chapter Topics

Hemic and Lymphatic
Systems

Endocrine System

Nervous System

Eye and Ocular Adnexa

Auditory System

Chapter Review

Quick Check Answers

Learning Objectives

After completing this chapter you should be able to

1   Review the Hemic and Lymphatic Systems subsection format.

2   Understand the Hemic and Lymphatic Systems subheadings.

3   Demonstrate the ability to code Hemic and Lymphatic System services.

4   Review the Endocrine System subsection format.

5   Understand the Endocrine System subheadings.

6   Demonstrate the ability to code Endocrine System services.

7   Review the Nervous System subsection format.

8   Understand the Nervous System subheadings.

9   Demonstrate the ability to code Nervous System services.

10 Review the Eye and Ocular Adnexa subsection.

11 Understand the Eye and Ocular Adnexa subheadings.

12 Demonstrate the ability to code Eye and Ocular Adnexa services.

13 Review the Auditory System subsection format.

14 Understand Auditory System subheadings.

15 Demonstrate the ability to code Auditory System services.

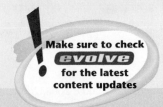
Make sure to check
evolve
for the latest
content updates

HEMIC AND LYMPHATIC SYSTEMS

Format

The Hemic and Lymphatic Systems subsection (38100-38999) is divided into subheadings: Spleen, General, and Lymph Nodes/Lymphatic channels (Fig. 10–1). Further division is based on type of procedure (i.e., excision, incision, repair). The codes for spleen and lymph nodes are located in the CPT manual index under main terms such as Spleen, Lymph Nodes, or Bone Marrow.

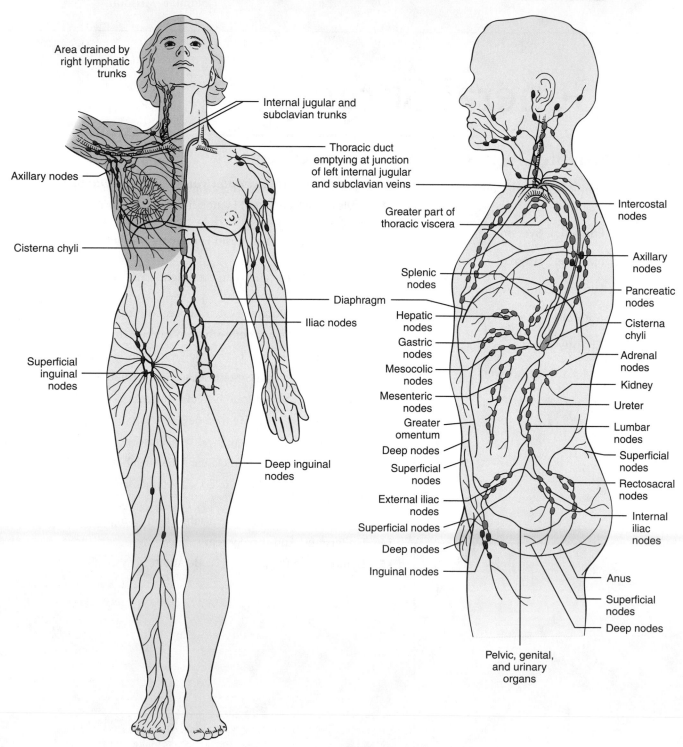

FIGURE 10–1 Lymphatic System.

Coding Highlights

Spleen. The spleen is composed of lymph tissue and is located in the left upper quadrant of the abdomen. The spleen is easily ruptured and can cause massive hemorrhage. It initiates an immune response, filters and removes bacteria from the bloodstream, and destroys worn out blood cells. A person can live without a spleen because the bone marrow, liver, and lymph nodes take over the work of the spleen after a total splenectomy.

Codes in the subheading Spleen (38100-38200) are further divided into categories for excision, repair, laparoscopy, and introduction. Codes in the Excision category are based on the type of splenectomy: total, partial, or total with extensive disease. The splenectomy, total and partial, carries the designation "(separate procedure)" behind the code description (38100-38101). This means that if the splenectomy is an integral part of another procedure, it is bundled into the main procedure code and not reported separately.

CODING SHOT If a repair of a ruptured spleen was performed and the surgeon removed a portion of the spleen as a part of the repair, you would report only the repair code (38115).

General. A marrow or blood cell transplant is a treatment for patients with blood diseases, such as leukemia or lymphoma, in which the patient's marrow or blood cells are replaced with healthy marrow or blood cells from a donor. There are three sources for blood cell formation: bone marrow, bloodstream, and umbilical cord. Bone marrow is the inner core of bones that manufactures most blood cells. Immature blood cells, called stem cells, originate in the marrow of bones. Leukemia is a malignant disease of the bone marrow in which excessive white blood cells are produced. Treatment often includes total-body irradiation or aggressive chemotherapy followed by transplantation of normal bone marrow. **Bone marrow aspiration** (38220) is a procedure in which a sample of the bone marrow is taken by means of a needle that is inserted into the marrow cavity. Marrow is then aspirated (pulled) through the needle and into the syringe. Usually the marrow is taken from the iliac crest, pelvic bone, or sternum. **Bone marrow biopsy** (38221) is a procedure in which small pieces of the marrow are obtained. These small chips are then processed in the laboratory by dissolving the pieces in a decalcification solution. The resulting substance is then analyzed and the service reported with a Pathology/Laboratory code (88305). **Bone marrow harvesting** (38230) is a procedure in which a larger amount of marrow is aspirated from a donor by means of a large aspiration needle. The marrow is then transplanted into the recipient patient. **Transplantation**, as represented in 38240-38242, is the procedure in which the donor bone marrow or stem cells are injected into the patient. The preparation and storage of the cells prior to transplantation are reported with 38207-38215. **Allogenic** bone marrow comes from the same species (human), such as a cadaver, a close relative, or a non-related donor. Testing is done to determine as close of a genetic match for the recipient as possible. **Autologous** bone marrow is collected from the patient, processed, and later transplanted or reinfused back to the patient, so there is a genetic match. **Stem cell harvesting** is the collection of stem cells from the blood system through a process termed apheresis. A needle is placed into a vein in one arm of the donor and the blood is removed. It is then filtered to remove the stem cells. The blood, with the stem cells removed, is returned to the donor through the other arm. Usually this process takes 4-6 hours and is usually completed in two sessions. The harvesting and return of the blood to the donor (replantation) is reported with codes 38205-38206.

QUICK CHECK 10-1

According to the notes in the CPT, the Bone Marrow/Stem Cell Services (38207-38215) may be reported only once per day.
True or False?

Lymph Nodes. The lymphatic system is a transportation system to take fluids, proteins, and fats through the lymphatic channels and back to the bloodstream. Stations along the lymphatic system are called lymph nodes. The nodes fight disease when lymphocytes from the nodes produce antibodies. The subheading of Lymph Nodes is divided on the basis of the various procedures (i.e., incision, excision, resection, and introduction). The majority of the Excision codes (38500-38555) are for biopsy or excision based on the **method** (open or needle) and the **location** (e.g., axillary or cervical). For the open procedures, the choice of codes depends on whether the procedure was superficial (38500) or deep (38510-38530).

Within the Lymph Node and Lymphatic Channels subheading are two categories of codes for lymphadenectomies that are based on whether the lymphadenectomy is limited or radical. A **limited lymphadenectomy** (38562-38564) is the removal of the lymph nodes only; a **radical lymphadenectomy** (38700-38780) is the removal of the lymph nodes, gland(s), and surrounding tissue. Sometimes, a limited lymphadenectomy will be bundled into a more major procedure, such as prostatectomy. If this is the case, you would not report the lymphadenectomy separately. Rather, you would report only the more major procedure, such as the prostatectomy code from the Male Genital System subsection of the Surgery section.

QUICK CHECK 10-2

Review the Radical Lymphadenectomy codes (38700-38780). According to the parenthetical statements, what modifier may be used under appropriate circumstances? _____

EXERCISE 10–1 *Hemic and Lymphatic Systems*

Using the CPT manual, code the following:

1 Excision of an axillary cystic hygroma, which the patient record indicates involved no deep neurovascular dissection

   Code: _____

2 Total removal of the spleen

   Code: _____

3 Injection procedure for a radiographic view of the portal vein of the spleen

   Code: _____

4 Bone marrow transplant, autologous

   Code: _____

ENDOCRINE SYSTEM

Format

The Endocrine System subsection includes the subheadings Thyroid Gland and Parathyroid, Thymus, Adrenal Glands, Pancreas, and Carotid Body. Within the Thyroid Gland subheading there are the categories of Incision and Excision. Within the Parathyroid, Thymus, Adrenal Glands, Pancreas, and Carotid Body there are the categories Excision, Laparoscopy, and Other Procedures.

CODING SHOT *Carotid body* is tissue rich in capillaries that act as receptors located near the bifurcation (splitting into two) of the carotid arteries. The receptors monitor arterial oxygen content and pressure. Tumors that develop in this tissue may need to be excised (60600).

The endocrine system has the important job of producing and releasing hormones into the bloodstream. The endocrine glands are located throughout the body (Fig. 10–2) and regulate a wide range of body functions. (Your anatomy and physiology background is very important to you as you code.)

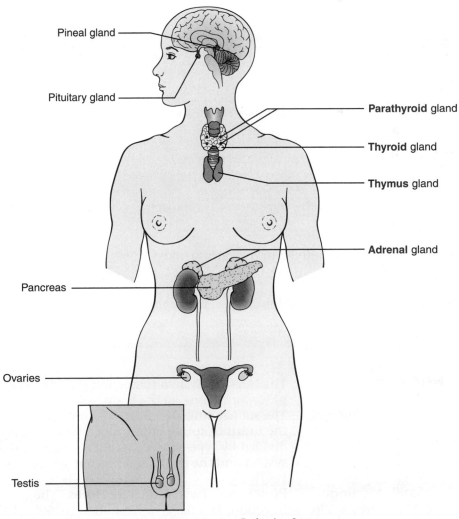

FIGURE 10–2 Endocrine System.

From the Trenches

"If someone expresses an interest in becoming a medical coder, I'd advise them to take a position in a physician's office or billing area first, so that they can get a feel for the field. Any experience in the field helps."

ELLEN

Coding Highlights

There are nine glands in the endocrine system, but only four are included in the Endocrine subsection (60000-60699) of the CPT manual—thyroid, parathyroid, adrenal, and thymus. The pituitary and pineal gland procedures are in the Nervous System subsection of the CPT manual, the pancreas is in the Digestive System subsection, and the ovaries and testes are in the respective Female or Male Genital System subsections.

The CPT manual lists only one thyroid incision code (60000) and one unlisted procedure code (60699) in the Endocrine System subsection; the remaining codes are for excisions/removal or laparoscopy. There is also a biopsy code (needle core, 60100), which is under the excision category. Partial/total or subtotal/total appear in many of the descriptions. Codes 60252 and 60254 include thyroidectomy for malignancy with neck dissection.

EXERCISE 10–2 *Endocrine System*

Using the CPT manual, code the following:

1 Excision of an adenoma from posterior aspect of the thyroid gland

   Code: _____

2 Surgical removal of a thyroglossal duct cyst

   Code: _____

3 Thymectomy using the transthoracic approach, with radical mediastinal dissection

   Code: _____

4 Removal of tumor affixed to the carotid body

   Code: _____

5 Partial unilateral thyroid lobectomy, with isthmusectomy

   Code: _____

NERVOUS SYSTEM

The Nervous System subsection (61000-64999) contains codes describing procedures done on the brain, spinal cord, nerves, and all associated parts.

Format

The subheadings are divided according to anatomic site—whether a part of the **brain** or **spinal column** or a type of **nerve**. The subheadings are further divided by type of procedure. The codes deal with both the central nervous system and the peripheral nervous system.

Skull, Meninges, and Brain

Punctures, Twists, or Burr Holes. The first two categories of codes Injection, Drainage, or Aspiration (61000-61070) and Twist Drill, Burr Hole(s), or Trephine (61105-61253) deal with conditions that may require that holes or openings be made into the brain to relieve pressure, to insert monitoring devices, to place tubing, or to inject contrast material or drain hemorrhage. Twist or burr holes are made through the skull to accomplish many of these procedures. Using twist or burr holes means that the skull stays intact except for the small openings (holes) that are made.

Craniectomy/Craniotomy. Codes in the category Craniectomy or Craniotomy describe procedures (61304-61576) that deal with an actual incision of the skull with possible removal of a portion of the skull to open the operative site to the surgeon for correction of the condition. Use of these codes is determined by site and condition (e.g., evacuation of hematoma, supratentorial, subdural, 61312).

As in other subsections, many procedures are bundled into one code. Only by careful attention to code description can you keep from unbundling surgical procedures and incorrectly report bundled components separately. Carefully review the descriptions in these codes before coding.

When craniectomies are performed, it is not uncommon that additional grafting must take place to repair the surgical defect caused by opening the skull. These grafting procedures would be coded separately, in addition to the major surgical procedure.

Coding Highlights

Surgery of Skull Base. The **skull base** is the area at the base of the cranium where the lobes of the brain rest. When lesions are found within the skull base, it often takes the skill of several surgeons working together to perform surgery dealing with these conditions. The operations found in the category Surgery of Skull Base are very involved, taking many hours to complete. The procedures are divided on the basis of the approach procedure, the definitive procedure, and the reconstruction/repair procedure.

The **approach procedure** (61580-61598) is the method used to obtain exposure of the lesion (e.g., anterior cranial fossa, middle cranial fossa, posterior cranial fossa). The **definitive procedure** (61600-61616) is what was done to the lesion (e.g., biopsy, excision). If one physician did both the approach and the definitive procedures, both would be coded. For example, a neoplasm is excised at the base of the anterior cranial fossa, extradural using a craniofacial approach to the anterior skull base. This would be coded 61600 for the procedure (definitive procedure) and 61580 for the approach (approach procedure). Because two procedures were done by the same physician—61600 and 61580—the lesser procedure, the approach, would have modifier -51. Modifier -62 (two surgeons) or -66 (surgical team) is used as appropriate.

Reconstruction or repair procedures (61618, 61619) are the various repairs that will be made to the skull on closure so as to rebuild the area used for entry. This last step of reconstruction or repair is reported separately **only** if it is extensive and documented in the medical record.

At any given point, one or more physicians may be performing distinctly different portions of these complex procedures. When one surgeon performs the approach procedure, another surgeon performs the definitive procedure, and another surgeon performs the reconstruction/repair procedure, each surgeon's services would be reported with the code for the specific procedure he or she individually performed. Again, if one surgeon performs more than one procedure (e.g., the approach procedure, the definitive procedure, and the reconstruction/repair procedure), they are reported separately, adding modifier -51 to the secondary procedures. For example, one surgeon performs the approach procedure (61580), definitive procedure (61600), and reconstruction/repair (61619). The services are reported as 61600 (the most resource intense), 61619-51, and 61590-51.

Aneurysm, Arteriovenous Malformation, or Vascular Disease.

Aneurysms may develop in the brain, requiring surgical repair. Also present in the brain may be arteriovenous malformations, which means the arteries and veins are not in the correct anatomic position. Codes to indicate the definitive procedure or repair of these conditions are found in the category Surgery for Aneurysm, Arteriovenous Malformation, or Vascular Disease (61680-61711) and are divided on the basis of the **approach** and **method** of procedure.

CODING SHOT   An electroencephalograph (EEG) is used to monitor currents emanating from the brain. It is usually done any time a procedure on the brain is being performed. Report the EEG with 95950.

Cerebrospinal Fluid Shunts (CFS).

A **shunt** can be considered a draining device that enables fluids to be drained from one area into another when the body is not able to perform this function on its own. In the case of cerebrospinal fluid (CSF) shunts (62180-62258), the CSF that is produced in the ventricles of the brain may not drain properly but may continue to accumulate in the brain, building pressure and causing brain damage. Drains or shunts are placed from the area of collection to a drainage area to keep the fluid level within normal ranges. For instance, code 62223 describes the creation of a shunt from the ventricle to the peritoneal space (ventriculoperitoneal), as illustrated in Fig. 10–3. This means that the shunt

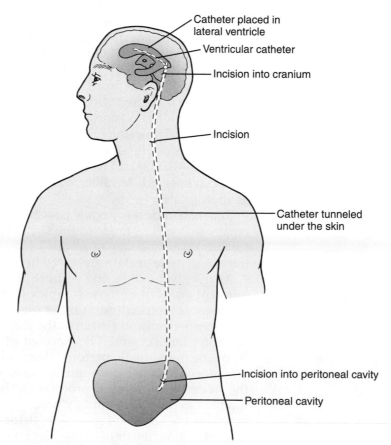

FIGURE 10-3   Ventriculoperitoneal shunt placed for chronic hydrocephalus.

starts in the ventricle of the brain and ends in the peritoneum. Codes in the CSF Shunt category describe all the various types of shunting procedures, including placement of shunting devices and subsequent repair, replacement, and removal.

Shunt systems may also be placed to drain obstructed CSF from the spine. As in the previously described shunt procedures, codes from the category Cerebrospinal Fluid (CSF) Shunt identify the creation, replacement, removal, or insertion of a shunt system.

Spine and Spinal Cord

The subheading Spine and Spinal Cord (62263-63746) includes codes for injections, laminectomies, excisions, repairs, and shunting. You should be familiar with the terminology for parts of the spinal column (Fig. 10–4). A medical dictionary will help you become familiar with the other parts of the vertebral column, including the lamina, foramina, vertebral bodies, disks, facets, and nerve roots. The basic distinction among the codes in these ranges deals with the **condition** (a herniated intervertebral disk versus a neoplastic lesion of the spinal cord) as well as the **approach** (e.g., anterior, posterior, costovertebral).

The complexity of the procedure is determined by the condition and approach. For example, a patient with a herniated disk at L5-S1 would

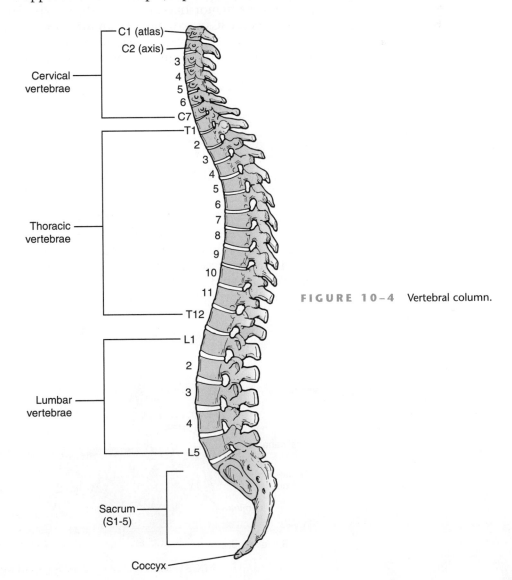

FIGURE 10–4 Vertebral column.

require less time in surgery for the removal of the disk and decompression of the nerve root than would a patient with a neoplastic growth intertwined in the same area, because removal of a piece of disk would not be as involved as separating a lesion from multiple components of the spinal column. The approaches differ in the amount of expertise and time required. Codes vary based on approach. A posterior approach means a surgical opening was formed from the back. An anterior approach means a surgical opening was formed from the front.

When coding spinal procedures, you should look for the condition, the approach, whether the procedure was unilateral or bilateral, and whether multiple procedures were performed.

Often when a laminectomy (removal of a lamina) (Fig. 10–5) is performed, an arthrodesis (surgical fusion of joints) is also performed. In some cases spinal instrumentation procedures (the use of rods, wires, and screws to create fusions) are also performed. Review the operative reports and confirm all procedures performed when coding multiple procedures.

A **lumbar puncture** (62270), or spinal tap, obtains cerebrospinal fluid by insertion of a needle into the subarachnoid space in the lumbar region, as illustrated in Fig. 10–6. The CSF is used to diagnose various conditions. For example, if the CSF is pinkish in color and contains erythrocytes, the patient could have a hemorrhage. A yellowish, cloudy CSF with numerous white blood cells (WBCs) may indicate an infection.

Notes throughout the Spine and Spinal Cord subsection refer you to other code ranges for commonly performed additional procedures (e.g., arthrodesis codes are in the Musculoskeletal subsection). Remember to use the modifier -51 for multiple procedures if more than one procedure is performed.

CODING SHOT A sensory evoked study, which monitors the central nervous system, is usually done with spinal surgery and reported with 95925.

Extracranial Nerves, Peripheral Nerves, and Autonomic Nervous System. Nerves are our sensing devices, and they carry stimuli to and from all parts of the body. Some common procedures done on nerves include injection, destruction, decompression, and suture/repair and are reported with codes from the Extracranial Nerves, Peripheral Nerves, and Autonomic Nervous System subheading (64400-64999).

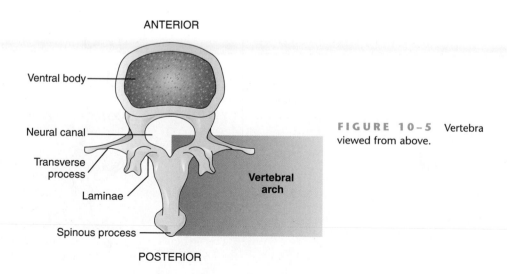

ANTERIOR

Ventral body

Neural canal

Transverse process

Laminae

Spinous process

Vertebral arch

POSTERIOR

FIGURE 10–5 Vertebra viewed from above.

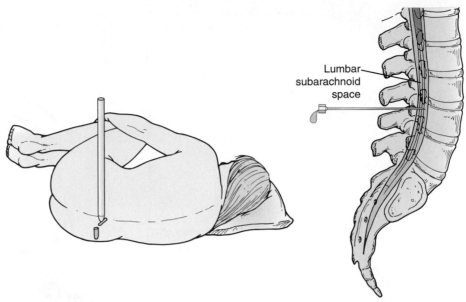

FIGURE 10–6 Lumbar puncture, or spinal tap, in which the cerebrospinal fluid is obtained by inserting a needle into the subarachnoid space. The patient lies laterally with knees drawn up so as to increase the spaces between the vertebrae.

The space around the nerves can be injected with anesthetic agents to cause a temporary loss of feeling (64400-64530). The code is chosen according to the type of nerve being injected. Nerves may also be injected to cause destruction of the nerve and permanent loss of feeling in a specific area of the body (64600-64640, 64680-64681). Persons with debilitating pain may undergo this type of procedure.

QUICK CHECK 10-3

1. List the code ranges for:

Nerves injected to cause temporary loss of feeling: _____
Nerves injected to cause permanent loss of feeling: _____

2. Within each subheading in Question 1, what are the two headings that further divide the codes? _____ Nerves, _____ Nerves

Neuroplasty is the decompression (freeing) of intact nerves (e.g., from scar tissue). If nerves receive excessive pressure from a source, such as scar tissue or displacement of intervertebral disk material, severe pain may occur. Movement or freeing of nerves is reported with codes from the Neuroplasty (Exploration, Neurolysis, or Nerve Decompression) category (64702-64727). Perhaps the most commonly known neuroplasty procedure is a carpal tunnel release, coded to 64721, in which the median nerve and flexor tendons of the wrist are surgically released (Fig. 10–7).

Nerves can also be removed or they can be repaired (sutured). Remember, the notes found before the repair codes in the Integumentary subsection state that if repair of nerves is necessary, codes from the Nervous System are used. The codes in the Neurorrhaphy (64831-64876) and the Neurorrhaphy with Nerve Graft (64885-64911) categories describe nerve repairs on the basis of the specific nerve being repaired. This category also includes codes that describe grafting on the basis of the size of the graft.

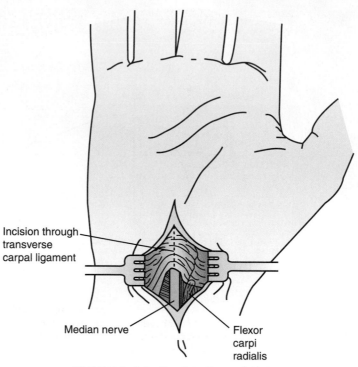

FIGURE 10-7 Carpal tunnel release.

EXERCISE 10-3 *Nervous System*

Using the CPT Manual, code the following:

1 Drainage of subdural hematoma using burr holes

   Code: _____

2 Drainage of subdural hematoma with craniectomy, supratentorial

   Code: _____

3 Resection of neoplasm, midline skull base, extradural, using infratemporal preauricular approach to middle cranial fossa

   Code(s): _____ and _____

4 Removal of complete cerebrospinal fluid shunt system, with replacement

   Code: _____

EYE AND OCULAR ADNEXA

Format

The Eye and Ocular Adnexa subsection (65091-68899) includes the subheadings Eyeball, Anterior Segment, Posterior Segment, Ocular Adnexa, and Conjunctiva. There are the typical incision, excision, repair, and destruction categories, but also some that are a little different. For example, the subheading Eyeball has categories for both Removal of Eye (65091-65114) and Removal of Foreign Bodies (65205-65265), although you would expect to find all removal codes in a category under one heading.

CODING SHOT Remember to use modifier -50 (bilateral procedure) when the procedure is done on both eyes.

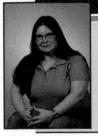

Some code groups have different codes for patients who have been operated on before. For example, in the subheading Ocular Adnexa, 67331 is used for a patient who has undergone previous eye surgery or injury. Also, the category Prophylaxis (means preventive treatment) (67141, 67145) under the subheading Posterior Segment has notes regarding the bundling in the codes. The Prophylaxis codes include all the sessions in a treatment period. The Destruction codes in this subcategory also include "one or more sessions." Be certain to read carefully so you know which elements are part of the code.

As in all sections of the CPT manual, there are directional notes throughout that will help you think about what defines a particular code. For example, code 67850 is for the "Destruction of lesion of lid margin (up to 1 cm)." Under this description is a note in parentheses: "(For Mohs' micrographic surgery, see 17311-17315)." This helpful note gives you the category of codes to refer to if the lesion destruction was done using Mohs' micrographic surgery.

Refer to Figs. 10–8 through 10–11 as you prepare for coding practice.

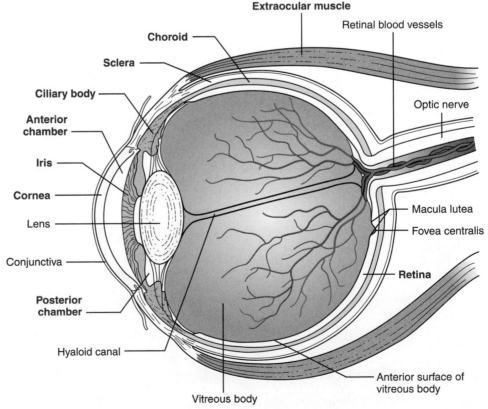

FIGURE 10-8 Eye and ocular adnexa.

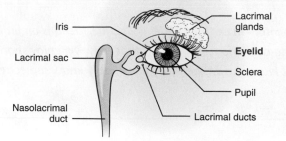

Iris

Lacrimal sac

Nasolacrimal duct

Lacrimal glands

Eyelid

Sclera

Pupil

Lacrimal ducts

FIGURE 10–9 Lacrimal apparatus.

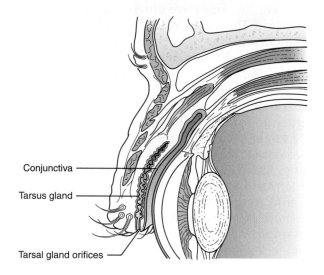

FIGURE 10–10 Eyelid.

Conjunctiva

Tarsus gland

Tarsal gland orifices

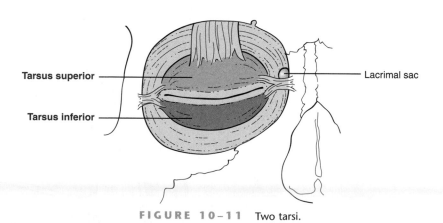

Tarsus superior

Tarsus inferior

Lacrimal sac

FIGURE 10–11 Two tarsi.

QUICK CHECK 10-4

Match the term with the correct description:

a. Evisceration
b. Enucleation
c. Exenteration

1. Removal of the eye, adnexa, bony structure
2. Removal of the contents of eyeball, structure intact
3. Removal of eyeball only, other structures intact

Eyeball

Removal of Eye. The **Removal of Eye** category codes contain codes to report **evisceration**, which is removal of the contents of the globe but leaving the extraocular muscles and sclera intact (65091, 65093); **enucleation**, which is removal of the eye while leaving the orbital structures intact, (65101-65105); and **exenteration**, which is removal of the eye, adnexa, and part of the bony orbit (65110-65114). The codes in the Removal of Eye category are divided based on which of these procedures was performed, if an implant was inserted, and in the case of the exenteration, if the bony orbit was removed or a muscle or myocutaneous flap was performed. These codes do not report skin grafting to the orbit. If the operative report indicates skin grafting, report the service separately with codes from the Integumentary System (15120/15121 or 15260/15261). If the type of repair was more than a muscle, myocutaneous, or skin graft, refer to the reconstruction codes 67930/67935 (partial or full thickness repair).

Secondary Implant(s) Procedures. Implants may be inside the muscular cone (ocular implant or fake eye) or outside the muscular cone (orbital implant) as illustrated in Fig. 10–12. The ocular implant is the artificial eye, and the orbital implant replaces the orbit that was occupied by the eyeball before removal. With some implants, the muscles are attached to the implant to enable the artificial eye to move and thus appear more natural. The codes in the 65125-65155 range report a subsequent implantation of ocular implants based on the type of service provided with the implant, such as grafting or attachment of muscles to implant. Removal of an ocular implant is reported with 65175. An orbital implant is a cosmetic device that covers the outer portion of the eye and is also known as a scleral shell prosthesis. Orbital implant insertion is reported with 67550 and removal with 67560.

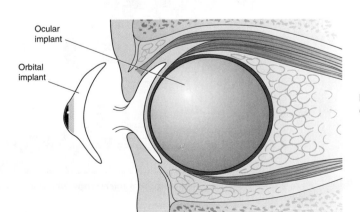

Ocular implant
Orbital implant

FIGURE 10–12
Ocular and orbital implants.

Removal of Foreign Body. Note the extensive list of parenthetical notes preceding 65205. Take time now to read these notes as they list important concepts that you need to know. The removal codes are for foreign bodies that are either located in the external eye or the intraocular eye. A **slit lamp** is a low-powered microscope with a high intensity light source that focuses the light as a long narrow beam or slit and is used to examine eyes (Fig. 10–13). Note that the only difference between 65220 and 65222 is whether a slit lamp is or is not utilized.

Repair of Laceration. The repair codes are assigned to report repair of laceration based on where the laceration is located on the conjunctiva, cornea, and/or sclera. Code 65286 reports the application of tissue glue for a perforation of the eyeball. The glue is used to repair a laceration as are other types of tissue glue that are used on the skin (topical skin adhesive).

Anterior Segment

The anterior segment includes the cornea, anterior chamber, anterior sclera, iris, ciliary body, and lens.

Cornea. The cornea is the transparent part of the eye. The cornea may be the site of a superficial lesion that is completely removed and reported with 65400. If only a portion of the lesion was removed from the cornea for pathology analysis, report the service as a biopsy with 65410.

A **keratoplasty** is repair of the cornea. Codes 65710-65756 are used to report keratoplasty based on the type of procedure performed. A penetrating keratoplasty (65730-65755) is one in which a full thickness of the cornea is removed and replaced with donor cornea. A lamellar keratoplasty (65710) is a procedure in which only a thin layer of the cornea is removed and replaced with donor cornea. **Aphakia** is absence of the lens of the eye, and **pseudophakia** is the presence of an artificial lens after cataract surgery and these terms are used in many of the keratoplasty code descriptions.

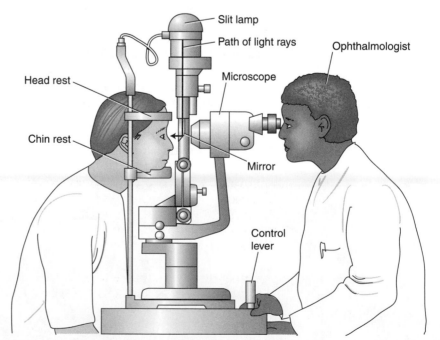

FIGURE 10–13 A slit lamp is a microscope with a light attached. The name is derived from the adjustable light beam.

Anterior Chamber. The anterior chamber of the eye is a fluid-filled (aqueous humor) space behind the cornea and in front of the iris. The categories of Incision (65800-65880), Removal (65900-65930), and Introduction (66020-66030) are for procedures performed on the anterior chamber of the eye.

Paracentesis is the removal of fluid. When a physician performs paracentesis of the anterior chamber of the eye, a needle is inserted into the anterior chamber and fluid withdrawn. The fluid may be withdrawn for diagnostic purposes (65800) or for therapeutic purposes (65805-65815). If an injection procedure is performed, report 66020 or 66030.

Goniotomy is a surgical procedure that utilizes an instrument called a goniolens. This procedure may be performed for congenital glaucoma, which is a condition in which the optic nerve at the back of the eye may be damaged and cause a loss of vision, especially peripheral vision. Code 65820 reports a goniotomy, and this code is not reported with modifier -63 (performed on infants less than 4 kg).

Codes in the Other Procedures category report severing of adhesions or scar tissue from the anterior chamber of the eye and are based on the location of the adhesion or scar tissue (65865-65880). These procedures are performed through an incision. **Posterior synechiae** are adhesions of the iris to the lens of the eye, and **anterior synechiae** are adhesions of the iris to the cornea.

Anterior Sclera. The sclera is the white, fibrous outer layer of the eyeball and the anterior sclera is the front part of the eye. The anterior sclera may be the site of lesions that are excised (66130) by incision of the conjunctiva to gain access to the lesion. Depending on the size of the lesion, the area of the sclera may not even require sutures, but rather only application of antibiotic ointment.

Sometimes, the flow of the aqueous humor is not absorbed or too much is being produced and a surgeon may perform a fistulization (creation of a passage) of the sclera to increase the flow. The fistulization can be created by means of removal of a portion of the sclera and iris (e.g., 66150), thermocauterization (e.g., hot probe, 66155), punch or scissor removal (e.g., 66160). A **trabeculectomy ab externo** (e.g., 65850, 66170, 66172) is a surgical procedure in which the trabecular meshwork (iris-scleral junction, drains aqueous humor) is reshaped or punctured. This procedure may be performed as a treatment for glaucoma or trauma.

Iris, Ciliary Body. The ciliary body is located behind the iris (colored part of the eye) and produces the aqueous humor. The smooth muscle of the ciliary body attaches to the lens. An iridectomy is usually performed for removal of a lesion (66600) or as a treatment for glaucoma (66625, 66630) by creation of an opening to drain aqueous humor. If the iridotomy is performed by means of laser, report the procedure with 66761 and if it is performed by means of photocoagulation, report the procedure with 66762.

Lens. A common procedure of the lens of the eye is cataract removal. Cataract removal and lens replacements (66830-66990) use one of three different approaches:

- Extracapsular cataract extraction (ECCE) is partial removal. It removes the hard nucleus in one piece, then removal of the soft cortex in multiple pieces. The posterior lens capsule is left in place.

- Intracapsular cataract extraction (ICCE) is total removal that removes the cataract in one piece (66983).
- Phacoemulsification dissolves the hard nucleus by ultrasound then removes the soft cortex in multiple pieces.

The most common procedure is the ECCE, represented by code 66984.

Extraocular Muscles. Under the subheading of Ocular Adnexa are codes for strabismus surgery, which corrects muscle misalignment. The codes are divided based on repair of vertical (67314, 67316) or horizontal (67311, 67312) muscle and are reported by the number of muscles repaired. Vertical muscles move the eye up and down, while the horizontal muscles move the eye side to side.

EXERCISE 10-4 *Eye and Ocular Adnexa*

Using the CPT manual, code the following:

1 Emboli removal from anterior segment of the left eye

Code: _____

2 New patient strabismus surgery involving the superior oblique muscle of the right eye

Code: _____

3 Xenon arc used in three sessions to prevent retinal detachment of left eye

Code: _____

4 Corneal incision for revision of earlier procedure that resulted in astigmatism of right eye

Code: _____

5 Removal of left eye, with implant, muscles attached to implant

Code: _____

AUDITORY SYSTEM

Format

The Auditory System subsection (69000-69979) is divided into the subheadings External Ear, Middle Ear, Inner Ear, and Temporal Bone/Middle Fossa Approach. The first three subheadings represent the anatomic divisions of the auditory system: external, middle, and inner ear (Fig. 10–14). The categories below each subheading include introduction, incision, excision, removal of foreign body, repair, and/or other procedures, depending on the particular subheading. The subheading Temporal Bone/Middle Fossa Approach (69950-69970) contains codes that describe various surgical procedures in which the surgeon makes an incision in front of the ear. Using this incision,

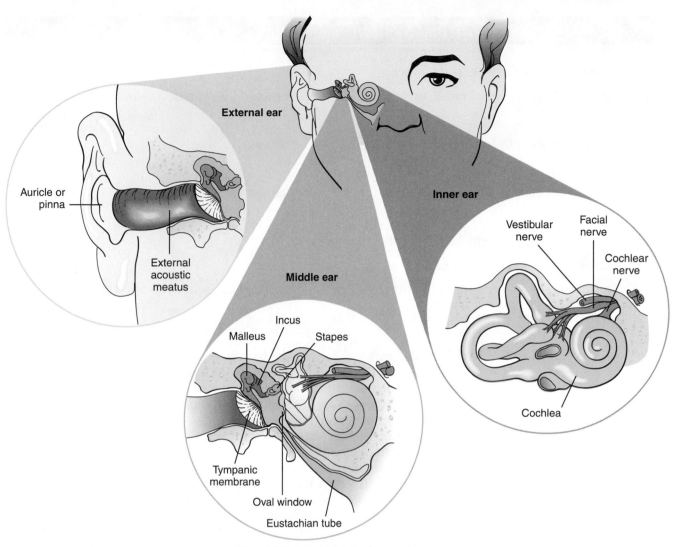

External ear

Auricle or pinna

External acoustic meatus

Inner ear

Vestibular nerve

Facial nerve

Cochlear nerve

Middle ear

Incus

Malleus

Stapes

Tympanic membrane

Oval window

Eustachian tube

Cochlea

FIGURE 10–14 Auditory system.

the surgeon performs a craniotomy and exposes the brain. The surgeon then repairs the nerve, removes a tumor, or otherwise repairs the area.

Common ear procedures are tympanostomy (69433, 69436, ventilation tubes) and myringotomy (69420, 69421, fluid removal from the middle ear).

The code for reporting the use of an operating microscope, 69990, is also in the Auditory System subsection. This code is an add-on code and is never reported alone; rather, it is reported with the procedure in which the operating microscope was used.

EXERCISE 10–5 *Auditory System*

Using the CPT manual, code the following:

1 Left labyrinthotomy with cryosurgery with multiple perfusions, transcanal

Code: _____

2 Bilateral insertion of ventilating tubes, using general anesthesia

Code(s): _____ and _____

3 Transcranial approach with sectioning of the left vestibular nerve

Code: _____

4 Reconstruction of the right auditory canal, due to injury

Code: _____

5 Establishment of an opening in the inner wall of the right inner ear, semicircular canal

Code: _____

External Ear

Incision. The external ear may be the site of an abscess or hematoma and incision and drainage may be simple (69000) or complicated (69005). If the abscess drained is within the auditory canal, report the service with 69020. Be careful when reporting this code as it would be included in more major procedures and not reported separately.

Excision codes for the external ear include codes that report biopsy by location of external ear (69100) or external auditory canal (69105), excision of the external ear, either partially or totally (69110, 69120). If the external ear was reconstructed after the excision, report the repair with split thickness autograft codes (15120, 15121) from the Integumentary System based on the square centimeters used in the repair.

Exostosis is a bony growth. When exostosis is present in the external auditory canal it is termed "surfer's ear," because it is associated with chronic cold water exposure. An incision is made behind the ear to gain access to the canal, and the bony growth is excised (69140).

Removal of Foreign Body. With the shape of the ear, it is easy to see how foreign bodies and cerumen (earwax) can become lodged in the external ear. When a foreign body is removed from the ear, the code reported is based on whether general anesthesia was or was not used (69200, 69205). If impacted cerumen is removed from both ears, report 69210 only once because the code states "one or both ears."

Repair. An **otoplasty** is a procedure performed for protruding ears that may or may not include a decrease in the size of the ear. This procedure is usually performed with the use of conscious sedation, and this sedation is included in code 69300. If both ears are repaired, add modifier -50.

Reconstruction of the external auditory canal may be performed for conditions such as stenosis due to injury or infection (69310) or for a congenital defect (69320). This procedure is a **canalplasty** and is bundled into some other middle ear repair codes, such as 69631-69646. Be careful not to unbundle other more complex repair procedures that include the canalplasty by reporting the canalplasty separately.

Middle Ear

Myringotomy and Tympanostomy. The eustachian tube connects the middle ear to the back of the throat and allows for drainage of fluid. When a eustachian tube dysfunctions, fluid collects in the middle ear. The tube can become inflamed from allergies or infection. Eustachian tube dysfunction is a fairly common condition in children, because the eustachian tube does not always mature to the level of normal function and therefore does not work as well as it does in adults. The condition prevents air from entering the middle ear, and pressure builds up in the middle ear. Surgical intervention is an inflation of the eustachian tube through the nose (transnasal, 69400, 69401). **Myringotomy** is the incision into the tympanic membrane (69420, 69421) and reinflation of the eustachian tube. Tympanostomy is the insertion of a small plastic or metal tube (PE [pressure equalization] tube) that allows the fluid to drain (69433, 69436). The tubes may later be removed, fall out naturally, or sometimes left in place. Surgical removal of a ventilation tube is reported with 69424, which is a procedure that requires general anesthesia. Ventilation tube removal is included in many other more major procedures, in which case the removal is not reported separately. The removal is also unilateral, so if the tubes were removed bilaterally, add modifier -50.

Excision. Middle ear excision procedures include antrotomy (simple mastoidectomy, 69501), mastoidectomy (complete, modified radical, or radical, 69502-69511), polyp removal (69540), and tumor removal (69550-69554). Also included in the Excision category is a petrous apicectomy. The petrous apex of the temporal bone may be the site of infection (petrous apicitis) that can lead to more complicated infection, such as brain abscess or meningitis. Sometimes, to remove the infected bone, a mastoidectomy is performed and is included in the petrous apicectomy code 69530.

Repair. Middle ear repair procedures include revision mastoidectomies based on the extent of the procedure. For example, a simple mastoidectomy is performed on a patient with cholesteatoma of the middle ear. A cholesteatoma is a benign growth of skin in an abnormal location, in this case in the middle ear. The growth may reoccur and the surgeon performs a complete mastoidectomy reported with 69601. If the disease has progressed to the point where the tympanic membrane is damaged and also excised, the procedure is reported with 69604. If a tympanoplasty is planned at the time of the initial surgery and subsequently performed, the procedure is reported with 69631 or 69632, depending on the extent of the repair.

The two major divisions in the tympanoplasty codes are with or without removal of the mastoid bone (mastoidectomy). When no mastoidectomy is performed, choose the code from the 69631-69633 range, based on the extent of the procedure. When a mastoidectomy is performed, report the service with codes from the 69641-69646 range, based on the extent of the procedure. The **ossicular chain** is the malleus (hammer), incus (anvil), and stapes (stirrup). The chain may be eroded and repaired as a part of a tympanoplasty, reported with 69632 or 69642. The repair may be so extensive that it may require the use of prosthesis, such as a partial ossicular replacement prosthesis (PORP, incus and malleus are absent or damaged) or total ossicular replacement prosthesis (TORP, incus and arch of the stapes are damaged, or the malleus, incus and arch of the stapes are absent). PORP and TORP are reported with 69633 or 69637 depending upon other repairs performed during the tympanoplasty.

Inner Ear

Incision and/or Destruction. A **labyrinth** is a cavelike structure, and in the inner ear the labyrinth is dominated by two fluid-filled spaces that contain endolymph and perilymph. These spaces contain the nervous tissue responsible for hearing and balance. When the pressure within a space is altered, vertigo, ringing in the ears and hearing loss may occur. A **labyrinthotomy** is a procedure in which the labyrinth is surgically incised, and various procedures performed to return the labyrinth to functional condition. Codes 69801 and 69802 are reported for a labyrinthotomy based on whether or not a mastoidectomy was performed.

Excision. A **labyrinthectomy** is a procedure in which the incus and stapes are removed. If a transcanal approach is used, report 69905 and if a postauricular incision (behind the ear) is used as the approach, report the procedure with 69910.

Introduction. A **cochlear device implant** (Fig. 10–15) is a computerized device that restores partial hearing in those who are profoundly hearing impaired. A receiver on the outside of the skin behind the ear picks up sound waves. The receiver is placed over the transmitter which is surgically implanted under the skin behind the ear. A sound processor, which is connected to an electrode that is implanted between the processor and the cochlea, receives a signal from the transmitter and transfers the signal to the cochlear nerve that is then stimulated. The implantation of the cochlear device is reported with 69930.

Temporal Bone, Middle Fossa Approach. The middle fossa approach is used by surgeons to excise acoustic neuromas, to decompress the facial nerve (proximal temporal), and repair nerves in the vestibular labyrinth. The codes in the Temporal Bone, Middle Fossa Approach subheading report removal of the vestibular nerve (69950), relief of pressure (decompression) of the facial nerve and/or repair (69955), decompression of the internal auditory canal (69960), and removal of tumors of the temporal bone (69970).

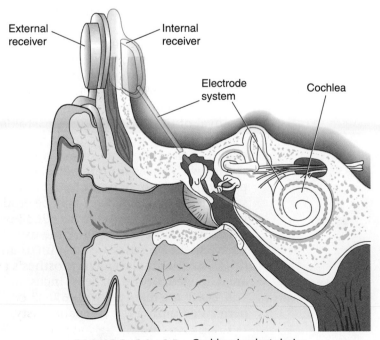

FIGURE 10–15 Cochlear implant device.

Operating Microscope. An operating microscope (Fig. 10–16) is used in microsurgical procedures and is reported separately with add-on code 69990, unless the code indicates the inclusion of use of an operating microscope. This does not include magnifying loupes (Fig. 10–17) that are used to enlarge the area being viewed.

QUICK CHECK 10-5

Use of the operating microscope is used only with procedures on the ear. True or False?

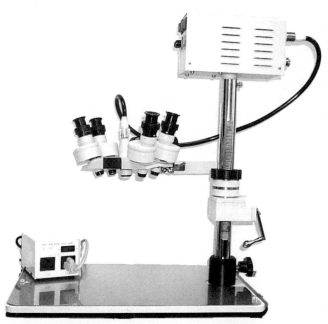

FIGURE 10–16 The operating microscope allows for visualization of minute structures, such as nerve fibers and blood vessels. (From Microsurgery Instruments Inc.: *The Economic Operating Microscope* (website): http://www.microsurgeryusa.com/EOM.htm. Accessed June 1, 2006.)

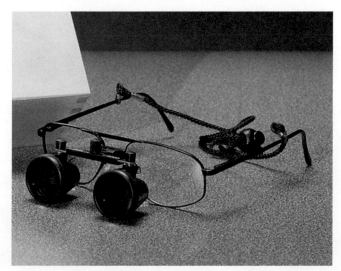

FIGURE 10–17 Magnifying loupes are produced in a range of powers. (From Mopec: *Magnifying Loupe* (website): http://www.mopec.com/chapter1/ch1_Magnifying_Loupe.htm. Accessed February 20, 2008.)

CHAPTER REVIEW

CHAPTER 10, PART I, THEORY

Complete the following:

1 The surgical removal of the spleen is a(n)

_____ .

2 Partial or total removal of the spleen is reported separately, even if it is a part of a more major procedure.

   True   False

3 A person can live only a short time without a spleen, so every effort is made to do only a partial removal.

   True   False

4 A(n) _____ lymphadenectomy is the removal of the lymph nodes, gland(s), and surrounding tissue.

5 How many endocrine glands are included in the Endocrine subsection of the CPT manual?

   _____

6 The pituitary and pineal gland procedure codes are in what subsection of the Surgery

   section? _____

7 The codes for pancreatic procedures are located in what subsection of the Surgery section?

   _____

8 Both subtotal and partial mean something less

   than _____ .

9 Twist or _____ holes are made through the skull to accomplish procedures of the brain.

10 The _____ procedure is the method used to obtain exposure to a lesion of

   the skull base, and the _____ procedure is what is done to the lesion.

11 CSF means _____ .

12 The most commonly known neuroplasty

   procedure is a _____ release.

CHAPTER 10, PART II, PRACTICAL

Code the following cases:

13 Using a cervical approach, ligation of the thoracic duct was accomplished.

 Code(s): _____

14 Surgical laparoscopy with bilateral total pelvic lymphadenectomy

 Code(s): _____

15 Superficial inguinofemoral lymphadenectomy with pelvic lymphadenectomy including the external iliac, hypogastric, and obturator nodes

 Code(s): _____

16 Total thyroidectomy

 Code(s): _____

17 Surgical laparoscopy with partial adrenalectomy using a transabdominal approach

 Code(s): _____

18 Parathyroidectomy with mediastinal exploration

 Code(s): _____

19 Excision of corneal lesion of right eye

 Code(s): _____

20 Iridectomy with corneal section for removal of lesion from left eye

 Code(s): _____

QUICK CHECK ANSWERS

QUICK CHECK 10-1
True

QUICK CHECK 10-2
Modifier -50

QUICK CHECK 10-3
1. Temporary: 64400-64530, Permanent: 64600-64681
2. Somatic, Sympathetic

QUICK CHECK 10-4
1. c
2. a
3. b

QUICK CHECK 10-5
False

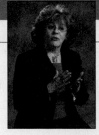

"Try not to stay in just one specialty. Become educated and learn other specialties so you can grow in all types of coding."

Patricia Champion, CPC
Licensed PMCC Instructor,
    Educator/Trainer
AAPC National Advisory Board
Nashville, Tennessee

Radiology Section

Chapter Topics

Format

Radiology Terminology

Procedures

Planes

Guidelines

The Radiology Subsections

Chapter Review

Quick Check Answers

Learning Objectives

After completing this chapter you should be able to

1   Demonstrate an understanding of Radiology terminology.

2   Analyze the elements of component coding in reporting radiology services.

3   Identify elements of the global procedure.

4   State the appropriate coding of contrast material.

5   Explain the format of the Radiology section.

6   Demonstrate the ability to code Radiology services and procedures.

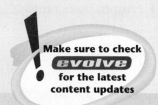

Make sure to check **evolve** for the latest content updates

FORMAT   **Radiology** is the branch of medicine that uses radiant energy to diagnose and treat patients. The term originally referred to the use of x-rays to produce radiographs but is now commonly applied to all types of medical imaging. A physician who specializes in radiology is a **radiologist.** Radiologists can provide services to patients independent of or in conjunction with another physician of a different specialty. The Radiology section of the CPT manual is divided into subsections:

- Diagnostic Radiology
- Diagnostic Ultrasound
- Radiologic Guidance
- Breast Mammography
- Bone/Joint Studies
- Radiation Oncology
- Nuclear Medicine

RADIOLOGY TERMINOLOGY   The suffix *-graphy* means "making of a film" using a variety of methods. **Radiography** is a broad term used to indicate any number of methods used by radiologists to do diagnostic testing. The following exercise will familiarize you with some of the numerous radiographic procedures in the CPT manual.

EXERCISE 11–1 *Radiology Terminology*

The following words end in "-graphy," meaning "making of a film." For example, in angiocardiography, "angio" means vessels and "cardio" means heart, so angiocardiography is the making of a film of the heart and vessels. What do the other "-graphy" words mean?

angiocardiography _____ heart and vessels _____

1 aortography _____

2 arthrography _____

3 cholangiopancreatography _____

4 cholangiography _____

5 cystography _____

6 dacryocystography _____

7 duodenography _____

8 echocardiography _____

9 encephalography _____

10 epididymography _____

11 hepatography _____

12 hysterosalpingography _____

13 laryngography _____

14 lymphangiography _____

15 myelography _____

16 pyelography _____

17 sialography _____

18 sinography _____

19 splenography _____

20 urography _____

21 venography _____

22 vesiculography _____

PROCEDURES   Here are just a few more radiographic procedures for your review:

1. **Fluoroscopy** is an x-ray procedure that allows the visualization of internal organs in motion. It uses real-time video images. After x-rays pass through the patient, instead of using film, the images are captured by a device called an image intensifier and converted into light. The light is then captured by a camera and diplayed on a video monitor. Fluoroscopy allows for the study of the function of the organ (physiology) as well as the structure of the organ (anatomy).

2. **Magnetic resonance imaging (MRI)** is a radiology technique that uses magnetism, radio waves, and a computer to produce images of body structures. The MRI scanner is a tube surrounded by a giant circular magnet. The patient is placed on a moveable bed that is inserted into the magnet. The magnet creates a strong magnetic field that aligns the protons of hydrogen atoms, which are then exposed to a beam of radio waves. This spins the various protons of the body and produces a faint signal that is detected by the receiver portion of the MRI scanner. The received information is processed by a computer, and an image is then produced.

3. **Tomography** is the process of producing a tomogram, a two-dimensional image of a slice or section, through a three-dimensional object. Tomography achieves this result by simply moving an x-ray source in one direction as the x-ray film is moved in the opposite direction. The tomogram is the picture, the tomograph is the apparatus, and the tomography is the process.

4. **Biometry** is the application of a statistical method to a biologic fact.

PLANES   Terminology referring to planes of the body and the positioning of the body is often used in the Radiology section. A **position** is how the patient is placed during the x-ray examination, and a **projection** is the path of the x-ray beam. An example of a projection is anteroposterior, which denotes that the x-ray beam enters the patient's body at the front (anterior) and exits from

From the Trenches

"We have a very strong camaraderie. Through networking, when coders have problems with their notes or some questions they may have in coding, they can always call someone they have networked with to get an answer."

PATRICIA

the back (posterior). An example of a position is **prone**, which means the patient is lying on his or her anterior (front), but the sides of entrance and exit of the x-ray beam are not specified. Familiarity with this terminology will aid you as you review the Radiology section and begin to choose the correct codes for physician services. Fig. 11–1 illustrates the major planes and the surfaces of the body that can be accessed by positioning the body.

Fig. 11–2 shows proximal and distal body references. **Proximal** and **distal** are directional body references that mean closest to (proximal) or farthest from (distal) the trunk of the body. These terms are relative, meaning they are used to describe the position of the part as compared with another part. Therefore, the term "proximal" describes a part as being closer to the body trunk than another part, and the term "distal" describes a part as being farther away from the body than another part. The knee would be described as being proximal to the ankle, and it would also be described as being distal to the thigh or hip.

Fig. 11–3 illustrates the **anteroposterior (AP)** (front to back) position, in which the patient has his or her front (anterior) closest to the x-ray machine, and the x-ray travels through the patient from the front to the back. In Fig. 11–4, the **posteroanterior (PA)** position, the patient has his or her back

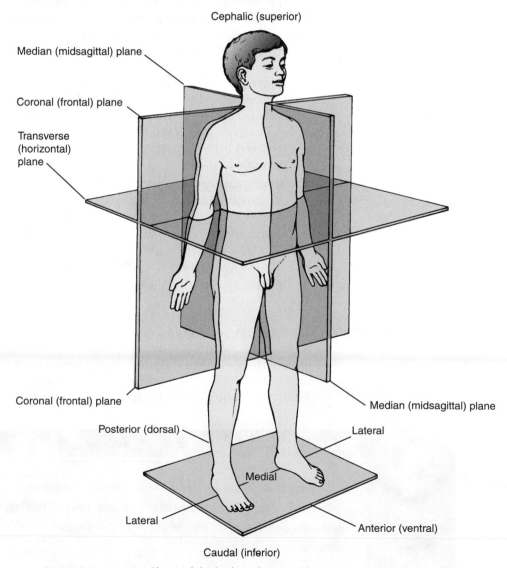

FIGURE 11–1   Planes of the body and terms of location and position of the body.

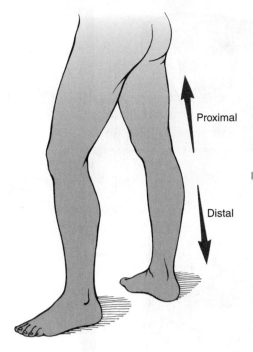

FIGURE 11–2   Proximal and distal.

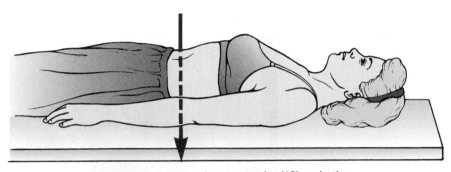

FIGURE 11–3   Anteroposterior (AP) projection.

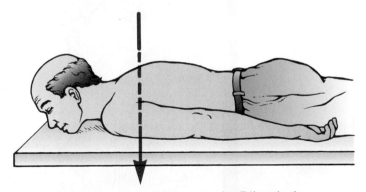

FIGURE 11–4   Posteroanterior (PA) projection.

(posterior) located closest to the machine, and the beam travels through the patient from back to front.

Lateral positions are side positions. When the patient's right side is closest to the film, it is called *right lateral*. When the patient's left side is closest to the film, it is called *left lateral*. For example, Fig. 11–5 shows a left lateral position, and Fig. 11–6 shows a right lateral position. The use of these various positions allows the physician to view the body from a variety of

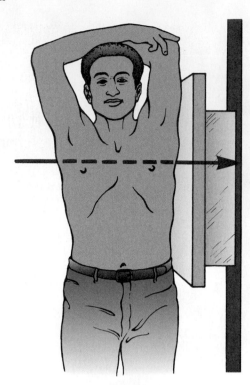

FIGURE 11–5 Left lateral projection.

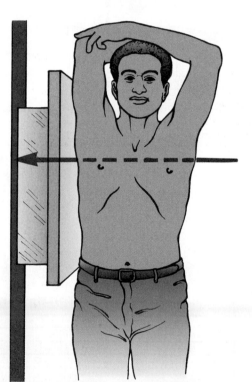

FIGURE 11–6 Right lateral projection.

angles. Fig. 11–7 shows posteroanterior and lateral positions used to view a patient with emphysema.

Dorsal (more commonly refers to the "back" but may be stated to mean "supine") means lying on the back; **ventral** (more commonly refers to the "anterior" but may be stated as "prone") means lying on the stomach; and **lateral** means lying on the side.

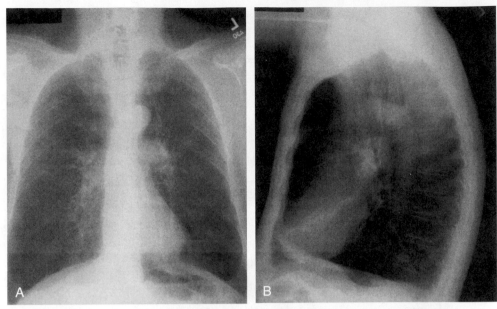

FIGURE 11–7 **(A)** Posteranterior and **(B)** lateral radiographs of the thorax in a patient with emphysema. (From Goldman L, Ausiello D, editors: *Cecil Medicine*, ed 23, Philadelphia, 2008, Saunders.)

Decubitus positions are recumbent positions; the x-ray beam is placed horizontally. *Ventral decubitus* (prone) is the act of lying on the stomach (Fig. 11–8, *A*), and *dorsal decubitus* (supine) is the act of lying on the back (Fig. 11–8, *B*). The term "decubitus," generally shortened to "decub," has a special meaning in radiology. The simple act of lying on one's back would be referred to as lying supine, but if a horizontal x-ray beam is used, the position becomes decubitus. The type of decubitus is determined by the body surface the patient is lying on.

Recumbent means lying down. Thus, *right lateral recumbent* means the patient is lying on the right side (Fig. 11–8, *C*), and *left lateral recumbent* means the patient is lying on the left side (Fig. 11–8, *D*). In the ventral decubitus position, the patient is positioned prone and the x-ray beam comes into the patient from the right side and exits on the left (Fig. 11–8, *E*).

In the *left lateral decubitus* position, the patient is lying on the left side with the beam coming from the front and passing through to the back (anteroposterior) (Fig. 11–8, *F*).

When the patient is positioned on his or her back (dorsal decubitus) and the x-ray beam comes into the left side of the patient, the positioning is dorsal decubitus, but the view obtained is a right lateral (because the right side is closest to the film) (Fig. 11–8, *G*).

Oblique views refer to those obtained while the body is rotated so it is not in a full anteroposterior or posteroanterior position but somewhat diagonal. Oblique views are termed according to the body surface on which the patient is lying. The *left anterior oblique (LAO)* position is depicted in Fig. 11–8, *H* with the patient's left side rotated forward toward the table. The patient is lying on the left anterior aspect of his or her body. The *right anterior oblique (RAO)* position has the patient on his or her right side rotated forward toward the table, as in Fig. 11–8, *I*.

Two more oblique views are left posterior oblique and right posterior oblique. In the *left posterior oblique (LPO)* view, the patient is rotated so that

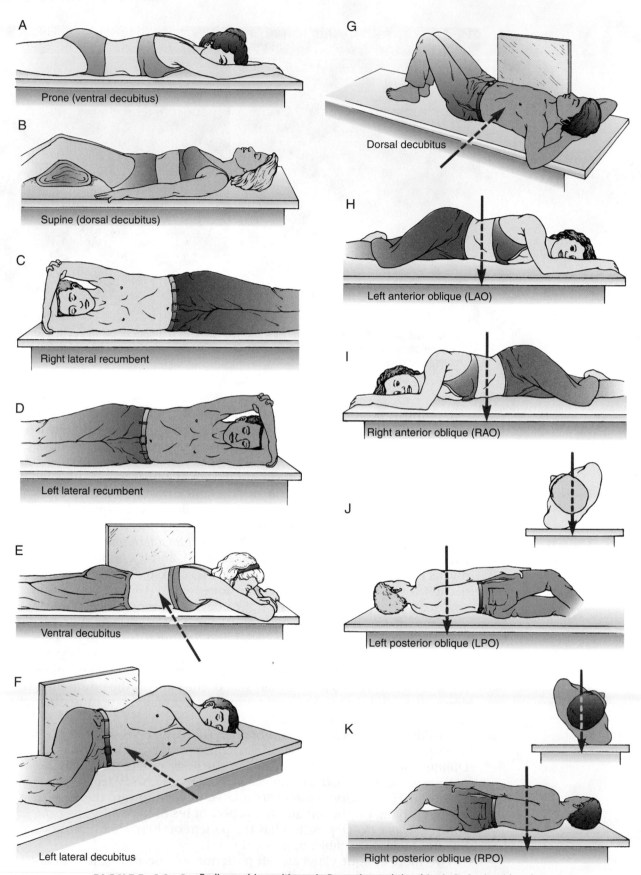

FIGURE 11–8 Radiographic positions. **A**, Prone (ventral decubitus). **B**, Supine (dorsal decubitus). **C**, Right lateral recumbent. **D**, Left lateral recumbent. **E**, Ventral decubitus. **F**, Left lateral decubitus. **G**, Dorsal decubitus. **H**, Left anterior oblique (LAO). **I**, Right anterior oblique (RAO). **J**, Left posterior oblique (LPO). **K**, Right posterior oblique (RPO).

the left posterior aspect of his or her body is against the table, as in Fig. 11–8, *J*. The *right posterior oblique (RPO)* view has the patient with the right side rotated back, as in Fig. 11–8, *K*.

The last two terms that are used to describe projections are tangential and axial. **Tangential** is the patient position that allows the beam to skim the body part, which produces a profile of the structure of the body (Fig. 11–9, *A*). Fig. 11–9, *B* illustrates the **axial** projection, which is any projection that allows the beam to pass through the body part lengthwise.

EXERCISE 11–2 *Planes*

Fill in the blanks with the correct words:

1 What is the word that indicates how the patient is placed during the x-ray examination?

_____

2 What is the term that indicates the path the x-ray beam travels? _____

_____

What do the following abbreviations mean?

3 AP _____

4 PA _____

5 RAO _____

6 LPO _____

7 What term indicates that a patient is lying supine, or on his or her back? _____

8 What term indicates that a patient is lying prone, or on his or her stomach?

_____

9 What term indicates that a patient is lying on his or her right side? _____

10 What is the term that indicates when a patient is on his or her back and the x-ray beam comes into the right side of the patient? _____

GUIDELINES   As with all Guidelines, the Radiology Guidelines should be read carefully before radiologic procedures or services are coded. The Guidelines contain the unique instructions used within the section and the indications for multiple procedures, separate procedures, unlisted radiology procedure codes, and applicable modifiers.

Guidelines that are used more commonly in this section than in others are those explaining the professional, technical, and global components of a procedure. These components are as follows:

1. **Professional:** describes the services of the physician, including the supervision of the taking of the x-ray film and the interpretation with report of the x-ray films.

2. **Technical:** describes the services of the technologist, as well as the use of the equipment, film, and other supplies.

3. **Global:** describes the combination of the professional and technical components (1 and 2).

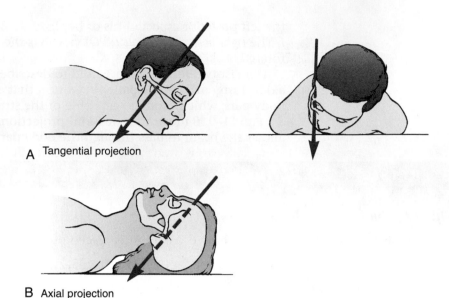

A Tangential projection

B Axial projection

FIGURE 11-9 Radiographic projections. **A,** Tangential projection. **B,** Axial projection.

For example, if a patient undergoes a radiology procedure in a clinic that owns its own equipment, employs its own technologist(s), and also employs the radiologist who supervises, interprets, and reports on the radiologic results, the global procedure is reported. But if the radiologist is reading and interpreting films that were taken at another facility, only the professional component would be reported for physician services.

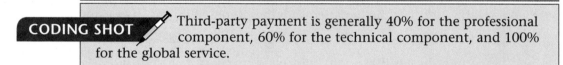

CODING SHOT Third-party payment is generally 40% for the professional component, 60% for the technical component, and 100% for the global service.

When only the professional component of the service is provided, the modifier -26 is placed after the CPT code. Modifier -26 alerts the third-party payer to the fact that only the professional component was provided. If, for example, an independent radiology facility takes a complete chest x-ray (71030) and sends the x-rays to an independent radiologist who reads the x-rays and writes a report of the findings in the x-rays, the coding for the independent radiologist would be

71030-26   Complete chest x-ray, four views
            Professional component only

There is no CPT modifier to indicate the technical component of radiologic services. The modifier most commonly used is the HCPCS Level II modifier -TC, which stands for technical component. HCPCS codes are for use with Medicare and Medicaid claims, which you will be learning about in Chapter 13 of this text; some commercial payers may also recognize some HCPCS codes such as those for drugs and supplies. When submitting claims for radiologic services in which only the technical component was provided, use a CPT code followed by -TC. For example, if you were the coder for the independent radiology facility that took the complete chest x-ray (71030), you would code as follows:

71030-TC   Complete chest x-ray, four views
            Technical component only

> **CODING SHOT** ✎ -TC (Technical Component) and -26 (Professional Component) are terms used by third-party payers. When contacting a payer regarding payment of a service, first determine if there is a separate allowance for the -TC and -26.

Supervision and Interpretation

The other coding practice most commonly used in the Radiology section is called **component** or **combination coding**, which means that a code from the Radiology section as well as a code from one of the other sections must be used to fully describe the procedure. For example, interventional radiologists may inject contrast material; place stents, catheters, or guide wires; or perform any number of procedures found throughout the CPT manual. Many times, before radiology procedures can be performed, a contrast material must be injected into the patient to make certain organs or vessels stand out more clearly on the radiographic image. When this contrast material is injected into the patient by the radiologist, a CPT code from the Surgery section must be used to indicate the injection procedure.

> **CODING SHOT** ✎ Codes in the Radiology section describe only the radiology procedures, not the injections or placement of other material necessary to perform the procedure.

Suppose, for example, a voiding urethrocystography with contrast medium enhancement is performed. In this procedure, a physician injects a radioactive material into the bladder. An x-ray of the bladder (cystography) is then obtained; the x-rays show filling, voiding, and post-voiding. The injection portion of the procedure is coded with a surgery code (51600: Injection procedure for cystography or voiding urethrocystography) and the cystography is coded with a radiology code (74455: Urethrocystography, voiding, radiologic supervision and interpretation).

As a new coder, you will need to pay special attention to the information in parentheses below the codes in the Radiology section. This parenthetic material gives you information about other components of procedures. Previous editions of the CPT manual had combination codes that were used when the physician did both components of some procedures. Using the combination code replaced the use of one code from surgery and one code from radiology; but many of these combination codes have been deleted. One reason they were deleted is to allow the physicians to more specifically indicate the services provided to the patient. There are many parenthetic phrases such as this throughout the Radiology section and you will want to refer to them when coding component procedures.

Odds and Ends

Many of the code descriptions state "radiologic supervision and interpretation" and alert you to component coding. Always read the parenthetic information that follows these component codes.

Some codes are divided based on the extent of the radiologic examination, such as procedures that "specify with KUB" (kidney, ureter, and bladder). You must read the radiologist's report or the details in the medical record so as to understand the full extent of the procedure.

Codes are also often divided on the basis of whether contrast materials were used. The phrase "with contrast" in the CPT manual means contrast that was administered intravascularly, intra-articularly, or intrathecally (into the subarachnoid space). If the procedure indicates that contrast was administered orally or rectally, the service is coded as "without contrast."

> **CODING SHOT** ✎ Report the supply of contrast material with Medicine section code 99070, supplies. Injection of contrast material is included in the "with contrast" radiology procedure code, unless guidelines state that a surgical code should also be used to report the injection procedure.

There are new guidelines issued by the CMS that were originally titled Medically Unbelievable Edits (MUEs). CMS changed the name to Medically Unlikely Edits. This information is included in a software system that allows Medicare to reduce the number of claims that contain medically improbable information, such as a hysterectomy on a male patient. There are approximately 3,000 edits in the software and 60 of those directly relate to radiology service. For example, one type of edit is the maximum number of units that can be reported. For example, if the MUE indicated that the maximum number of units for a particular radiology service was two for particular service and you submitted for three units, the claim would be automatically edited. Unlike some edits, you cannot override the MUEs by addending a modifier. Denied claims must be appealed with supporting documentation that indicates the service was medically necessary, was administered in a separate session, or was a repeat procedure by the same physician. Pay special attention to the parenthetical information following the codes in the CPT because this material provides necessary information about the components of the procedure. Radiographic procedures are located in the CPT manual index under the main term "X-ray," with subterms for the anatomic part (e.g., hand, spine).

EXERCISE 11–3 *Guidelines*

Fill in the blanks using the Radiology Guidelines of your CPT manual:

1 What procedure is one that is "performed independently of, and is not immediately related to, other services"? _____

2 What is the name of the Medicare edit software?

_____

3 Using your CPT manual, list at least four of the subsections of the Radiology section.

_____

_____

_____

_____

THE RADIOLOGY SUBSECTIONS

Diagnostic Radiology

The most standard radiographic procedures are contained in the Diagnostic Radiology subsection (70010-76499) of the Radiology section. This subsection describes diagnostic imaging, including plain x-ray films, the use of computed axial tomography (CAT or CT) scanning, magnetic resonance imaging (MRI), magnetic resonance angiography (MRA), and angiography. CT scanning uses an x-ray beam that rotates around the patient, as illustrated in Fig. 11–10. Fig. 11–11 shows the detail that can be obtained

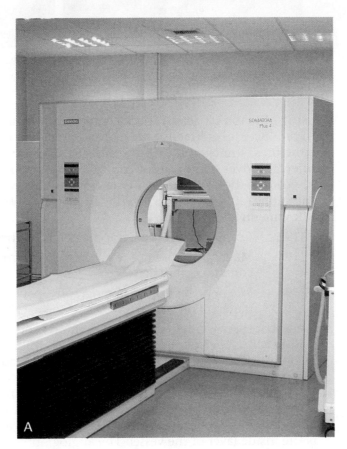

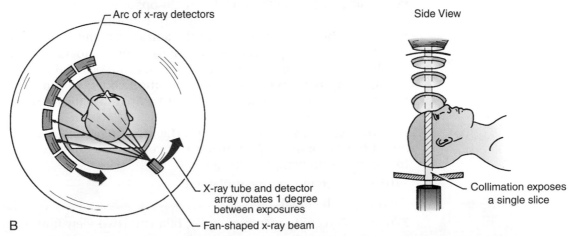

FIGURE 11–10 **A,** Computed tomography scanner. **B,** Principles of computed tomographic (CT) scanning. The x-ray tube produces a fan-shaped beam that passes through a section (slice) of the patient. This fan-shaped beam is received by a circular array of detectors at the opposite side. These detectors receive x-rays along the path through the patient's body. The detector and x-ray source rotate around the axis, producing exposures at 1-degree intervals of rotation. (From Drake RL, Vogl W, Mitchell AWM: *Gray's Anatomy for Students,* Philadelphia, 2005, Elsevier Inc. **B** from Stimac GK: *Introduction to Diagnostic Imaging,* Philadelphia, WB Saunders, 1992, p 5.)

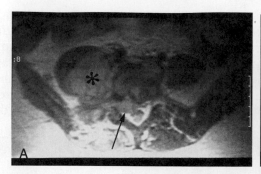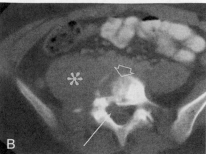

FIGURE 11–11 **(A)** and **(B)** Axial MRI frame. *Arrows* highlight the descending aorta. (From Bragg DG, Rubin P, Hricak H: *Oncologic Imaging,* ed 2, Philadelphia, 2002, Saunders.)

using MRI and CT scans. Special computer software is used with CT scanners to produce three-dimensional images, which are used to study internal structures. Tomography, CT scanning, and MRI may include the use of injectable dyes (radiographic contrast) to aid in imaging, and the codes are divided on the basis of whether or not contrast was used. For example, under the subheading Spine and Pelvis (72010-72295), the codes for CAT, MRI, and MRA are divided as follows:

72192   Computerized tomography, pelvis; without contrast material

72195   Magnetic resonance (e.g., proton) imaging, pelvis; without contrast material(s)

72198   Magnetic resonance angiography, pelvis, with or without contrast material(s)

Note that there is one code for the CAT, one code for the MRI, and one code for the MRA. The codes are divided by CAT, MRI, and MRA throughout the Diagnostic Radiology subsection. So you must read the code carefully to ensure that you are using the code that represents the correct type of imaging. Fig. 11–12 is an example of a magnetic resonance image.

In **angiography**, dyes are injected into the vessels to add contrast that facilitates the visualization of vessels' lumen size and condition. The lumen is the inside layer of the vessel. The angiography is performed to view blood vessels after injecting them with a radio-opaque dye that outlines the vessels on x-ray. Angiography is used to identify abnormalities inside the vessels. Fig. 11–13 shows an angiogram of the aortic arch and brachiocephalic vessels. The radiologist studies the vessels using angiography to detect conditions such as malformations, strokes, or myocardial infarctions.

Angiography allows for some combination codes; so you must carefully read the complete procedure descriptor and parenthetical information to assure correct coding.

Mammography (77051-77059) is the use of diagnostic radiology to detect breast tumors or other abnormal breast conditions, such as these codes used to report mammography services:

77055   Mammography; unilateral

77056   bilateral

77057   Screening mammography, bilateral (two-view film study of each breast)

Codes 77055 and 77056 are for use when the mammography is performed to detect a suspected tumor. For example, a patient who upon examination has demonstrated an abnormality in a breast would appropriately have the service reported with 77055. If, however, a patient has presented for the usual screening mammography, you would report the service with 77057.

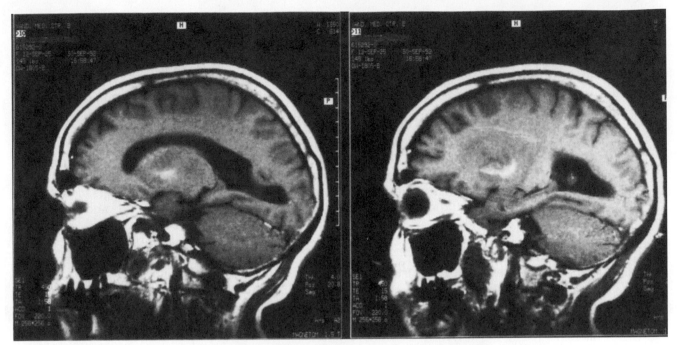

FIGURE 11-12 Magnetic resonance imaging (MRI) scan slices into the axial, coronal, and sagittal planes from a patient with subcortical aphasia. The lesion is an infarction involving the anterior caudate, putamen, and anterior limb of the left internal capsule. (From Bradley WG, Daroff RB, Fenichel GM, Jankovic J: *Neurology in Clinical Practice*, ed 5, Philadelphia, 2008, Butterworth-Heinemann.)

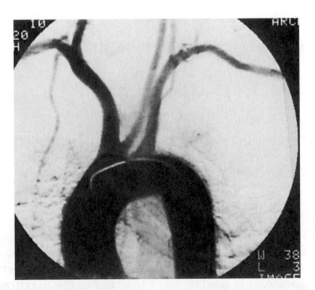

FIGURE 11-13 Angiography of the aortic arch and brachiocephalic vessels. (From Stimac GK: *Introduction to Diagnostic Imaging*, Philadelphia, WB Saunders, 1992, p 447.)

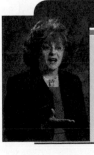

From the Trenches

What are the benefits to working in medical coding?

"Feeling that you have not just helped doctors improve their bottom line, but you also have helped patients not to have to worry about their bills."

PATRICIA

Note that the description for the usual screening mammography indicates "bilateral," because screening mammography is done on both breasts.

When new codes are published, such as 77055-77057, new in 2007, the submission of the new codes may require special attention. Under radiology guidelines, if a service is rarely provided, unusual, variable, or new, when submitting for reimbursement of the service a special report may be necessary. The report would include the complexity of symptoms, final diagnosis, pertinent physical findings, diagnostic/therapeutic procedures, concurrent problems, and follow up care.

Codes in the Diagnostic Radiology subsection are divided according to anatomic site, from the head down. Some of the codes indicate a specific number of views, such as a minimum of three views or a single view. You should pay special attention to the description in each code and understand clearly how many views are specified in the code.

CODING SHOT If fewer than the total number of views specified in the code are taken, modifier -52 would be used to indicate to the third-party payer that less of the procedure was performed than is described by the code, unless a code already exists for the smaller number of views.

EXERCISE 11-4 *Diagnostic Radiology*

Code the radiology portion of the procedures unless otherwise directed:

1 What is the code for a diagnostic mammography, bilateral?

Code: _____

2 What is the code for an unlisted diagnostic radiologic procedure?

Code: _____

3 What is the code for the supervision and interpretation of an aortography, thoracic, by serialography?

Code: _____

Diagnostic Ultrasound

The second subsection (76506-76999) in Radiology is Diagnostic Ultrasound. **Diagnostic ultrasound** is the use of high-frequency sound waves to image anatomic structures and to detect the cause of illness and disease. It is used by the physician in the diagnosis process. Ultrasound moves at different speeds through tissue, depending on the density of the tissue. Forms and outlines of organs can be identified by ultrasound as the sound waves move through or bounce back (echo) from the tissues.

QUICK CHECK 11-1

According to the information in Diagnostic Ultrasound, Obstetrical, the studies of multiple gestation pregnancies are reported with an add-on code or modifier _____.

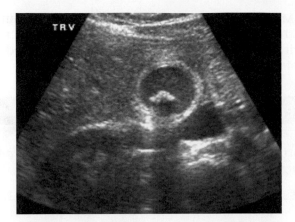

FIGURE 11–14 Ultrasound showing a gallstone. (From Goldman L, Ausiello D, editors: *Cecil Medicine,* ed 23, Philadelphia, 2008, Saunders.)

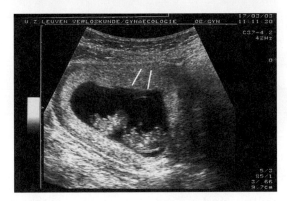

FIGURE 11–15 Twins (indicated by *arrows*) on first trimester ultrasound scan. (From James DK, Steer PJ, Weiner CP, Gonik B: *High Risk Pregnancy: Management Options,* ed 3, Philadelphia, 2006, Saunders.)

There are many uses for ultrasound in medicine, such as showing a gallstone (Fig. 11–14) and showing twins in the first trimester (Fig. 11–15). You may think that these ultrasound procedures do not produce a picture clear enough to be of use to the physician in the diagnosis process, but a professional trained in the interpretation of ultrasound images is able to read them clearly.

Codes for ultrasound procedures are found in three locations:

- Radiology section, Diagnostic Ultrasound subsection, 76506-76999, is usually divided on the basis of the anatomic location of the procedure (chest, pelvis)

- Medicine section, Non-Invasive Vascular Diagnostic Studies subsection, 93875-93990, divided on the basis of the anatomic location of the procedure (cerebrovascular, extremity)

- Medicine section, Echocardiography (ultrasound of the heart and great arteries), 93303-93350

An **interventional radiologist** is a physician who is skilled in both the surgical procedure and the radiology portion of an interventional radiologic service. The interventional radiologist is a board-certified physician who specializes in minimally invasive, targeted treatments performed using image guidance. These procedures have less risk, pain, and recovery time compared with open surgery. For example, an interventional radiologist who performed a liver biopsy using CT guidance to locate the lesion would report the services by using a surgery code (47000) and a radiology code (77012). Neither code would have a modifier because the interventional radiologist provided the surgical portion of the service, reporting it with a surgery code, and provided the CT guidance service, reporting it with a code from the Radiology section.

Most of the services in the Diagnostic Ultrasound subsection are located in the index of the CPT manual under the main term "Ultrasound." These terms are subdivided anatomically and by procedure, e.g., guidance or drainage.

EXERCISE 11–5 *Diagnostic Ultrasound*

In the CPT manual, Diagnostic Ultrasound is usually divided into subheadings. Locate and list the subheadings:

1 _____

2 _____

3 _____

4 _____

5 _____

6 _____

7 _____

8 _____

9 _____

An ultrasound is a radiology technique that uses high frequency sound waves to produce images of the organs and structures of the body. The sound waves are sent through body tissues with a device called a transducer. The transducer is placed directly on the skin to which a gel has been applied. The sound waves that are sent by the transducer through the body are then reflected by internal structures that return an echo to the transducer. The echoes are then transmitted electronically to the viewing monitor. The echo images are recorded on film or video tape. After the ultrasound, the gel is wiped off. The technical term for ultrasound testing and recording is sonography. Ultrasound testing is painless and involves no radiation and produces no harmful side effects.

Ultrasound examinations can be used in various areas of the body for a multitude of purposes. These purposes can include examination of the chest, abdomen, and blood vessels (such as to detect blood clots in veins). Ultrasound can obtain detailed images of the size and function of the heart and detect abnormalities of the valves (such as mitral valve prolapse and aortic stenosis) and endocarditis (infection of the heart). Ultrasound is commonly used to guide fluid withdrawal (aspiration) from the chest, lung, or heart. Other uses of ultrasound include gallstone detection and viewing of the ureter, liver, spleen, pancreas, and aorta within the abdomen. Ultrasound can detect fluid, cysts, tumors, or abscesses in the abdomen or liver, aortic aneurysms, evaluate the structure of the thyroid gland in the neck, arteriosclerosis in the legs, and evaluation of the size, gender, movement, and position of the growing baby during pregnancy.

Modes and Scans. There are four different types of ultrasound listed in the CPT manual: A-mode, M-mode, B-scan, and real-time scan.

A-mode: one-dimensional display reflecting the time it takes the sound wave to reach a structure and reflect back. This process maps the outline of the structure. "A" is for amplitude of sound return (echo).

M-mode: one-dimensional display of the movement of structures. "M" stands for motion.

B-scan: two-dimensional display of the movement of tissues and organs. "B" stands for brightness. The sound waves bounce off tissue or organs and are projected onto a black and white television screen. The strong signals display as black and the weaker signals display as lighter shades of gray. B-scan is also called gray-scale ultrasound.

Real-time scan: two-dimensional display of both the structure and the motion of tissues and organs that indicates the size, shape, and movement of the tissue or organ.

These modes and scans are used to describe the codes throughout the Diagnostic Ultrasound subsection. Codes are often divided on the basis of the scan or mode that was used. The medical record will indicate the scan or mode used.

Several codes within the subsection include the use of Doppler ultrasound. **Doppler ultrasound** is the use of sound that can be transmitted only through solids or liquids and is a specific version of ultrasonography, or ultrasound. Doppler ultrasound is named for an Austrian physicist, Johann Doppler, who discovered a relationship between sound and light waves—a relationship upon which ultrasound technology was built. Doppler ultrasound is used to measure moving objects and so is ideal for measuring bloodflow. Codes often state "with or without Doppler." Doppler ultrasound can be standard black and white or color. Color Doppler translates the standard black and white into colored images. Just imagine how much easier it is to see a leak in a vessel when the vessel is yellow and the blood is red. The code descriptions will specifically state "color-flow Doppler."

There is some component coding necessary, but it occurs mostly under the subheading of Ultrasonic Guidance Procedures (76930-76999). The parenthetic information will refer you to the surgical procedure code. For example, code 76945 is for the radiologic supervision and interpretation of ultrasonic guidance for chorionic villus sampling. The physician guides the insertion of a needle to withdraw the sample. If the physician performed both the radiologic portion of the procedure and the surgical procedure, you would report 59015 from the Surgery section and 76945 from the Radiology section.

EXERCISE 11–6 *Modes and Scans*

Fill in the codes for the following:

1 An ultrasound of the spinal canal

Code: _____

2 An ultrasound of the chest and mediastinum, real time

Code: _____

3 A complete abdominal ultrasound in real time with image documentation

Code: _____

4 A repeat uterine ultrasound in real time with image documentation of a 32-week pregnant female

Code: _____

5 A fetal profile, biophysical, with nonstress testing

Code: _____

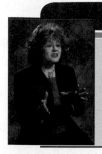

From the Trenches

"There are so many opportunities and not enough skilled coders to fill the positions for physician's offices, clinics, hospitals, as health care consultants, and also in colleges to teach coding at a college level."

PATRICIA

Radiation Oncology

The Radiation Oncology subsection (77261-77799) of the Radiology section deals with both professional and technical treatments utilizing radiation to destroy tumors. The subsection is divided on the basis of treatment. In this subsection, special attention must be given to reporting the professional and technical components. Read all of the definitions carefully to make certain you know what the code includes. Many third-party payers have developed strict guidelines determining the number of times certain procedures are allowed within each treatment course. You should work closely with third-party payers to understand their preferred reporting system.

The service codes within this subheading include codes for the initial consultation through the management of the patient throughout the course of treatment. When the initial consultation occurs, the code for the service would come from the E/M section. For example, the patient might be an inpatient when the therapeutic radiologist first sees the patient for evaluation of treatment options and before a decision for treatment is made. You would code this consultation service with an Inpatient Consultation code from the E/M section.

Clinical Treatment Planning. Clinical Treatment Planning (77261-77263) reflects professional services by the physician. It includes interpretation of special testing, tumor localization, treatment volume determination, treatment time/dosage determination, choice of treatment modality (method), determination of number and size of treatment ports, selection of appropriate treatment devices, and any other procedures necessary to adequately develop a course of treatment. A treatment plan is set up for all patients requiring radiation therapy.

There are three types of clinical treatment plans: simple, intermediate, and complex.

Simple planning requires that there be a single treatment area of interest that is encompassed by a single port or by simple parallel opposed ports with simple or no blocking.

Intermediate planning requires that there be three or more converging ports, two separate treatment areas, multiple blocks, or special time/dose constraints.

Complex planning requires that there be highly complex blocking, custom shielding blocks, tangential ports, special wedges or compensators, three or more separate treatment areas, rotational or special beam consideration, or a combination of therapeutic modalities.

Simulation. Simulation (77280-77299) is the service of determining treatment areas and the placement of the ports for radiation treatment, but it does not include the administration of the radiation. A simulation can be performed on a simulator designated for use only in simulations in a radiation therapy treatment unit, or on a diagnostic x-ray machine. Codes are divided to indicate four levels of service:

- **Simple** simulation of a single treatment area, with either a single port or parallel opposed ports and simple or no blocking
- **Intermediate** simulation of three or more converging ports, with two separate treatment areas and multiple blocks
- **Complex** simulation of tangential ports, with three or more treatment areas, rotation or arc therapy, complex blocking, custom shielding blocks, brachytherapy source verification, hyperthermia probe verification, and any use of contrast material
- **Three-dimensional (3D)** computer-generated reconstruction of tumor volume and surrounding critical normal tissue structures based on direct CT scan and/or MRI data in preparation for non-coplanar or coplanar therapy; this is a simulation that utilizes documented three-dimensional beam's-eye view volume dose displays of multiple or moving beams. Documentation of three-dimensional volume reconstruction and dose distribution is required.

After the initial simulation and treatment plan has been established for a patient, if any change is made in the field of treatment, a new simulation billing is required. When coding for a treatment period, you will have codes for planning, simulation, the isodose plan, devices, treatment management (the number of treatments determines the number of times billed), and the radiation delivery.

The codes in Clinical Treatment Planning are located in the index of the CPT manual under the main term "Radiation Therapy." Codes can also be located under the main term of the specific service, such as "Port Film."

EXERCISE 11–7 *Clinical Treatment Planning*

Using the CPT manual, code the following:

1 Complex therapeutic radiology simulation-aided field setting

   Code: _____

2 Therapeutic radiology treatment planning; simple

   Code: _____

Medical Radiation Physics, Dosimetry, Treatment Devices, and Special Services. Medical Radiation Physics, Dosimetry, Treatment Devices, and Special Services (77300-77370, 77399) deals with the decision making of the physicians as to the type of treatment (modality), dose, and development of treatment devices. It is common to have several dosimetry or device changes during a treatment course. **Dosimetry** is the calculation of the radiation dose and placement.

Codes in this subheading are divided mostly on the basis of the level of treatment (simple, intermediate, complex). The codes are located in the index of the CPT manual under the main term "Radiation Therapy" and the subterm of the specific service, such as dose plan or treatment.

EXERCISE 11–8 *Medical Radiation, Physics, Dosimetry, Treatment Devices, and Special Services*

Using the CPT manual, code the following:

1 Design and construction of a bite block, intermediate

    Code: _____

2 Calculation of an isodose for brachytherapy, single plane, two sources, simple

    Code: _____

3 Teletherapy, isodose plan, to one area, simple

    Code: _____

Radiation Treatment Delivery. Stereotactic Radiation Treatment Delivery (77371-77373) and Radiation Treatment Delivery (77401-77423) reflect the **technical components** only. These codes are used to report the actual delivery of the radiation. Radiation treatment is delivered in units called megaelectron volts (MeV). A megaelectron volt is a unit of energy. The radiation energy **delivered** by the machine is measured in megaelectron volts; the energy that is **deposited** in the patient's tissue is measured in Gray (1 Gray = 100 rads; 1 centigray [cGy] = 1 rad). A rad is a radiation absorbed dose. The therapy dose in a cancer treatment would typically be in the thousands of rads.

To code Radiation Treatment Delivery services, you need to know the amount of radiation delivered (6-10 MeV, 11-19 MeV) and the number of

- **Areas** treated (single, two, three or more),
- **Ports** involved (single, three or more, tangential), and
- **Blocks** used (none, multiple, custom).

EXERCISE 11–9 *Radiation Treatment Delivery*

Using the CPT manual, code the following:

The patient receives radiation treatment delivery:

1 To a single area at 4 MeV

    Code: _____

2 With superficial voltage only

    Code: _____

3 To four separate areas with a rotational beam at 4 MeV

    Code(s): _____

4 For two separate areas, using three or more ports with multiple blocks at 5 MeV

    Code(s): _____

5 For three or more separate areas using custom blocks, wedges, rotation beams, up to 5 MeV

    Code(s): _____

Radiation Treatment Management. Radiation Treatment Management codes (77427-77499) reflect the reporting of the **professional component.** The codes are used to report weekly management of radiation therapy. The notes under the heading Radiation Treatment Management state that clinical management is based on five fractions or treatment sessions regardless of the time interval separating the delivery of treatment. This means that these codes may be used if the patient receives a treatment at least five times within a 7-day week; it also means that if the patient receives five treatments at any time during this week (i.e., skipping a day or two between treatments), these codes may still be used.

If the patient receives five treatments and then receives an additional one or two fractions, you do not code for the additional fractions. Only if three or more fractions beyond the original five are delivered would you code using 77427 to indicate the additional treatment.

Bundled into the Radiation Treatment Management codes are the following physician services:

■ Review of port films

■ Review of dosimetry, dose delivery, and treatment parameters

■ Review of patient treatment setup

■ Examination of the patient for medical evaluation and management (e.g., assessment of the patient's response to treatment, coordination of care and treatment, review of imaging and/or lab test results).

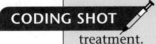 **CODING SHOT** Services covered under Radiation Treatment Management are bundled up to **90 days** after the end of radiation treatment.

The following can be reported in addition to the 77427 (treatment management) because none of the following are bundled into the treatment management:

■ 77417 Port films can be reported at two per week per treatment course

■ 77300 Basic plan calculation at the onset of treatment

■ 77263 Complex planning reported at the beginning of treatment

■ E/M code Usually on the first day of treatment as either an office visit or a consultation code

The 77427 is reported once per week (once every seventh day of treatment) and the physics maintenance code 77336 is reported once per every fifth fraction.

It would be inappropriate to report these items individually. For example, the physician sees the patient in the office to evaluate the patient's response to treatment. You might think you should use an E/M code to report the office visit, but that would be incorrect because the management codes already include the office visit service.

Proton Beam Treatment Delivery. The delivery of radiation treatment (77520-77525) using a proton beam utilizes particles that are positively charged with electricity. The use of the proton beam is an alternative delivery method for radiation in which proton (electromagnetic) radiation would traditionally be used.

The codes in the subheading are divided according to whether there was simple, intermediate, or complex delivery.

Hyperthermia. Hyperthermia (77600-77615) is an increase in body temperature; it is used as a treatment for cancer. The heat source can be ultrasound, microwave, or another means of increasing the temperature in an area. When the temperature of an area is increased, metabolism increases, which boosts the ability of the body to eradicate cancer cells. The location of the heat source can be external (to a depth of greater or less than 4 cm), interstitial (within the tissues), or intracavitary (inside the body). External treatment would be the application to the skin of a heat source such as ultrasound. Interstitial treatment is the insertion of a probe that delivers heat directly to the treatment area. Codes 77600-77615 are used to report external or interstitial treatment delivery.

Intracavitary hypothermia treatment delivery requires the insertion of a heat-producing probe into a body orifice, such as the rectum or vagina. Code 77620 is used to report intracavitary treatment and is the only code listed under Clinical Intracavitary Hyperthermia.

QUICK CHECK 11-2

Hyperthermia is used as an independent treatment modality.
True or False?

EXERCISE 11–10 *Clinical Treatment Management*

Using the CPT manual, code the following management services:

1 Five radiation treatments

Code: _____

2 Unlisted procedure code for therapeutic radiation clinical treatment management (Submission of this unlisted procedure code would necessitate a special report and assumes that no Category III code exists for the procedure.)

Code: _____

Clinical Brachytherapy. Clinical **brachytherapy** (77750-77799) is the placement of radioactive material directly into or surrounding the site of the tumor. Placement may be **intracavitary** (within a body cavity) or **interstitial** (within the tissues), and material may be placed permanently or temporarily.

The terms "source" and "ribbon" are used in the Clinical Brachytherapy codes. A **source** is a container holding a radioactive element that can be inserted directly into the body where it delivers the radiation dose over time. Sources come in various forms, such as seeds or capsules, and are placed in a cavity (intracavitary) or permanently placed within the tissue (interstitial). Fig. 11–16 illustrates the results of a single permanent seed implanted into

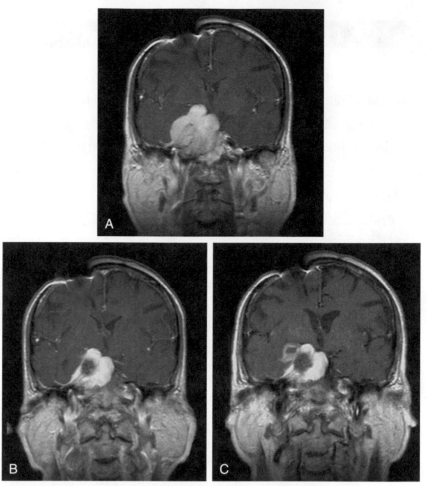

FIGURE 11–16 **A,** MR image scan of 80-year-old man with large petroclival meningioma previously treated with radiosurgery 6 years earlier. **B,** Results 3 months after placement of single permanent I-125 seed. **C,** Results 9 months after placement of single seed. (From Crownover RL, ed: *Hematology/Oncology Clinics of North America,* Vol 13, Number 3, June 1999, p 645.)

the cranial posterior fossa of a patient with a meningioma. **Ribbons** are seeds embedded on a tape. The ribbon is cut to the desired length to control the amount of radiation the patient receives. Ribbons are inserted temporarily into the tissue.

Codes are divided on the basis of the number of sources or ribbons used in an application:

- Simple   1-4
- Intermediate   5-10
- Complex   11 or more

The Clinical Brachytherapy codes include the physician's work related to the patient's admission to the hospital as well as the daily hospital visits.

CODING SHOT The add-on code for coronary intravascular brachytherapy is 92974 and can be indexed in the CPT manual under "Coronary Artery, Placement, Radiation Delivery Device."

EXERCISE 11–11 *Clinical Brachytherapy*

Using the CPT manual, code the following:

1 A simple application of a radioactive source, intracavitary

Code: _____

2 A simple application of a radioactive source, interstitial

Code: _____

3 Surface application of a radiation source

Code: _____

Nuclear Medicine

Nuclear medicine (78000-79999) deals with the placement of radionuclides within the body and the monitoring of emissions from the radioactive elements. Nuclear medicine is used not only for diagnostic studies but also for therapeutic treatment, such as treatment of thyroid conditions.

Stress tests are an example of nuclear medicine techniques. Radioactive material may be used during stress tests to monitor coronary artery bloodflow. Radioactive material (called a tracer) adheres to red blood cells (such as thallium or technetium sestamibi [Cardiolite]). The radioactive materials on the red blood cells allow an image of the heart to be seen and indicate areas where the blood is flowing. The radioactive materials are injected 1 minute before the end of a stress test and then again 24 hours later for a comparison study. If the bloodflow is decreased or absent, the image will show a blank area. If the coronary arteries are clear and allow blood to flow to the heart muscle, the image will show blood dispersement to all areas. If the arteries are partially blocked, the flow may be decreased but adequate during rest. During exercise, however, the necessary amount of oxygenated blood may not be adequate to keep the heart going, and that is when chest pain may occur. During a stress test, if radionuclide dispersement is absent during exercise (showing inadequate blood supply to the area during peak demand) but is present during resting periods (showing adequate flow at rest), this is called **reversible ischemia**, meaning that heart muscle death has not occurred. With intervention, arteries may be opened or bypassed to increase the supply of blood to the muscle before heart muscle death does occur. If the radionuclide is absent during rest and exercise, the ischemia is considered **irreversible**, meaning that heart muscle death has already occurred. A stress test is one of the many uses of nuclear medicine for diagnostic purposes. As you code, you will become familiar with these various diagnostic tests and how they are reported.

None of the codes in the subsection includes the radiopharmaceutical(s) used for diagnosis or therapy services. When radiopharmaceutical(s) are supplied for diagnostic purposes, report 79005 (oral), 79101 (intravenous), 79440 (intra-articular) or 79445 (intra-arterial) or use the specific Level II HCPCS code. The oral and intravenous administration codes include the administration service. For intra-arterial, intra-cavity, and intra-articular administration also report the appropriate injection/procedure codes as well as the imaging guidance and radiological supervision/interpretation when appropriate.

There are two subheadings within the Nuclear Medicine subsection—Diagnostic (78000-78999) and Therapeutic (79005-79999). The subheading Diagnostic is further divided into category codes based on system, such as the endocrine system and the cardiovascular system.

EXERCISE 11–12 *Nuclear Medicine*

Under which subheading in the Nuclear Medicine subsection would you look to locate codes for the following?

1 Liver _____

2 Thyroid _____

3 Spleen _____

4 Bone _____

5 Brain _____

CHAPTER REVIEW

CHAPTER 11, PART I, THEORY

Without the use of the CPT manual, complete the following:

1 What is a branch of medicine that uses radiant energy to diagnose and treat patients?

_____

2 The CPT manual divides the Radiology section into subsections of Radiologic Guidance, Breast Mammography, Bone/Joint Studies, Diagnostic Radiology,

_____, _____, and Nuclear Medicine.

3 What type of procedure is "performed independently of, and is not immediately related to, other services"?

_____

4 One Gray equals how many rads?

_____

5 The modifier used to indicate the Professional Component is _____

6 The two words that mean supervising the taking of the x-rays and reading/reporting the

results of the films are _____ and

_____.

7 The name for the use of high-frequency sound waves in an imaging process that is used to diagnose patient illness is

_____.

8 The Radiation Oncology section of the CPT manual is divided into subsections based on

the _____ of service provided to the patient.

9 The scientific study of energy is

_____.

10 The scientific calculation of the radiation emitted from various radioactive sources is

_____.

11 Radiation treatment delivery codes are based on the treatment area involved and further divided based on levels of what?

_____

12 MeV stands for _____.

13 Radiation Treatment Management is reported

in units of _____ fractions.

14 Nuclear Medicine uses these to image organs for diagnosis and treatment:

_____

Identify the planes of the body on the figure on the next page:

15 _____

16 _____

17 _____

CHAPTER 11, PART II, PRACTICAL

The coding exercise that follows uses codes from a variety of CPT sections.

Using the CPT manual, code the following:

18 An established patient is seen in the physician's office with the chief complaint of a persistent cough. Otherwise, the patient claims to be in good health. The physician collects a history, including the chief complaint and the history of the present illness. The physical examination performed focuses on the respiratory tract. The decision making is straightforward because the physician wants to evaluate the patient for a possible case of bronchitis.

🌐 Code(s): _____

The patient is sent to the clinic's radiology department for a two-view chest x-ray study, frontal and lateral.

🌐 Code(s): _____

The radiologist sends the x-ray results to the physician, who reviews them and decides to order a consultation with a pulmonologist from another clinic. The patient sees the other clinic's pulmonologist, who performs a comprehensive history and a comprehensive examination with moderate complexity.

🌐 Code(s): _____

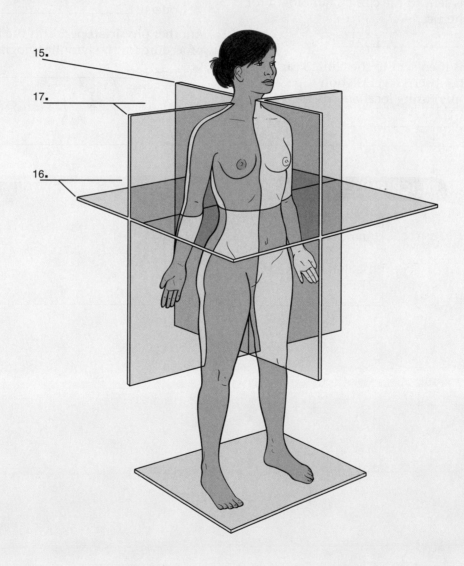

15. _____

17. _____

16. _____

A bronchoscopy with transbronchial lung biopsy is performed.

✿ Code(s): _____

Then there is radiologic supervision and interpretation of a unilateral bronchography.

✿ Code(s): _____

19 A new patient is seen in the office for unilateral ear pain. In the expanded problem focused history and the physical examination, the physician focuses his attention on the head, ears, nose, and throat. The physician's provisional diagnoses include otalgia and possible ear infections. The decision making is straightforward for the physician.

✿ Code(s): _____

The patient is sent to the clinic's radiologist for an x-ray of the ear.

✿ Code(s): _____

The patient is then sent to the clinic's ear specialist, who inserts a ventilation tube (tympanostomy) using local anesthesia.

✿ Code(s): _____

20 A new patient is seen in the office for a variety of complaints, but in particular a swelling and heaviness of his right leg. The physician documents the patient's complaints, collects a comprehensive history of the present illness, performs a comprehensive review of systems, and inquires about the patient's past, family, and social history. A complete multisystem physical examination is performed. The physician's working diagnosis is edema of the lower extremity, cause to be determined. Given the nature of the problem, the physician considers the decision making process to be highly complex.

✿ Code(s): _____

The patient is sent to radiology for a unilateral lymphangiography of one extremity.

✿ Code(s): _____

Another physician performs the injection procedure for the lymphangiography.

✿ Code(s): _____

QUICK CHECK ANSWERS

QUICK CHECK 11-1
modifier -59

QUICK CHECK 11-2
False

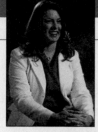

"Continuing education is vital. Gain as much knowledge and experience in other specialties, fields, or branches of HIM as possible."

Cynthia Stahl, CPC, CCS-P, CPC-H
Reimbursement and Coding Specialist
Lebanon, Indiana

Pathology/Laboratory Section

Chapter Topics

Format

Subsections

Chapter Review

Quick Check Answers

Learning Objectives

After completing this chapter, you should be able to

1 Explain the format of the Pathology and Laboratory section.

2 Demonstrate an understanding of Pathology and Laboratory terminology.

3 Understand the use of venipuncture with Pathology and Laboratory services.

4 Define a facility indicator.

5 Understand the information in the Pathology and Laboratory Guidelines.

6 Demonstrate the ability to code Pathology and Laboratory services.

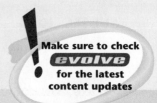

Make sure to check *evolve* for the latest content updates

Most Pathology and Laboratory subsections contain notes. Whenever notes are available, be sure to read them before assigning codes from the subsection because specific information pertinent to the codes is contained in these notes.

FORMAT The Pathology and Laboratory section of the CPT manual is formatted according to type of tests performed—automated multichannel, panels, assays, and so forth. An example of some of the subsections are as follows.

- Organ or Disease Oriented Panels
- Drug Testing
- Therapeutic Drug Assays
- Evocative/Suppression Testing
- Consultations (Clinical Pathology)
- Urinalysis
- Chemistry
- Hematology and Coagulation
- Immunology
- Transfusion Medicine
- Microbiology
- Anatomic Pathology
- Cytopathology
- Cytogenetic Studies
- Surgical Pathology
- Transcutaneous Procedures
- Other Procedures
- Reproductive Medicine Procedures

Laboratories have built-in **indicators** that allow additional tests to be performed without a written order from the physician. These standards are set by the medical facility and imply that when a certain test is found to be positive, it is assumed that the physician would want further information on the condition. For example, if a routine urinalysis is performed, a culture is performed if the test is positive for bacteria. If a culture is performed to identify the organism, a sensitivity test is performed if the bacteria are of a certain type or count, as predetermined by the medical facility to warrant the additional laboratory studies. You will code only after the tests are done. This ensures that all laboratory tests performed are reported. Remember that what the physician ordered may not be all the laboratory work performed, depending on the facility's policy concerning further tests.

The services in the Pathology and Laboratory section include the laboratory **tests** only. The **collection** of the specimen is coded separately from the analysis of the test. For example, if a patient had a technician in a clinic laboratory withdraw blood by means of a venipuncture of the arm, and the blood sample was then analyzed in the laboratory, you would code 36415 for the venipuncture in addition to a code to report the test performed on the blood.

SUBSECTIONS The codes in the Organ or Disease Oriented Panels subsection (80047-80076) are grouped according to the usual laboratory work ordered by a physician for the diagnosis of or screening for various diseases or conditions. Groups of tests may be performed together, depending on the situation or disease. For example, during the first obstetric visit, a mother is commonly asked to have baseline laboratory tests performed to ensure that appropriate antepartum care can be provided. CPT code 80055 describes an obstetric panel that would typically be used for the first obstetric visit. To assign a panel code, each test listed in the panel description must be performed. Additional tests are reported separately. The development of panels saves the facility from having to report each test separately, and it is often more economical for the patient. If you list a panel, each test must have been performed to qualify for use of the code. You cannot use modifier -52 (reduced service) with a panel. For example, if all of the tests in the obstetric panel were done except the syphilis test, you could not report 80055 (Obstetrical Panel) with modifier -52. You would instead list each of the tests separately.

CODING SHOT Be careful when coding multiple panels on the same day for the same patient. Sometimes several panels include some of the same tests. For example, a hepatitis B surface antigen test is included in both the obstetric panel and the hepatitis panel. It would be inappropriate to code the same test twice, as it would not be performed on the same patient more than once in a single day.

The laboratory and pathology reports in the patient record will contain the method by which the test was done. There are many different methods of performing the various tests that you will find in this subsection. For example, a urinalysis can be automated or nonautomated and can include microscopy or exclude microscopy. It is necessary to know these details if you are to choose the correct urinalysis code. If the details you need are not in the medical record, ask the laboratory staff or physician for further clarification.

EXERCISE 12–1 *Organ or Disease Oriented Panels*

Complete the following:

1 Hepatic function panel code

   Code: _____

2 How many laboratory tests must be included in a hepatic function panel? _____

3 Does an obstetric panel include a rubella antibody test? _____

4 Is blood typing ABO included in an obstetric panel? _____

Drug Testing Laboratory drug testing (80100-80103) is done to identify the presence or absence of a drug. Testing that determines the presence or absence of a drug is qualitative (the drug is either present or not present in the specimen).

When the presence of a drug is detected in the qualitative test, a confirmation test is usually performed by using a second testing method. Code 80102 is used to describe this confirmation test. Codes from the Therapeutic Drug Assay and Chemistry subsections are used to further identify the exact amount of the drug that is present (quantitative). For example, a patient who has been on a medication for a long time might need to undergo testing to determine whether the drug level is therapeutic.

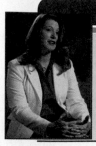

From the Trenches

"Don't be afraid of developing your coding network in both directions. Include advanced coders as well as beginning coders. I often find that a fresh point of view on a topic brings forth as many solutions as advice from a seasoned coder."

CYNTHIA

The CPT manual lists the drugs most commonly tested for, although the use of the codes is not limited to the drugs listed. Modifier -51 is not used with pathology or laboratory codes; instead, each test is listed separately. For example, if a confirmation test was conducted for both alcohol and cocaine, code 80102 twice and append modifier -91, repeat clinical diagnostic laboratory test, to the second code.

QUICK CHECK 12-1

What is the repeat clinical laboratory test modifier? _____

Therapeutic Drug Assays

Drug assays (80150-80299) test for a specific drug and for the amount of that drug. If qualitative information is not enough, quantitative information is needed. **Quantitative** information determines not only the presence of a drug but also the exact amount present (or quantity present). Many types of drugs are listed in this subsection. If the drug is not listed, it is possible that quantitative analysis may be listed under the methodology (e.g., immunoassay, radioassay).

Therapeutic drug assays are performed to help the physician monitor the level of medication in the patient's system or to monitor compliance. For example, levels may be measured to make certain the patient is getting the correct level of antibiotics. Blood specimens for drug monitoring are usually taken during the drug's highest therapeutic concentration (peak level) and at the drug's lowest therapeutic concentration (trough or residual level). Peak and trough levels should fall within the therapeutic range directed by the physician.

The drugs are listed by their generic names, not their brand names. For example, 80152 is for the generic drug amitriptyline, also sold under the brand names of Elavil and Endep. A *Physician's Desk Reference* that lists pharmaceuticals by the generic and brand name will be helpful as you code drug testing and assays.

One location of Drug Testing codes in the index of the CPT manual is under the main term "Drug," subtermed by the reason for the tests—analysis or confirmation. Therapeutic Drug Assay subsection codes can be found under the main term "Drug Assay" and subterms of the material examined, for example, amikacin, digoxin.

EXERCISE 12-2 *Therapeutic Drug Testing and Drug Assays*

Choose the correct CPT code for the following drug tests:

1 Confirmation of cocaine (qualitative)

Code: _____

2 Identify the amount of digoxin in the blood (quantitative)

Code: _____

3 Quantitative examination of blood for amikacin

Code: _____

4 Examination of blood, quantitative for lithium

Code: _____

Evocative/Suppression Testing

Evocative/Suppression (80400-80440) testing is performed to determine measurements of the effect of evocative or suppressive agents on chemical constituents. For example, code 80400 is reported when a patient undergoes testing to determine whether adrenocorticotropic hormone (ACTH) is being produced in the body. The physician may suspect that the patient suffers from adrenal gland insufficiency. Note that following each of the code descriptions is a statement of the services that must have been provided for the code to be applicable. For example, the requirement to report 80400 ACTH stimulation panel is "Cortisol (82533 × 2)" or two cortisol tests, as described in 82533. You will have to read the description for code 82533 to ensure that it is the correct test before you can report 80400.

 CAUTION *Remember that the codes from the Pathology and Laboratory section are only for the tests performed and do not reflect the complete service.*

To code the components of Evocative/Suppression Testing:

- If the physician **supplied** the agent, report the supply using 99070 from the Medicine section.
- If the physician **administered** the agent, report the infusion or injection using codes 96360-96379 from the Medicine section.
- If the test involved **prolonged attendance** by the physician, report the service using the appropriate E/M code.

Consultations (Clinical Pathology)

A clinical pathologist, upon request from a primary care physician, will perform a consultation to render additional medical interpretation regarding test results. For example, a primary care physician reviews lab test results and requests a clinical pathologist to review, interpret, and prepare a written report on the findings.

There are two codes under the subsection Consultations (80500, 80502) that are reserved for clinical pathology consultations. These consultations are based on whether the consultation is limited or comprehensive. A **limited consultation** is one that is done without the pathologist's reviewing the medical record of the patient, and a **comprehensive consultation** is one in which the medical record is reviewed as a part of the consultative services. When either of these consultation codes is submitted to a third-party payer, it is accompanied by a written report.

These are not the only pathology consultation codes in the Pathology and Laboratory section of the CPT manual. There are also consultation codes toward the end of the section in the Surgical Pathology subsection (88321-88334) that are used to report the services of a pathologist who reviews and gives an opinion or advice concerning pathology slides, specimens, material, or records that were prepared elsewhere or for pathology consultation during surgery.

Pathology consultations during surgery are provided to examine tissue removed from a patient during a surgical procedure. If the pathologist did not use a microscope to examine the tissue, report 88329. If a microscope was used to examine the tissue, report 88331 or 88332, depending on the number of samples that were examined.

A **specimen** is a sample of tissue from a suspect area; a **block** is a frozen piece of a specimen; and a *section* is a slice of a frozen block. A pathologist prepares a specimen by cutting it into blocks and taking sections from the blocks. The number of sections taken depends on the judgment of the pathologist as to the number of areas of the specimen that need to be examined. The frozen section is placed (mounted) on a slide or held by other means that allow the pathologist to view the tissue under a microscope.

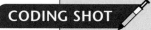

CODING SHOT Each specimen may be reported separately, but each slide from that specimen may not.

When one block is sectioned and examined, the service of examining that first section is reported using 88331. The second and subsequent sections of the same block are included in the reporting of 88331. If another block from another area was sectioned, the first section would be reported using 88331, and subsequent sections from the second block using 88332. You cannot use 88332 without first using 88331. Although 88332 is not marked as an add-on code (one that is used only with another code), its function is that of an add-on code as it indicates that subsequent sections were examined.

Urinalysis and Chemistry

Many types of tests are located under the Urinalysis and Chemistry subsections (81000-84999). Urinalysis codes are for **nonspecific** tests done on urine. Chemistry codes are for **specific** tests done on material from any source (e.g., urine, blood, breath, feces, sputum). For example, a urinalysis using a dipstick (81000-81003) would report the presence and quantity of the following constituents: bilirubin, glucose, hemoglobin, ketones, leukocytes, nitrite, pH, protein, specific gravity, and urobilinogen. Any number of these constituents may be analyzed and reported using a code from the Urinalysis subsection (81000-81099). However, if the physician ordered an analysis of the urine specifically to determine the presence of urobilinogen (reduced bilirubin) and the exact amount of urobilinogen present (quantitative analysis), you would choose a code (84580) from the

Chemistry subsection. The main things to remember when coding from these two subsections are

1. The identification of specific tests
2. Whether the test is automated (by machine) or nonautomated (manually)
3. The number of tests performed
4. The identification of combination codes for similar types of tests
5. Whether the results are qualitative or quantitative
6. The methodology of testing

EXERCISE 12–3 *Urinalysis and Chemistry*

Code the following:

1 An automated urinalysis without microscopy

Code: _____

2 Urinalysis, microscopic only

Code: _____

3 Albumin, serum

Code: _____

4 Total bilirubin

Code: _____

5 Gases, blood pH only

Code: _____

6 Sodium, urine

Code: _____

7 Uric acid, blood

Code: _____

Hematology and Coagulation

The Hematology and Coagulation subsection contains codes (85002-85999) based on the various blood-drawing methods and tests. The method used to do the test is often what determines the code assignment. Blood counts can be manual or automated, with many variations of the tests.

There are codes within the Hematology and Coagulation subsection for bone marrow smear and smear interpretations (85060, 85097). Codes to report the procurement of the bone marrow through the use of aspiration are located in the Hemic and Lymphatic Systems subsection of the Surgery section.

There are many blood coagulation tests located in the Hematology and Coagulation subsection. The codes are divided based on the particular factor being tested. Great care must be taken to ensure that the correct factor has been coded based on the information in the medical record.

Most of the tests in the Hematology and Coagulation subsection can be located in the index of the CPT manual under the name of the test, such as prothrombin time, coagulation time, or hemogram.

EXERCISE 12–4 *Hematology and Coagulation*

Code the following:

1 Blood count by an automated hemogram (RBC, WBC, Hgb, Hct, and platelet count)

Code: _____

2 Blood count by an automated hemogram and platelet count with complete differential white blood cell count

Code: _____

3 Automated RBC

Code: _____

4 Interpretation of a bone marrow smear

Code: _____

As you can see, there are many variations of just one test! So read the patient record and code descriptions carefully before assigning the codes.

Immunology Immunology codes (86000-86804) deal with the identification of conditions of the immune system caused by the action of antibodies (e.g., hypersensitivity, allergic reactions, immunity, and alterations of body tissue).

EXERCISE 12–5 *Immunology*

Code the following:

1 ANA (antinuclear antibody) titer

Code: _____

2 ASO (antistreptolysin O) screen

Code: _____

3 Cold agglutinin screen

Code: _____

Transfusion Medicine The Transfusion Medicine subsection (86850-86999) deals with tests performed on blood or blood products. Tests include screening for antibodies, Coombs testing, autologous blood collection and processing, blood typing, compatibility testing, and preparation of and treatments performed on blood and blood products.

EXERCISE 12–6   *Transfusion Medicine*

Code the following:

1 ABO and Rh blood typing

 Code(s): _____

2 Irradiation of blood product, 3 units

 Code(s): _____

Microbiology

Microbiology (87001-87999) deals with the study of microorganisms and includes bacteriology (study of bacteria), mycology (study of fungi), parasitology (study of parasites), and virology (study of viruses). Culture codes for the identification of organisms as well as the identification of sensitivities of the organism to antibiotics (called culture and sensitivity) are found in this subsection. Culture codes must be read carefully because some codes are used to indicate screening only to detect the presence of an organism; some codes indicate the identification of specific organisms; and others indicate additional sensitivity testing to determine which antibiotic would be best for treatment of the specified bacteria. You should code all tests performed on the basis of whether they are quantitative or qualitative and/or a sensitivity study.

QUICK CHECK 12-2

According to the Microbiology Guidelines, what modifier is used for reporting multiple specimens/sites?

_____

EXERCISE 12–7   *Microbiology*

Code the following:

1 HIV-1, quantification

Code: _____

2 Streptococcus, group A, using an amplified probe method

Code: _____

3 Quantification of *Gardnerella vaginalis,* herpes simplex, and *Candida* species

Code(s): _____, _____, and _____

4 Direct probe method of mycobacterial tuberculosis, herpes simplex virus, and *Chlamydia trachomatis*

   🔬 Code(s): _____

5 Bacterial culture of urine, quantitative with colony count

   🔬 Code(s): _____

6 If code 87116 indicates that a TB organism is present, what is code 87118 used for?

_____

Anatomic Pathology

Anatomic Pathology (88000-88099) deals with examination of the body fluids or tissues in postmortem (after death) examination. Postmortem examination involves the completion of gross microscopic and limited autopsies. Codes are divided according to the extent of the examination. This subsection also contains codes for forensic examination and coroners' cases.

Cytopathology and Cytogenic Studies

The Cytopathology subsection (88104-88199) deals with the laboratory work performed to determine whether any cellular changes are present. For example, a very common cytopathology procedure is the Papanicolaou smear (Pap smear). Cytopathology may also be performed on fluids that have been aspirated from a site to identify cellular changes. Cytogenetic Studies (88230-88299) include tests performed for genetic and chromosomal studies.

QUICK CHECK 12-3

Where are the modifiers for cytogenic studies located? _____

Surgical Pathology

Surgical Pathology codes (88300-88399) describe the evaluation of specimens to determine the pathology of disease processes. When choosing the correct code for pathology, you must identify the source of the specimen and the reason for the surgical procedure. The Surgical Pathology subsection contains codes that are divided into six levels (Levels I through VI) based on the specimen examined and the level of work required by the pathologist. Pathology testing is performed on all tissue removed from the body. The surgical pathology classification level is determined by the complexity of the pathologic examination.

> **Level I** pathology code 88300 identifies specimens that normally do not need to be viewed under a microscope for pathologic diagnosis (e.g., a tooth)—those for which the probability of disease or malignancy is minimal.

> **Level II** pathology code 88302 deals with those tissues that are usually considered normal tissue and have been removed not because of the

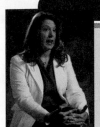

From the Trenches

"Many student coders believe that as soon as they earn their coding certification they'll be making the 'big bucks.' The certification is proof that you have the basic knowledge needed to code, but experience is still needed. Be patient, build your knowledge base, and the increase in pay will follow."

CYNTHIA

probability of the presence of disease or malignancy, but for some other reason (e.g., a fallopian tube for sterilization, foreskin of a newborn).

Level III pathology code 88304 is assigned for specimens with a low probability of disease or malignancy. For example, a gallbladder may be neoplastic (benign or malignant), but when the gallbladder is removed for cholecystitis (inflammation of the gallbladder), it is usually inflamed from chronic disease and not because of cancerous changes.

Level IV pathology code 88305 carries a higher probability of malignancy or decision making for disease pathology. For example, a uterus is removed because of a diagnosis of prolapse. There is a possibility that the uterus is malignant or that there are other causes of disease pathology.

Level V pathology code 88307 classifies more complex pathology evaluations (e.g., examination of a uterus that was removed for reasons other than prolapse or neoplasm).

Level VI pathology code 88309 includes examination of neoplastic tissue or very involved specimens, such as a total resection of a colon.

CODING SHOT A specimen is defined as tissue submitted for examination. If two specimens of the same area are received and examined, each specimen is coded. For example, if two anus tags are received and each is examined, code 88304 × 2. If one anus tag is received and two different areas of the tag are examined, code 88304 only once.

The remaining codes at the end of the subsection classify specialized procedures, utilization of stains, consultations performed, preparations used, and/or instrumentation needed to complete testing.

The surgical pathology codes are located in the index under the main term "Pathology" and subterms "Surgical" and "Gross and Micro Exam."

EXERCISE 12–8 *Surgical Pathology*

Code the following using one of the six surgical pathology codes in the CPT manual:

1 The specimen is a uterus, tubes, and ovaries. The procedure was an abdominal hysterectomy for ovarian cancer.

🔵 Code(s): _____

2 The specimen is a portion of a lung. The procedure was a left lower lobe segmental resection.

🔵 Code(s): _____

3 The specimen is the prostate. The procedure was a transurethral resection of the prostate.

🔵 Code(s): _____

4 What is the surgical pathology code for the following pathology report?

🔵 Code(s): _____

PATHOLOGY DEPARTMENT

Patient:	Alice C. Fisher	**Date Collected:**	02/09/0X
DOB:	12/06/37	**Date Received:**	02/09/0X
Sex	F	**Date Examined:**	02/10/0X
Record Number:	5909890	**Access Number:**	P4218
Account:	MP8352	**Surgeon:**	Dr. White

CLINICAL HISTORY: UMBILICAL HERNIA, INFLAMED

TISSUE RECEIVED: UMBILICAL HERNIA

GROSS DESCRIPTION: The specimen is labeled with the patient's name and "umbilical hernia" and consists of yellow-white fibrofatty tissue approximately 3.5 × 2 × 1 cm. Representative sections are processed in two slides.

MICROSCOPIC DIAGNOSIS: Mature adipose tissue with fibrovascular and fibrotendinous tissue with focal reactive fibrous tissue consistent with umbilical hernia.

Alberto Matusa, MD

Alberto Matusa, MD
Head, Pathology Department
Merry Brook Hospital

Other Procedures   Other Procedures includes miscellaneous testing on body fluids, the use of special instrumentation, and testing performed on oocytes and sperm.

CHAPTER REVIEW

CHAPTER 12, PART I, THEORY

Without the use of the CPT manual, complete the following:

1 The Pathology and Laboratory section of the CPT manual is formatted according to the type of _____ performed.

2 Laboratories have built-in _____ that allow additional tests to be performed without the written order of the physician.

3 Codes that are grouped according to the usual laboratory work ordered by a physician for diagnosis or screening of various diseases or conditions are

_____.

4 Can you use a reduced service modifier with pathology or laboratory codes?

Yes   No

5 Will the medical record contain the method used to perform the test done?

Yes   No

CHAPTER 12, PART II, PRACTICAL

Answer the following:

6 The Hematology and Coagulation subsections contain codes based on the various testing methods and tests. The method used to do the test is often the code determiner. Blood cell counts can be manual or automated, with many variations of the tests. What would the code be for an automated blood count (hemogram) with automated differential WBC count? A manual blood count (hemogram) with manual cell count?

Automated code: _____

Manual code: _____

Code the following three cases with the correct pathology code from the CPT manual:

7 The specimen is tonsils and adenoids. The procedure is a tonsillectomy with adenoidectomy.

🌐 Code(s): _____

8 The specimen is an appendix. The procedure is an incidental appendectomy.

🌐 Code(s): _____

9 The specimen is a tooth. The procedure is an odontectomy, gross examination only.

🌐 Code(s): _____

Code the following:

10 Western Blot of blood, with interpretation and report

🌐 Code(s): _____

11 Vitamin K analysis of blood

🌐 Code(s): _____

12 Quantitative analysis of urine for alkaloids

🌐 Code(s): _____

13 Three specimens of gastric secretions for total gastric acid

🌐 Code(s): _____

14 Blood analysis for HGH

🌐 Code(s): _____

15 Total insulin

🌐 Code(s): _____

16 LDL cholesterol using direct measurements

🌐 Code(s): _____

17 Blood count: one manual cell count

🌐 Code(s): _____

18 Blood smear interpretation

🌐 Code(s): _____

19 PTT of whole blood

🌐 Code(s): _____

20 Sedimentation rate, automated

🌐 Code(s): _____

21 Lee and White coagulation time

🌐 Code(s): _____

22 Clotting factor XII (Hageman factor)

🌐 Code(s): _____

23 Blood typing for paternity test, ABO, Rh, and MN

🌐 Code(s): _____

24 Culture of urine for bacteria with colony count

🌐 Code(s): _____

25 Schlichter test

🌐 Code(s): _____

26 Postmortem examination, gross only, with brain and spinal cord

🌐 Code(s): _____

27 Therapeutic drug assay for digoxin and vancomycin

🌐 Code(s): _____

28 Pathology consultation during surgery

🌐 Code(s): _____

QUICK CHECK ANSWERS

QUICK CHECK 12-1
Modifier -91

QUICK CHECK 12-2
Modifier -59

QUICK CHECK 12-3
Appendix I

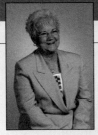

"Teamwork is an essential requirement in our profession. We learn from each other...then pass the knowledge on. It is an unbroken cycle."

Nancy Maguire, ACS, PCS, FCS, CPC, CPC-H, HCS-D, CRT
Physician Coding
Consultant/Auditor
San Antonio, Texas

The Medicine Section and Level II National Codes

Chapter Topics

Diagnostic and Therapeutic Services

History of National Level Coding

Chapter Review

Quick Check Answers

Learning Objectives

After completing this chapter, you should be able to

1. Analyze the format of the Medicine section.
2. Understand the coding of immunizations.
3. Identify major subsection information.
4. List the major features of Level II National Codes, HCPCS.
5. Demonstrate the ability to assign HCPCS codes.
6. Demonstrate the ability to assign Medicine section codes.

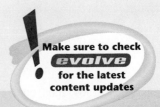

Make sure to check **evolve** for the latest content updates

DIAGNOSTIC AND THERAPEUTIC SERVICES

The Medicine section (90281-99607) is for coding diagnostic and therapeutic services that are generally **non-invasive** (not entering a body cavity), but there are invasive procedures in the section, such as cardiac catheterization. The section begins with Guidelines applicable to all of the Medicine section codes (i.e., multiple procedures, add-on codes, separate procedures, subsection information, unlisted service/procedure, special reports, modifiers, and materials supplied by the physician).

The various subsections of Medicine contain many specific notes to be used with certain groups of codes, so be sure to read all notes that pertain to the group of codes with which you are working.

Format

AN EXAMPLE OF MEDICINE SUBSECTIONS:

- Immune Globulins
- Immunization Administration for Vaccines/Toxoids
- Vaccines, Toxoids
- Psychiatry
- Dialysis
- Gastroenterology
- Ophthalmology
- Special Otorhinolaryngologic Services
- Cardiovascular
- Intracardiac Electrophysiological Procedures/Studies
- Peripheral Arterial Disease Rehabilitation
- Non-Invasive Vascular Diagnostic Studies
- Cerebrovascular Arterial Studies
- Pulmonary
- Allergy and Clinical Immunology
- Neurology and Neuromuscular
- Routine Electroencephalography
- Electromyography and Nerve Conduction Tests
- Neurostimulators, Analysis-Programming
- Functional Brain Mapping
- Medical Genetics and Genetic Counseling Services
- Central Nervous System Assessments/Tests
- Health and Behavior Assessment/Intervention
- Chemotherapy Administration
- Special Dermatological Procedures
- Physical Medicine and Rehabilitation
- Acupuncture
- Osteopathic Manipulative Treatment
- Chiropractic Manipulative Treatment
- Special Services, Procedures, and Reports
- Education and Training for Patient Self-Management
- Moderate (Conscious) Sedation
- Home Health Procedures/Services
- Medication Therapy Management Services

Many specialized types of testing can be found in the Medicine section (e.g., biofeedback, audiologic function tests, electrocardiograms). Codes in this section do not usually include the supplies used in the testing, therapy, or diagnostic treatments unless specifically stated in the code description. For example, there are codes for the prescription and fitting of an artificial eye—one code includes the supply of an artificial eye and one code does not include the supply of an artificial eye. Reading the entire code description is critical to ensure that you do not unbundle the services by reporting services already included in the code. You should code supplies, including drugs, separately unless otherwise instructed in the code information. CPT code 99070 is the supplies and materials code used to identify the supplying of drugs, trays, supplies, or materials needed to provide the service or the specific HCPCS supply code. For example, Fig. 13–1 shows the code for the service of a prescription for corneal contact lenses (92310). When the lenses and the prescription services are provided, both the lenses and the prescription service are reported.

Subsections

Introduction to Immunization. There are two types of immunization—active and passive. Active immunization is the type given when it is anticipated that the person will be in contact with the disease. Active immunization agents can be toxoids or vaccines. Toxoids are bacteria that have been made nontoxic; when injected, they produce an immune response that builds protection against a disease. Vaccines are viruses that are given in small doses and cause an immune response. **Passive immunization** does not cause an immune response; rather, the injected material contains a high level of antibodies against a disease (e.g., rabies, hepatitis B, tetanus), called immune globulins.

The first three subsections in the Medicine section are

- Immune Globulins
- Immunization Administration for Vaccines/Toxoids
- Vaccines, Toxoids

QUICK CHECK 13-1

The administration codes for immune globulins are:

a. 90465-90474
b. 96365-96368
c. 96372, 96374, 96375
d. b and c

One code for the prescription; second code for lenses

92310   Prescription of optical and physical characteristics of and fitting of contact lens, with medical supervision of adaptation; corneal lens, both eyes, except for aphakia.

FIGURE 13–1   Some codes are for the supply only.

Immune Globulins. The Immune Globulins subsection (90281-90399) is a relatively new subsection in the CPT manual. Many of the codes in the subsection were located throughout the Medicine section, but with the creation of the Immune Globulins subsection, the codes are now grouped together. The codes in this subsection identify only the immune globulin **product** and must be reported in addition to the appropriate administration code.

Codes in the Immune Globulins subsection are categorized according to the type of immune globulin (rabies, hepatitis B, etc.), the method of injection (IM, IV, SQ, etc.), and the type of dose (full dose, mini dose, etc.).

Immunization Administration for Vaccines, Toxoids. The Immunization Administration subsection codes (90465-90474) are reported in conjunction with the Vaccines, Toxoids subsection codes (90476-90749). The codes in the Immunization Administration subsection are reported for the administration—injection, intranasal, or oral. A variety of administration methods are used to deliver the vaccine/toxoid: percutaneous, intradermal, subcutaneous, intramuscular, intranasal, and oral administration. The administration codes are divided based on the method of administration— intranasal or oral; *or* percutaneous, intradermal, subcutaneous, and intramuscular and in some codes, the patient age. Report each dose administered—single or combination. Codes 90465-90468 report immunization administration for patients under the age of 8 and for which the physician has counseled the patient's family regarding the injection. 90465 and 90466 report percutaneous, intradermal, subcutaneous, or intramuscular injection and 90467 and 90468 report intranasal or oral routes of administration.

For example, you can report multiple administration for a patient over 8 years of age by using 90471 for the first administration and then listing 90472 for each administration after the first.

Example

90471	Administration service for tetanus
90703	Tetanus toxoid (substance injected, IM)
90472	Administration service for rubella
90706	Rubella virus (substance injected, SQ)
90472	Administration service for diphtheria
90719	Diphtheria toxoid (substance injected, IM)

Or you can report the first administration with 90471, as you would always do, and then list 90472 times the number of injections after the first one.

Example

90471	Administration service for tetanus
90472 × 2	Administration service, rubella and diphtheria

If a combination vaccine was used, you would report the service as:

Example

90471	Administration service for tetanus and diphtheria
90702	Tetanus and diphtheria toxoids (substances injected, IM)
90472	Administration service for rubella
90706	Rubella virus (substance injected, SQ)

CODING SHOT The injection codes 90465-90468 can also be reported for patients under 8 years of age if the documentation shows counseling by the physician, nurse practitioner, or physicians assistant.

Vaccines, Toxoids. The Vaccines, Toxoids subsection (90476-90749) lists vaccine products given in immunizations. The subsection contains many codes for a single disease (e.g., 90703 for tetanus toxoid) as well as codes for a combination of diseases (e.g., 90701 for diphtheria, tetanus, and pertussis [DTP]). In many of the code descriptions, specific ages are identified. For example, 90658, influenza vaccine, specifies age 3 and above, whereas code 90657, influenza vaccine, specifies ages 6 to 35 months. The vaccines have pediatric or adult listed on the label of the vial. You must carefully review the description of the vaccine product code to determine which disease is specified. When one code is available to describe multiple products given, the combination code must be used. If each vaccine were to be listed separately when a combination vaccine was administered, it would be considered unbundling.

CAUTION *When coding diphtheria, there are eight codes with combinations of diphtheria. Read all descriptions carefully before assigning a code.*

There are codes that describe schedules for a vaccine, such as a three-dose or four-dose schedule. For example, 90633 is a two-dose hepatitis A vaccine that is intended to be given on a two-dose schedule. Each time the vaccine is administered, 90633 is reported along with the date of the injection. A schedule is the number of doses provided and the timing of the administration. However, the doses and timing must be exactly as specified in the code; otherwise, you should use multiple codes to identify the vaccine.

Usually, you do not use modifier -51 (multiple procedures) with the Vaccines/Toxoid codes; however, in 2008 the description for modifier -51 added the use with vaccines and toxoid codes. Most payers want you to list the codes multiple times or use the "times" symbol (×) and indicate the

From the Trenches

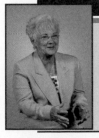

"Coding requires patience, persistence, good communication skills, and the ability to research and follow billing and coding rules. Coders usually have an investigative mind and like to put pieces of a puzzle together."

NANCY

number of injections given, as described in the Immunization Administration for Vaccines, Toxoids information described earlier.

If a patient is given a vaccine in the course of an E/M service, the administration and vaccine/toxoid codes are assigned in addition to the E/M code. Some third-party payers require a -25 modifier on the E/M code, so be sure to check with your local carrier on how to submit the E/M code.

> **CODING SHOT** If the only service is administration of a vaccine and no other service is provided, do not code an E/M. Rather only code for the administration of the vaccine and the vaccine product.

Influenza and Pneumococcal Immunizations. Two vaccinations that are commonly provided are those for influenza and pneumococcal infections. You report a code for the substance injected (vaccine) and a code for the administration of the vaccine. The third-party payer may require you to submit CPT codes or CPT with HCPCS codes for the service. The following identifies the codes that you would report.

CPT INFLUENZA VACCINE CODES:

90657   Influenza virus vaccine split, virus when administered to children **6-35 months of age,** for intramuscular use

90658   Influenza virus vaccine, split virus when administered to individuals **3 years of age and older,** for intramuscular use

HCPCS CODE USED TO REPORT THE ADMINISTRATION OF AN INFLUENZA VACCINE:

G0008   Administration of an influenza virus vaccine

CPT CODES USED TO REPORT THE ADMINISTRATION OF AN INFLUENZA VACCINE:

90471   Intramuscular **administration,** one vaccine

90472   Intramuscular **administration,** each additional vaccine

CPT PNEUMOCOCCAL VACCINE CODE:

90732   Pneumococcal polysaccharide **vaccine,** 23-valent, 2 years of age and older, for subcutaneous or intramuscular use

HCPCS CODE TO REPORT THE ADMINISTRATION OF A PNEUMOCOCCAL VACCINE:

G0009   **Administration** of a pneumococcal vaccine

CPT CODES USED TO REPORT THE ADMINISTRATION OF A PNEUMOCOCCAL VACCINE:

90471   Intramuscular **administration,** one vaccine

90472   Intramuscular **administration,** each additional vaccine

> **CODING SHOT** For Medicare patients, you would only report an administration code for an immunization when no office service code was reported. Medicare policy states that if an office service is reported, the office service code includes the administration of an immunization.

EXERCISE 13–1   *Immunization Injections*

Using the CPT manual, code the following:

1 A parent takes a 9-year-old child to the child's physician for an oral poliomyelitis vaccine. The physician's assistant evaluates the child (established patient) and administers the vaccine orally to the child.

   Code(s): _____, _____ and _____.

2 The following series of vaccines is indicated as having been administered to a variety of patients; a brief history and examination are performed to assess vaccine needs and general health status. How would you code these vaccinations and E/M services?

   a. An established patient (10 years old); the only service for the visit is an injection of DTP (diphtheria, tetanus toxoid, pertussis) and oral poliovirus. Services were provided by the nurse, at the direction of the physician.

   🔵 Code(s): _____

   b. An established patient, a 1-year-old, is brought in for a well-baby checkup (separate service) by the physician, and the following are given: DT and IM injectable poliomyelitis. The physician counseled the parent on the vaccines. An initial comprehensive preventative medicine evaluation was provided by the physician.

   🔵 Code(s): _____

   c. A 64-year-old established patient comes in for an influenza virus (not preservative-free) vaccine that is administered intramuscularly by the nurse. The vaccine is the only service provided at that visit.

   🔵 Code(s): _____

   d. A new patient, 30 years old, comes for an office visit at which the physician does an expanded problem focused history and physical examination (separate service) and also administers a DTP and *Haemophilus influenzae* B (Hib) vaccine.

   🔵 Code(s): _____

3 A parent brings an 18-month-old infant (established patient) for a well-baby examination at which the physician administers a vaccine intramuscularly for diphtheria and tetanus toxoid (DT) after counseling the parent on the vaccines.

   🔵 Code(s): _____

Hydration. Codes 96360 and 96361 report hydration services. The physician's work related to these services usually involves oversight of the treatment plan and staff supervision. When the physician provides a significant separately identifiable E/M service, report the service with an appropriate E/M service using modifier -25. Modifier -25 must be added to the E/M code or the E/M service will be assumed to be related to the physician's service for the hydration, injection, or infusion service.

Bundled into the hydration, injection, and infusion services are local anesthesia, placing the intravenous line, accessing an indwelling access line/catheter/port, flushing at the end of the infusion, and all standard supplies.

The codes 96360 and 96361 report intravenous hydration infusions that include the prepackaged fluid and electrolytes. If other than a prepackaged substance is used, that substance would be reported separately. Saline is reported separately if administered separately. If the drugs are mixed into the saline, then only the drug is reported and the saline is bundled into the cost of the drug and not reported separately. Included in these codes are the physician supervision and oversight of the staff providing the service. Code 96360 is reported for 31 minutes to one hour of intravenous infusion hydration service and 96361, the add-on code, reports each additional hour. You can only report 96361 if the service is at least 30 minutes. Time under 30 minutes is not reported.

Therapeutic, Prophylactic, and Diagnostic Injections and Infusions.

Codes 96365-96379 report the administration of a therapeutic, prophylactic, or diagnostic intravenous infusion or injection. Intravenous **infusions** are reported with 96365-96368 and are divided based on the time and type of infusion. The initial infusion is reported with 96365 (up to 1 hour) and each additional hour (over 31 minutes) is reported with 96366. Sometimes one infusion is provided **followed by** another infusion (sequential infusions), in which case the initial infusion is listed first and the additional sequential infusion (96367) is listed second. There are times when more than one infusion is provided at the **same** time. A concurrent infusion is when there is one site and two lines infusing. Report the initial infusion first and then the additional concurrent infusion (96368).

Subcutaneous infusions are reported with codes 96369-96371. Initial set up and first hour is reported with 96369. Each additional hour is reported with 96370. Additional set up for a new infusion site is reported with 96371.

Therapeutic, prophylactic, and diagnostic **injections** are divided based on the method used for the administration (Fig. 13–2). *Subcutaneous* and *intramuscular* injections are reported with 96372 in addition to a code to report the substance injected. For example, if the injection was a subcutaneous human rabies immune globulin, report 90375 for the substance and 96372 for the administration. The vaccines/toxoids are reported with 90465/90466 or 90471/90472. Code 96372 is not used to report chemotherapy administration (see 96401-96549). Injections for allergen immunotherapy are reported with 95115/95117, not with therapeutic, prophylactic, or diagnostic injection codes. *Intra-arterial* (96373) and *intravenous push* (96374/96375/96376) are reported with therapeutic, prophylactic, and diagnostic injection codes.

EXERCISE 13–2 *Injections*

Using the CPT manual, code the following injections:

1 An established patient is seen in the office for pernicious anemia. The nurse gives the patient an injection of vitamin B_{12}.

   Code(s): _____

2 An established patient (50 years old) presents to the nurse for a flu shot.

   Code(s): _____

Psychiatry.

The Psychiatry subsection (90801-90899) has a lengthy note under the heading detailing the use of psychiatric codes in conjunction with hospital and clinic E/M services. If psychiatric treatments are rendered on the same day as E/M services, both the E/M service and the psychiatric treatment are reported with one code from the Psychiatry subsection. For

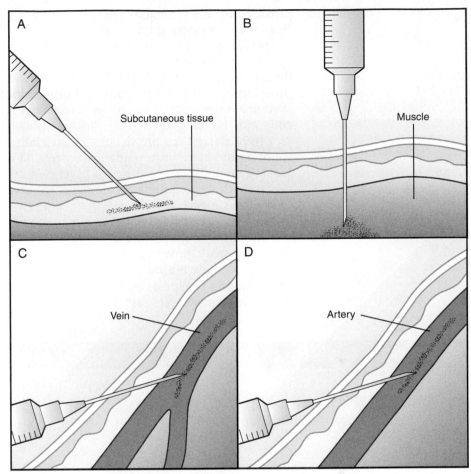

FIGURE 13-2 Injection methods. **A,** Subcutaneous (SQ). **B,** Intramuscular (IM). **C,** Intravenous (IV). **D,** Intra-arterial.

example, if a patient is admitted to the hospital with a drug overdose secondary to depression, and the physician spends 25 minutes in supportive psychotherapy with the patient several hours after he was admitted to the hospital, services to be coded would be 90817 (Individual Medical Psychotherapy) for the psychiatric treatment and medical evaluation/ management on the same day. The code includes the development of orders, the review and interpretation of laboratory work or other diagnostic studies, and the review of therapy reports and other information from the medical record. You will work closely with third-party payers to determine any specific regional instructions for coding psychiatric services.

Partial hospitalization refers to a hospital setting in which the patients are in the hospital during the day and return to their homes in the evenings and on weekends. The facilities may be open only during the day, 5 days a week, although there are also facilities that are open 7 days a week. When a physician admits a patient to a partial hospital facility, the physician is responsible for preparing all of the same admission paperwork that is prepared for admission to an acute care hospital. E/M Initial Hospital Care and Subsequent Hospital Care codes (99221-99233) are used to report inpatient stays. The psychiatric services the physician provides to the patient are listed separately unless the E/M service and psychiatric service are provided on the same day. These same-day services are reported with codes from the Psychiatry subsection.

Specific descriptions dealing with services included in each of the codes appear in the Psychiatry subsection. Some codes reflect evaluation or diagnostic services, such as CPT code 90801; some reflect therapeutic procedures, such as 90804; and still others, located in the Central Nervous System Assessments/Tests, are used to report psychological testing, such as code 96101.

A **psychiatrist** is a physician who specializes in psychiatry. A **psychologist** is not a physician but is a qualified specialist in psychiatry. States have varying regulations about how a psychologist reports services to patients, and some states require a psychologist to provide and report services only under the supervision of a psychiatrist. Third-party payers may also restrict the types of service a psychologist may report for reimbursement.

Time is the major billing factor in the Psychiatry subsection. Diagnostic and therapeutic time must be clearly documented in the patient's record to provide accurate billing.

Psychiatric Diagnosis and Psychiatric Treatment are two CPT manual index locations for the psychiatric service codes.

EXERCISE 13–3 *Psychiatry*

Using the CPT manual, code the following:

1 Individual medical psychotherapy in office for 30 minutes

   Code: _____

2 Psychological testing, 2 hours, administered by a physician

   🌐 Code(s): _____

3 Psychiatric evaluation of tests, medical records, or hospital data to make appropriate diagnosis

   Code: _____

4 Initial psychiatric interview examination

   Code: _____

Biofeedback. **Biofeedback** is the process of giving a person self-information. The information can be used by patients to gain some control over their physiologic processes, such as blood pressure, heart rate, or pain. Patients are trained to use biofeedback by a professional and then continue the use of the therapy on their own. Biofeedback training is often incorporated in individual psychophysiologic therapy. When biofeedback is part of the individual psychophysiologic therapy, a code is listed for both the biofeedback training and the individual psychophysiologic therapy (90875).

Biofeedback codes (90901, 90911) are located in the CPT manual index under the main terms "Training" and "Biofeedback."

EXERCISE 13–4 *Biofeedback*

Using the CPT manual, code the following:

1 A 40-year-old woman has been seen by the physician for several individual psychiatric sessions as the patient attempts to give up a two-pack-a-day cigarette addiction of 15 years' duration. The patient is experiencing increased anxiety and insomnia. As a part of the last 30-minute psychiatric session, the physician teaches the patient to use biofeedback in an attempt to help her alleviate the anxiety and insomnia. The patient is instructed to use the biofeedback techniques three times a day until the next session.

   Code: _____

2 A 52-year-old man is referred to the physician by his primary care physician for biofeedback to help regulate his blood pressure. The physician conducts a 60-minute session during which the patient is trained in the use of biofeedback.

   Code: _____

Dialysis. Dialysis is the cleansing of the blood of waste products when it is not possible for the body to perform the cleansing function adequately on its own. Dialysis may be temporary, as in the case of a patient who has acute renal failure from which he or she recovers, or permanent, as in the case of a patient with end-stage renal disease (ESRD) who will not recover without a kidney transplant.

The Dialysis subsection of the Medicine section (90935-90999) is divided into types of patient services. The subheading End Stage Renal Disease Services deals with dialysis of a permanent nature. The codes reflect all services included in treating a patient with ESRD and are listed according to patient age (e.g., younger than 2 years of age, 2-11 years of age) and the number of services provided (1, 2-3, 4). Dialysis services are usually billed as a monthly fee. For those cases in which a patient may be, for example, visiting the area and will not require a full month of dialysis, daily fees may be billed using codes 90967-90970. Few third-party payers allow E/M codes to be reported in addition to dialysis service codes. Most payers consider the dialysis codes to be bundled to include all the treatment necessary for a patient with renal disease, including the E/M services. To report a separate E/M service, the condition would have to be unrelated to the renal condition and -25 must be added to the E/M code.

Dialysis is usually performed in an outpatient setting at a hospital. The physician services are reported based on the type of dialysis the patient is receiving, the complexity of the service, and the number of visits the physician provides to the patient. One code covers all physician visits to the dialysis laboratory during that month to assess the patient while the patient is receiving dialysis. As with all people, dialysis patients must sometimes be admitted to the hospital, and while in the hospital must continue to receive dialysis treatments. When the physician sees the inpatient while the patient is undergoing dialysis, you would code 90935 (single visit) or 90937 (multiple visits) for hemodialysis. Code 90937 may include a significant revision of the dialysis prescription. If a hospitalized patient receiving peritoneal dialysis is seen by the physician, the physician services are reported with 90945 (single visit) and 90947 (multiple visits). Code 90947 may include a significant revision of the dialysis prescription. Modifier -26 is not used on these codes, as the code descriptions describe only the physician service to the dialysis patient.

When a patient does not receive a full month of dialysis in the outpatient setting because of a kidney transplant, relocation, or death, report the number of days on which the patient had dialysis. For example, a 50-year-old patient receives peritoneal dialysis from March 1 through 10. On March 11, the patient receives a kidney transplant. The 10 days of service are reported with 90970 × 10.

Hemodialysis is the routing of blood and its waste products to the outside of the body where it is filtered. After the blood is cleansed, it is returned to the body. Hemodialysis codes are reported for each day the service is provided. The codes in the hemodialysis category are based on the number of times the physician evaluates the patient during the procedure.

Peritoneal dialysis involves using the peritoneal cavity as a filter. Dialysis fluid is introduced into the cavity and left there for several hours so cleansing can take place (Fig. 13–3). The dialysis fluid is then drained from the peritoneal cavity. Peritoneal dialysis is reported on the basis of each day the service is provided. Some patients learn how to perform dialysis for themselves. Dialysis teaching codes are located under Other Dialysis Procedures.

"Dialysis" is the main term to be referenced in the CPT manual index.

CODING SHOT Temporary HCPCS codes are used for reporting monthly dialysis services for Medicare patients. Instead of 90951-90962, for hemodialysis use G0308-G0319 and for peritoneal dialysis use G0320-G0327.

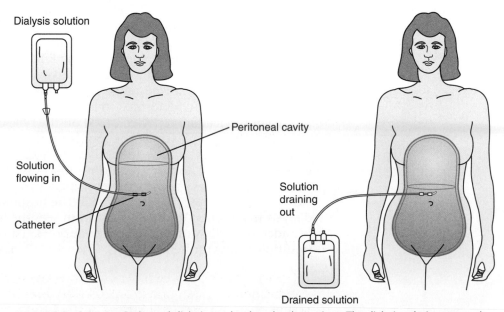

FIGURE 13–3 Peritoneal dialysis can be done by the patient. The dialysis solution enters the peritoneal cavity by a catheter. After the solution has been inside the patient for several hours, it is drained out through the catheter.

EXERCISE 13–5 *Dialysis*

Using the CPT manual, code the following dialysis services:

1 A 10-year-old patient with end-stage renal disease has three encounters during a full month of hemodialysis treatment

   Code: _____

2 Hemodialysis with a single physician evaluation, inpatient

   Code: _____

3 Peritoneal dialysis with repeated physician evaluations, inpatient

   Code: _____

Define the following subsection words or abbreviations:

4 peritoneal _____

5 hemofiltration _____

6 ESRD _____

Gastroenterology. The Gastroenterology subsection (91000-91299) contains many types of tests and treatments that are performed on the esophagus, stomach, and intestine. Several intubation codes are listed in the Gastroenterology subsection. You must carefully review the code descriptions to determine which services are bundled into the code. For example, CPT code 91055 includes intubation, collection, and preparation of specimens. Because these three services are bundled into one code, it would be incorrect to code each service individually.

EXERCISE 13–6 *Gastroenterology*

Using the CPT manual, code the following:

1 A gastroesophageal reflux test with nasal catheter intraluminal impedence electrode for detection of reflux, 2 hours

   Code: _____

2 Gastric intubation and aspiration for treatment of ingested poison

   Code: _____

3 Gastric intubation with washings and slide preparation for cytology

   Code: _____

Define the following subsection words:

4 motility study _____

5 manometric studies _____

Ophthalmology. The notes located at the beginning of the Ophthalmology subsection (92002-92499) describe the services included in the various types of ophthalmologic services. Ophthalmology is a very specialized field and ophthalmologists can treat patients for a variety of diseases and injuries. Often the services provided and documented do not adequately fall into an E/M definition. Therefore, the AMA developed specialized codes that deal specifically with ophthalmology services. There are extensive subsection notes that are required reading before you code in the subsection. The notes explain the levels of service and present excellent examples to clarify the use of the codes. The general ophthalmologic services (e.g., routine yearly eye examinations) are located in the subheading General Ophthalmological Services. The codes in this subsection are based on whether the patient is a new or an established patient and on the complexity of service provided. There are two levels of service (intermediate and complex). Of special note are the definitions of new and established patients. The definitions of the terms "new" and "established" patient are the same as those used in the E/M section. You will recall that those definitions are as follows:

New patient: one who has not received any face-to-face professional service from the physician, or another physician of the same specialty who belongs to the same group practice, within the past 3 years.

Established patient: one who has received face-to-face professional services from the physician, or another physician of the same specialty who belongs to the same group practice, within the past 3 years.

The subheading Special Ophthalmological Services contains mostly **bilateral codes.** Each service in this subheading is performed on both eyes (unless otherwise stated), and these codes do not require a modifier to indicate that two eyes were examined or tested. In fact, should you need to report only one eye from these codes, you would need to use modifier -52 to indicate a reduced service. It is a good idea to make a note next to the codes that are bilateral codes in the CPT manual and also to make a note of modifier -52, which you would use to reduce the service if it was performed for only one eye. As always, the code description and/or notes indicate the way in which the code is to be reported.

Special Ophthalmological Service codes are those services that are not normally performed in a general eye examination. Services in this group are performed for medically indicated reasons. The definitions of the codes are very comprehensive in detailing the services involved with each code.

Other codes that are found in the Ophthalmology subsection under the subheading Spectacle Services, category Supply of Materials, deal with the provision of materials to the patient (e.g., spectacles, contact lenses, or ocular prostheses). The refraction that is done to determine the lens prescription may be billed separately, depending on the policies set by third-party payers.

From the Trenches

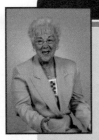

"Beginners think that if you have the coding books (CPT, ICD-9-CM) you're good to go. I tell them there is a story and history behind every code...They must investigate codes, modifiers, HCPCS codes, and more before a final decision can be made. It is never boring!"

NANCY

QUICK CHECK 13-2

Many of the codes for Contact Lens and Spectacle services are selected based on the diagnosis of aphakia. Define aphakia. _____

EXERCISE 13–7 *Ophthalmology*

Using the CPT manual, code the following:

1 Established patient, comprehensive ophthalmologic examination

Code: _____

2 Fitting of contact lens for treatment of a cataract, including the lens

Code: _____

3 Tonography (procedure to check the intraocular pressure of the eye, indention method) with interpretation and report

Code: _____

4 New patient, comprehensive ophthalmologic examination

Code: _____

Special Otorhinolaryngologic Services. The services in this subsection (92502-92700) deal with special testing or studies for the ears, nose, and larynx. Audiology (hearing) testing is found in the Special Otorhinolaryngologic Services subsection, too. An audiology test may be performed by a physician or an audiologist trained in this area.

CODING SHOT Otorhinolaryngologic diagnostic and treatment services are usually reported using codes from the Surgery section. Special services are reported using these otorhinolaryngologic codes from the Medicine section. For example, a nasopharyngoscopy with endoscopy service provided during an office visit would be reported using 92511 and an office visit code from the E/M section.

EXERCISE 13–8 *Special Otorhinolaryngologic Services*

Using the CPT manual, code the following:

1 Hearing aid check in one ear (monaural: "mon" is one and "aural" is ear)

Code(s): _____

2 Screening test, pure tone, air only

Code(s): _____

3 A nasopharyngoscopy with endoscope

Code(s): _____

4 Nasal function study

Code(s): _____

Cardiovascular. The Cardiovascular subsection is discussed in Chapter 7.

CONGRATULATIONS! Keep up the hard work; you will soon be finished with the entire CPT manual!

Therapeutic Services. Under this heading you will find noninvasive cardiovascular service codes (92950-92998), such as cardiopulmonary resuscitation (CPR) and cardio-conversions. You will also locate percutaneous translumeninal coronary angioplasty (PTCA) codes 92982, 92984. For PTCA, two catheters are placed; one a central venous catheter inserted through the femoral or brachial artery and a second catheter with a balloon tip is threaded up to the heart. The balloon is inflated in the area of occlusion and the occlusive material is pressed back, thereby widening the vessel.

Echocardiography. (93303-93350) is an ultrasound examination of the heart chambers/valves, the adjacent vessels, and the pericardium.

Cardiac Catheterization. Codes 93501-93581 report cardiac catheterization, which is a diagnostic medical procedure performed of the heart. In this section you report the catheter placement, injection, and guidance services with the following codes:

- Catheter placement 93501-93533
- Injection 93539-93545
- Guidance 93555-93556

Noninvasive Vascular Diagnostic Studies. The codes in this subsection (93875-93993) are used to identify procedures that are conducted to study veins and arteries other than the heart and great vessels. These studies use the same devices as are used in heart and great-vessel echocardiography, discussed previously, except that the divisions are based on the location of the vein or artery being studied.

EXERCISE 13-9 *Noninvasive Vascular Diagnostic Studies*

Using the CPT manual, code the following:

1 A patient is referred for a single-level, bilateral venous occlusion plethysmography of the legs.

Code: _____

2 A 34-year-old patient presents with a history of inability to sustain an erection. The physician uses a duplex scan to conduct a complete study of the arterial and venous flow of the penis.

Code: _____

Pulmonary. Codes found in the Pulmonary subsection (94002-94799) include codes for therapies, such as nebulizer treatments and incentive spirometry (illustrated in Fig. 13–4), and for diagnostic tests, such as pulmonary function tests. A nebulizer is a device that produces a spray, which is inhaled; it is used to treat patients with, for example, asthma. Pulmonary function tests are used to monitor the function of the pulmonary system; they examine the lung capacity of patients with, for example, emphysema. In most cases, several pulmonary function tests are performed together. The data are then compiled, and a diagnosis is made. Several indicators must be present from a variety of tests, and those tests must be performed many times and produce the same result each time for

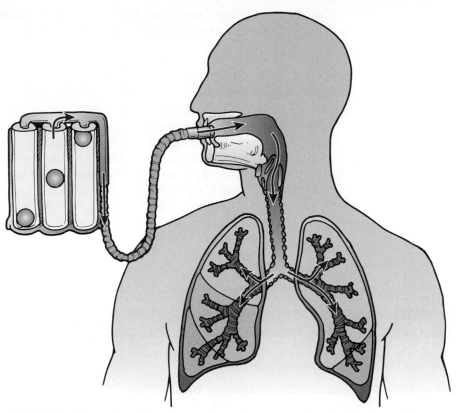

FIGURE 13–4   Incentive spirometry is used to promote alveolar inflation and lung capacity.

the results to be considered conclusive. In most cases, each type of test may be reported separately, unless it is specifically stated otherwise in the code description. Add -26 to the code when reporting the physician interpretation of the test if the physician does not own the testing equipment.

EXERCISE 13–10   *Pulmonary*

Using the CPT manual, code the following:

1 Pulmonary stress test, simple

Code: _____

2 Vital capacity, total

Code: _____

3 Bronchodilation responsiveness evaluation with spirometry before and after bronchodilator treatment

Code: _____

Allergy and Clinical Immunology.   You are strongly encouraged to read the notes that appear at the beginning of the Allergy and Clinical Immunology subsection (95004-95199). The subsection is divided into two parts. The first is Allergy Testing, which describes allergy testing by various methods (percutaneous, intracutaneous, inhalation) and the type of tests (allergenic extracts, venoms, biologicals, food). The number of tests must always be specified for billing purposes because for most of these codes, payment is made per test.

The second subheading is Allergen Immunotherapy. Allergen Immunotherapy codes specify three types of services:

1. Injection only
2. Prescription and injection
3. Provision of antigen only

All the codes in Allergen Immunotherapy have specific notes that you must read to know whether the code is for injection, prescription and injection, or antigen only. For example, code 95115 covers the injection of antigen only and does not include the antigen or the prescription, but code 95120 covers the injection, antigen, and prescription. So careful reading of the descriptions is a necessity.

The professional service necessary to provide the immunotherapy is bundled into the code, so an office visit code would not usually be reported. If the physician provided another identifiable service at the time of the immunotherapy, an office visit could be reported. But for the patient who has only the injection, prescription, antigen, or any combination of these three, the codes already contain the professional service.

EXERCISE 13–11 *Allergy and Clinical Immunology*

Using the CPT manual, code the following:

1 Direct nasal mucous membrane allergy test

   Code(s): _____

2 Percutaneous test using allergen extracts, immediate type reaction, 10 tests

   Code(s): _____

3 Single injection of allergen using extract provided by the patient

   Code(s): _____

Endocrinology. This subsection contains only codes used to report glucose monitoring (95250, 95251). The monitoring is a minimum of 72 hours, using continuous recording. The service includes the initial hookup, calibration of the monitor, patient training, recording, and downloading of data with printout of results.

Neurology and Neuromuscular Procedures. There are codes in the Neurology and Neuromuscular Procedures (95805-96020) subsection for sleep testing, muscle testing (electromyography), range of motion measurements, cerebral seizure monitoring, and a variety of neurologic function tests. The codes in this subsection are usually used by physicians who specialize in neurology, called neurologists. A neurologist usually is a consultant to a physician who needs the advice and input of another physician concerning a patient with suspected neurologic problems.

One of the specialized tests conducted in the neurology specialty area is sleep studies (95805-95811). **Sleep studies** are the monitoring of a patient's sleep for 6 or more hours. The studies include the tracing (technical component) and the physician's review, interpretation, and report (professional component). If a physician performs only the professional component, modifier -26 is used along with the CPT code.

Sleep studies are used to diagnose various sleep disorders and to measure a patient's response to therapy. An electroencephalogram (EEG) is a procedure that is used to record changes in brain waves. **Polysomnography** is the measurement of the brain waves during sleep but with the added feature of recording the various stages of sleep (i.e., excited, relaxed, drowsy, asleep, or deep sleep). During each of these stages, the rate and amplitude (height) of the brain waves are measured and compared with normal ranges. Certain neurologic conditions can be identified by the degree to which brain waves vary from normal ranges.

QUICK CHECK 13-3

According to the Sleep Testing Guidelines, Polysomnography includes sleep staging with:

a. EEG, EOG, EMG, ECG
b. Monitoring snoring, continuous blood pressures, and body positions
c. ECG, Extended EEG, NCPAP
d. EEG, EOG, EMG

Parameters are what are being measured while the sleep testing is being conducted. For example, parameters include the measurement of snoring. Another parameter is blood pressure. The parameters are listed under the subheading of Sleep Testing. Be certain to read these parameters before coding in this area. The patient's record will contain the parameters, or measurements, recorded during the test. Several of the codes in the category are based on the number of parameters being measured.

To code sleep tests accurately, you must know the parameters and stages of testing. Additionally, many codes include a time component.

The electromyographic (EMG) studies use needles and electric current to stimulate nerves and record the results. Assessments of dysphasia, developmental testing, neurobehavior status, and neuropsychological test codes are also found in this subsection.

EXERCISE 13–12   *Neurology and Neuromuscular Procedures*

Using the notes under the Sleep Testing subheading and the code descriptions following the notes, identify the following abbreviations:

1 NCPAP _____

2 EEG _____

3 EMG _____

4 EOG _____

Using the CPT manual, code the following:

5 Awake and drowsy EEG and photic stimulation in clinic

   ✿ Code(s): _____

6 Needle electromyography, three extremities and related paraspinal areas

   ✿ Code(s): _____

7 Range of motion measurement and report on both legs

   ✿ Code(s): _____

Central Nervous System Assessments/Tests. The Central Nervous System Assessments/Tests codes (96101-96125) identify psychological testing, speech/language (aphasia) assessment, developmental progress assessments, and thinking/reasoning status examination (neurobehavioral). Except for the basic developmental testing, the codes are defined on a per-hour basis. The results of all the tests are to be developed into a report that is included in the patient record.

EXERCISE 13-13   *Central Nervous System Assessments/Tests*

Using the CPT manual, code the following (code all cases at 60 minutes in length):

1 A mother presented to the office of a psychiatrist with a 10-year-old who had been referred by the child's pediatrician for his nonconformist behavior. At the psychiatric office visit, the mother expressed great concern about the child's inability to behave as she and the child's father believed appropriate. One week later the psychiatrist conducted several limited developmental tests of this patient. The psychiatrist then discussed the results of the tests with the mother. Code only the developmental testing.

   Code(s): _____

2 A young executive is referred for an 80-minute Minnesota Multiphasic Personality Inventory (MMPI) test by his employer. The employer requests the testing for all newly hired executives who will be working with highly sensitive government documents.

   Code(s): _____

3 A 14-year-old is seen in the office for a 70-minute assessment of the child's attention span. The child is experiencing increasingly severe episodes of daydreaming. The physician conducts a clinical assessment of the child's cognitive function.

   Code(s): _____

Health and Behavior Assessment/Intervention. The codes in this subsection (96150-96155) are not used to report preventive medicine services, nor are they used to report psychiatric treatments. Instead, these codes are used to report assessment and/or intervention for behavioral, emotional, social, psychological, or knowledge factors that are affecting the patient's health.

CODING SHOT These services are provided to prevent, treat, or manage a medical condition, for example, behavior modification for chronic pain.

Examples of assessments are clinical interview, behavior observation, and questionnaires. Examples of interventions are individual, group, or family sessions. All services are based on 15-minute increments. These services are not performed by a physician. If these services are performed by a physician they are reported with E/M codes.

Chemotherapy Administration. The chemotherapy codes 96401-96549 are used to report a variety of chemotherapy services. The Injection and Intravenous Infusion Chemotherapy codes (96401-96417) are used to report subcutaneous/intramuscular, intralesional, and intravenous chemotherapy.

Intra-Arterial Chemotherapy codes (96420-96425) are used to report various forms of chemotherapy administered via the arteries. Other Chemotherapy codes (96440-96549) are used to report various types of chemotherapy, such as pleural (96440), peritoneal (96445), and central nervous system (96450), in addition to refilling/maintenance of portable or implantable pumps or reservoirs (96521, 96522).

There are two other sets of codes that are used when reporting chemotherapy services: Hydration (96360-96361) and Therapeutic, Prophylactic, and Diagnostic Injections and Infusions (96365-96379). In addition to these CPT codes, HCPCS "J" codes report the medications.

Included (not reported separately) with chemotherapy infusion or injection codes 96401-96549 are the following:

1. Use of local anesthesia

2. IV start

3. Access to indwelling intravenous, subcutaneous catheter or port

4. Flush at the conclusion of infusion

5. Standard tubing, syringes, and supplies

6. Preparation of the chemotherapy agent(s)

If other services are provided, they can be reported separately.

The initial intravenous infusion (the treatment) is reported with 96365 and each additional hour of infusion, up to 8 hours, is reported with 96366. If a sequential (one after another) intravenous therapy is provided, the service is reported with 96367. When a concurrent (at the same time as another) intravenous therapy is provided the service is reported with 96368. A concurrent infusion is one in which multiple infusions are provided through the same intravenous line. A concurrent infusion can be billed once per patient encounter.

If more than one substance is placed in the same bag, it is considered one infusate and one infusion. The practice would bill one administration code and a Level II HCPCS J code for each substance or drug.

Any administration that is 15 minutes or less is considered a push, not an infusion. The administration of an initial or single intravenous push is reported with 96374 and each additional push is reported with 96375. Only bill one push per drug. For example, if a patient is given a push of morphine 2 mg at the beginning of a service and morphine 2 mg later in the service, bill one administration code for the two IV pushes of morphine. The appropriate units of the J code (J2270—morphine 10 mg × 1) would also be billed for the total dose.

If two drugs are mixed in the same bag and administered for 15 minutes or less, the service is reported with the appropriate push CPT code (initial or subsequent) × 1 unit. The drug(s) or substance would be separately reported with the appropriate J code.

A patient will often receive hydration and ancillary medications before or after chemotherapy. *Only one initial administration code can be reported* for each encounter, so these other services are reported with **secondary** or **subsequent** codes.

Example

A patient presents for a chemotherapy session and is given hydration prior to chemotherapy. The hydration service is reported with 96361 if the time is greater than 30 minutes. If the patient receives hydration before and after chemotherapy, calculate the entire time of hydration infusion and code the appropriate number of units for 96361. For example, a patient received 1 hour of hydration before chemotherapy and ½ hour of hydration after chemotherapy. The total hydration time is 90 minutes. Code 96361 × 1 unit. A second unit of 96361 can only be reported after 30 minutes beyond 1-hour increments.

The -59 modifier should be used to indicate that hydration was provided prior to or following chemotherapy. Hydration provided at the same time as chemotherapy to facilitate drug delivery is not separately reportable. All infusions must have a documented start and stop time.

The patient may also receive medications before and/or after chemotherapy, such as anti-nausea medications. These medications are reported in addition to the chemotherapy. Chemotherapy is always the primary service. For example, a patient is given intravenous Benadryl reported with J1200. When the patient receives multiple intravenous infusions of medications and these medications are administered individually, each is reported separately; but if the medications are mixed together and given in one infusion, they are reported as one infusion.

Example

A patient received Aloxi (J2469), Benadryl (J1200), and Decadron (J1100) in three separate infusions of less than 15 minutes (pushes). The J codes are reported along with 96375 × 3.

If the medications are all mixed together and administered in one infusion of less than 15 minutes, the J codes are reported along with 96375 × 1.

Example

A patient presents for chemotherapy and receives two pushes, one of Aloxi, 0.25 mg, and one of Benadryl, 50 mg. Chemotherapy with Rituximab, 100 mg, is administered for 3 hours by means of an intravenous infusion. After therapy, the patient is administered Decadron, 1 mg, by intravenous push. The services are reported as follows:

Pre and post-medications: 96375 × 3 (three total IV pushes); J2469 (Aloxi) × 10 units; J1200 (Benadryl) × 1 unit; and J1100 (Decadron) × 1 unit. NOTE: 1 unit of Aloxi = 25 mcg, therefore, 0.25 mg = 250 mcg = 10 units.

Chemotherapy: 96413 (initial hour); 96415 × 2 (two additional hours); J9310 × 1 (Rituximab). Chemotherapy is the initial infusion and the hydration and pushes are secondary/subsequent.

If a significant identifiable office visit service was provided, in addition to the chemotherapy administration, report that service with an E/M code adding -25 to indicate the service was separate and significant.

CODING SHOT Chemotherapy administration codes (96401-96459) include the use of local anesthesia, initiating the intravenous therapy, access to an indwelling port, flush at conclusion, tubing/supplies/syringes, and preparation of the chemotherapy agent(s) and are not reported separately.

EXERCISE 13–14 *Chemotherapy Administration*

Using the CPT manual, code only the chemotherapy administration:

1 Chemotherapy injected into the pleural cavity with thoracentesis

Code: _____

2 Refilling and maintenance of a patient's portable pump

Code: _____

3 Chemotherapy administered subcutaneously with local anesthesia

Code: _____

4 Chemotherapy administered intravenously using the infusion technique for 50 minutes

Code: _____

5 Chemotherapy injected into the central nervous system using a lumbar puncture

Code: _____

Photodynamic Therapy. The photodynamic therapy codes (96567-96571) are used in conjunction with the codes for bronchoscopy or endoscopy. An agent is injected into the patient and remains in cancerous cells longer than in normal cells. After the agent has dissipated from the normal cells, the patient is exposed to laser light. The agent absorbs the light and the light produces oxygen, destroying the cancerous cells.

Codes for endoscopic application are divided on the basis of time—the first 30 minutes and each additional 15 minutes. External application is based on each exposure session.

Special Dermatological Procedures. The dermatology codes (96900-96999) are usually used by a dermatologist who sees a patient in an office on a consultation basis. The dermatology codes for special procedures would typically be used in addition to the E/M consultation codes. For example, if a patient is referred by his family physician to a dermatologist for treatment of acne, the dermatologist conducts a history and examination and treats the patient with ultraviolet light (actinotherapy). The codes would be an Office or Other Outpatient Consultation code, depending on the level of service provided, *and* 96900 for the actinotherapy.

EXERCISE 13–15 *Special Dermatological Procedures*

Using the CPT manual, code the following:

1 A 16-year-old patient sees a dermatologist in consultation, at which time the physician does a problem focused history and physical examination regarding the patient's acne. The physician prescribes and provides a treatment of ultraviolet light therapy.

Code(s): _____ and _____

2 Photochemotherapy is provided for a 34-year-old consultative patient with severe dermatosis. The patient receives 8 hours of treatment. The physician provides a comprehensive history and physical examination with moderately complex medical decision making.

Code(s): _____

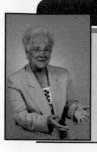

From the Trenches

What advice do you give to a coder looking to advance or move up?
"Enlarge your circle of influence, investigate other specialties, look to areas of coding compliance, attend workshops, become certified, and continue to learn."
NANCY

Physical Medicine and Rehabilitation. The codes in the Physical Medicine and Rehabilitation subsection (97001-97799) can be used by a physician or therapist. The subsection includes codes dealing with different modalities of treatments (e.g., traction, whirlpool, electrical stimulation) as well as various types of patient training (e.g., functional activities, gait training, massage). The codes are reported on the basis of time or treatment area, as stated in the description of the code. Codes are divided by supervision or constant attendance. Unit coding is necessary if the time spent administering the treatment exceeds the time listed in the code.

Example

Coding for patient's prosthetic training of 60 minutes would be:

97761 × 4   Prosthetic training, each 15 minutes

Test and measurement codes are listed by the type of testing and the time the testing takes. The type of test would be items such as orthoses, prostheses, and musculoskeletal or functional capacity. Note the use of type and time in the following CPT code.

Example

97750   Physical performance test or measurement (e.g., musculoskeletal, functional capacity, with written report, each 15 minutes)

Time must be noted in the documentation that is placed in the patient's medical record.

The codes in Physical Medicine and Rehabilitation are used for physical medicine and therapy as well as for other rehabilitation, for example, community/work reintegration (97537).

Active Wound Care Management. Nonphysician personnel perform the procedures (97597-97606) described in Active Wound Care Management codes. The codes are not used with or to replace the surgical debridement represented by codes 11040-11044; a physician performs the procedures reported with codes 11040-11044.

These wound management codes are based on nonselective or negative pressure procedures. **Nonselective** debridement is that in which healthy tissue is removed along with necrotic tissue. The tissue is gradually loosened with water (hydrotherapy). Loosened tissue may be cut away with sharp instruments. Nonselective debridement is usually done over the course of several office visits.

Negative Pressure Wound Therapy (97605, 97606) may include vacuuming the drainage and tissue from the wound area, application of topical medications or ointments, assessment of the wound, and directions to the patient for continued care of the wound. Choice of codes is dependent on the square centimeters treated.

EXERCISE 13–16 *Physical Medicine and Rehabilitation*

Using the CPT manual, code the following:

1 Application of cold packs to one area (modality)

   Code(s): _____

2 Initial prosthetic training, 30 minutes

   Code(s): _____

3 Physical medicine treatment procedure, gait training, 30 minutes

   Code(s): _____

Medical Nutrition Therapy. These codes (97802-97804) are used by nonphysician personnel for medical nutritional therapy assessment or intervention. If a physician provides the service, the service is reported using E/M codes or Preventive Medicine codes.

Osteopathic Manipulative Treatment (OMT). Osteopathic manipulative treatment (98925-98929) is a form of manual treatment applied by a physician to eliminate somatic (body) dysfunction and related disorders. The codes are listed according to body regions. The body regions considered are the head; cervical, thoracic, lumbar, sacral, and pelvic regions; lower extremities; upper extremities; rib cage; and abdomen and viscera. Codes are separated on the basis of the number of body regions treated. These codes are usually used by osteopathic physicians (doctors of osteopathy, D.O.).

Chiropractic Manipulative Treatment (CMT). The Chiropractic Manipulative Treatment subsection (98940-98943) is divided by the number of regions manipulated. For this subsection, the **spine** is divided into five regions (cervical, thoracic, lumbar, sacral, and pelvic), and the **extraspinal** regions are divided into five regions (head, lower extremities, upper extremities, rib cage, and abdomen). Chiropractic manipulation is the manipulation of the spinal column and other structures. Each of the codes in the Chiropractic Manipulative Treatment subsection has a professional assessment bundled into the code. An office visit code is used only if the patient had a significant separately identifiable service provided; otherwise, the service of the office visit is bundled into the code.

Non-Face-to-Face Nonphysician Services. This subsection is divided into Telephone Services (98966-98968) and On-Line Medical Evaluation (98969) and is used to report services provided by qualified health care professionals. The notes and the code descriptions for these codes indicate that the telephone or online service cannot originate from a related assessment that was provided within the previous seven days or result in an appointment within the next 24 hours or the soonest available appointment. The telephone services are reported based on the documented time, and the online service is per incident.

EXERCISE 13–17 *Manipulative Treatment*

Using the CPT manual, code the following therapies:

1 Sally, a 43-year-old woman, presents with the complaint of a seizing pain in the area of her lower left hip. The chiropractor conducts an assessment of the patient and provides a chiropractic alignment to two spinal regions.

   ❧ Code(s): _____

2 Osteopathic lumbar manipulation (OMT), one region

   ❧ Code(s): _____

Special Services, Procedures, and Reports. Special Services, Procedures, and Reports (99000-99091) is a miscellaneous subsection that includes codes that do not fit into other sections. Codes that reflect services rendered at unusual hours of the day or on holidays, for example, are considered adjunct codes and are to be used in addition to the codes for the major service. For example, if a physician goes to the office on a Sunday to meet an established patient and provide urgent, but not emergency, service, the correct E/M service code for the office visit would be used in addition to 99050 to indicate the unusual time at which the service was provided.

An often used code is 99024, which is used to report an office visit provided during a global period.

You have used 99070, supplies, from this subsection often. One of the big advantages of the HCPCS coding system is that you specifically identify the supply reported with 99070. For example, you may use 99070 to report a body sock that was given to a patient. With the HCPCS coding system, you can specify the body sock with a specific code, L0984. It is best to use HCPCS codes when reporting supplies since most third-party payers will request additional information when 99070 is reported.

The subsection also contains codes for medical testimony, the completion of complicated reports, education services, unusual travel, and supplies. Although this subsection is small, it contains codes that are used often. Take a few minutes to become familiar with the kinds of codes listed within Special Services, Procedures, and Reports and then mark the subsection for future use.

The codes for Special Services are located in the CPT manual index under the main term "Special Services."

EXERCISE 13–18 *Special Services, Procedures, and Reports*

Using the CPT manual, code the following:

1 What Medicine code is reported in addition to the basic service code when a service is provided after hours on Sunday?

   Code: _____

2 Conveyance of a specimen from the physician's office to a laboratory

   Code: _____

3 Supplies provided for an office visit exceeding those usually used

   Code: _____

Qualifying Circumstances for Anesthesia. Anesthesia is discussed in Chapter 3.

Moderate Sedation. Sedation reported with 99143-99150 is discussed in Chapter 3.

Other Services and Procedures. A wide variety of codes (99170-99199) is found in this subsection of the Medicine section. For example, you will find codes for anogenital examination with a colposcope of a child in a case of suspected trauma, visual function screenings, pumping poison from the stomach, and therapeutic phlebotomy treatments. Because the codes are so varied, the way in which they are divided is also varied. For example, the code range 99190-99192 is divided on the basis of time, whereas other codes are divided according to the extent of the service.

Home Health Procedures/Services. These codes (99500-99602) are used to report nonphysician services provided at the patient's residence. The residence may be an assisted living apartment, custodial care facility, group home, or other nontraditional residence. The codes are divided based on the reason for the service (e.g., injection, hemodialysis).

Home Infusion Procedures Services. The codes 99601 and 99602 represent services of administration of a variety of therapies (e.g., nutrition, chemotherapy, pain management). The services are provided by nonphysician allied health professionals. Codes are divided based on the time spent.

Medication Therapy Management Services. These codes (99605-99607) are for patient assessments and interventions by a pharmacist, upon request. These codes do not describe the product-specific information that a pharmacist would ordinarily provide to a patient regarding a medication; but rather to assist in the management of treatment-related medication complications or interactions. The codes are reported by the pharmacist based on the patient status (new or established) and the time spent in assessment and intervention.

HISTORY OF NATIONAL LEVEL CODING

CPT coding is only one of a two-part coding system called HCPCS (pronounced hick-picks). The Centers for Medicare and Medicaid Services (CMS), formerly the Health Care Financing Administration, developed the Healthcare Common Procedure Coding System in 1983. The HCPCS is a collection of codes that represent procedures, supplies, products, and services that may be provided to Medicare and Medicaid beneficiaries and to individuals enrolled in private health insurance programs.

Three Levels of Codes

HCPCS is divided into two levels or groups.

Level I codes are CPT codes in the CPT manual, which was developed and is maintained and copyrighted by the AMA. The CPT is the primary coding system used in the outpatient setting to code professional services provided to patients.

Level II codes (National Codes) are approved and maintained jointly by the Alpha-Numeric Workgroup, consisting of the CMS, the Health Insurance Association of America, and the Blue Cross and Blue Shield Association. Level II codes are five-position alphanumeric codes representing physician and nonphysician services that are not represented in the Level I codes.

There used to be **Level III** codes (Local Codes) that were developed by Medicare carriers or state payers for use at the local (carrier) level. These were five-position alphanumeric codes representing physician and nonphysician services that were not represented in the Level I or Level II codes. Local codes are no longer available since the implementation of HIPAA (Health Insurance Portability Accountability Act). Some local codes were integrated into the national codes (HCPCS).

Level II National Codes. CPT codes do not cover all services that are provided to patients. Allied health care professionals—such as dentists, orthodontists, and various technical support services, such as ambulance services—are not covered by the CPT coding system. There are also no codes in the CPT system for many of the supplies that are used in patient care (e.g., drugs, durable medical equipment, and orthoses). Use of national codes is mandatory on all Medicare and Medicaid claims submitted for payment for services of the previously listed professionals. Although many of the national codes were developed for use when reporting for services rendered to Medicare patients, many third-party payers now require that providers use the national codes when submitting bills for non-Medicare patients too, because the system allows for continuity and specificity when billing. This uniformity also helps the effort to collect uniform health service data.

QUICK CHECK 13-4

1. What is the code range for Drugs? _____
2. In what publication are these codes (from Question 1) published?
   a. HCPCS
   b. CPT
   c. CDT
   d. ICD

The first digit in a national code is a letter—A, B, C, D, E, G, H, J, K, L, M, P, Q, R, S, T, or V—that is followed by four numbers. Codes beginning with the letters K, G, Q, and S are for temporary assignment until a definitive decision can be made about appropriate code assignment. The K codes are temporary codes for durable medical equipment, the G codes are temporary codes for procedures and professional services, and the Q codes are temporary codes for procedures, services, and supplies. S codes are temporary Blue Cross/Blue Shield codes that are not valid for Medicare or Medicaid patients. All codes and descriptions are updated annually by the CMS. The alphanumeric listing contains headings of groups of codes, as illustrated in Fig. 13–5.

QUICK CHECK 13-5

Match the temporary code heading with the correct alpha category:

Alpha Category: G K Q S

1. Temporary National Codes (not CMS)   _____
2. Temporary procedure and professional services _____
3. DME (Durable Medical Equipment)   _____
4. Procedures, services, and supplies

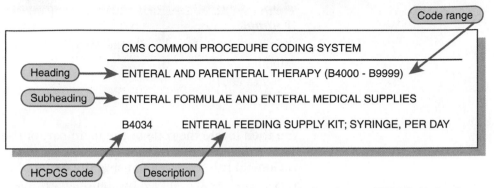

FIGURE 13–5   CMS's Healthcare Common Procedure Coding System (HCPCS), National Codes. (Courtesy U.S. Department of Health and Human Services, Centers for Medicare and Medicaid Services.)

> **Note:** In Figures 13–5 through 13–11, and 13–14, the HCPCS codes are samples for the purpose of illustration only. They may not be displayed as such in the current HCPCS manual.

Note that following the heading is listed the range of codes available for assignment in the category. There are also subheadings preceding the codes and the description of the codes to identify the type of codes that follow.

CODES	USED BY OR FOR
C	Report items used in the hospital outpatient departments for Medicare patients
G	Professional health care procedures and services not identified in CPT
H	State Medicaid agencies
K	DMERC, durable medical equipment regional carriers
Q	Drugs, biologicals, and medical equipment
S	Developed by BC/BS (Blue Cross/Blue Shield) to report drugs, services, and supplies. Not valid for Medicare or Medicaid programs.
T	Medicaid agencies and third-party payers. Not valid for Medicare services.

National codes are not used by health care facilities to code for the services provided to inpatients. Inpatient health care facilities use the diagnosis (from ICD-9-CM) as the basis of payment for their services and assign codes from ICD-9-CM, Volume 3, for inpatient procedures. The two levels of national codes are used in outpatient settings (including physicians' offices) where the basis of payment is the service rendered, not the diagnosis.

General Guidelines. The HCPCS manual includes the general guidelines for use of the national codes, a list of modifiers, the codes, a Table of Drugs, and an index. We begin our study of the HCPCS manual at the index. You have to be able to locate items in the index in order to be able to identify the correct code. The main index terms include tests, services, supplies, orthoses, prostheses, medical equipment, drugs, therapies, and some medical and surgical procedures. The subterms of the index are listed under the main term to which they apply, along with the code.

> *Example*
>
> *Apnea monitor* is found under the entry:
>
> Monitor
>
>   apnea E0618

You then locate the code in the main part of the manual and read any notes that are listed with the code.

General rules for coding using the national codes are as follows:

1. Never code directly from the index. Always use both the alphanumeric listing and the index.
2. Analyze the statement or description provided that designates the item that needs a code.
3. Identify the main term in the index.
4. Check for relevant subterms under the main term. Verify the meaning of any unfamiliar abbreviations.
5. Note the code or codes found immediately after the selected main term or subterm.
6. After locating the term and the code in the index, verify the code and its full description in the alphanumeric listing to ensure the specificity of the code.
7. In most cases, for each entry a specific code is provided. In some cases, you are referred to a range of codes among which you can locate the exact code desired. You must review the entire range in the numeric listing to find the correct entry.

   If the code is a single number, locate that code number in the alphanumeric listing. Verify the code number and the description to be sure that you have selected the correct code to describe the item you are coding. You must review the alphanumeric listing to select the appropriate code number in this case.
8. In all cases, when locating an entry in the index, it is necessary to look at all descriptors under the main term and subterms in order to choose the correct entry.

QUICK CHECK 13-6

In the HCPCS Index, locate the main term Aerosol.

Identify the sub-terms that represent:

a. Compressor E0571, E0572
b. Compressor Filter K0178-K0179
c. Mask K0180

1. A single code   _____
2. A range of codes   _____
3. Multiple codes   _____

CODE GROUPINGS

- **A Codes** — Transportation Services, including Ambulance
  Medical and Surgical Supplies
  Administrative, Miscellaneous, and Investigational
- **B Codes** — Enteral and Parenteral Therapy
- **C Codes** — Hospital Outpatient Prospective Payment System (OPPS)
- **D Codes** — Dental Procedures (published in Current Dental Terminology, CDT)
- **E Codes** — Durable Medical Equipment
- **G Codes** — Temporary (Procedures/Professional Services)
- **H Codes** — Alcohol and/or Drug Services
- **J Codes** — Drugs Administered Other Than Oral Method
- **K Codes** — Temporary (Durable Medical Equipment)
- **L Codes** — Orthotics and Prosthetics
- **M Codes** — Medical Services
- **P Codes** — Pathology and Laboratory Services
- **Q Codes** — Temporary (Procedures, Services, and Supplies)
- **R Codes** — Diagnostic Radiology Services
- **S Codes** — Temporary National Codes (developed by BC/BS)
- **T Codes** — State Medicaid Agencies
- **V Codes** — Vision/Hearing Services

Index. The index is in alphabetical order and includes main terms and subterms (Fig. 13–6). The entries in the index of the national codes may be listed under more than one main term. For example, surgical kits can be found under the two entries "Kits" and "Surgical," as illustrated in Fig. 13–7.

From the index, you turn to the code in the alphanumeric listing. The entries in the alphanumeric listing further explain what is included in the code. The dialysis kit code numbers are shown as they appear in the alphanumeric listing in Fig. 13–8. Note that A4918 specifies "each."

There are more than 50 alphabetical modifiers available for assignment to add further specificity to the five-digit national code. For example, modifiers can be used to specify the service provider, specify the anatomic site, or add specificity (Fig. 13–9). Appendix A of the CPT contains some of the Level II, HCPCS/National modifiers.

 CAUTION *HCPCS manuals can vary considerably depending on publisher.*

Table of Drugs. J codes are used to identify the drugs administered and the amounts or dosages given. The national codes contain a Table of Drugs (Fig. 13–10) to direct the user to the appropriate drug titles and the corresponding codes. J codes refer to drugs only by generic name. However, if a drug is known only by a brand or trade name, you will be directed to the generic name of the drug and then to the associated J code by a cross-reference system within the table. A *Physicians' Desk Reference* (PDR) is a valuable resource for the coder when using the Table of Drugs.

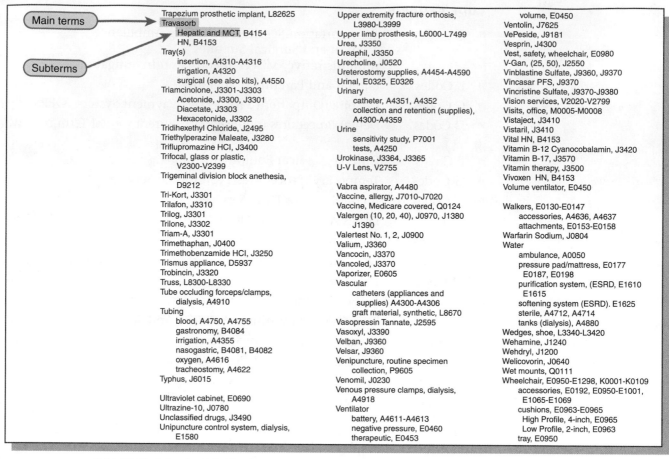

FIGURE 13–6 HCPCS index, National Codes. (Courtesy U.S. Department of Health and Human Services, Centers for Medicare and Medicaid Services.)

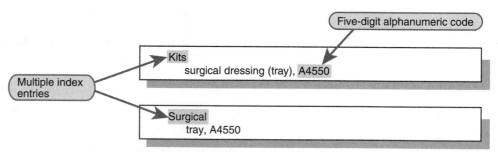

FIGURE 13–7 HCPCS index entries. (Courtesy U.S. Department of Health and Human Services, Centers for Medicare and Medicaid Services.)

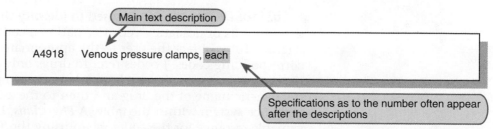

FIGURE 13–8 HCPCS main text display. (Courtesy U.S. Department of Health and Human Services, Centers for Medicare and Medicaid Services.)

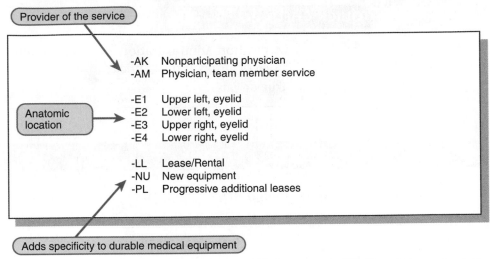

FIGURE 13–9 HCPCS modifiers. (Courtesy U.S. Department of Health and Human Services, Centers for Medicare and Medicaid Services.)

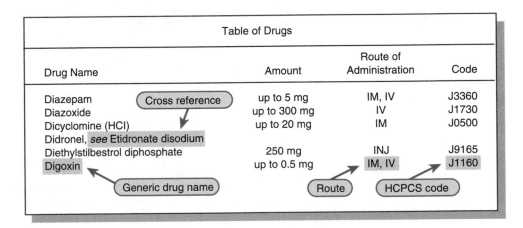

FIGURE 13–10 Example from Table of Drugs. (Courtesy U.S. Department of Health and Human Services, Centers for Medicare and Medicaid Services.)

The Route of Administration column (see Fig. 13–10) lists the most common methods of delivering the referenced generic drug. The official definitions for Level II J codes generally describe administration other than by the oral method. Orally given drugs are not usually provided in a physician's office but are bought at a pharmacy after the visit. Therefore, with a few exceptions, orally delivered drugs are omitted from the Route of Administration column. The following abbreviations and listings are used in the Route of Administration column:

INJ	Injection
IT	Intrathecal
IV	Intravenous
IM	Intramuscular
SC	Subcutaneous
INH	Inhalant solution
VAR	Various routes
OTH	Other routes

QUICK CHECK 2-2

Medication Administration Route information is provided with the Table of Drugs and Chemicals.
True or False?

EXERCISE 13-19 *Table of Drugs*

Define the following routes of administration for drugs:

1 Intrathecal _____

_____

2 Intravenous _____

_____

3 Intramuscular _____

_____

4 Subcutaneous _____

_____

5 Inhalant solution _____

_____

Routes of Administration of Drugs. Intravenous administration includes all methods, such as gravity infusion, injections, and timed pushes. When several routes of administration are listed, the first listing is the most common method. A "VAR" posting denotes various routes of administration and is used for drugs that are commonly administered into joints, cavities, or tissues, and as topical applications. Listings posted with "OTH" alert the coder to other administration methods, for example, suppositories or catheter injections. A dash (—) in a column signifies that no information is available for that particular listing. Fig. 13–11 illustrates J code information as listed in the alphanumeric listing to which you refer after locating the drug in the Table of Drugs.

Durable Medical Equipment. Durable medical equipment (DME) is equipment used by a patient with a chronic disabling condition, and the term also includes some equipment that is used only temporarily until the

CMS Healthcare Common Procedure Coding System

J1120	INJECTION, ACETAZOLAMIDE SODIUM, UP TO 500 MG
J1160	INJECTION, DIGOXIN, UP TO 0.5 MG
J1165	INJECTION, PHENYTOIN SODIUM, PER 50 MG
J1170	INJECTION, HYDROMORPHONE, UP TO 4 MG
J1180	INJECTION, DYPHYLLINE, UP TO 500 MG
J1190	INJECTION, DEXRAZOXANE HYDROCHLORIDE, PER 250 MG
J1200	INJECTION, DIPHENHYDRAMINE HCL, UP TO 50 MG
J1205	INJECTION, CHLOROTHIAZIDE SODIUM, PER 500 MG

FIGURE 13-11 HCPCS J codes. (Courtesy U.S. Department of Health and Human Services, Centers for Medicare and Medicaid Services.)

patient has healed. Claims for DME and related supplies can be paid only if the items meet the Medicare definition of covered DME and are medically necessary. The determination of medical necessity is made using documentation written by the physician. The documentation can include medical records, a plan of care, discharge plans, and prescriptions or forms explicitly designed to document medical necessity. These forms are referred to as Certificates of Medical Necessity (CMN). An example of a CMN is CMS-848 for a transcutaneous electrical nerve stimulator (Fig. 13–12).

Claims for other items require the use of the CMN, for example, power-operated vehicles, air-fluidized beds, decubitus care pads, seat-lift mechanisms, and paraffin baths.

Physician completion of the required medical documentation ensures that the DME items furnished to a Medicare beneficiary are those specifically needed for the unique medical condition of the patient. The CMS also requires the use of form CMS-484 for the Certification of Medical Necessity—Oxygen (Fig. 13–13).

National Physician Fee Schedule. Each fall, the Centers for Medicare and Medicaid Services produces the National Physician Fee Schedule, which lists all HCPCS and CPT codes along with the amount allocated for each services and the covered/noncovered status of each service. A list of fees for drugs is produced on a quarterly basis based on the current Average Sales Price (ASP) of each drug. Fig. 13–14 illustrates a portion of the National Physician Fee Schedule for 2002. You will learn more about CMS allocations in Chapter 16 of this text.

DEPARTMENT OF HEALTH AND HUMAN SERVICES
CENTERS FOR MEDICARE & MEDICAID SERVICES

Form Approved
OMB No. 0938-0679

CERTIFICATE OF MEDICAL NECESSITY

DME 06.03B

CMS-848 — TRANSCUTANEOUS ELECTRICAL NERVE STIMULATOR (TENS)

SECTION A Certification Type/Date: INITIAL ___/___/___ REVISED ___/___/___ RECERTIFICATION ___/___/___

PATIENT NAME, ADDRESS, TELEPHONE and HIC NUMBER

SUPPLIER NAME, ADDRESS, TELEPHONE and NSC or applicable NPI NUMBER/LEGACY NUMBER

(___ ___ ___) ___ ___ ___ - ___ ___ ___ ___ HICN _____

(___ ___ ___) ___ ___ ___ - ___ ___ ___ ___ NSC or NPI # _____

PLACE OF SERVICE_____	HCPCS CODE	PT DOB ___/___/___ Sex ____ (M/F) Ht. ____(in) Wt ____(lbs.)
NAME and ADDRESS of FACILITY *if applicable (see reverse)*	_____ _____ _____ _____	PHYSICIAN NAME, ADDRESS, TELEPHONE and applicable NPI NUMBER or UPIN (___ ___ ___) ___ ___ ___ - ___ ___ ___ ___ UPIN or NPI # _____

SECTION B Information in this Section May Not Be Completed by the Supplier of the Items/Supplies.

EST. LENGTH OF NEED (# OF MONTHS): _____ 1-99 *(99=LIFETIME)* DIAGNOSIS CODES (ICD-9): _____ _____ _____ _____

ANSWERS	ANSWER QUESTIONS 1-6 for purchase of TENS (Circle Y for Yes, N for No,)
Y N	1. Does the patient have chronic, intractable pain?
_____ Months	2. How long has the patient had intractable pain? (Enter number of months, 1 - 99.)
1 2 3 4 5	3. Is the TENS unit being prescribed for any of the following conditions? (Circle appropriate number) 1 - Headache 2 - Visceral abdominal pain 3 - Pelvic pain 4 - Temporomandibular joint (TMJ) pain 5 - None of the above
Y N	4. Is there documentation in the medical record of multiple medications and/or other therapies that have been tried and failed?
Y N	5. Has the patient received a TENS trial of at least 30 days?
____/____/____	6. What is the date that you reevaluated the patient at the end of the trial period?

NAME OF PERSON ANSWERING SECTION B QUESTIONS, IF OTHER THAN PHYSICIAN (Please Print):
NAME: _____ TITLE: _____ EMPLOYER: _____

SECTION C   Narrative Description of Equipment and Cost

(1) Narrative description of all items, accessories and options ordered; (2) Supplier's charge; and (3) Medicare Fee Schedule Allowance for each item, accessory, and option. (see instructions on back)

SECTION D   PHYSICIAN Attestation and Signature/Date

I certify that I am the treating physician identified in Section A of this form. I have received Sections A, B and C of the Certificate of Medical Necessity (including charges for items ordered). Any statement on my letterhead attached hereto, has been reviewed and signed by me. I certify that the medical necessity information in Section B is true, accurate and complete, to the best of my knowledge, and I understand that any falsification, omission, or concealment of material fact in that section may subject me to civil or criminal liability.

PHYSICIAN'S SIGNATURE _____ DATE ____/____/____

Form CMS-848 (09/05) EF 08/2006

FIGURE 13-12 CMS Certificate of Medical Necessity. (Courtesy U.S. Department of Health and Human Services, Public Health Service, Centers for Medicare and Medicaid Services.)

DEPARTMENT OF HEALTH AND HUMAN SERVICES
CENTERS FOR MEDICARE & MEDICAID SERVICES

Form Approved
OMB No. 0938-0534

CERTIFICATE OF MEDICAL NECESSITY
CMS-484 — OXYGEN

DME 484.03

SECTION A	Certification Type/Date: **INITIAL** __/__/__ **REVISED** __/__/__ **RECERTIFICATION** __/__/__

PATIENT NAME, ADDRESS, TELEPHONE and HIC NUMBER	SUPPLIER NAME, ADDRESS, TELEPHONE and NSC or applicable NPI NUMBER/LEGACY NUMBER
(___) ___ - ___ HICN _____	(___) ___ - ___ NSC or NPI #_____

PLACE OF SERVICE_____	HCPCS CODE	PT DOB __/__/__ Sex ___ (M/F)
NAME and ADDRESS of FACILITY *if applicable (see reverse)*	_____ _____ _____ _____	PHYSICIAN NAME, ADDRESS, TELEPHONE and applicable NPI NUMBER or UPIN (___) ___ - ___ UPIN or NPI #_____

SECTION B	**Information in This Section May Not Be Completed by the Supplier of the Items/Supplies.**

EST. LENGTH OF NEED (# OF MONTHS): _____ 1-99 *(99=LIFETIME)*   DIAGNOSIS CODES (ICD-9): _____ _____ _____ _____

ANSWERS	ANSWER QUESTIONS 1-9. (Circle Y for Yes, N for No, or D for Does Not Apply, unless otherwise noted.)
a)_____mm Hg b)_____% c)___/___/___	1. Enter the result of most recent test taken on or before the certification date listed in Section A. Enter (a) arterial blood gas PO2 and/or (b) oxygen saturation test; (c) date of test.
1 2 3	2. Was the test in Question 1 performed (1) with the patient in a chronic stable state as an outpatient, (2) within two days prior to discharge from an inpatient facility to home, or (3) under other circumstances?
1 2 3	3. Circle the one number for the condition of the test in Question 1: (1) At Rest; (2) During Exercise; (3) During Sleep
Y N D	4. If you are ordering portable oxygen, is the patient mobile within the home? If you are not ordering portable oxygen, circle D.
_____LPM	5. Enter the highest oxygen flow rate ordered for this patient in liters per minute. If less than 1 LPM, enter a "X".
a)_____mm Hg b)_____% c)___/___/___	6. If greater than 4 LPM is prescribed, enter results of most recent test taken on 4 LPM. This may be an (a) arterial blood gas PO2 and/or (b) oxygen saturation test with patient in a chronic stable state. Enter date of test (c).
	ANSWER QUESTIONS 7-9 **ONLY** IF PO2 = 56–59 OR OXYGEN SATURATION = 89 IN QUESTION 1
Y N	7. Does the patient have dependent edema due to congestive heart failure?
Y N	8. Does the patient have cor pulmonale or pulmonary hypertension documented by P pulmonale on an EKG or by an echocardiogram, gated blood pool scan or direct pulmonary artery pressure measurement?
Y N	9. Does the patient have a hematocrit greater than 56%?

NAME OF PERSON ANSWERING SECTION B QUESTIONS, IF OTHER THAN PHYSICIAN (Please Print):
NAME: _____ TITLE: _____ EMPLOYER:_____

SECTION C	**Narrative Description of Equipment and Cost**

(1) Narrative description of all items, accessories and options ordered; (2) Supplier's charge and (3) Medicare Fee Schedule Allowance for each item, accessory and option. (See instructions on back.)

SECTION D	**Physician Attestation and Signature/Date**

I certify that I am the treating physician identified in Section A of this form. I have received Sections A, B and C of the Certificate of Medical Necessity (including charges for items ordered). Any statement on my letterhead attached hereto, has been reviewed and signed by me. I certify that the medical necessity information in Section B is true, accurate and complete, to the best of my knowledge, and I understand that any falsification, omission, or concealment of material fact in that section may subject me to civil or criminal liability.

PHYSICIAN'S SIGNATURE _____ DATE ____/____/____

Form CMS-484 (09/05) EF 08/2006

FIGURE 13–13 CMS Certificate of Medical Necessity—Oxygen. (Courtesy U.S. Department of Health and Human Services, Public Health Service, Centers for Medicare and Medicaid Services.)

HCPCS	Description	Status Code	Conversion Factor
A0021	Outside state ambulance serv	I	$36.1992
A0080	Noninterest escort in non er	I	$36.1992
A0090	Interest escort in non er	I	$36.1992
A0100	Nonemergency transport taxi	I	$36.1992
A0110	Nonemergency transport bus	I	$36.1992
A0120	Noner transport mini-bus	I	$36.1992
A0130	Noner transport wheelch van	I	$36.1992
A0140	Nonemergency transport air	I	$36.1992
A0160	Noner transport case worker	I	$36.1992
A0170	Noner transport parking fees	I	$36.1992
A0180	Noner transport lodgng recip	I	$36.1992
A0190	Noner transport meals recip	I	$36.1992
A0200	Noner transport lodgng escrt	I	$36.1992
A0210	Noner transport meals escort	I	$36.1992
A0380	Basic life support mileage	X	$36.1992
A0382	Basic support routine suppls	X	$36.1992
A0384	Bls defibrillation supplies	X	$36.1992
A0390	Advanced life support mileag	X	$36.1992
A0392	Als defibrillation supplies	X	$36.1992

FIGURE 13–14 CMS's National Physician Fee Schedule Relative Value File indicates HCPCS code and description along with the conversion factor for that code for the following year. (Courtesy U.S. Department of Health and Human Services, Centers for Medicare and Medicaid Services.)

EXERCISE 13–20 *National Codes*

With information provided in this chapter, complete the following:

1 HCPCS is divided into two levels. List the names of the levels, in order, and the level numbers:

a. _____

Level _____

b. _____

Level _____

2 There are four groups of codes that are used by CMS for temporary assignment until a definitive decision can be made about the correct code assignment. What are the alphabetic letters of these four groups of codes? _____, _____, _____, and

_____.

3 Are all HCPCS modifiers numeric? _____

4 What alphabetic group of codes is used to reference drugs in the HCPCS? _____

5 The term "route of administration" generally describes the administration of drugs by methods other than _____.

6 What group of codes is used to reference durable medical equipment in the national codes?

_____

Use Fig. 13–6 through Fig. 13–11 to answer the following questions:

7 What is the modifier for each of the following (Fig. 13–9)?

a. New equipment _____

b. Lower left eyelid _____

c. The services of a physician who was a member of a team that provided service _____

8 What is the route of administration of dicyclomine (Fig. 13–10)?

_____

9 What is the amount of diazepam for code J3360 (Fig. 13–10)?

_____

10 What is the J code for an injection of diazoxide (Fig. 13–10)?

_____

11 What is the code available for a wheelchair tray (Fig. 13–6)?

_____

CHAPTER REVIEW

CHAPTER 13, PART I, THEORY

Without the use of the CPT manual, answer the following questions:

1 There are two types of services in the Medicine section. One is diagnostic and the other is

_____.

2 What do the following abbreviations mean?

a. IV _____

b. IM _____

c. SQ _____

3 The routing of blood, including the waste products, outside of the body for cleansing is

_____.

4 The dialysis that involves using the peritoneal cavity as a filter is known as what kind of

dialysis? _____

5 What is the name of the test that checks the intraocular pressure of the eye?

_____

6 What is the name of the scope that is used to examine color vision?

_____

7 What is the word that means the body of knowledge about the ear, nose, and larynx?

_____

8 In what subsection of the Medicine section would you find CPR, coronary atherectomies, and heart valvuloplasties?

_____

9 What kind of scanning uses ultrasonic technology with a display of both structure and motion with time?

_____

10 What is the name of the ultrasonic documentation that records velocity mapping and imaging?

_____

11 In what Medicine subsection would you find therapies such as nebulizer treatments?

_____

12 Percutaneous, intracutaneous, and inhalation are examples of what from the Allergy subsection?

_____

13 Allergenic extracts, venoms, biologicals, and food are examples of what from the Allergy subsection?

_____

14 If you were looking for the code number to indicate the circumstance in which a physician sees a patient between the hours of 10 pm and 8 am, in what subsection of the Medicine section would you find that code?

_____

CHAPTER 13, PART II, PRACTICAL

Using the CPT manual, code the following:

15 An 18-month-old established patient receives a DT that is administered intramuscularly by the physician, after the physician counseled the parents on the vaccine.

⚛ Code(s): _____

16 A 30-year-old established patient receives a tetanus toxoid that is administered intramuscularly by the physician's assistant.

⚛ Code(s): _____

17 A DTP and an oral poliomyelitis vaccine (live) are administered to a new 10-year-old patient. A problem focused history and examination are done, and the medical decision making is straightforward.

⚛ Code(s): _____

18 An established, 40-year-old patient presents to the nurse for a pneumonia and a flu immunization (2 injections).

⚛ Code(s): _____

19 A patient brings his allergy medication into the office, and a single injection service is provided by the nurse.

⚛ Code(s): _____

20 A patient receives the initial 30-minute training for her prosthetic arm.

⚛ Code(s): _____

21 A patient has a bronchospasm evaluation before and after a spirometry that is administered to monitor his lung capacity.

⚛ Code(s): _____

22 Nasopharyngoscopy with endoscope

⚛ Code(s): _____

23 A 30-year-old with end-stage renal disease receives a full month of dialysis that included six encounters.

⚛ Code(s): _____

24 Ophthalmology Clinic Progress Note

Today, I saw a new patient who is a 46-year-old white female who was diagnosed with Graves' hypothyroidism early last year. She had some swelling of the eyes and was originally told she had an allergy; then the same person, after he found out she had Graves', put her on prednisone. It was unknown what the dose was, but the patient showed me her bottles and it is obvious that she was on 20 mg a day, taken at suppertime. She has now come down from this. She was also on prednisone acetate eye drops. The patient denies any history of any problems except that she became quite depressed and her head felt funny on the steroids. The patient had a history of an ulcer problem in the past, which was treated with diet. The patient allegedly had a positive Mantoux test years ago, but her chest x-rays have always been negative.

Today when I saw her, she was 20/80 in the right and 20/40 in the left with her refraction. The lids are markedly swollen, and she has marked inferior ptosis from the sagging lids, the water collection, and the redness. There is marked chemosis of the conjunctivae and thickening of the lids. The patient has full extraocular motility, except she cannot converge. There is marked swelling of the globes on the retropulsion exam. The pressures are 21 and 20 in primary gaze and 30 and 24 in up gaze. The disks are flat. The patient has pseudoexfoliation in the right eye and nuclear sclerotic cataracts in both eyes, right greater than left.

I counseled the patient about the treatment of this and offered her radiation therapy along with the proper dose of steroids of 100 mg a day for a week and then taper down from the 100 mg. I will send her to see Dr. Zapata for consultation radiation therapy, and then I think we would see her weekly as we get this problem under control. I did not feel she needed any topical medication, and she definitely does not need surgery now since there is no proptosis at this time. We will see her again in 1 week. I counseled her about the side effects of the high dose of steroids and how to take them.

⚛ Code(s): _____

QUICK CHECK ANSWERS

QUICK CHECK 13-1
d. b and c

QUICK CHECK 13-2
Aphakia—absence of the lens of the eye

QUICK CHECK 13-3
d. EEG, EOG, EMG

QUICK CHECK 13-4
1. J0120-J9999

2. a. HCPCS

QUICK CHECK 13-5
1. S

2. G

3. K

4. Q

QUICK CHECK 13-6
1. c

2. b

3. a

QUICK CHECK 13-7
True

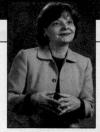

"Qualities that best describe a successful coder would include meticulous attention to detail, a strong sense of honesty and integrity, and perseverance."

Patricia Cordy Henricksen, CPC, CCP

Approved PMCC Instructor

President, Lexington Local Chapter of AAPC

Bluegrass Medical Managers Association

Lexington, Kentucky

An Overview of the ICD-9-CM

Chapter Topics

What Is the ICD-9-CM?

ICD-9-CM Format and Conventions

Alphabetic Index, Volume 2

Tabular List, Volume 1

The Appendices in the Tabular List, Volume 1

Procedures, Volume 3

Chapter Review

Quick Check Answers

Learning Objectives

After completing this chapter you should be able to

1 List the uses of the ICD-9-CM.

2 Explain the uses of coding conventions when assigning codes.

3 Identify the characteristics of the Alphabetic Index, Volume 2.

4 Identify the characteristics of the Tabular List, Volume 1.

5 Identify the characteristics of the Procedures Index and Tabular List, Volume 3.

6 Demonstrate use of ICD-9-CM.

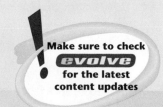

Make sure to check **evolve** for the latest content updates

WHAT IS THE ICD-9-CM?

The International Classification of Diseases, 9th Revision, Clinical Modification (ICD-9-CM) is designed for the classification of patient morbidity (sickness) and mortality (death) information for statistical purposes and for the indexing of health records by disease and operation for data storage and retrieval.

The ICD-9-CM is based on the ICD-9—the 9th revision of the official version of the International Classification of Diseases compiled by the World Health Organization (WHO). In February 1977, a committee was convened by the National Center for Health Statistics (NCHS) to provide advice and counsel concerning the development of a clinical modification of the ICD-9. The ICD-9-CM is the resulting clinical modification (CM). The term "clinical" was used to emphasize the intent of the modification to serve as a tool in the area of classification of morbidity data for indexing of disease, medical care review, ambulatory care, other medical care programs, and basic health statistics.

Through the years, the use of the ICD-9-CM (often called the ICD-9) has grown. The Medicare Catastrophic Coverage Act of 1988 (P.L. 100-330) required the submission of the appropriate ICD-9-CM diagnosis codes, with charges billed to Medicare Part B (outpatient services). The law was later repealed, but the coding requirement still stands.

Although coding was originally designed to provide access to medical records through retrieval for medical research, education, and administration, today codes are used to:

- Facilitate payment of health services
- Evaluate patients' use of health care facilities (utilization patterns)
- Study health care costs
- Research the quality of health care
- Predict health care trends
- Plan for future health care needs

The use and results of coding are widespread and evident in our everyday lives. Many people hear the results of coding on a regular basis and don't even know it. Anytime you listen to the news and hear the newscaster refer to a specific number of AIDS cases in the United States or read a newspaper article about an epidemic of measles, you are seeing the results of ICD-9-CM coding. The ICD-9-CM classification system is totally compatible with its parent system, ICD-9, thus meeting the need for comparability of morbidity and mortality statistics at the international level. This classification system is used to track morbidity and mortality. A classification system means that each condition or disease can be coded to only one code as much as possible to ensure the validity and reliability of data.

Coding must be performed correctly and consistently to produce meaningful statistics. (Refer to Fig. 14–1 for the Standards of Ethical Coding.) To code accurately, it is necessary to have an in-depth knowledge of medical terminology, anatomy, disease conditions, and pharmacology along with an understanding of the guidelines, terminology, and conventions of the ICD-9-CM. Transforming verbal or narrative descriptions of diseases, injuries, conditions, and procedures into numeric designations is a complex activity and should not be undertaken without proper training. Learning to use the ICD-9-CM codes will be a valuable tool to you in any health care career.

Medical Coding Code of Ethics

Members of the American Academy of Professional Coders shall be dedicated to providing the highest standard of professional coding and billing services to employers, clients and patients. Professional and personal behavior of AAPC members must be exemplary.

AAPC members shall maintain the highest standard of personal and professional conduct. Members shall respect the rights of patients, clients, employers and all other colleagues.

Members shall use only legal and ethical means in all professional dealings and shall refuse to cooperate with, or condone by silence, the actions of those who engage in fraudulent, deceptive or illegal acts.

Members shall respect and adhere to the laws and regulations of the land and uphold the mission statement of the AAPC.

Members shall pursue excellence through continuing education in all areas applicable to their profession.

Members shall strive to maintain and enhance the dignity, status, competence and standards of coding for professional services.

Members shall not exploit professional relationships with patients, employees, clients or employers for personal gain.

Above all else we will commit to recognizing the intrinsic worth of each member.

This code of ethical standards for members of the AAPC strives to promote and maintain the highest standard of professional service and conduct among its members. Adherence to these standards assures public confidence in the integrity and service of professional coders who are members of the AAPC.

Failure to adhere to these standards, as determined by AAPC, will result in the loss of credentials and membership with the American Academy of Professional Coders.

FIGURE 14–1 Medical Coding Code of Ethics. (From American Academy of Professional Coders: *Medical Coding Code of Ethics* [website]: http://www.aapc.com/aboutus/code-of-ethics.aspx. Accessed February 20, 2008.)

EXERCISE 14–1 *What Is the ICD-9-CM?*

Using the information presented in this text, complete the following:

1 The ICD-9-CM is designed for the classification of patient _____

   or _____.

2 The ICD-9-CM manual is based on what text developed by the World Health Organization?

   _____

3 The CM in ICD-9-CM stands for _____.

4 List four of the six reasons why the ICD-9-CM codes are used today.

   _____

   _____

   _____

   _____

5 The ICD-9-CM is used to translate what descriptive information into numeric codes?

   _____ and _____

ICD-9-CM FORMAT AND CONVENTIONS

Several publishing companies produce editions of the ICD-9-CM manual. All editions are based on the official government version of the ICD-9-CM, as is this text.

There are four groups whose function it is to deal with in-depth coding principles and practices: Centers for Medicare and Medicaid Services (CMS), which was formerly known as the Health Care Financing Administration (HCFA); National Center for Health Statistics (NCHS); American Health Information Management Association (AHIMA); and American Hospital Association (AHA).

Format

The ICD-9-CM manual is published in a three-volume set:

Volume 1   Diseases: Tabular List

Volume 2   Diseases: Alphabetic Index

Volume 3   Procedures: Tabular List and Alphabetic Index

Volume 1 contains the disease and condition codes and the code descriptions (nomenclature) as well as the Supplementary Classification of Factors Influencing Health Status and Contact with Health Services (V codes) and External Causes of Injury and Poisoning (E codes). Volume 2 is the Alphabetic Index for Volume 1. Volumes 1 and 2 are used in inpatient and outpatient settings to substantiate medical services (medical necessity) by assigning diagnosis codes. Volume 3, used for coding procedures, contains codes for surgical, therapeutic, and diagnostic procedures and is used primarily by hospitals. ICD-9-CM codes are reported on the CMS-1500 insurance claim form used in physician's offices and on the CMS-1450 form used in hospitals (Fig. 14–2). Private insurance carriers also require ICD-9-CM codes on forms submitted for payment for services.

To begin the study of ICD-9-CM codes, you will be introduced to the format and content of the volumes. When the review has been completed, you will begin to practice locating codes for various diseases and illnesses using the ICD-9-CM manual, because the only way to learn to code is to practice. For now, just relax, and let's take a look at the conventions that are used in the ICD-9-CM.

Conventions

The ICD-9-CM manual contains symbols, abbreviations, punctuation, and notations called conventions. Some conventions are used in all three volumes of the ICD-9-CM manual, and others are used in only one or two of the volumes. The ICD-9-CM manual contains a list of the conventions and definitions to be used when assigning codes, usually in the front matter of the manual. It is important that you be familiar with the conventions as you prepare to use the ICD-9-CM codes.

Although the maintenance of the ICD-9-CM is the responsibility of the NCHS (National Center for Health Statistics) and CMS (Centers for Medicare and Medicaid Services), many private companies publish editions of the ICD-9-CM, and each publisher has its own conventions in addition to the standard conventions. For example, some publishers indicate that a fifth digit is required by placing a special symbol next to the code. These additional symbols are helpful to coders but are not a recognized convention. For example, Elsevier's ICD-9-CM uses the symbols illustrated in Figure 14-3.

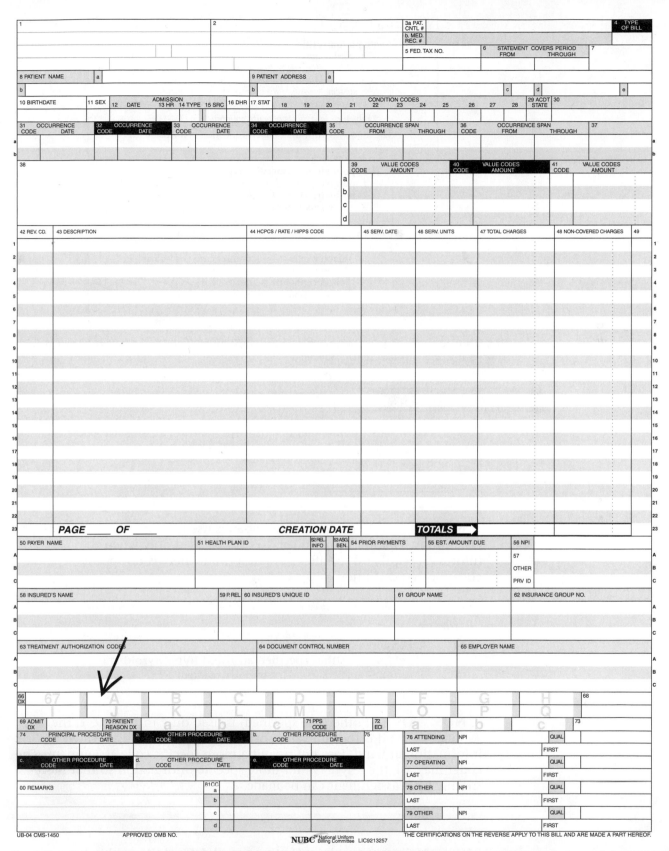

FIGURE 14–2 CMS-1450 was updated from the UB-92 to the UB-04 paper form effective May 23, 2007. (Courtesy U.S. Department of Health and Human Services, Public Health Service, Centers for Medicare and Medicaid Services.)

● 045 **Acute poliomyelitis**
Also called infantile paralysis and is caused by the poliovirus, which enters the body orally and infects the intestinal wall and then enters the blood stream and central nervous system, causing muscle weakness and paralysis. This disease has been nearly eradicated with the polio vaccine.

Excludes *late effects of acute poliomyelitis (138)*

The following fifth-digit subclassification is for use with category 045:

■ 0 **poliovirus, unspecified type**
1 **poliovirus type I**
2 **poliovirus type II**
3 **poliovirus type III**

● 045.0 **Acute paralytic poliomyelitis specified as bulbar**
[0–3] ◄
Infantile paralysis (acute) specified as bulbar
Poliomyelitis (acute) (anterior) specified as bulbar
Polioencephalitis (acute) (bulbar)
Polioencephalomyelitis (acute) (anterior) (bulbar)

FIGURE 14–3 Example of symbols in Elsevier's ICD-9-CM. (From Buck CJ: *2009 ICD-9-CM, Volumes 1, 2, & 3*, St. Louis, 2009, Saunders.)

QUICK CHECK 14-1

What two places could you find information regarding the coding conventions in your publication of ICD-9-CM?
1. _____
2. _____

NEC. NEC (not elsewhere classifiable) is used in Volume 1, the Tabular List, and in Volume 2, the Index. NEC to be used only when the information at hand specifies a condition but there is no specific separate code for that condition in the coding manual.

Example

244   Acquired hypothyroidism
    244.8   **Other specified acquired hypothyroidism**
        Secondary hypothyroidism NEC

NOS. NOS (not otherwise specified) is used only in Volume 1, the Tabular List, and is the equivalent of "unspecified." It is used when the information at hand does not permit a more specific code assignment. The coder may ask the physician for more specific information so that more specific code assignment can be made.

Example

159   **Malignant neoplasm of other and ill-defined sites within the digestive organs and peritoneum**
    159.0   **Intestinal tract, part unspecified**
        Intestine NOS

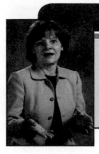

From the Trenches

"Study and understand the guidelines that are included in the resources, and learn the meaning and correct application of each code."

PATRICIA

Brackets [ ]. Brackets are used to enclose synonyms, alternative wording, or explanatory phrases. They are found in the Tabular List and the Index.

Example

426.8   **Other specified conduction disorders**
 426.89   **Other**
        Dissociation:
            atrioventricular [AV]
            interference
            isorhythmic
        Nonparoxysmal AV nodal tachycardia

Parentheses ( ). Parentheses are used to enclose supplementary words (nonessential modifiers) that may be present or absent in the statement of a disease or procedure without affecting the code number to which it is assigned. Parentheses are found in both the Alphabetic Index and the Tabular List.

Example

158   **Malignant neoplasm of retroperitoneum and peritoneum**
 158.8   **Specified parts of peritoneum**
        Cul-de-sac (of Douglas)
        Mesentery

Colon :. Colons are used in the Tabular List after an incomplete term that needs one or more of the modifiers that follow in order to make it assignable to a given category.

Example

628   **Infertility, Female**
 628.4   **Of cervical or vaginal origin**
        Infertility associated with:
            anomaly of cervical mucus
            congenital structural anomaly
            dysmucorrhea

Brace }. A brace is used to enclose a series of terms, each of which is modified by the statement appearing at the right of the brace.

Example

473   **Chronic sinusitis**

        Includes: abscess

                    empyema   (chronic) of sinus

                    infection   (accessory) (nasal)

                    suppuration

Lozenge □. In some versions of the ICD-9-CM, the lozenge symbol is printed in the left margin preceding the disease code to denote a four-digit number unique to the ICD-9-CM manual. The content of these codes in the ICD-9-CM is not the same as those in ICD-9. The lozenge symbol is used only in Volume 1, the Tabular List. Coders seldom concern themselves with the differences between ICD-9-CM and ICD-9; however, these differences are important to researchers.

Example

□   295.90   **Unspecified schizophrenia**

Section Mark §. In some versions of the ICD-9-CM, the section mark in the Tabular List indicates that a footnote is located at the bottom of the page.

Example

§   E807   **Railway accident of unspecified nature**

The footnote on the page states:

§   Requires fourth digit.

Bold Type. Bold type is used for all codes and titles in the Tabular List in Volume 1.

Example

244.8   **Other specified acquired hypothyroidism**

                Secondary hypothyroidism NEC

Italicized Type. Italicized type is used for all exclusion notes and to identify those codes that are not usually sequenced as the first-listed diagnosis. Italicized type codes cannot be assigned as a principal diagnosis because they always follow another code. Italicized codes are to be sequenced in the order specified in the Alphabetic Index, Volume 2, or according to specific coding instructions in the Tabular List, Volume 1, such as "code first . . ."

> ### Example
>
> **420.0** **Acute pericarditis in diseases classified elsewhere**
>
> *Code first underlying disease, as:*
>   actinomycosis (039.8)
>   amebiasis (006.8)
>   chronic uremia (585.9)
>   nocardiosis (039.8)
>   tuberculosis (017.9)
>   uremia NOS (586)

Slanted Brackets [ ]. Slanted brackets used in the Alphabetic Index, Volume 2, are used to enclose the manifestation of the underlying condition. When a code is listed inside the slanted brackets, you must sequence that code **after** the underlying condition code.

> ### Example
>
> Diabetic retinal hemorrhage
>
> Hemorrhage, hemorrhagic (nontraumatic) 459.0
>   retina, retinal (deep) (superficial) (vessels) 362.81
>   diabetic 250.5 *[362.01]*

You would sequence the code 250.5X (the appropriate fifth digit would have to be included) and then 362.01 to indicate that the retinal hemorrhage (the manifestation) was due to diabetes (the underlying disease).

Includes. Includes notes appear in the Tabular List, Volume 1; they further define or provide examples and can apply to the chapter, section, or category. The notes at the beginning of a **chapter** apply to that entire chapter; the notes at the beginning of the **section** apply to that entire section; and the notes at the beginning of the **category** apply to that entire category. You have to refer to the beginning of the chapter or section for any Includes notes that refer to an entire chapter or section because the Includes notes are not repeated within the chapter or section. Includes notes can also be found before or after category codes.

> ### Example
>
> Includes and Excludes notes that apply to codes 001-139 at the beginning of a chapter:
>
> **1. INFECTIOUS AND PARASITIC DISEASES (001-139)**
> Note: Categories for "late effects" of infectious and parasitic diseases are to be found at 137-139.
>
> diseases generally recognized as communicable or transmissible as well as a few diseases of unknown but possibly infectious origin
>
> *acute respiratory infections (460-466)*
> *carrier or suspected carrier of infectious organism (V02.0-V02.9)*
> *certain localized infections*
> *influenza (487.0-487.8, 488)*

Example

Includes notes that apply to codes 010-018 at the beginning of a section:

TUBERCULOSIS (010-018)

> INCLUDES infection by Mycobacterium tuberculosis (human) (bovine)

> EXCLUDES *congenital tuberculosis (771.2)*
> *late effects of tuberculosis (137.0-137.4)*

Example

Includes notes that apply to code 006 at the beginning of a category:

006 Amebiasis

> INCLUDES infection due to Entamoeba histolytica

> EXCLUDES *amebiasis due to organisms other than Entamoeba histolytica (007.8)*

Excludes. *Excludes* notes appear in the Tabular List, Volume 1, and indicate terms that are to be coded elsewhere. *Excludes* notes can be located at the beginning of a chapter or section or below a category or subcategory. *Excludes* notes can be used for three reasons:

Example

1. The condition may have to be coded elsewhere.

861 Injury to heart and lung

> EXCLUDES *injury to blood vessels of thorax (901.0-901.9)*

This Excludes note indicates that injuries to the blood vessels of the thorax are assigned within the codes 901.0-901.9 and are not assigned within the codes in 861.

Example

2. The code cannot be assigned if the associated condition is present.

§ 463 Acute tonsillitis

> EXCLUDES *streptococcal tonsillitis (034.0)*

If the tonsillitis is caused by a streptococcal organism, it would be coded 034.0, not 463.

Example

3. Additional codes may be required to fully explain the condition. For example, the following appears at the beginning of Chapter 4 in the ICD-9-CM.

4. DISEASES OF BLOOD AND BLOOD-FORMING ORGANS (280-289)

> EXCLUDES *Anemia complicating pregnancy or the puerperium (648.2)*

This *Excludes* note tells you that you should code 648.2X (the appropriate fifth digit would have to be included) to indicate the complication of pregnancy, followed by an additional code to specify the type of anemia.

Use Additional Code. You add information (by assigning an additional code) to provide a more complete picture of the diagnosis or procedure. The use of an additional code is mandatory **if** supporting physician documentation is found in the record.

Example

510   Empyema
         Use additional code to identify infectious organism (041.0-041.9)

For example, if you are coding empyema due to pseudomonas, the codes would be Empyema (510.9), due to pseudomonas (041.7). If no organism has been identified, no additional code is assigned.

Code First Underlying Disease. The phrase "Code first underlying disease" is used in the categories in the Tabular List, Volume 1, and is not intended to indicate the principal diagnosis. In such cases, the code, title, and instructions appear in italics. The note requires that the underlying disease (etiology) be sequenced first.

Example

366.4   Cataract associated with other disorders
            366.41   Diabetic cataract
                          Code first diabetes (250.5X)

By following this convention, diabetes 250.5X is sequenced first, followed by the diabetic cataract code 366.41.

Code, if Applicable, Any Causal Condition. A code with this note may be the principal diagnosis if no causal condition is applicable or known.

Example

707   Chronic ulcer of skin
            707.1   Ulcer of lower limbs, except pressure ulcer
                        Ulcer, chronic, of lower limb:
                            neurogenic of lower limb
                            trophic of lower limb
                        Code, if applicable, any causal condition first:
                            atherosclerosis of the extremities with ulceration (440.23)
                            chronic venous hypertension with ulcer (459.31)
                            chronic venous hypertension with ulcer and
                                inflammation (459.33)
                            diabetes mellitus (249.80-249.81, 250.80-250.83)
                            postphlebitic syndrome with ulcer (459.11)
                            postphlebitic syndrome with ulcer and inflammation
                                (459.13)

A postphlebitic syndrome with ulcer of the lower limb is coded 459.11 (postphlebitic syndrome with ulcer) and 707.10 (ulcer of lower limb, unspecified).

And and With. Although the two words "and" and "with" have similar meanings in everyday language, in ICD-9-CM terminology they have special significance and meanings. "And" means and/or, whereas "with" indicates that two conditions are included in the code and both conditions must be present.

And

Example

474   Chronic disease of tonsils and adenoids

The code 474 is used to identify the disease as one of tonsils and/or adenoids.

With

Example

   Diabetes, diabetic (brittle) (congenital) (familial) (mellitus) (poorly
    controlled) (severe) (slight) (without complication) 250.0
  with
   coma (with ketoacidosis) 250.3
    hyperosmolar (nonketotic) 250.2
   complication NEC 250.9
    specified NEC 250.8
   gangrene 250.7 *[785.4]*
   hyperosmolarity 250.2
   ketosis, ketoacidosis 250.1
   osteomyelitis 250.8 *[731.8]*

The "Diabetes" entry in the Index of the ICD-9-CM illustrates the use of "with" to direct the coder to the correct codes and sequence of codes for conditions that may present with diabetes.

EXERCISE 14–2 *Conventions*

Match the abbreviations, punctuation, symbols, and words to the correct descriptions:

1 [ ] _____

2 NOS _____

3 : _____

4 § _____

5 italics _____

6 *Excludes* _____

7 Includes _____

8 } _____

9 NEC _____

10 ( ) _____

11 *[ ]* _____

12 bold type _____

a. must be modified by an additional term to complete the code description

b. used in Volume 2 to enclose the disease manifestation codes that are sequenced after the underlying disease

c. typeface used for all codes and titles in Volume 1

d. indicates the use of code assignment for "other" when a more specific code does not exist

e. encloses a series of terms that modify the statement to the right

f. encloses synonyms, alternative words, or explanatory phrases

g. equals unspecified

h. typeface used for all exclusion notes or diagnosis codes not to be used for principal diagnosis

i. footnote or section mark

j. appears under a three-digit code title to further define or explain category content

k. encloses supplementary words that do not affect the code assignment

l. indicates terms that are to be coded elsewhere

Answer the following questions about conventions:

13 Includes and *Excludes* notes have no bearing on the code selection.

   True   False

14 Brackets enclose synonyms, alternative wordings, or explanatory phrases.

   True   False

ALPHABETIC INDEX, VOLUME 2

The Alphabetic Index is Volume 2 of the ICD-9-CM. Your study will begin with the Index because, as a coder, you will reference the Index first and then locate the diagnosis code identified in the Index in the Tabular List, Volume 1.

 CAUTION *There are terms in the Index that do not appear in the Tabular. For example, Anton's syndrome, 307.9, is listed in the Index but not in the Tabular. Even though the term is not listed in the Tabular description for the code, the code is correct because of the Index direction.*

So, let's begin with the modifiers used in the Index.

Modifiers

A main term in the Index may be followed by a series of terms in parentheses. The presence or absence of these parenthetic terms in the diagnosis has no effect on the selection of the code listed for the main term. These are called **nonessential modifiers.**

> **Example**
>
> **Ileus** (adynamic) (bowel) (colon) (inhibitory) (intestine) (neurogenic) (paralytic) 560.1
>
> The nonessential modifiers are the words "(adynamic) (bowel) (colon)," and so forth. Nonessential modifiers are words that may be used to clarify the diagnosis but do not affect the code assignment. The code for ileus is 560.1, and the code for adynamic ileus is also 560.1. The addition of the modifier "adynamic" does not affect the code assignment.

A main term may also be followed by a list of **subterms** that *do* have an effect on the selection of the appropriate code for a given diagnosis. These subterms are indented under the main term and offer additional specificity.

> **Example**
>
> **Incoordination**
>   esophageal-pharyngeal (newborn) 787.24
>   muscular 781.3
>   papillary muscle 429.81
> The term in parentheses (newborn) is nonessential and merely supplementary. The indented subterms are essential modifiers, such as muscular or papillary muscle.

General adjectives such as "acute," "chronic," "epidemic," or "hereditary" and references to anatomic site, such as "arm," "stomach," and "uterus," will appear as main terms, but they will have a "*see*" or "*see also* condition" reference.

> **Example**
>
> **Hereditary**—*see* condition
>
> **Uterus**—*see* condition

You will now learn more about the "*see*" cross references.

Cross References   Cross references provide the coder with possible alternatives for a term or its synonyms. There are three types of cross references:

1. *see*
2. *see* also
3. *see* category

The "*see*" cross reference is an explicit direction to look elsewhere. It is used for anatomic sites and many general adjective modifiers not normally used in the Alphabetic Index. The "*see*" cross reference is also used to reference the appropriate main term under which all the information concerning a specific disease will be found.

Example

Encephalomeningitis—*see* Meningoencephalitis

Endamebiasis—*see* Amebiasis

Kidney—*see* condition

Leukosis—*see* Leukemia

Lipofibroma (M8851/0)—*see* Lipoma, by site

The "*see also*" cross reference directs you to look under another main term if all the information being searched for cannot be located under the first main term entry.

Example

Laryngoplegia—(*see also* Paralysis, vocal cord) 478.30

The "*see* **category**" cross reference directs you to Volume 1, Tabular List, for important information governing the use of the specific code.

Example

Late—*see also* condition
 effect(s) (of)—*see also* condition
  abscess
   intracranial or intraspinal (conditions classifiable to 324)—*see* category 326

Notes   Certain main terms are followed by notes that are used to define terms and give coding instructions.

Example

Amputation
 traumatic (complete) (partial)
  arm 887.4
   at or above elbow 887.2
    complicated 887.3

Note: "Complicated" includes traumatic amputation with delayed healing, delayed treatment, foreign body, or infection.

Mandatory Fifth Digit

Three-digit codes (250) are category codes, four-digit codes (250.4) are subcategory codes, and five-digit codes (250.42) are subclassification codes.

Notes are also used to list the fifth-digit subclassifications for subcategories—such as the entries "Tuberculosis" or "Diabetes." Only the four-digit code is given for the individual entry, and you must refer to the note following the main term to locate the appropriate fifth-digit subclassification. For example, Fig. 14–4 shows the fifth digit's use when coding diabetes.

Eponyms

Eponyms (diseases, procedures, or syndromes named for persons) are listed both as main terms in their appropriate alphabetic sequence and under the main terms "Disease" or "Syndrome." A description of the disease or syndrome is usually included in parentheses following the eponym.

Example

Crigler-Najjar disease or syndrome
(congenital hyperbilirubinemia) 277.4

Disease
Crigler-Najjar (congenital hyperbilirubinemia) 277.4

Syndrome
Crigler-Najjar (congenital hyperbilirubinemia) 277.4

The cross-reference feature will be very helpful to you as you code using the ICD-9-CM.

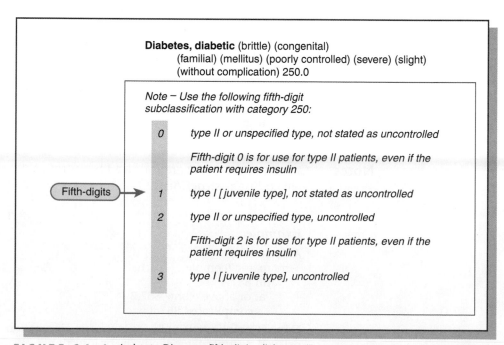

FIGURE 14–4 Index to Diseases, fifth digit, diabetes. (From International Classification of Diseases, 9th Revision, U.S. Department of Health and Human Services, Public Health Service, Centers for Medicare and Medicaid Services.)

EXERCISE 14–3   *More Conventions*

Match the convention to the definition:

1 *see* category _____

2 subterms _____

3 *see* _____

4 Notes _____

5 modifiers _____

6 *see also* _____

7 eponym _____

a. terms in parentheses or following main terms; they may or may not be essential

b. terms indented under main terms, considered essential modifiers

c. explicit direction to look elsewhere

d. follows code descriptions to define and give instructions

e. directs coder to look under another term if all information isn't found under the first term

f. directs coder to use Volume 1, Tabular List, for additional information

g. disease, procedure, or syndrome named for a person

Fill in the blank in the following question:

8 What directs you to look under another main term? _____

Etiology and Manifestation of Disease

For certain conditions it is important to record both the **etiology** (cause) and the **manifestation** (symptom) of the disease. In many cases, the recording of the etiology and manifestation can be accomplished by using a single four- or five-digit code. The single four- or five-digit code is termed a **combination code.** For example, Fig. 14–5 shows the etiology and manifestation combined in one code. The etiology is gonococcal, and the manifestation is cystitis; both are represented by the code 098.11.

For some conditions it is not possible to provide specific fifth-digit subclassifications that indicate both etiology and manifestation. Multiple coding is then required. In such cases the two facets of the disease—etiology and manifestation—are coded individually, as in Fig. 14–6.

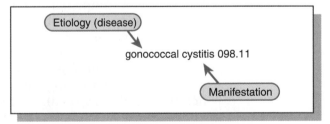

FIGURE 14–5 Manifestation and etiology, combination code. (From International Classification of Diseases, 9th Revision, U.S. Department of Health and Human Services, Public Health Service, Centers for Medicare and Medicaid Services.)

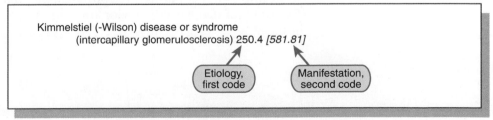

FIGURE 14–6 Manifestation and etiology, multiple coding. (From International Classification of Diseases, 9th Revision, U.S. Department of Health and Human Services, Public Health Service, Centers for Medicare and Medicaid Services.)

CAUTION *It is important to record the multiple codes on the insurance form in the same sequence as that used in the Alphabetic Index.*

Chapter 15 provides more information about the use of combination and multiple codes.

Hypertension Table

The Hypertension Table is found in the Alphabetic Index under the main term "Hypertension." The table contains a complete list of all conditions due to or associated with hypertension. The table classifies the hypertension conditions according to malignant, benign, or unspecified. Hypertension codes will be discussed in greater detail in the hypertension guidelines in Chapter 15.

Neoplasms

Neoplasms are tumors. Two steps are needed to locate the neoplasm code in the Alphabetic Index. The first step is to locate the neoplasm by its name or its morphology (form and structure). For example, glioma, lymphoma, and adenoma are considered histologic (minute structure, composition, and function) types and are found in the Alphabetic Index. This is where hospital coders will locate the M codes to classify the morphology of the tumor. You follow the instructions in the Index to reach the proper code in the Tabular List. If you wanted to locate the correct neoplasm code for adenocarcinoma, you would find the following entry in the Index.

Example

Adenocarcinoma (M8140/3)—*see also*
Neoplasm, by site, malignant

This *"see also"* instruction means you are to refer to the Neoplasm Table to locate the appropriate code.

The second step is to locate the Neoplasm Table in the Alphabetic Index under "N" for neoplasm. The Neoplasm Table is organized on the basis of anatomic site. A comprehensive list of anatomic sites with subterms for greater specificity is found in this table under the main term, "Neoplasm." The table contains six columns, as indicated in Fig. 14–7. For each site there are six possible code numbers; the proper code is determined by whether the neoplasm in question is malignant, and then by further specifying the malignancy as primary (originating site of neoplasm), secondary (site to which the neoplasm spread), or in situ (confined to the original site without invasion of neighboring tissue); benign (not malignant); of uncertain behavior (behavior cannot be determined at this time); or of unspecified nature (behavior is not stated). A malignant tumor is aggressive and invasive of other body tissue, and a benign tumor is one that is not.

Examples of neoplasms are epithelial, papillary, basal cell, and adenoma. Examples of neoplasm behavior are benign, malignant, and carcinoma in situ.

Neoplasm INDEX TO DISEASES

Neoplasm, neoplastic—*continued*	Primary	Secondary	Ca in situ	Benign	Uncertain Behavior	Unspecified
breast (connective tissue) (female) (glandular tissue) (soft parts)	174.9	198.81	233.0	217	238.3	239.3
areola	174.0	198.81	233.0	217	238.3	239.3
male	175.0	198.81	233.0	217	238.3	239.3
axillary tail	174.6	198.81	233.0	217	238.3	239.3
central portion	174.1	198.81	233.0	217	238.3	239.3
contiguous sites	174.8	—	—	—	—	—
ectopic sites	174.8	198.81	233.0	217	238.3	239.3
inner	174.8	198.81	233.0	217	238.3	239.3
lower	174.8	198.81	233.0	217	238.3	239.3
lower-inner quadrant	174.3	198.81	233.0	217	238.3	239.3
lower-outer quadrant	174.5	198.81	233.0	217	238.3	239.3
male	175.9	198.81	233.0	217	238.3	239.3
areola	175.0	198.81	233.0	217	238.3	239.3
ectopic tissue	175.9	198.81	233.0	217	238.3	239.3
nipple	175.0	198.81	233.0	217	238.3	239.3
mastectomy site (skin)	173.5	198.2	—	—	—	—
specified as breast tissue	174.8	198.81	—	—	—	—
midline	174.8	198.81	233.0	217	238.3	239.3
nipple	174.0	198.81	233.0	217	238.3	239.3

FIGURE 14–7 M Codes, Section 1, Index to Disease, breast. (From International Classification of Diseases, 9th Revision, U.S. Department of Health and Human Services, Public Health Service, Centers for Medicare and Medicaid Services.)

EXERCISE 14–4 *Neoplasms*

Referring to Fig. 14–7, fill in the codes for the following:

1 Primary malignant tumor of a male, breast, nipple

Code: _____

2 Benign neoplasm, breast, female, lower-outer quadrant

Code: _____

Morphology codes are used to supplement the appropriate ICD-9-CM neoplasm code. A complete listing of morphology codes is found in Appendix A of Volume 1, Morphology of Neoplasms, and is presented later in this chapter. M codes are optional; whether you assign these codes may depend on the particular facility's policy and are used in the inpatient setting.

Sections   Volume 2: Alphabetic Index serves as an index to Volume 1, Tabular List. Everything in the Index is listed by condition—meaning diagnosis, signs, symptoms, and conditions such as pregnancy, admission, encounter, or complication. Volume 2: Alphabetic Index contains three sections, as illustrated in Fig. 14–8.

Section 1 contains terms referring to diseases and injuries in alphabetic order.

Section 2 is the Table of Drugs and Chemicals and it includes codes for poisonings and external causes of injury by drugs or chemicals.

Section 3 is the Index to External Causes (E Codes); it is an alphabetic index of the causes of accidents and injuries.

Section 1: Index to Diseases and Injuries. Section 1 is the largest portion of the Alphabetic Index. To locate a code in the Tabular List, you must first locate the possible code in the Alphabetic Index. In the Index, main terms (conditions) are in bold type, and indented subterms (modifying words for additional specificity) are in regular type.

Main Terms and Subterms. Main terms in the Alphabetic Index are in bold type, and subterms are indented two spaces to the right.

Example

Fracture
styloid process
metacarpal (closed) 815.02
open 815.12

TABLE OF CONTENTS

Volume 2

FIGURE 14–8   Volume 2, Table of Contents. (From International Classification of Diseases, 9th Revision, U.S. Department of Health and Human Services, Public Health Service, Centers for Medicare and Medicaid Services.)

From the Trenches

"A medical coding career is a continuing process of education. Learning the basics of medical terminology, anatomy, utilization guidelines . . . and correct coding applications are all fundamental elements to a successful coding career."

PATRICIA

Each term is followed by the code or codes that apply to the term (Fig. 14–9). The Alphabetic Index includes most diagnostic terms currently in use. Some types of codes may be a little difficult to find, such as those dealing with complications, late effects, and V codes.

Section 2: Table of Drugs and Chemicals. Section 2, Table of Drugs and Chemicals, contains a classification of drugs and other chemical substances associated with poisoning and adverse effects. An **adverse effect** occurs when a substance, usually a prescribed medication, is taken correctly, but there is a **negative response** to the substance. For example, a physician prescribes penicillin for a patient with pneumonia. The patient takes the medication as prescribed, but develops a rash. The patient has taken the medication correctly but has had a negative response. A **poisoning** occurs when a substance, including medications, has been **incorrectly taken.** For example, a physician prescribes a sedative to an anxious patient. The patient takes ten times the dose prescribed and becomes comatose. The patient has taken the medication incorrectly and this is a poisoning.

In Fig. 14–10, the Table of Drugs and Chemicals shows that column 1 (Substance) contains the name of the drug or chemical. Column 2 (Poisoning) contains the list of poisoning codes. The remaining five columns are the E codes that are assigned to indicate how the poisoning or adverse effect occurred. *Remember, E codes are never reported as the principal diagnosis.* The table headings pertaining to external causes are defined as follows:

Accident (E850-E869): instances of accidental overdose of a drug, wrong substance given or taken, drug taken inadvertently, accidents in the use of drugs and biological agents during medical and surgical procedures, and external causes of poisonings classifiable to 980-989.

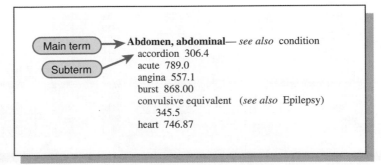

Main term → **Abdomen, abdominal**— *see also* condition
Subterm → accordion 306.4
 acute 789.0
 angina 557.1
 burst 868.00
 convulsive equivalent (*see also* Epilepsy)
  345.5
 heart 746.87

FIGURE 14–9 Volume, 2, Format. (From International Classification of Diseases, 9th Revision, U.S. Department of Health and Human Services, Public Health Service, Centers for Medicare and Medicaid Services.)

TABLE OF DRUGS AND CHEMICALS

Substance	Poisoning	Accident	Therapeutic Use	Suicide Attempt	Assault	Undetermined
			External Cause (E-Code)			
Acrolein (gas)	987.8	E869.8	—	E952.8	E962.2	E982.8
liquid	989.89	E866.8	—	E950.9	E962.1	E980.9
Actaea spicata	988.2	E865.4	—	E950.9	E962.1	E980.9
Acterol	961.5	E857	E931.5	E950.4	E962.0	E980.4
ACTH	962.4	E858.0	E932.4	E950.4	E962.0	E980.4
Acthar	962.4	E858.0	E932.4	E950.4	E962.0	E980.4
Actinomycin (C) (D)	960.7	E856	E930.7	E950.4	E962.0	E980.4
Adalin (acetyl)	967.3	E852.2	E937.3	E950.2	E962.0	E980.2
Adenosine (phosphate)	977.8	E858.8	E947.8	E950.4	E962.0	E980.4
Adhesives	989.89	E866.6	—	E950.9	E962.1	E980.9
ADH	962.5	E858.0	E932.5	E950.4	E962.0	E980.4
Adicillin	960.0	E856	E930.0	E950.4	E962.0	E980.4
Adiphenine	975.1	E855.6	E945.1	E950.4	E962.0	E980.4
Adjunct, pharmaceutical	977.4	E858.8	E947.4	E950.4	E962.0	E980.4
Adrenal (extract, cortex or medulla) (glucocorticoids) (hormones) (mineralocorticoids)	962.0	E858.0	E932.0	E950.4	E962.0	E980.4
ENT agent	976.6	E858.7	E946.6	E950.4	E962.0	E980.4
ophthalmic preparation	976.5	E858.7	E946.5	E950.4	E962.0	E980.4
topical NEC	976.0	E858.7	E946.0	E950.4	E962.0	E980.4
Adrenalin	971.2	E855.5	E941.2	E950.4	E962.0	E980.4
Adrenergic blocking agents	971.3	E855.6	E941.3	E950.4	E962.0	E980.4
Adrenergics	971.2	E855.5	E941.2	E950.4	E962.0	E980.4
Adrenochrome (derivatives)	972.8	E858.3	E942.8	E950.4	E962.0	E980.4
Adrenocorticotropic hormone	962.4	E858.0	E932.4	E950.4	E962.0	E980.4
Adrenocorticotropin	962.4	E858.0	E932.4	E950.4	E962.0	E980.4
Adriamycin	960.7	E856	E930.7	E950.4	E962.0	E980.4
Aerosol spray - *see* Sprays	—	—	—	—	—	—
Aerosporin	960.8	E856	E930.8	E950.4	E962.0	E980.4
ENT agent	976.6	E858.7	E946.6	E950.4	E962.0	E980.4
ophthalmic preparation	976.5	E858.7	E946.5	E950.4	E962.0	E980.4
topical NEC	976.0	E858.7	E946.0	E950.4	E962.0	E980.4
Aethusa cynapium	988.2	E865.4	—	E950.9	E962.1	E980.9
Afghanistan black	969.6	E854.1	E939.6	E950.3	E962.0	E980.3
Aflatoxin	989.7	E865.9	—	E950.9	E962.1	E980.9
African boxwood	988.2	E865.4	—	E950.9	E962.1	E980.9
Agar (-agar)	973.3	E858.4	E943.3	E950.4	E962.0	E980.4
Agricultural agent NEC	989.89	E863.9	—	E950.6	E962.1	E980.7
Agrypnal	967.0	E851	E937.0	E950.1	E962.0	E980.1
Air contaminant(s), source or type not specified	—	—	—	—	—	—
specified type - *see* specific substance	987.9	E869.9	—	E952.9	E962.2	E982.9
Akee	988.2	E865.4	—	E950.9	E962.1	E980.9
Akrinol	976.0	E858.7	E946.0	E950.4	E962.0	E980.4
Alantolactone	961.6	E857	E931.6	E950.4	E962.0	E980.4
Albamycin	960.8	E856	E930.8	E950.4	E962.0	E980.4
Albumin (normal human serum)	964.7	E858.2	E934.7	E950.4	E962.0	E980.4
Albuterol	975.7	E858.6	E945.7	E950.4	E962.0	E980.4
Alcohol	980.9	E860.9	—	E950.9	E962.1	E980.9
absolute	980.0	E860.1	—	E950.9	E962.1	E980.9
beverage	980.0	E860.0	E947.8	E950.9	E962.1	E980.9
amyl	980.3	E860.4	—	E950.9	E962.1	E980.9
antifreeze	980.1	E860.2	—	E950.9	E962.1	E980.9
butyl	980.3	E860.4	—	E950.9	E962.1	E980.9
dehydrated	980.0	E860.1	—	E950.9	E862.1	E980.9
beverage	980.0	E860.0	E947.8	E950.9	E962.1	E980.9
denatured	980.0	E860.1	—	E950.9	E962.1	E980.9
deterrents	977.3	E858.8	E947.3	E950.4	E962.0	E980.4
diagnostic (gastric function)	977.8	E858.8	E947.8	E950.4	E962.0	E980.4
ethyl	980.0	E860.1	—	E950.9	E962.1	E980.9
beverage	980.0	E860.0	E947.8	E950.9	E962.1	E980.9
grain	980.0	E860.1	—	E950.9	E962.1	E980.9
beverage	980.0	E860.0	E947.8	E950.9	E962.1	E980.9

Drug/chemical name

How adverse effect occurred

Poisoning code + How the poisoning occurred

FIGURE 14–10 Section 2, Table of Drugs and Chemicals. (From Buck CJ: *2009 ICD-9-CM, Volumes 1, 2, & 3, Professional Edition,* St. Louis, 2009, Saunders.)

> ### Example: Accident
>
> A 35-year-old male is brought to the emergency department with memory disturbance after an accidental exposure to lead paint.
>
> | | |
> |---|---|
> | Lead paint | 984.9 |
> | memory disturbance | 780.93 |
> | Accident, intention | E861.5 |

Therapeutic Use (E930-E949): instances in which a correct substance properly administered in a therapeutic (treatment) or prophylactic (preventive) dosage has been the external cause of adverse effects.

> ### Example: Therapeutic Use
>
> A 2-year-old male is taken by his mother to the pediatrician for a routine vaccination. That evening the child's temperature is 104°F, and he is taken by the mother to the emergency department.
>
> | | |
> |---|---|
> | Fever | 780.6 |
> | Unspecified vaccine | E949.9 |

Suicide Attempt (E950-E959): instances in which self-inflicted injuries or poisonings have been involved.

> ### Example: Suicide
>
> Rachael broke up with her boyfriend of 6 years. She became so despondent in the days that followed that she wrote a note indicating she was ending her life and took the entire bottle of her mother's prescription of Valium. She was found unconscious later by her mother.
>
> | | |
> |---|---|
> | Poisoning, Valium (diazepam) | 969.4 |
> | Unconscious | 780.09 |
> | Suicide, intention | E950.3 |

Assault (E961-E969): instances in which injury or poisoning has been inflicted by another person with the intent to injure or kill.

> ### Example: Assault
>
> A 42-year-old male presents to his physician with complaints of severe abdominal cramping and pain. After extensive laboratory tests, the physician identifies the source of the problem as high levels of arsenic in the patient's system. The patient's wife was later charged with the attempted murder of her husband.
>
> | | |
> |---|---|
> | Poisoning, arsenic | 985.1 |
> | Abdominal pain and cramps | 789.00 |
> | Assault, intention | E962.1 |

Undetermined (E980-E989): instances in which it cannot be determined whether the poisoning or injury was intentional or accidental.

Example: Undetermined

A transient is found comatose under a freeway overpass. Later at the emergency department the patient is found to have high levels of heroin in his system. It is unknown at this time if the overdose was intentional or accidental.

Poisoning, heroin	965.01
Coma	780.01
Undetermined, intention	E980.0

(*Coding Clinic,* 1996, 4th quarter, pgs 41 and 42)

A thorough review of the documentation would be done to identify any indication of drug addiction and code if documented in the medical record.

The table also contains the American Hospital Formulary Service (AHFS) List numbers, which can be used to classify new drugs not listed in the table by name. The AHFS List numbers are found in the Table of Drugs and Chemicals under the main term "Drug." For example, under "Drug" in the table, "24.04, cardiac drugs," is listed. The number 24.04 is an AHFS number. The AHFS List numbers and their ICD-9-CM equivalents are also found in Appendix C of Volume 1, Tabular List. The Formulary is a listing of drugs, dosage forms, package sizes, and drug strengths stocked by hospitals and pharmacies. Usage of the drugs is then tracked by means of these numbers. For example, the following were the top five drugs dispensed in Manitoba, Canada, in 1996*:

AHFS CLASSIFICATION	NO. OF CLAIMS
1. 24:04.00 Cardiac Drugs	690,884
2. 08:12.16 Penicillins	479,336
3. 28:08.04 Nonsteroidal Anti-Inflammatory Agents	363,463
4. 28:08.08 Opiate Agonists	338,537
5. 28:24.08 Benzodiazepines	331,469

The AHFS codes are not assigned by coders, but by pharmacy personnel.

Although certain substances are indexed in the Table of Drugs and Chemicals with one or more subentries, the majority are listed according to one use or state (i.e., solid, liquid, or gas). It is recognized that many substances may be used in various ways, in medicine and in industry, and may cause adverse effects or poisoning, whatever the state of the agent. In cases in which the reported data indicate a use or state not in the table, or one that is clearly different from those listed, an attempt should be made to classify the substances in the category that most nearly expresses the reported facts.

EXERCISE 14–5   *Table of Drugs and Chemicals*

Using the ICD-9-CM manual, code the following:

1 Poisoning by the ingestion of the beverage grain alcohol

    Code(s): _____

2 Undetermined poisoning by antifreeze

    Code(s): _____

---

*www.umanitoba.ca/centers/mchp/concept/dict/admin_data.htm.

3 Accidental overdose due to therapeutically prescribed valium

    🔗 Code(s): _____

Manifestations (symptoms or signs) of poisonings and adverse effects of drugs and chemicals are found in Section 1, under the specific symptom or disease. For example, Fig. 14–11 illustrates the location of the symptom Rash in Volume 2, the Alphabetic Index. If the symptom of the drug poisoning or adverse effect is a rash, the subterm "drug (internal use)" directs you to 693.0.

    Turn to code 693.0 in Volume 1, Tabular List.

4 What does the description of the code state?_____

Note the statement below the code: "Use additional E code to identify drug." In this case the condition is a rash. So when you see this statement, you know you have to identify the drug that caused the rash.

Section 3: Alphabetic Index to External Causes of Injuries and Poisonings (E Code). Section 3: Alphabetic Index to External Causes of Injuries and Poisonings is the **index** for the E codes. The index classifies environmental events (tornadoes, floods), circumstances, and other conditions as the cause of injury and other adverse effects alphabetically. **E codes are never used as a principal diagnosis.** Rather, E codes are used to clarify the cause of an injury or adverse effect.

    E code terms describe the external circumstances under which an accident, injury, or act of violence occurred. The main terms in this section usually represent the type of accident or violence (e.g., assault, collision), with the specific agent or other circumstance listed below the main term. "Collision" in Fig. 14–12 is the type of accident, and listed below Collision are the circumstances of the accident.

    You must be sure to read all the information under a term in the E code index, then locate the code in the E code section of Volume 1, Tabular. Be sure to check for fourth-digit specificity for railway accidents, motor vehicle traffic and nontraffic accidents, other road vehicle accidents, water transport accidents, and air and space transport accidents shown in the Index of the External Causes section. See an example of fifth digits above E810 in the ICD-9-CM.

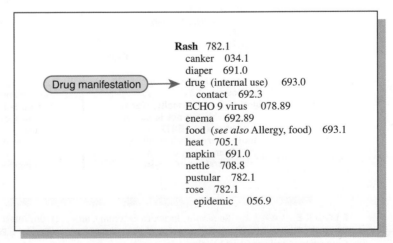

FIGURE 14–11 Index to Diseases, Rash. (From International Classification of Diseases, 9th Revision, U.S. Department of Health and Human Services, Public Health Service, Centers for Medicare and Medicaid Services.)

INDEX TO EXTERNAL CAUSES   **Collision**

Type ——▶ **Collision** (accidental) — *continued*

Circumstance

motor vehicle (on public highway) (traffic
   accident) — *continued*
  and — *continued*
    fallen — *continued*
      tree E815
    guard post or guard rail E815
    inter-highway divider E815
    landslide, fallen or not moving E815
      moving E909
    machinery (road) E815
    nonmotor road vehicle NEC E813
    object (any object, person, or vehicle
      off the public highway resulting
      from a noncollision motor vehicle
      nontraffic accident) E815
      off, normally not on, public
       highway resulting from a
       noncollision motor vehicle
       traffic accident E816
    pedal cycle E813
    pedestrian (conveyance) E814
    person (using pedestrian conveyance)
      E814
    post or pole (lamp) (light) (signal)
      (telephone) (utility) E815
    railway rolling stock, train, vehicle
      E810
    safety island E815
    street car E813
    traffic signal, sign, or marker
      (temporary) E815
    tree E815
    tricycle E813
    wall of cut made for road E815
  due to cataclysm — *see* categories E908,
    E909
  not on public highway, nontraffic
    accident E822
    and
      animal (carrying person, property)
      (herded) (unattended) E822
      animal-drawn vehicle E822
      another motor vehicle (moving),
       except off-road motor vehicle
       E822
       stationary E823
      avalanche, fallen, not moving
       E823
       moving E909
      landslide, fallen, not moving E823
       moving E909
      nonmotor vehicle (moving) E822
       stationary E823
      object (fallen) (normally) (fixed)
       (movable but not in motion)
       (stationary) E823
       moving, except when falling
        from, set in motion by,
        aircraft or cataclysm E822

Collision (accidental) — *continued*

motor vehicle (on public highway) (traffic
   accident) — *continued*
  not on public highway, nontraffic
    accident — *continued*
    and — *continued*
      pedal cycle (moving) E822
       stationary E823
      pedestrian (conveyance) E822
      person (using pedestrian
       conveyance) E822
      railway rolling stock, train, vehicle
       (moving) E822
       stationary E823
      road vehicle (any) (moving) E822
       stationary E823
      tricycle (moving) E822
       stationary E823
  off-road type motor vehicle (not on public
    highway) E821
    and
      animal (being ridden) (-drawn vehicle)
       E821
      another off-road motor vehicle, except
       snow vehicle E821
      other motor vehicle, not on public
       highway E821
      other object or vehicle NEC, fixed or
       movable, not set in motion by
       aircraft, motor vehicle on
       highway, or snow vehicle, motor-
       driven E821
      pedal cycle E821
      pedestrian (conveyance) E821
      railway train E821
  on public highway — *see* Collision,
    motor vehicle
pedal cycle E826
  and
    animal (carrying person, property)
      (herded) (unherded) E826
    animal-drawn vehicle E826
    another pedal cycle E826
    nonmotor road vehicle E826
    object (fallen) (fixed) (movable)
      (moving) not falling from or set
      in motion by aircraft, motor
      vehicle, or railway train NEC
      E826
    pedestrian (conveyance) E826
    person (using pedestrian conveyance)
      E826
    street car E826
pedestrian(s) (conveyance) E917.9
  with fall E886.9
    in sports E886.0
  and
    crowd, human stampede (with fall)
      E917.1
    machinery — *see* Accident, machine

FIGURE 14–12   Section 3, Index to External Causes. (From International Classification of Diseases, 9th Revision, U.S. Department of Health and Human Services, Public Health Service, Centers for Medicare and Medicaid Services.)

TABULAR LIST, VOLUME 1

The Tabular List is Volume 1 in the ICD-9-CM. After referencing the Index (Volume 2), you will locate the code(s) identified in the Tabular. You can never code directly from the Index. Rather, you must always reference the Index and then verify the code number in the Tabular. Let's begin by learning about the divisions in the Tabular.

Divisions

Volume 1: Tabular List is the listing of all the code numbers available for assignment, including their descriptions. When the exact word is not found in the code description in the Tabular List but the descriptive word is found in the Alphabetic Index, you must trust the code provided in the Alphabetic Index to be correct because the Index contains descriptive words that the Tabular List **does not**. Not listing all possible descriptive terms in the Tabular List saves space.

Anything that can happen, in the way of injury or disease, to a human body has a code number in Volume 1. Although there are certainly many things that can happen to us, the people who developed the ICD-9-CM not only included them all but organized them in a systematic way. Volume 1 is separated into two major divisions:

1. Classification of Diseases and Injuries
2. Supplementary Classification

Classification of Diseases and Injuries. The Classification of Diseases and Injuries is the main part of the ICD-9-CM, Volume 1, Tabular List; it consists of 17 chapters with codes ranging from 001 to 999. Fig. 14–13 illustrates that most chapters are based on body system (e.g., nervous system [Chapter 6], respiratory system [Chapter 8], or digestive system [Chapter 9]). Some chapters are based on the cause or type of disease (e.g., infectious and parasitic diseases [Chapter 1] or neoplasms [Chapter 2]). Fig. 14–14 indicates the format of each chapter.

Chapter
A chapter is the main division in the ICD-9-CM manual.

Section
A section is a group of three-digit categories that represent a group of conditions or related conditions.

Category
A three-digit category is a code that represents a single condition or disease. There are approximately 100 codes at the category level; most others require a fourth or fifth digit.

Subcategory
A four-digit subcategory code provides more information or specificity as compared to the three-digit code in terms of the cause, site, or manifestation of the condition. You must assign the fourth digit if it is available. Always code to the highest level of specificity based on the documentation in the medical record.

Subclassification
A five-digit subclassification code adds even more information and specificity to a condition's description. You must assign the fifth digit if it is available.

TABLE OF CONTENTS

FIGURE 14-13 Volume 1, Diseases: Table of Contents. (From International Classification of Diseases, 9th Revision, U.S. Department of Health and Human Services, Public Health Service, Centers for Medicare and Medicaid Services.)

Chapter → **10. DISEASES OF THE GENITOURINARY SYSTEM (580-629)**

NEPHRITIS, NEPHROTIC SYNDROME, AND NEPHROSIS ← **Section**
(580-589)

Excludes: hypertensive chronic kidney disease (403.00-403.91, 404.00-404.93)

580 Acute glomerulonephritis ← **Category, 3 digit**
Includes: acute nephritis

580.0 With lesion of proliferative glomerulonephritis
Acute (diffuse) proliferative glomerulonephritis
Acute poststreptococcal glomerulonephritis

580.4 With lesion of rapidly progressive glomerulonephritis
Acute nephritis with lesion of necrotizing
glomerulitis

580.8 With other specified pathological lesion in kidney ← **Subcategory, 4 digit**

580.81 *Acute glomerulonephritis in diseases* ← **Subclassification, 5 digit**
classified elsewhere

FIGURE 14–14 Volume 1, Diseases: format. (From International Classification of Diseases, 9th Revision, U.S. Department of Health and Human Services, Public Health Service, Centers for Medicare and Medicaid Services.)

EXERCISE 14–6 *ICD-9-CM Chapter Format*

Using ICD-9-CM, Volume 1, Tabular List, locate the first page of Chapter 3 and answer the following questions about the chapter:

1 The name of the chapter: _____

2 The name of the first section: _____

3 The description of the first category: _____

4 The description of the first subcategory: _____

The information in this activity was important to your learning because it will enable you to communicate effectively about information in the ICD-9-CM manual using common terminology.

Fig. 14–15 illustrates the indented format used in Volume 1, Tabular List, for ease of reference.

The basic ICD-9-CM code is a three-digit code, as shown in Fig. 14–16. Each code is a rubric (something under which something else is classed). Both the code number and the entry are in bold type. Diagnosis codes always contain at least three digits before the decimal point. If the diagnosis code is "1," it is written 001. Procedure codes from Volume 3 always consist of two digits, both placed before the decimal point. You can always tell a procedure code from a diagnosis code by noting the number of digits before the decimal point.

Example

496	Diagnosis code
27.54	Procedure code
461.9	Diagnosis code
21.1	Procedure code

Five-Digit Specificity. The addition of the fourth and fifth digits to the basic three-digit code provides greater specificity to the numeric designation of the patient's condition and reduces third-party payer (insurance company) returns of claims for further clarification of the diagnosis code(s). When four digits (one digit after the decimal point) are used, they are called *subcategory* codes. If five digits are used (two digits after the decimal point), they are called *subclassification* codes. Fig. 14–17 shows the first three digits of the code used to identify the disease "Osteomyelitis, periostitis, and other infections involving bone"; the fourth digit provides further specificity by distinguishing between acute and chronic osteomyelitis.

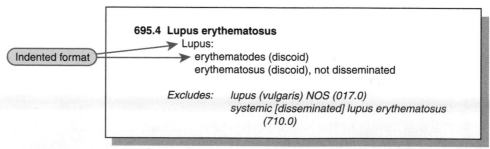

FIGURE 14–15   Indented format. (From International Classification of Diseases, 9th Revision, U.S. Department of Health and Human Services, Public Health Service, Centers for Medicare and Medicaid Services.)

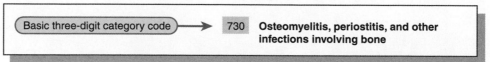

FIGURE 14–16   ICD-9-CM three-digit category code. (From International Classification of Diseases, 9th Revision, U.S. Department of Health and Human Services, Public Health Service, Centers for Medicare and Medicaid Services.)

Not all codes have fourth or fifth digits, but when a fourth or fifth digit is available, it must be used. It is a good idea to highlight the codes with which a fifth digit is listed. This will serve as a reminder to you to always use that fifth digit. As an example of the fifth digit: Code 730 appears with a list of fifth digits that are used to identify the location of acute osteomyelitis as

0 site unspecified

1 shoulder region

2 upper arm

3 forearm

4 hand

5 pelvic region and thigh

6 lower leg

7 ankle and foot

8 other specified sites

9 multiple sites

You indicate that acute osteomyelitis is located in the patient's shoulder by adding the fifth digit 1 to the 730.0 code (Fig. 14–18), 730.01.

CODING SHOT Remember that the goal is to be as accurate, as complete, and as specific as possible. The code(s) selected must be supported by physician documentation. ***If it isn't documented, it can't be coded.***

If a coder notes an abnormal x-ray result, the physician should be queried before additional codes are added. Fig. 14–19 illustrates how adding the fourth and fifth digits adds specificity to the information about the patient's condition.

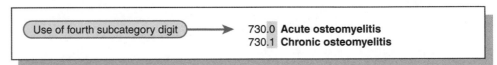

FIGURE 14–17 ICD-9-CM four-digit subcategory code.

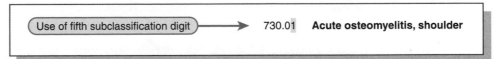

FIGURE 14–18 ICD-9-CM five-digit subclassification code.

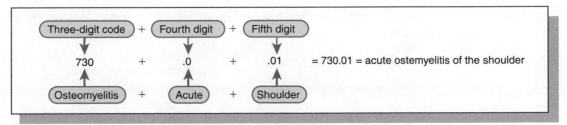

FIGURE 14–19 Specificity in ICD-9-CM codes.

The addition of a fourth or fifth digit to a three-digit code provides greater specificity to the diagnosis. Greater specificity decreases the number of third-party-payer returns for further clarification of the diagnosis code(s). Delayed claims result in delayed payment to the practice or hospital.

EXERCISE 14–7 *Five-Digit Specificity*

Locate the first page of Chapter 13, Diseases of the Musculoskeletal System and Connective Tissues, in the ICD-9-CM manual. Notes immediately following the chapter title indicate the fifth-digit subclassifications and the specific categories with which these fifth digits are used. Read the notes for Chapter 13.

The following is a part of the fifth-digit subclassifications used with categories 711-712, 715-716, 718-719, and 730:

0 site unspecified
1 shoulder region
   Acromioclavicular joint(s)
   Clavicle
   Glenohumeral joint(s)
   Sternoclavicular
   Scapula joint(s)
2 upper arm
   Elbow joint
   Humerus

The various joints of the shoulder region or the elbow joint and humerus of the upper arm are the specific anatomic terms to which the main term refers. The use of the 2 indicates the elbow joint, the humerus, and so forth. These anatomic terms serve to provide further specificity to the code selection.

Locate code 711 in the ICD-9-CM manual, then answer the following:

The patient record states: Pyogenic arthritis in lower leg.

1 What would the correct five-digit code be?

   Code: _____

2 Is the use of the fifth digit optional? _____

3 How is specificity added to ICD-9-CM codes?

   _____

   _____

QUICK CHECK 14-2

1. Locate code 719 in the Tabular. Read the notes there. The code for effusion of the knee would be 719.0_. You choose the fifth digit.

   a. 6
   b. 7
   c. 8
   d. 9

2. By reading the notes, how could you identify which of the fifth digits represents "knee"? _____

Supplementary Classification. The Supplementary Classification in Volume 1 contains the following:

1. Supplementary Classification of Factors Influencing Health Status and Contact with Health Services (V codes)

2. Supplementary Classification of External Causes of Injury and Poisoning (E codes)

V Codes: Supplementary Classification of Factors Influencing Health Status and Contact with Health Services. V codes from the Supplementary Classification of Factors Influencing Health Status and Contact with Health Services are found under such main term references as admission, examination, history, observation, and problem. V codes are used under the following circumstances:

- When a person who is not currently sick encounters health services for some specific purpose, such as to act as a donor or receive a vaccination

- When a person with a known disease or injury presents for specific treatment of that condition—such as dialysis, chemotherapy, or cast change

- When a circumstance may influence a patient's health status

- To indicate the birth status and outcome of delivery of a newborn

The Supplementary Classification is located near the back of Volume 1, Tabular List, and contains three- or four-digit code numbers preceded by the letter V. The codes in this section are called V codes, and are used in these two ways.

1. When a person who is currently not sick encounters the health services for some specific purpose, such as to act as donor of an organ or tissue, to receive a preventive vaccination, or to discuss a problem that is in itself not a disease or injury. Occurrences such as these will be fairly rare among hospital inpatients but common among outpatients at health clinics.

Example

Code V59.4 indicates a donor of a kidney; the donor is not sick but encounters health care:

V59   Donors

    V59.4   Kidney

V59 is the category and V59.4 is the subcategory. You would first locate Donor, kidney, in the Index (Volume 2), and then verify code V59.4 in the V codes in the Tabular List.

Example

A well child receives a polio vaccination:

V04   Need for prophylactic vaccination and inoculation against certain diseases

    V04.0   Poliomyelitis

Code V04.0 indicates a patient who is not ill but encounters health care for a polio vaccination. V04 is the category and V04.0 is the subcategory.

The Index (Volume 2) entry is Vaccination, poliomyelitis. If you want to indicate that a child had been in contact with poliomyelitis, assign code V01.2, which has an Index location of Contact, poliomyelitis.

Example

A student seeks health care to discuss a problem with school:

V62	**Other psychosocial circumstances**
	V62.3 **Educational circumstances**
	Dissatisfaction with school environment

V62 is the category code and V62.3 is the subcategory code.

Code V62.3 indicates a patient who is not ill but encounters health care for a psychosocial circumstance. Index location is Dissatisfaction with, education.

2. When some circumstance or problem is present that influences the person's health status but is not in itself a current illness or injury. For example, a family history of malignant neoplasms is significant to the patient's health care.

Example

V16	**Family history of malignant neoplasm**
	V16.0 **Gastrointestinal tract**

V16 is the category and V16.0 is the subcategory. The Index location is always the main term for starting your search of the Index. The main term here is History, family, malignant neoplasm, gastrointestinal tract. If, however, the diagnosis was a personal history of malignant neoplasm, the Index location would be History, malignant, neoplasm, gastrointestinal tract, and the code would be V10.00.

Example

V45	**Other postprocedural states**
	V45.01 **Cardiac pacemaker**

V45 is the category, V45.0 is the subcategory, and V45.01 is the subclassification code. The Index location would be Cardiac, device, pacemaker, in situ.

EXERCISE 14–8 *V Codes*

Locate the V codes in the ICD-9-CM manual in Volume 2, Alphabetic Index, and then in Volume 1, Tabular List. Code the following:

1 A person who has been in contact with smallpox

Index location: _____

Code: _____

2 Prophylactic vaccination against smallpox

Index location: _____

Code: _____

3 Personal history of malignant neoplasm of the tongue

Index location: _____

Code: _____

E Codes: Supplementary Classification of External Causes of Injury and Poisoning. The E codes are located in Supplementary Classification of External Causes of Injury and Poisoning (E800-E999), behind the V codes in the ICD-9-CM manual. The E codes are alphanumeric designations of external causes of injuries, poisonings, and adverse effects.

 CAUTION *Coding guidelines direct the coder to assign the appropriate E code for the initial encounter, not for subsequent treatment, with the exception of acute fracture coding.*

The E code section permits the classification of environmental events, circumstances, and conditions as the cause of injury, poisoning, and other adverse effects. With E codes, anything that can injure or have an adverse effect on a human body can be coded. The E codes can supply a code if a person is injured while pearl diving (E910.3), injured when a window of a railroad car falls on someone's head (E806.9), or hurt when pecked by a bird (E906.8). They are all in the E codes! These are rather far-fetched examples, granted, but they show how extensive and specific the codes are.

CODING SHOT Place of occurrence E codes are reported to provide further specificity as to where the accident/external cause occurred. If the place of occurrence is unknown, no code is assigned.

When a code from the E section is used, it is used **in addition** to a code from the Tabular List of the ICD-9-CM. The E code classification is used as an additional code for greater detail. Most groups of E codes have Includes or *Excludes* notes that provide further detail about using the codes in the group. For example, the E845, Accident involving spacecraft, the Includes note states that launching-pad accidents are included and the *Excludes* note states that the effects of weightlessness in a spacecraft are not included. Be sure to read these notes as you begin to code.

E codes have their own index. You can locate the E code index term in Volume 2, Section III, Index to External Causes of Injury, and then turn to the codes you're directed to in the E code Supplementary Classification of Volume 1.

The following information presents the E codes available in each group and an example of the type of code located in each range. The use of the fourth digit adds specificity as to who was injured in the accident. For example, if the injured person was the driver of a car involved in a motor vehicle accident, the fifth digit would be 0. If the injured person was a passenger in the vehicle, the fifth digit would be 1.

Some states have made the assignment of E codes mandatory, and the general use of E codes has increased significantly. At the beginning of Chapter 17, Injury and Poisoning (800-999), the note tells you to "Use E code(s) to identify the cause and intent of the injury or poisoning (E800-E999)." The Occupational Safety and Health Administration (OSHA) and Workers' Compensation are two entities that track the data from E codes to identify the causes of accidents. In states where E code assignment is not mandatory, each facility decides if it will or will not require assignment of E codes.

EXERCISE 14–9   *E Codes*

Using the ICD-9-CM manual, locate the correct E code for each of the following in Volume 2, Alphabetic Index, and then in Volume 1, Tabular List.

1 Railway (E800-E807)
Railway accident involving derailment without antecedent collision, injuring a porter

E code index term(s): _____

Code: _____

2 Motor Vehicle Traffic (E810-819)
Motor vehicle traffic accident due to tire blowout; driver of the car was injured

E code index term(s): _____

Code: _____

3 Motor Vehicle Nontraffic (E820-E825)
Nontraffic accident of two bicyclists; pedal cyclist injured

E code index term(s): _____

Code: _____

4 Other Road Vehicle (E826-E829)
Horse being ridden, rider injured, and non-motor vehicle collision

E code index term(s): _____

Code: _____

5 Water Transport (E830-E838)
Accident to watercraft causing other injury; occupant of small powered boat injured due to collision

E code index term(s): _____

Code: _____

You are ready to move on to the appendices. There is much interesting information waiting for you in the appendices.

THE APPENDICES IN THE TABULAR LIST, VOLUME 1

Volume 1, Tabular List, contains five appendices:

Appendix A	Morphology of Neoplasms
Appendix B	Glossary of Mental Disorders (Deleted in 2004)
Appendix C	Classification of Drugs by American Hospital Formulary Service List Number and Their ICD-9-CM Equivalents
Appendix D	Classification of Industrial Accidents According to Agency
Appendix E	List of Three-Digit Categories

(Note that in some commercially published ICD-9-CM texts, Appendix E or F is a listing of complications and comorbidities for the Medicare Severity Diagnosis Related Groups.)

Appendices are included as a reference for the coder so it is possible to

- provide further information about the patient's clinical picture
- further define a diagnostic statement
- aid in classifying new drugs
- reference three-digit categories

The appendices are titled Appendix A, B, C, D, and E to indicate their positions in the back of Volume 1 of the ICD-9-CM manual.

Appendix A: Morphology of Neoplasms

The World Health Organization has published an adaptation of the International Classification of Diseases for Oncology (ICD-O). The ICD-O contains codes for the **location** (topography) and morphology of tumors. **Morphology** is the study of neoplasms. The morphology codes consist of five digits: the first four identify the histologic type of the neoplasm and the fifth indicates the behavior of the neoplasm.

Examples of **types** of neoplasm are epithelial, papillary, basal cell, and adenoma. Refer to a medical dictionary if you are not familiar with the types of neoplasms presented in Appendix A of the ICD-9-CM.

Examples of the **behaviors** of neoplasms are the terms "benign," "malignant," and "carcinoma in situ." "In situ" means the neoplasm has not spread from another site and is located in its original place without invasion of neighboring tissue. ICD-O codes are used to gather data about the behavior, type, and location of tumors. For example, the coder would assign an ICD-9-CM code from Chapter 2, Neoplasms (140-239); the Certified Tumor Registrar (CTR) would receive a listing of code data for all neoplasm codes. The CTR would then assign an M code for the morphology (histological type) along with an ICD-O code to indicate the location of the tumor. For example, the coder indicates a breast tumor (basal cell) of the upper-outer quadrant as the diagnosis, using ICD-9-CM code 174.4. The CTR then researches the patient's medical record and applies an M code to indicate infiltrating ductal (M8500/3) and an ICD-O code to indicate the location of the tumor as C50.4 (upper-outer quadrant).

The one-digit morphology behavior code is as follows:

/0 Benign

/1 Uncertain whether benign or malignant
Borderline malignancy

/2 Carcinoma in situ
Intraepithelial (within the epithelial cells, those cells that cover the internal organs and vessels of the body)
Noninfiltrating (cancer that has not spread to other, adjacent areas)
Noninvasive (cancer that has not spread outside the original area)

/3 Malignant, primary site

/6 Malignant, metastatic site (secondary site, or site spread to)
Secondary site

/9 Malignant, uncertain whether primary or metastatic site (secondary site, or site spread to)

A primary site is the originating site of the tumor, and a secondary site is the metastatic site (a spread from the primary to the secondary site).

Appendix B: Glossary of Mental Disorders

The psychiatric terms that appear in ICD-9-CM, Chapter 5, Mental Disorders, used to be listed in alphabetic order in Appendix B. Appendix B was deleted in 2005. Most psychiatric disorders are classified using the Diagnostic and Statistical Manual of Mental Disorders (DSM-IV).

Appendix C: Drugs

This alphabetized subsection is entitled Classification of Drugs by American Hospital Formulary Services List Number and Their ICD-9-CM Equivalents. (Have you noticed how few short titles there are in the ICD-9-CM!) A division of the American Hospital Formulary Service (AHFS) regularly publishes a coded listing of drugs. These AHFS codes have as many as five digits. Each has a number, then a colon, and then up to four additional digits to provide specificity.

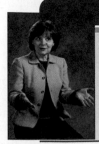

From the Trenches

"Certified coders are in high demand in many areas, not only as coders for physician offices, but for claims review by insurance companies, contract auditing, out-source billing, and educators."

PATRICIA

Example

AHFS		ICD-9-CM
8:12.04	Antifungal Antibiotics	960.1

Note that the ICD-9-CM code and the AHFS poisoning codes mean the same thing. For example, both AHFS 8:12.04 and ICD-9-CM 960.1 are poisoning by Antifungal Antibiotics.

Appendix D: Industrial Accidents

The subsection Classification of Industrial Accidents According to Agency contains three-digit codes to identify occupational hazards. The subsection is divided into the following categories:

1. Machines
2. Means of Transport and Lifting Equipment
3. Other Equipment
4. Materials, Substances, and Radiations
5. Working Environment
6. Other Agencies, Not Elsewhere Classified (NEC)
7. Agencies Not Classified for Lack of Sufficient Data

The identification of occupational hazards is especially important in coding injury or death that is job-related. Statisticians analyze the data and make statements about the risks involved in various occupations based on the data collected from the forms completed by health care workers. Occupational hazard codes **are not** placed on the insurance or billing forms. Instead, these specialized codes are used by state and federal organizations to summarize data concerning industrial accidents.

Appendix E: Three-Digit Categories

Appendix E is a list of all the three-digit categories in the ICD-9-CM, presented by chapter. The categories are labeled 1 through 17.

Example

1. **INFECTIOUS AND PARASITIC DISEASES**
   Intestinal infectious diseases (001-009)

001	Cholera
002	Typhoid and paratyphoid fevers
003	Other salmonella infections
004	Shigellosis
005	Other food poisoning (bacterial)
006	Amebiasis
007	Other protozoal intestinal diseases
008	Intestinal infections due to other organisms
009	Ill-defined intestinal infections

Reviewing Appendix E is a good way to get a quick overview of all of the codes in the ICD-9-CM manual.

EXERCISE 14–10 *The Five Appendices in Volume 1*

Fill in the following:

1 In which appendix of the ICD-9-CM manual would you find the following information?

a. Glossary of Mental Disorders _____

b. Classification of Industrial Accidents According to Agency _____

c. Morphology of Neoplasms _____

d. List of Three-Digit Categories _____

e. Classification of Drugs by American Hospital Formulary Service List

_____

2 In which appendix of the ICD-9-CM manual would you find the code to identify an injury resulting from a job-related accident involving a machine?

_____

PROCEDURES, VOLUME 3

Procedure codes are located in Volume 3 of the ICD-9-CM. These codes are used only in hospital settings. You can purchase the ICD-9-CM with or without Volume 3.

History

An important new development occurred with the publication of the ICD-9-CM manual—a Classification of Procedures in Medicine was added. Although some countries, notably the United States, had included classifications of surgical procedures in their adaptations of the ICD-9-CM since 1959, international agreement about classification of procedures was never reached. The classification of procedures has never been included in the ICD-9-CM manual itself but has always been a separate volume.

The WHO had recognized the growing need for a classification of procedures used in medicine and in 1971 sponsored an international working party that was convened by the American Hospital Association to coordinate the recommendations for a classification of procedures, with the primary emphasis on surgery. The International Conference for the 9th Revision of the International Classification of Diseases was convened at WHO Headquarters in Geneva in 1975. From that gathering, a proposal for a classification of procedures was submitted. The recommendations of the working party were to publish the provisional procedures classification as a supplement to the ICD-9. When the ICD-9 manual was published, a series of separate sections called fascicles (supplements) was also published. Each fascicle provides a classification of a different mode (type) of therapy (e.g., surgery, radiology, and laboratory procedures).

Subsequently, the ICD-9-CM was published in a three-volume set, including Volume 3, Procedures. Volume 3 was drawn primarily from WHO's Fascicle V, Surgical Procedures. At the same time, the codes in Volume 3 were expanded from three to four digits to allow for greater detail.

Volume 3 of the ICD-9-CM manual did not maintain compatibility with the ICD-9 as Volumes 1 and 2 had done. A different approach was taken in the development of Volume 3 that was deemed more appropriate to a classification system that would deal with surgical and therapeutic procedures.

Format Volume 3 contains two parts—the Tabular List and the Alphabetic Index. Approximately 90% of the codes in Volume 3 refer to surgical procedures (Fig. 14–20). The remaining 10% of the codes are diagnostic (to diagnose) and therapeutic (to treat) procedures, as shown in Fig. 14–21. For the most part, nonsurgical procedures are segregated from surgical procedures and confined to the codes 87 to 99.

Surgical procedure ──▶ **81.2 Arthrodesis of other joint**

Includes: arthrodesis with:
bone graft
external fixation device
excision of bone ends and compression

81.20 Arthrodesis of unspecified joint

81.21 Arthrodesis of hip

81.22 Arthrodesis of knee

81.23 Arthrodesis of shoulder ◀── Anatomic divisions

81.24 Arthrodesis of elbow

FIGURE 14–20 Volume 3, Surgical procedures. (From International Classification of Diseases, 9th Revision, U.S. Department of Health and Human Services, Public Health Service, Centers for Medicare and Medicaid Services.)

Therapeutic procedure ──▶ **88.4 Arteriography using contrast material**

Includes: angiography of arteries
arterial puncture for injection of
contrast material
radiography of arteries (by fluoroscopy)
retrograde arteriography

Note: The fourth-digit subclassification identifies the site to be viewed, not the site of injection.

Excludes: *arteriography using:*
radioisotopes or radionuclides (92.01-92.19)
ultrasound (88.71-88.79)
fluorescein angiography of eye (95.12)

88.40 Arteriography using contrast material, unspecified site

FIGURE 14–21 Volume 3, Therapeutic procedures. (From International Classification of Diseases, 9th Revision, U.S. Department of Health and Human Services, Public Health Service, Centers for Medicare and Medicaid Services.)

Volume 3 is **not** used in physicians' offices because procedures done by physicians are coded using the CPT codes. Hospitals use Volume 3 extensively to code services provided to inpatients and outpatients, including surgery, therapy, and diagnostic procedures. Hospitals use the ICD-9-CM codes to bill for facility fees (e.g., operating room, room and board, nurses, supplies). For example, a patient is admitted for a total abdominal hysterectomy. The physician would report his or her services and bill for the service of the total abdominal hysterectomy using the CPT code 58150. The hospital would report and bill for facility services for the hysterectomy procedure using the ICD-9-CM procedure code 68.49. The physician and the hospital would report the patient's diagnosis using an ICD-9-CM diagnosis code. If the patient in this example had a diagnosis of chronic endometriosis, both the physician and the hospital would indicate the patient's diagnosis and the reason for their services due to endometriosis of the uterus using the ICD-9-CM code of 617.0.

Example

Physician Codes
Diagnosis: ICD-9-CM, Vols. 1 and 2
Procedure: CPT

Inpatient Hospital Codes
Diagnosis: ICD-9-CM, Vols. 1 and 2
Procedure: ICD-9-CM, Vol. 3

Outpatient Hospital Codes
Diagnosis: ICD-9-CM, Vols. 1 and 2
Procedure: CPT

EXERCISE 14–11 *Table of Contents*

The Table of Contents, Volume 3 (Fig. 14–22) indicates the 16 chapters in Volume 3. Note that each chapter is based on a body system, except for Chapters 13 and 16.

1 What is Chapter 13? _____

2 What is Chapter 16? _____

3 What is Chapter 00? _____

Tabular List, Volume 3

Volume 3 has abbreviations, punctuation, symbols, and words similar to those used in Volumes 1 and 2. The following are the conventions, which are the same in all volumes:

1. Abbreviations of NEC and NOS
2. Punctuation symbols brackets, parentheses, colons, and braces
3. Bold type for all codes and titles
4. Italicized type for all exclusion notes
5. Instructional notations of Includes and Excludes

The term "Code also" has two purposes in Volume 3:

A. To allow the coding of each component of a procedure
B. To allow the coding of the use of special adjunctive (at the same time) procedures or equipment

These instructions are not mandatory, but they serve as a reminder to code these additional procedures if they were performed.

TABLE OF CONTENTS

FIGURE 14–22   Volume 3, Table of Contents. (From International Classification of Diseases, 9th Revision, U.S. Department of Health and Human Services, Public Health Service, Centers for Medicare and Medicaid Services.)

Using the following ICD-9-CM code as an example, let us take a closer look at the code to make sure you understand what the procedure is and how the term "Code also" is used.

Example

42.6   **Antesternal anastomosis of esophagus**
          Code also any synchronous:
             esophagectomy (42.40-42.42)
             gastrostomy (43.1)

The word "antesternal" will not be located in most medical dictionaries. It is at this time that your skill in medical terminology will help you out. The prefix "ante" means before, and "sternal" refers to sternum. Anastomosis is the joining together of two openings; in this case it is an opening into the esophagus. The location of the opening into the esophagus is above the sternum, which stated in medical terms is antesternal anastomosis of esophagus. **"Synchronous"** means occurring at the same time; "esophagectomy" is the removal of a part of the esophagus, and "gastrostomy" is the creation of an opening into the stomach. The statement from code 42.6 is translated into "Code also any [esophagectomy or gastrostomy] occurring at the same time." The medical coder needs excellent skills in medical terminology, anatomy, and persistence in the search for accurate definitions of the words used in the medical records. The study of terminology is a lifelong endeavor. There are always new words to be discovered. Just remember to always look up any word you are not certain of and take the time to understand the word in the context in which it is used. If you make a practice of doing this, you will soon find that you have a very dependable medical terminology vocabulary. Coders need excellent medical terminology skills.

An example of the second use of the instruction notation "Code also," which is a reminder to code the use of special adjunctive (accessory) procedures or equipment, follows. If the procedure or equipment is not used, no additional code is assigned.

Example

39.21	**Caval-pulmonary artery anastomosis**
	Code also cardiopulmonary bypass (39.61)

The "Code also" note below code 39.21 directs you to code 39.61, which is the code for extracorporeal (outside the body) circulation. Extracorporeal circulation is an auxiliary procedure performed during heart surgery.

EXERCISE 14–12   *Terminology*

State the definitions of the following terms:

1 cava(l) _____

2 pulmonary _____

3 anastomosis _____

4 cardiopulmonary _____

5 extracorporeal _____

6 What is a caval-pulmonary artery anastomosis?

_____

_____

7 What does a heart-lung machine do for a patient who is having a caval-pulmonary artery anastomosis?

_____

_____

**Alphabetic Index,
Volume 3**

The Index of Procedures is an important complement to the Tabular List of Procedures because the index contains many procedure terms that do not appear in the Tabular List of Procedures. The list of procedures included in the two-digit category code of the Tabular List of Procedures is not meant to be exhaustive; the terms serve as examples of the content of the category. The Index to Procedures, however, includes most procedure terms currently in use in North America. When the exact word is not found in the Tabular List of Procedures but is found in the Index to Procedures, you must trust that the code given in the Index to Procedures is correct.

Example

In the Index to Procedures, you will find the entry Gastrostomy, subterm Janeway, which is a type of gastrostomy. The entry directs you to code 43.19. When you then verify the code 43.19 in the Tabular List of Procedures, there is no mention of the term Janeway.

Never code directly from the Index to Procedures. After locating a code in the index, refer to that code in the Tabular List of Procedures for important instructions. Instructions in the form of notes suggesting the use of additional codes and exclusion notes that indicate the circumstances under which a procedure would be coded elsewhere are found only in the Tabular List of Procedures.

The Index to Procedures is arranged primarily by procedure (Fig. 14–23). Procedure codes are numbers only, with no alphabetic characters. The classification is based on a two-digit structure with two additional digits when necessary for greater specificity.

Fig. 14–24 indicates the two-digit category codes, the three-digit subcategory codes, and the four-digit subclassification codes contained in the Tabular List of Procedures. All category codes in Volume 3, Procedures, are **two-digit codes**, whereas all category codes in Volume 1, Tabular List, Disease, are **three-digit codes.**

The sequence of the Index to Procedures is letter-by-letter alphabetic order. Letter-by-letter alphabetizing ignores single spaces and hyphens and produces sequences.

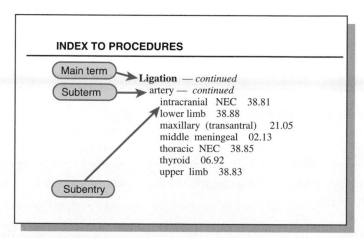

FIGURE 14–23 Index to procedures. (From International Classification of Diseases, 9th Revision, U.S. Department of Health and Human Services, Public Health Service, Centers for Medicare and Medicaid Services.)

TABULAR LIST

Category ⟶ **27   Other operations on mouth and face**

Includes: operations on:
lips
palate
soft tissue of face and mouth, except tongue
and gingiva

Excludes: *operations on:*
gingiva (24.0-24.99)
tongue (25.01-25.99)

Subcategory ⟶ **27.0   Drainage of face and floor of mouth**
Drainage of:
facial region (abscess)
fascial compartment of face
Ludwig's angina

Excludes: *drainage of thyroglossal tract (06.09)*

27.1   Incision of palate

27.2   Diagnostic procedures on oral cavity

Subclassification ⟶ **27.21   Biopsy of bony palate**

27.22   Biopsy of uvula and soft palate

27.23   Biopsy of lip

27.24   Biopsy of mouth, unspecified structure

27.29   Other diagnostic procedures on oral cavity
Excludes: *soft tissue x-ray (87.09)*

27.3   Excision of lesion or tissue of bony palate

27.31   Local excision or destruction of lesion or tissue of bony palate
Local excision or destruction of palate by:
cautery
chemotherapy
cryotherapy
Excludes: *biopsy of bony palate (27.21)*

FIGURE 14–24   Volume 3, format. (From International Classification of Diseases, 9th Revision, U.S. Department of Health and Human Services, Public Health Service, Centers for Medicare and Medicaid Services.)

Example

opening

open reduction

Upon first consideration, you would think that these two words were not in correct alphabetical order; "open" should come before "opening." The old filer's rule of "nothing comes before something" does not apply here. To alphabetize "opening" and "open reduction," you consider the beginning of the two words as "o-p-e-n"; the fifth letter in "opening" is "i" and the fifth letter in "open reduction" is "r." For alphabetizing purposes, the terms are considered as

opening

openreduction

Numbers, whether Arabic (1, 2, 3), Roman (I, II, III), or ordinal (first, second, third), are all placed in numeric sequence *before* alphabetic characters. Simply stated, numbers come before letters (Fig. 14–25).

The **prepositions** as, by, and with immediately follow the main term to which they refer. When multiple prepositional references are present, they are listed in alphabetic sequence.

The Index to Procedures is organized according to main terms, which are printed in bold type. Main terms usually identify the type of procedure performed, rather than the anatomic site involved.

A main term may be followed by a series of terms in parentheses. The presence or absence of these parenthetic terms in the procedure description has no effect on the selection of the code listed for the main term. These parenthetic terms are called **nonessential modifiers**. For example, all of the following words in parentheses are nonessential modifiers.

Example

Clipping
aneurysm (basilar) (carotid) (cerebellar) (cerebellopontine) (communicating artery) (vertebral) 39.51

Operation
Beck I (epicardial poudrage) 36.39
Beck II (aorto-coronary sinus shunt) 36.39
Beck-Jianu (permanent gastrostomy) 43.19

FIGURE 14–25 Numbers.

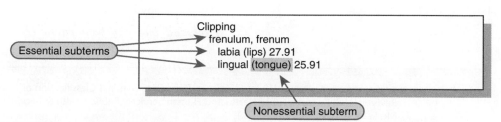

FIGURE 14–26 Essential and nonessential subterms. (From International Classification of Diseases, 9th Revision, U.S. Department of Health and Human Services, Public Health Service, Centers for Medicare and Medicaid Services.)

A main term may also be followed by a list of subterms (modifiers) that do have an effect on the selection of the appropriate code for a given procedure. These subterms form individual line entries and describe essential differences in site or surgical technique (Fig. 14–26).

Terms that identify incisions are listed as main terms in the Index to Procedures. If the incision was made only for the purpose of performing further surgery, the instruction "omit code" is given. The incision for the operative approach is bundled (included in) into the surgical code and would therefore not be coded separately. Closure of a surgical wound is not coded separately unless the closure takes place during a separate operative procedure.

Example

Arthrotomy 80.10
 as operative approach—*omit* code with
  arthrography—*see* Arthrogram
  arthroscopy—*see* Arthroscopy
  injection of drug 81.92
  removal of prosthesis (*see also* Removal, prosthesis, joint structures) 80.00
 ankle 80.17
 elbow 80.12

For some operative procedures it is necessary to record the individual components of the procedure. In these instances the Index to Procedures lists both codes.

Example

Code 57.87 describes the reconstruction of a urinary bladder, and 45.51 indicates the intestinal resection (cutting out of a portion of the intestine) necessary to create an ileal bladder.

Ileal bladder
 closed 57.87 [45.51]

 It is important to record these codes in the same sequence as that used in the Index to Procedures.

The cross references section provides you with possible modifiers for a term or its synonyms. There are three types of cross references:

1. The term *"see"* is an explicit direction to look elsewhere. It is used with terms that do not define the type of procedure performed.

Example

Bacterial smear—*see* Examination, microscopic

---

2. The term *"see also"* directs you to look under another main term because all of the information being searched for cannot be located under the first main term entry.

> ### Example
>
> Immunization—*see also* Vaccination

3. The term *"see category"* directs you to the Tabular List of Procedures for further information or specific site references.

> ### Example
>
> Osteolysis—*see* category 78.4

Notes are used in the Index to Procedures to list fourth-digit subclassifications for those categories that use the same fourth digit. In these cases, only the three-digit code is given for the individual entry; you must refer to the note following the main term to obtain the appropriate fourth digit. For an example of a note, see Fig. 14–27.

The fourth-digit subclassification codes also appear in the Tabular List of Procedures with the category codes 90 and 91.

90   Microscopic examination - I

The following fourth-digit subclassification is for use with categories in section 90 to identify type of examination:

1   bacterial smear
2   culture
3   culture and sensitivity
4   parasitology
5   toxicology
6   cell block and Papanicolaou smear
9   other microscopic examination

Fourth digit also appears in the tabular list under the categories

FIGURE 14–27   Volume 3, Notes, Alphabetic Index. (From International Classification of Diseases, 9th Revision, U.S. Department of Health and Human Services, Public Health Service, Centers for Medicare and Medicaid Services.)

Example

Operations named for persons (eponyms) are listed both as main terms in their appropriate alphabetic sequence and under the main term "Operation." A description of the procedure or anatomic site affected usually follows the eponym.

Under O:

Operation

Thompson
cleft lip repair 27.54
correction of lymphedema 40.9
quadricepsplasty 83.86
thumb opposition with bone graft 82.69

Under T:

Thompson operation
cleft lip repair 27.54
correction of lymphedema 40.9
quadricepsplasty 83.86
thumb opposition with bone graft 82.69

EXERCISE 14–13 *Procedures: Volume 3*

Code the following using Volume 3 of the ICD-9-CM manual:

1 Flexible sigmoidoscopy

Code: _____

2 Vasectomy

Code: _____

3 Closed reduction of maxillary fracture

Code: _____

4 Transfusion of 2 units packed cells

Code: _____

5 Control of epistaxis by cauterization

Code: _____

CONGRATULATIONS! You have now completed the study of the arrangement of the information in the ICD-9-CM manual. The knowledge you have gained will be used as the foundation that will be built upon in Chapter 15. In Chapter 15 you will begin further work with the correct assignment and sequencing of ICD-9-CM codes.

CHAPTER REVIEW

CHAPTER 14, PART I, THEORY

Match the appendix to the information contained in the appendix:

1 Appendix A _____
2 Appendix B _____
3 Appendix C _____
4 Appendix D _____
5 Appendix E _____

a. Industrial Accidents
b. Classification of Drugs
c. Morphology of Neoplasms
d. Three-Digit Categories
e. Was deleted in 2004

Circle the correct answer in each of the following:

6 The ICD-9-CM is designed to classify what two things?

  a. sickness and disease

  b. symptoms and illness

  c. causes of morbidity and mortality

  d. diagnosis and disease

7 Which of the following is not a stated use for the ICD-9-CM?

  a. facilitate payment of health services

  b. study health care costs

  c. plan for future health care needs

  d. evaluate appropriateness of treatment

Match the ICD-9-CM volume number to the correct name of the volume:

8 Volume 1 _____
9 Volume 2 _____
10 Volume 3 _____

a. Tabular List of Procedures and Alphabetic Index to Procedures
b. Diseases: Alphabetic Index
c. Diseases: Tabular List

Identify the format of the chapters in the ICD-9-CM Volume 1, Tabular List, in the proper sequence, from first to last:

11 _____
12 _____
13 _____
14 _____
15 _____

a. subcategory
b. chapter
c. subclassification
d. section
e. category

Are the following statements about V codes true or false?

16 V codes refer primarily to persons who are not ill but use health care. _____

17 V codes do not use fourth digits.

_____

18 V codes can indicate the place of birth as having been elsewhere, before admission, or after admission. _____

Circle the correct answer in the following:

19 The purpose of E codes is to describe

  a. external circumstances

  b. accidents

  c. acts of violence

  d. all of the above

20 Morphology is the science of

  a. human anatomy

  b. physiologic function

  c. neoplasms

  d. tissue

CHAPTER 14, PART II, PRACTICAL

Using an ICD-9-CM manual, answer the following questions:

21 What does the Excludes note state under category code 175? _____

_____

22 What does the Includes note state under category 444? _____

_____

23 Under category 805, which codes use the subclassification 0-8? _____

_____

24 Would code 362.72 be sequenced as the principal diagnosis? _____

_____

QUICK CHECK ANSWERS

QUICK CHECK 14-1
guidelines, introduction, or footnotes

QUICK CHECK 14-2
1. a. 6
2. Notes instruct to "See listing at the beginning of the chapter for definitions"

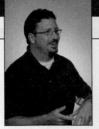

"Take some baby steps and figure out where you want to be—then as time progresses, you'll fall into your niche."

John R. Neumann III, RN, CPC
Account Executive
Durham, North Carolina

Using the ICD-9-CM

Learning Objectives

After completing this chapter you should be able to

1 Trace the development of the Official Guidelines for Coding and Reporting.
2 Apply the Official Guidelines for Coding and Reporting.
3 Define the steps to diagnosis coding.
4 Examine current Official Guidelines for Coding and Reporting.
5 Review infectious and parasitic diseases coding.
6 Analyze the neoplasms coding.
7 Examine the endocrine, nutritional, metabolic diseases, and immunity disorders coding.
8 Review the blood conditions, mental disorders, nervous system, and sense organs coding.
9 Review the circulatory system coding.
10 Review the respiratory system coding.
11 Examine the digestive system coding.
12 Analyze the genitourinary system coding.
13 Review the pregnancy, childbirth, and puerperium coding.
14 Review the skin and subcutaneous tissue coding.
15 Examine the congenital anomalies and certain conditions originating in the perinatal period coding.
16 Define the rules of symptoms, signs, and ill-defined conditions coding.
17 Review the outpatient coding guidelines.
18 Explain the format of the ICD-10-CM.

This Chapter is based on the Official Guidelines for Coding and Reporting. If clarifications have been made to the Guidelines by the author, they are in parentheses and in italic typeface to identify the material as being separate from, and not part of, the Official Guidelines for Coding and Reporting.

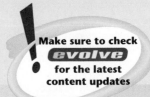

Make sure to check **evolve** for the latest content updates

SOME GENERAL INFORMATION ABOUT THE OFFICIAL GUIDELINES FOR CODING AND REPORTING

As was discussed in Chapter 14, Official Guidelines for Coding and Reporting have been developed and approved for coding and reporting by the Cooperating Parties for ICD-9-CM: the American Hospital Association (AHA), American Health Information Management Association (AHIMA), Centers for Medicare and Medicaid Services (CMS), and National Center for Health Statistics (NCHS).

Inpatient and Outpatient Coding

The complete Official Guidelines for Coding and Reporting appears in Appendix A of the text. The Guidelines are organized into sections. Section I includes the structure and conventions of the classification and general guidelines that apply to the entire classification, and chapter-specific guidelines that correspond to the chapters as they are arranged in the classification. Section II includes guidelines for selection of principal diagnosis for non-outpatient settings. Section III includes guidelines for reporting additional diagnoses in non-outpatient settings. Section IV is for outpatient coding and reporting. Appendix I includes Present on Admission Reporting Guidelines. Increasingly, coders are called upon to code a wider range of services in a variety of settings. In this text, Guidelines that apply to only one setting are identified as being "Inpatient" or "Outpatient."

QUICK CHECK 15-1

Examine your ICD-9-CM to determine if the Official Guidelines for Coding and Reporting are included in your publication. If so, where are they located?

_____

General Guidelines

The number that appears to the left of the guideline in this text is the number of the guideline as listed in the Official Guidelines for Coding and Reporting. For the purposes of this text, the Guidelines will sometimes appear out of order. Appendix A of this text presents the guidelines in their entirety, in numeric order.

In the examples in this text, main terms and subterms are often noted for you after the term enclosed in parentheses to help you locate the terms in the Alphabetic Index. For example, Hodgkin's (main term) disease (subterm) directs you to the location of Hodgkin's disease in the Alphabetic Index. Remember, the extensive indexing system in the ICD-9-CM allows you many options for locating codes in the Alphabetic Index. The examples and subsequent identification of main terms and subterms represent only one way a term can be located.

You will be practicing coding using the ICD-9-CM throughout this chapter. You need to practice using the steps that are always necessary to assign an ICD-9-CM code. If you begin your ICD-9-CM coding using these steps, you will develop good coding habits that will last throughout your career.

Steps to Accurate Coding

1. Identify the main term(s) in the diagnostic statement.

2. Locate the main term(s) in the Alphabetic Index (Volume 2) (referred to in this text as the Index).

3. Review any subterms under the main term in the Index.

4. Follow any cross-reference instructions, such as *see also*.

5. Verify the code(s) selected from the Index (Volume 2) in the Tabular List (Volume 1) (referred to in this text as the Tabular).

6. Refer to any instructional notations in the Tabular.

7. Assign codes to the highest level of specificity. For example, if a fourth digit is available, you cannot assign only a three-digit code, and if a fifth digit is available, you cannot assign only a four-digit code.

8. Code the diagnosis until all elements are completely identified.

Guidelines are presented and followed by examples or exercises to illustrate the rule(s).

OFFICIAL GUIDELINES FOR CODING AND REPORTING

SECTION I. B. General Coding Guidelines

1. Use of Both The Alphabetic Index and Tabular List
Use both the Alphabetic Index and the Tabular List when locating and assigning a code. Reliance on only the Alphabetic Index or the Tabular List leads to errors in code assignments and less specificity in code selection.

2. Locate each term in the Alphabetic Index
Locate each term in the Alphabetic Index and verify the code selected in the Tabular List. Read and be guided by instructional notations that appear in both the Alphabetic Index and the Tabular List.

inpatient/outpatient

Examples

Use of Both the Alphabetic Index and the Tabular List

Diagnosis: Hodgkin's Disease

Index: **Hodgkin's** (main term)

              disease (subterm) 201.9

Tabular: **201 Hodgkin's disease** [category code]

                           201.9 Hodgkin's disease, unspecified [subcategory code]

Code: 201.9X Hodgkin's Disease [subclassification code]

Verify 201.9 in the Tabular and note that the code requires a fifth-digit assignment of 0 to 8 to indicate the disease location. You would have missed the required fifth-digit subclassification indicated by the X in the example if you had used only the Index and not verified the code in the Tabular. You must also always go back to the beginning of the section and read any notes located there. In the case of 201, the section notes (above code 200) indicate the fifth digits to be used with codes 200-202.

Diagnosis:	Stroke, due to vertebral artery occlusion
Index:	**Stroke** (main term) 434.91
Tabular:	**434.9 Cerebral artery occulsion, unspecified**

As the occlusion is specified as due to vertebral artery occlusion, 434.9X, cerebral artery occlusion, unspecified, does not accurately describe the condition. Return to the Index and locate the term "occlusion" to see what other codes might more accurately describe this condition.

Index:	**Occlusion**
	artery (subterm), vertebral (subterm) 433.2
Tabular:	**433 Occlusion and stenosis of precerebral arteries**
	0 without mention of cerebral infarction
	1 with cerebral infarction
	433.2 Vertebral artery
Code:	433.21 Stroke, due to vertebral artery occlusion

The diagnosis statement "fits" or is classifiable to 433.21 and since the 436 category note indicates "Excludes any condition classifiable to categories 430-435," which 433.21 is, you cannot assign 436. You would have incorrectly coded the diagnosis to 436 if you had not verified the code in the Tabular. There are no shortcuts in this process: Always check the Tabular. The fifth digit is "1, with cerebral infarction" because a stroke is an infarction.

OFFICIAL GUIDELINES FOR CODING AND REPORTING

SECTION I. B. 3. Level of Detail in Coding

Diagnosis and procedure codes are to be used at their highest number of digits available.

ICD-9-CM diagnosis codes are composed of codes with 3, 4, or 5 digits. Codes with three digits are included in ICD-9-CM as the heading of a category of codes that may be further subdivided by the use of fourth and/or fifth digits, which provide greater detail.

A three-digit code is to be used only if it is not further subdivided. Where fourth-digit subcategories and/or fifth-digit subclassifications are provided, they must be assigned. A code is invalid if it has not been coded to the full number of digits required for that code. For example, Acute myocardial infarction, code 410, has fourth digits that describe the location of the infarction (e.g., 410.2, Of inferolateral wall), and fifth digits that identify the episode of care. It would be incorrect to report a code in category 410 without a fourth and fifth digit.

ICD-9-CM Volume 3 procedure codes are composed of codes with either 3 or 4 digits. Codes with two digits are included in ICD-9-CM as the heading of a category of codes that may be further subdivided by the use of third and/or fourth digits, which provide greater detail.

inpatient/outpatient

Examples

Level of Specificity

Three-Digit Category

Diagnosis: Subarachnoid hemorrhage

Index: **Hemorrhage**, subarachnoid, nontraumatic 430

Tabular: **430 Subarachnoid hemorrhage** [category code]

Code: 430 Subarachnoid hemorrhage

Diagnosis: AIDS

Index: **AIDS 042**

Tabular: **042 Human immunodeficiency virus (HIV) disease** [category code]

Code: 042 AIDS

Both of the preceding diagnostic statements are correctly assigned to three-digit category codes because there are no four-digit subcategory codes available within either code.

Four-Digit Subcategory

Diagnosis: Crohn's disease of large intestine

Index: **Crohn's disease** (see also Enteritis, regional) 555.9

Tabular: **555 Regional enteritis (Includes: Crohn's disease)** [category code]

555.1 Large intestine [subcategory code]

Code: 555.1 Crohn's disease of large intestine

Diagnosis: Cellulitis of the upper right leg

Index: **Cellulitis**, leg

Tabular: **682 Other cellulitis and abscess** [category code]

682.6 Leg, except foot [subcategory code]

Code: 682.6 Cellulitis of the upper right leg

Both of the preceding diagnostic statements are correctly assigned to four-digit subcategory codes because no five-digit subclassification codes are available.

Five-Digit Subclassification

Diagnosis: RUQ abdominal pain

Index: **Pain**, abdominal

Tabular: **789.0 Abdominal pain** [subcategory code]

789.01 Right upper quadrant [subclassification code]

Code: 789.01 RUQ abdominal pain

Diagnosis: Bilateral, congenital bowing of femur

Index: **Bowing**

femur 736.89

congenital 754.42

Tabular: **754 Certain congenital musculoskeletal deformities** [category code]

754.4 Congenital genu recurvatum and bowing of long bones of leg [subcategory code]

754.42 Congenital bowing of femur [subclassification code]

Code: 754.42 Bilateral, congenital bowing of femur

Both of the preceding diagnostic statements are correctly assigned to five-digit subclassification codes, having been carried out to the highest level of specificity available.

EXERCISE 15–1 *Level of Specificity in Coding*

Identify and fill in the category, subcategory, and subclassifications of the following:

1 Diagnosis: Recurrent right inguinal hernia, with obstruction

  Index: **Hernia**

  inguinal 550.9

  Tabular: **550 Inguinal hernia** _____

  550.1 Inguinal hernia, with obstruction, without mention of gangrene

  _____

  550.11 Inguinal hernia, with obstruction, without mention of gangrene, unilateral, recurrent _____

2 Diagnosis: Transient hypertension, 30 weeks' gestation, undelivered

  Index: **Hypertension**

  transient

  of pregnancy (soubrette) 642.3

  Tabular: **642 Hypertension complicating pregnancy, childbirth, and the puerperium**

  _____

  642.3 Transient hypertension of pregnancy _____

  642.33 Antepartum condition or complication _____

NEC and NOS

OFFICIAL GUIDELINES FOR CODING AND REPORTING

SECTION I. A. 2. Abbreviations

a. Index abbreviations

  NEC "Not elsewhere classifiable"
  This abbreviation in the index represents "other specified" when a specific code is not available for a condition the index directs the coder to the "other specified" code in the tabular.

b. Tabular abbreviations

  NEC "Not elsewhere classifiable"
  This abbreviation in the tabular represents "other specified." When a specific code is not available for a condition the tabular includes an NEC entry under a code to identify the code as the "other specified" code. *(See Section I.A.5.a."Other" codes).*

  NOS "Not otherwise specified"
  This abbreviation is the equivalent of unspecified. *(See Section I.A.5.b., "Unspecified" codes)*

inpatient/outpatient

Example

NEC

Diagnosis:	Pneumonia due to gram-negative bacteria
Index:	**Pneumonia**
	gram-negative bacteria NEC 482.83
Tabular:	**482.8 Pneumonia due to other specified bacteria**
	482.83 Other gram-negative bacteria
Code:	482.83 Pneumonia due to gram-negative bacteria

Code 482.83 identifies gram-negative bacterial pneumonia that cannot be classified more specifically into the other subclassifications. The other subclassifications within 482.8 are for anaerobes, *Escherichia coli [E. coli]*, "other than gram-negative" bacteria, Legionnaire's disease, and other specified bacteria. None of these other subclassifications can be assigned to the diagnostic statement; therefore, 482.83 is the most appropriate choice.

NEC can be used in two ways:

1. NEC directs the coder to look under other classifications if appropriate. Other subterms or *Excludes* notes may provide hints as to what the other classifications may be.

2. NEC is used when the ICD-9-CM does not have any codes that provide greater specificity.

Example

NOS

Diagnosis:	Bronchitis
Index:	**Bronchitis** 490
Tabular:	**490 Bronchitis, not specified as acute or chronic Bronchitis NOS**
Code:	490 Bronchitis

The diagnosis was not specified by the physician as acute or chronic; therefore, the "not otherwise specified" code 490 must be assigned. In this situation, it would be appropriate for the coder to request specificity from the practitioner.

CODING SHOT Third-party payers prefer specific codes and do not appreciate a coder's dependence on NOS codes. If the NOS code is the only correct code, you must use it, but only after thorough review of all available documentation.

Acute and Chronic

OFFICIAL GUIDELINES FOR CODING AND REPORTING

SECTION I. B. 10. Acute and Chronic Conditions

If the same condition is described as both acute (subacute) and chronic, and separate subentries exist in the Alphabetic Index at the same indentation level, code both and sequence the acute (subacute) code first.

See Fig. 15–1 for the format of acute pancreatitis and chronic pancreatitis. Both acute and chronic forms of pancreatitis are subcategorized under code 577. Acute pancreatitis is 577.0 and chronic pancreatitis is 577.1. If the same condition is described as acute and chronic pancreatitis, two codes are required and the acute code is listed first.

Examples

Acute and Chronic Conditions

Diagnosis: Acute and chronic thyroiditis

Index: **Thyroiditis**

        acute 245.0

        chronic 245.8

(Note: acute and chronic are at the same indention level.)

Tabular: **245 Thyroiditis**

        245.0 Acute thyroiditis

        245.8 Other and unspecified chronic thyroiditis

Sequence: 245.0, 245.8 Acute and chronic thyroiditis

Note that the acute form of thyroiditis is sequenced before the chronic form, as directed by Section I. B. 10.

Diagnosis: Acute and chronic pericarditis

Index: **Pericarditis**

        acute 420.90

        chronic 423.8

Tabular: **420 Acute pericarditis**

        420.9 Other and unspecified acute pericarditis

           420.90 Acute pericarditis, unspecified

Tabular: **423 Other diseases of pericardium**

        423.8 Other specified diseases of the pericardium

Sequence: 420.90, 423.8 Acute and chronic pericarditis

577.0 Acute pancreatitis

Abscess of pancreas	Pancreatitis:
Necrosis of pancreas:	NOS
acute	acute (recurrent)
infective	apoplectic
	hemorrhagic
	subacute
	suppurative

Excludes: mumps pancreatitis (072.3)

577.1 Chronic pancreatitis

Chronic pancreatitis:	Pancreatitis:
NOS	painless
infectious	recurrent
interstitial	relapsing

FIGURE 15–1   Indent level of acute and chronic. (From International Classification of Diseases, 9th Revision. U.S. Department of Health and Human Services, Public Health Service, Centers for Medicare and Medicaid Services.)

✋ **CAUTION** *Note that while the Index directs you to code 423.8 for chronic pericarditis, when the Tabular is verified, there is no mention of chronic pericarditis. This is an example of a common coding situation in which you must trust the Index to have more descriptive terms than the Tabular. When the condition is both acute and chronic, and both acute and chronic are listed in the Index as separate entries and at the same indentation level, the code for acute is sequenced first.*

Combination Codes

OFFICIAL GUIDELINES FOR CODING AND REPORTING

SECTION I. B. 11. Combination Code

A combination code is a single code used to classify:

> Two diagnoses, or
>
> A diagnosis with an associated secondary process (manifestation)
>
> A diagnosis with an associated complication

Combination codes are identified by referring to subterm entries in the Alphabetic Index and by reading the inclusion and exclusion notes in the Tabular List.

Assign only the combination code when that code fully identifies the diagnostic conditions involved or when the Alphabetic Index so directs. Multiple coding should not be used when the classification provides a combination code that clearly identifies all of the elements documented in the diagnosis. When the combination code lacks necessary specificity in describing the manifestation or complication, an additional code should be used as a secondary code.

(inpatient/outpatient)

Examples

Combination Codes

Diagnosis:	Acute cholecystitis with cholelithiasis
Index:	**Cholecystitis** with calculus (stones in the gallbladder) directs you to *See* Cholelithiasis
Index:	**Cholelithiasis** with, cholecystitis, acute 574.0
Tabular:	**574 Cholelithiasis**
	574.0 Calculus of gallbladder with acute cholecystis

A fifth-digit subclassification is indicated as 0 for a case without mention of obstruction and as 1 when there is obstruction; since there was no mention of obstruction, use the fifth digit 0.

Code:	574.00 Acute cholecystitis with cholelithiasis

The single code 574.00 fully describes the diagnosis of acute cholecystitis with cholelithiasis.

Another example of a diagnosis (streptococcal) and manifestation (pharyngitis or sore throat) assigned to a combination code is as follows:

Diagnosis:	Streptococcal pharyngitis
Index:	**Pharyngitis**, streptococcal 034.0

Tabular: **034 Streptococcal sore throat and scarlet fever**

          034.0 Streptococcal sore throat

Septic:	Streptococcal:
angina	angina
sore throat	laryngitis
	pharyngitis
	tonsillitis

The single code 034.0 fully describes the diagnosis of streptococcal pharyngitis.

Code(s):   034.0 Streptococcal pharyngitis

EXERCISE 15–2 *Combination Codes*

Fill in the codes for the following using combination coding:

1 Pneumonia due to *Hemophilus influenzae*

    Code(s): _____

2 Candidiasis of the mouth (thrush)

    Code(s): _____

3 Enteritis due to *Clostridium difficile*

    Code(s): _____

4 Hypertensive cerebrovascular disease

    Code(s): _____

5 Closed fracture of the tibia and fibula

    Code(s): _____

Multiple Coding

OFFICIAL GUIDELINES FOR CODING AND REPORTING

SECTION I. B. 9. Multiple coding for a single condition

In addition to the etiology/manifestation convention that requires two codes to fully describe a single condition that affects multiple body systems, there are other single conditions that also require more than one code. "Use additional code" notes are found in the tabular at codes that are not part of an etiology/manifestation pair where a secondary code is useful to fully describe a condition. The sequencing rule is the same as the etiology/manifestation pair-, "use additional code" indicates that a secondary code should be added.

    For example, for infections that are not included in chapter 1, a secondary code from category 041, Bacterial infection in conditions classified elsewhere and of unspecified site, may be required to identify the bacterial organism causing the infection. A "use additional code" note will normally be found at the infectious disease code, indicating a need for the organism code to be added as a secondary code.

    "Code first" notes are also under certain codes that are not specifically manifestation codes but may be due to an underlying cause. When a "code first" note is present and an underlying condition is present the underlying condition should be sequenced first.

inpatient/outpatient

"Code, if applicable, any causal condition first", notes indicate that this code may be assigned as a principal diagnosis when the causal condition is unknown or not applicable. If a causal condition is known, then the code for that condition should be sequenced as the principal or first-listed diagnosis.

Multiple codes may be needed for late effects, complication codes, and obstetric codes to more fully describe a condition. See the specific guidelines for these conditions for further instruction.

Examples

Multiple Coding (also known as dual coding)

Diagnosis: Diabetic retinopathy with type I diabetes

(Note: Retinopathy is the manifestation and diabetes is the etiology, or cause, of the retinopathy or retinal hemorrhage.)

Diagnosis: Index: **Retinopathy**, diabetic 250.5 *[362.01]*

The Index subterm "diabetic" identifies the code for the etiology as 250.5 and directs you to the code for the manifestation of [362.01] retinopathy. The italicized code is never sequenced first as the principal diagnosis but is used to identify a manifestation.

Tabular: **250 Diabetes mellitus**

250.5 Diabetes with ophthalmic manifestations

Use additional code to identify manifestation

250.51 Type I, not stated as uncontrolled

Note that the diagnosis of diabetes mellitus will always be reported with a five-digit code because the fifth digit indicates the type of diabetes. See the fifth-digit codes listed after code 250 in the Tabular of your ICD-9-CM.

Code 250.51 is the correct code to describe the diabetes (etiology). The statement "Use additional code to identify manifestation. . ." directs you to assign a code that identifies the manifestation (retinopathy).

Tabular: **362 Other retinal disorders**

362.0 Diabetic retinopathy

Code first diabetes (250.5)

362.01 Background diabetic retinopathy

Note that the *"Code first diabetes"* directs you to the etiology code.

Code: 250.51, 362.01 Diabetic retinopathy with type I diabetes

The multiple codes fully describe the diagnostic statement. The guideline directs you to place the etiology code first, followed by the manifestation code. Let's review another example of multiple coding.

Diagnosis: Staphylococcal cellulitis of the face

(Staphylococcal infection is the etiology and cellulitis is the manifestation.)

Index: **Cellulitis**, face (any part, except eye) 682.0

Tabular: **682 Other cellulitis and abscess**

682.0 Face

Code(s):   682.0 Cellulitis of the face

QUICK CHECK 15-2

When verifying 682.0 in the Tabular, what note pertaining to infections is given?

You now must identify the etiology (staphylococcal) code.

Index: **Infection**, staphylococcal NEC 041.10

Tabular: **041 Bacterial infection in conditions classified elsewhere and of unspecified site**

> *Note:* This category is to be used as an additional code to identify the bacterial agent in diseases classified elsewhere. This category is also used to classify bacterial infections of unspecified nature or site.

> **041.1 Staphylococcus**

> **041.10 Staphylococcus, unspecified**

Code: 682.0, 041.10 Staphylococcal cellulitis of the face

Note that it is acceptable to sequence the manifestation code first in this example because code 682.0 is not italicized in the Tabular, and the instructional notation listed under category 682 in the Tabular specifically states, "Use additional code to identify organism . . ."

EXERCISE 15–3   *Multiple Coding*

Using multiple codes, fill in the codes for the following diagnoses:

1 Chronic prostatitis due to *Streptococcus* species

  Code(s): _____   _____

2 Acute bronchitis due to *Pseudomonas* species

  Code(s): _____   _____

3 Gangrene due to diabetes mellitus, type I, not stated as uncontrolled

  Code(s): _____   _____

4 Urinary tract infection due to *Escherichia coli*

  🌐 Code(s): _____

5 Amyloid cardiomyopathy

  🌐 Code(s): _____

Uncertain Diagnosis

OFFICIAL GUIDELINES FOR CODING AND REPORTING

SECTION II. H. Uncertain Diagnosis

If the diagnosis documented at the time of discharge is qualified as "probable", "suspected", "likely", "questionable", "possible", or "still to be ruled out", or other similar terms indicating uncertainty, code the condition as if it existed or was established. The bases for these guidelines are the diagnostic workup, arrangements for further workup or observation, and initial therapeutic approach that correspond most closely with the established diagnosis.

  Note: This guideline is applicable only to inpatient admissions to short-term, acute, long-term care and psychiatric hospitals.

inpatient

The basis for this guideline is that the diagnostic workup and arrangements for further workup, observation, or therapies are the same whether treating the confirmed condition or ruling the condition out.

Because hospitals are paid a lump sum (diagnosis-related group amount) for each hospitalization for Medicare patients, the facility resources used are averaged across the entire patient stay in the hospital. In an outpatient setting, only confirmed diagnoses may be coded, and rule-out, possible, or probable diagnoses are coded to the chief complaint or sign or symptom that occasioned the visit. In an outpatient setting, each visit in the process of confirming a diagnosis is reported.

Examples

Uncertain Diagnosis

Hospital Inpatient

Diagnosis: <u>Probable</u> bronchitis (code as bronchitis)

Index: **Bronchitis 490**

Tabular: **490 Bronchitis**

Hospital Inpatient

Diagnosis: <u>Rule out</u> Graves' disease (code as Graves' disease)

Index: **Graves' Disease 242.0**

Tabular: **242.00 Toxic diffuse goiter** (Graves' disease)

Clinic Outpatient

Diagnosis: Chest pain, <u>rule out</u> myocardial infarction (code as chest pain)

Index: **Pain(s), chest 786.50**

Tabular: **786.50 Chest pain, unspecified**

Clinic Outpatient

Diagnosis: Cough and fever, <u>probably</u> pneumonia (code as cough and fever)

Index: **Cough 786.2**

Index: **Fever 780.6**

Tabular: **786.2 Cough**

780.6 Pyrexia of unknown origin (fever)

Impending or Threatened Condition

OFFICIAL GUIDELINES FOR CODING AND REPORTING

SECTION I. B. 13. Impending or Threatened Condition

Code any condition described at the time of discharge as "impending" or "threatened" as follows:

If it did occur, code as confirmed diagnosis.

If it did not occur, reference the Alphabetic Index to determine if the condition has a subentry term for "impending" or "threatened" and also reference main term entries for "Impending" and for "Threatened."

If the subterms are listed, assign the given code.

If the subterms are not listed, code the existing underlying condition(s) and not the condition described as impending or threatened.

inpatient

Examples

Impending or Threatened Condition

Diagnosis: Threatened abortion

Index: **Threatened, abortion 640.0**

Tabular:	**640 Hemorrhage in early pregnancy**
	640.0 Threatened abortion
Code:	640.03 Threatened abortion

Fifth digit 3 indicates an antepartum condition or complication

Diagnosis:	Impending myocardial infarction
Index:	**Impending,** myocardial infarction 411.1
Tabular:	**411 Other acute and subacute forms of ischemic heart disease**
	411.1 Intermediate coronary syndrome
	Impending infarction
	Preinfarction angina
	Preinfarction syndrome
	Unstable angina
Code:	411.1 Impending myocardial infarction

If the infarction had occurred, you would have coded it as a confirmed diagnosis by coding myocardial infarction (with the appropriate fifth digit to denote the episode of care).

EXERCISE 15–4 *Uncertain and Impending/Threatened Condition*

Fill in the codes for the following:

1 Evolving stroke

Code: _____

2 Impending delirium tremens

Code: _____

3 Threatened miscarriage

Code: _____

4 Threatened labor

Code: _____

5 Impending coronary syndrome

Code: _____

Selection of Principal Diagnosis

OFFICIAL GUIDELINES FOR CODING AND REPORTING

SECTION II. Selection of Principal Diagnosis

The circumstances of inpatient admission always govern the selection of principal diagnosis. The principal diagnosis is defined in the Uniform Hospital Discharge Data Set (UHDDS) as "that condition established after study to be chiefly responsible for occasioning the admission of the patient to the hospital for care."

The UHDDS definitions are used by hospitals to report inpatient data elements in a standardized manner. These data elements and their definitions can be found in the July 31, 1985, Federal Register (Vol. 50, No. 147), pp. 31038-40.

Since that time the application of the UHDDS definitions has been expanded to include all non-outpatient settings (acute care, short term, long

inpatient/outpatient

term care and psychiatric hospitals; home health agencies; rehab facilities; nursing homes, etc).

In determining principal diagnosis the coding conventions in the ICD-9-CM, Volumes I and II take precedence over these official coding guidelines *(See Section I. A., Conventions for the ICD-9-CM)*

The importance of consistent, complete documentation in the medical record cannot be overemphasized. Without such documentation the application of all coding guidelines is a difficult, if not impossible, task.

SECTION IV. H. ICD-9-CM code for the diagnosis, condition, problem, or other reason for encounter/visit

List first the ICD-9-CM code for the diagnosis, condition, problem, or other reason for encounter/visit shown in the medical record to be chiefly responsible for the services provided. List additional codes that describe any coexisting conditions. In some cases the first-listed diagnosis may be a symptom when a diagnosis has not been established (confirmed) by the physician.

The **principal diagnosis** is sequenced **first** in inpatient coding. In an outpatient setting, it is important to indicate as the primary diagnosis the main reason for the visit, as well as subsequent diagnoses to substantiate adjunct services (such as laboratory and radiology) and to sequence the **primary diagnosis first**. The terminology "principal diagnosis" refers only to an acute care setting such as a hospital and is used in conjunction with the MS-DRG payment scheme; "first-listed diagnosis" refers only to outpatient settings.

OFFICIAL GUIDELINES FOR CODING AND REPORTING

INTRODUCTION (Paragraph 3)

These guidelines are based on the coding and sequencing instructions in Volumes I, II and III of ICD-9-CM, but provide additional instruction. Adherence to these guidelines when assigning ICD-9-CM diagnosis and procedure codes is required under the Health Insurance Portability and Accountability Act (HIPAA). The diagnosis codes (Volumes 1-2) have been adopted under HIPAA for all healthcare settings. Volume 3 procedure codes have been adopted for inpatient procedures reported by hospitals.

Symptoms, Signs, and Ill-Defined Conditions

OFFICIAL GUIDELINES FOR CODING AND REPORTING

SECTION II. A. Codes for symptoms, signs, and ill-defined conditions

Codes for symptoms, signs, and ill-defined conditions from Chapter 16 are not to be used as a principal diagnosis when a related definitive diagnosis has been established.

OFFICIAL GUIDELINES FOR CODING AND REPORTING

SECTION IV. E. Codes that describe symptoms and signs

Codes that describe symptoms and signs, as opposed to diagnoses, are acceptable for reporting purposes when a diagnosis has not been established (confirmed) by the provider. Chapter 16 of ICD-9-CM, Symptoms, Signs, and Ill-defined conditions (codes 780.0-799.9), contains many, but not all codes for symptoms.

EXERCISE 15-5 *Symptoms, Signs, and Ill-Defined Conditions*

1 A 63-year-old male is admitted with chest pain. Cardiac enzyme levels are elevated and the ECG indicates an acute myocardial infarction. The principal diagnosis is acute myocardial infarction. Chest pain is not coded, because it is a symptom of the definitive diagnosis of acute myocardial infarction.

Let's code this case together.
   a. For an acute myocardial infarction, infarction is the **manifestation.** "Acute" indicates the **episode** of care and "myocardial" indicates the general **site** of the infarction.
   b. Locate the term "Infarct, infarction" in the Index.
   c. Under the term "Infarct, infarction" locate the subterm "myocardium." Note after "myocardium, myocardial" you find "(acute . . .)" and are directed to code 410.9. You can never stop at the Index. You must always refer to the Tabular, otherwise you will miss important notes, such as "a fifth digit is required."
   d. Now turn to 410.9 in the Tabular, Volume 1.
   e. Under "410.9 Unspecified site" you are presented with a notation that a fifth digit is required.
   f. Go back to the three-digit category code 410 where the fifth digits are listed. The fifth digit 0 is for an unspecified episode of care; the fifth digit 1 is for the initial episode of care; and the fifth digit 2 is for a subsequent episode of care. The myocardial infarction was diagnosed during this visit, so that would be the initial episode of care as defined in the ICD-9-CM. The correct fifth digit is 1.
   g. The complete, correct code is 410.91.

Now you try one.

2 A patient is admitted to the hospital with severe flank pain and hematuria. A urinalysis is done and it is positive for *Escherichia coli*. The discharge summary states acute pyelonephritis.

   a. What is the principal diagnosis? _____

   b. Locate the principal diagnosis in the Index. What code does the Index direct you to locate?

      Code(s): _____

   c. Locate the code in the Tabular. What is the three-digit category code and the title of the category you were directed to?

      Code(s) and title: _____

   d. Was there mention of a lesion in the case above? _____

   e. What is the correct five-digit code for this case? _____

   f. Why do you think "severe flank pain and hematuria" are noted on this patient's case?

      _____

 STOP *Wait, you're not finished with this case yet. Go back to the three-digit category code 590 and look at the entry immediately under "Infections of kidney." A note states, "Use additional code to identify organism, such as Escherichia coli [E. coli] (041.4)." You also code 041.4 to indicate the type of infection present. You have to be very careful to read all notes in the category before coding. If, in the end, you arrived at codes 590.10 (acute pyelonephritis) and 041.4 (Escherichia), you did a fine job.*

Codes in Brackets

OFFICIAL GUIDELINES FOR CODING AND REPORTING

SECTION I. A. 6. Etiology/manifestation convention ("code first", "use additional code" and "in diseases classified elsewhere" notes)

Certain conditions have both an underlying etiology and multiple body system manifestations due to the underlying etiology. For such conditions, the ICD-9-CM has a coding convention that requires that the underlying condition be sequenced first followed by the manifestation. Wherever such a combination exists, there is a "use additional code" note at the etiology code, and a "code first" note at the manifestation code. These instructional notes indicate the proper sequencing order of the codes, etiology followed by manifestation.

In most cases the manifestation codes will have in the code title, "in diseases classified elsewhere." Codes with this title are a component of the etiology/manifestation convention. The code title indicates that it is a manifestation code. "In diseases classified elsewhere" codes are never permitted to be used as first listed or principal diagnosis codes. They must be used in conjunction with an underlying condition code and they must be listed following the underlying condition.

There are manifestation codes that do not have "in diseases classified elsewhere" in the title. For such codes a "use additional code" note will still be present and the rules for sequencing apply.

In addition to the notes in the tabular, these conditions also have a specific index entry structure. In the index both conditions are listed together with the etiology code first followed by the manifestation codes in brackets. The code in brackets is always to be sequenced second.

The most commonly used etiology/manifestation combinations are the codes for Diabetes mellitus, category 250. For each code under category 250 there is a use additional code note for the manifestation that is specific for that particular diabetic manifestation. Should a patient have more than one manifestation of diabetes, more than one code from category 250 may be used with as many manifestation codes as are needed to fully describe the patient's complete diabetic condition. The category 250 diabetes codes should be sequenced first, followed by the manifestation codes.

"Code first" and "Use additional code" notes are also used as sequencing rules in the classification for certain codes that are not part of an etiology/manifestation combination. *See—Section I.B.9. "Multiple coding for a single condition"*.

inpatient

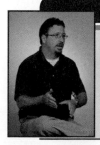

From the Trenches

"Coding is like solving a mystery . . . I think it is like detective work. There are some easy codes that you'll find very quickly, but there are others that take a great deal of intellect and research to determine whether or not you are actually getting it right."

JOHN

EXERCISE 15–6   *Codes in Brackets*

1 A patient is admitted with the diagnosis of malarial hepatitis.

  a. You might not be sure whether the principal diagnosis is hepatitis or malaria.

  b. Locate the term "malaria" in the Index. Under the subterm "any type, with" you will find "hepatitis 084.9 *[573.2]*." The slanted brackets alert you that *[573.2]* cannot be sequenced as the principal diagnosis.

  c. Locate the term "hepatitis" and then the subterm "malarial." You again find 084.9 *[573.2]*.

  d. Both Index entries direct you to the principal diagnosis of malaria. Hepatitis can be a manifestation of malaria. The slanted brackets in 084.9 *[573.2]* indicate that this hepatitis is a manifestation of the condition malaria. "Hepatitis" is the condition and "malarial" describes the hepatitis.

  e. Under the four-digit code of 084.9 locate "Malarial" and then "hepatitis." 084.9 Malaria is the principal diagnosis and *[573.2]* hepatitis is the complication, and you would record both, (084.9, 573.2) after checking 573.2 in the Tabular.

You do the next one.

2 The patient's record states: endocarditis due to disseminated lupus erythematosus.

  a. When you locate the term "Endocarditis, due to disseminated lupus erythematosus" in the

  Index, what do you find? _____

  _____

  b. Locate the main term (condition) "Lupus," the subterm "erythematosus," and the second subterm "systemic." What code are you directed to?

  Code: _____

  c. What is the title of 710 in the Tabular for the codes from b. above?

  _____

  d. What does the three-digit category code include, according to the Includes notes in the Tabular?

  _____

  _____

  e. Under the three-digit category code 710.0 you are also directed to "Use additional code to identify manifestation," which is endocarditis in this case. What code are you directed to?

  _____

That "Use additional code . . ." under 710.0 tells you that you are to use endocarditis (424.91) if the first-listed diagnosis is in the 710.0 category and further specified as "with endocarditis." This patient has heart involvement, so be alert to the use of the code in the brackets.

Again, the importance of verification in the Tabular is critical. This is where you receive instruction regarding the coding of endocarditis.

  f. What four-digit code designates the principal diagnosis of "systemic lupus erythematosus"?

  Code(s): _____

  g. What are the two codes for this case?

  Code(s): _____ and _____

Two or More Interrelated Conditions

OFFICIAL GUIDELINES FOR CODING AND REPORTING

SECTION II. B. Two or more interrelated conditions, each potentially meeting the definition for principal diagnosis.

When there are two or more interrelated conditions (such as diseases in the same ICD-9-CM chapter or manifestations characteristically associated with a

inpatient

certain disease) potentially meeting the definition of principal diagnosis, either condition may be sequenced first, unless the circumstances of the admission, the therapy provided, the Tabular List, or the Alphabetic Index indicate otherwise.

EXERCISE 15–7 *Two or More Interrelated Conditions*

1 A patient is admitted with chest pain, shortness of breath, and a heart murmur. The patient undergoes a diagnostic cardiac catheterization, which shows two-vessel coronary artery disease (native coronary arteries) and severe mitral (valve) stenosis. It is recommended that bypass surgery with mitral valve replacement be performed as soon as possible.

The patient has two conditions, each of which has the potential to be the principal diagnosis: mitral valve stenosis and coronary artery disease.

a. Locate stenosis in the Index: both "mitral" and "valve" indicate the site of the stenosis the patient has—the condition is stenosis. Under the main term "Stenosis," locate the subterm "mitral." The words in parentheses indicate the kinds of mitral stenosis, such as valve, chronic, or inactive. You are looking for valve, so the correct four-digit category code for the mitral valve stenosis is likely to be 394.0.

b. Locate coronary artery disease by locating the main term "Disease" and the subterms "artery" and "coronary." The entry directs you to "*see* Arteriosclerosis, coronary." Under the main term "Arteriosclerosis" and the subterm "coronary (native artery)" you will be directed to code 414.01. If the Tabular validates codes 394.0 (mitral valve stenosis) and 414.01 (coronary artery disease, native artery), either code could be sequenced first because none of the information indicates one condition is more the principal diagnosis than the other.

Now you do one.

2 A patient is involved in a car accident and is admitted with an open fracture of the right humerus and an open fracture of the distal femur. Both fractures require open reduction, which means that the fracture will be repaired using an open incision into the fracture site.

a. What are the two diagnoses?

_____

Either of these diagnoses may be principal, because both are addressed and plans are made to treat both surgically. They were equally the reason for admission to the hospital.

b. Under what main term in the Index would you locate both diagnoses?

_____

c. After the main term "Fracture," what would be the first subterm for the fracture of the right humerus?

_____

d. What is the word that appears in parentheses after humerus?

_____

Because the patient's case states "open," you know that 812.20 is not the correct code because 812.20 specifies "closed." Go farther down the list of subterms to "Fracture, humerus, open." What is the code for "open"?

Code(s): _____

e. In the Tabular, does the code you chose in the Index match the description?

_____

You still have to locate the code for the open fracture of distal femur.

f. After looking in the Index using the main term "Fracture," what is the subterm you would locate?

_____

g. What is the word in parentheses after the first subterm?

_____

h. What is the next subterm?

_____

i. What does this subterm direct you to do?

_____

j. When you take the subterm direction, what is the next subterm that you must use to locate the correct code?

_____

Note: If "open" or "closed" fracture is not stated, assume it is a "closed" fracture.

k. What is the code that you are directed to look up under "Fracture, femur, lower end, open"?

Code(s): _____

l. After checking the code in the Tabular, is the code correct?

_____

Two or More Diagnoses

If two or more diagnoses are equally responsible for the outpatient visit, either can be sequenced as the first-listed diagnosis.

OFFICIAL GUIDELINES FOR CODING AND REPORTING

SECTION II. C. Two or more diagnoses that equally meet the definition for principal diagnosis

In the unusual instance when two or more diagnoses equally meet the criteria for principal diagnosis as determined by the circumstances of admission, diagnostic workup and/or therapy provided, and the Alphabetic Index, Tabular List, or another coding guidelines does not provide sequencing direction, any one of the diagnoses may be sequenced first.

inpatient

EXERCISE 15–8 *Two or More Diagnoses*

1 A patient is admitted with weakness, diarrhea of 2 days' duration, diaphoresis, and abdominal pain. The attending physician lists the diagnoses as viral gastroenteritis and dehydration. Intravenous fluids with electrolyte supplements are ordered.

a. Locate "Gastroenteritis" as the main term in the Index and then the subterm "viral." When you do this you will be directed to code 008.8 (unspecified) because the record does not specify the organism type.

b. After you have located code 008.8 in the Tabular and made sure it is the correct code, look for any notes under the three-digit category code to see if there are any fifth digits that need to be assigned.

c. The correct code is 008.8 and there are no fifth digits to be assigned. Now you need to code the other diagnosis of dehydration. It seems almost too good to be true: There is only one word in the diagnosis. "Dehydration" is the main term. Dehydration appears in the Index, and it points to only one code. Check out the code 276.51 in the Tabular.

d. The Tabular confirms that 276.51 is for dehydration and there is no note regarding any *Excludes* that concern this case. The correct code is 276.51.

e. Remember, when two equally important diagnoses are indicated, it does not matter which code is sequenced first. So, the two codes for this case can be stated to be 008.8 and 276.51 *or* 276.51 and 008.8. The order of the codes may not seem too earth-shattering right now, but the order of the codes is significant. Later in this text, you will learn about how the hospital payment is made to the hospital by third-party payers based on the diagnosis codes. One of these diagnoses may be reimbursed at a higher rate than the other; therefore, selection of the principal diagnosis is critically important.

Now you have the opportunity to do the next case.

2 A patient is admitted with heavy menstrual bleeding of 2 days' duration, severe abdominal pain, and anemia due to acute blood loss. The patient is given medication intravenously to control the pain and bleeding. She also receives two units of packed cells for the anemia.

   a. What is the medical term for heavy menstrual/uterine bleeding?

   _____

   b. The medical term from the question above is the first-listed diagnosis that you will need to locate. What code does the Index indicate and the Tabular of the text confirm as a code for the first diagnosis?

      Code: _____

   c. What is the second diagnosis? _____

   d. Locate the second diagnosis code and confirm your finding in the Tabular. (Hint: The subterms for the second code are "blood loss" and "acute.") What is the code?

      Code: _____

Comparative or Contrasting Conditions

OFFICIAL GUIDELINES FOR CODING AND REPORTING

SECTION II. D. Two or more comparative or contrasting conditions.

In those rare instances when two or more contrasting or comparative diagnoses are documented as "either/or" (or similar terminology), they are coded as if the diagnoses were confirmed and the diagnoses are sequenced according to the circumstances of the admission. If no further determination can be made as to which diagnosis should be principal, either diagnosis may be sequenced first.

inpatient

EXERCISE 15-9 *Comparative or Contrasting Conditions*

1 A patient is admitted to the hospital with chest pain, nausea, and dyspnea. The patient has a history of a prior myocardial infarction 2 years earlier. The pain is atypical (irregular). An ECG and cardiac enzyme study (creatine phosphokinase) are ordered, as well as an upper gastrointestinal series to rule out esophageal reflux. The admitting diagnosis by the attending physician is myocardial infarction or esophageal reflux.

   a. Infarction is located by the main term "Infarct, infarction" and the subterm "myocardium." In the Tabular, there is a notation of five-digit subclassifications that are used with category 410 codes. You might think that the patient was having a subsequent episode of care until you read the definitions attached to the fifth digits for initial and subsequent. "Subsequent" refers to a patient who has received care for the condition within the past 8 weeks. This patient was diagnosed and treated 2 years earlier, so this episode is considered an initial episode of care and has the fifth digit 1. The correct code is 410.91.

b. The second diagnosis is reflux, esophageal, located in the Index under the main term "Reflux" and the subterm "esophageal." You are directed to code 530.81. After checking this in the Tabular to be sure this is the correct code and has no exclusions or additions, you have the second of the two contrasting conditions, 530.81. Only further evaluation by the physician will finally determine what the principal diagnosis is; but for now, the case has been coded to the greatest specificity possible with the information available in the patient record as 530.81 and 410.91 or 410.91 and 530.81. Either diagnosis may be selected as the principal diagnosis.

Here's a case for you to code.

2 A 75-year-old man is admitted with severe low back pain. He is known to have prostate cancer as well as severe spondylosis. Spine x-ray films and a bone scan are ordered. Differential diagnoses are compression fracture versus bone metastases from prostate cancer. (*Note:* The physician would have to be consulted to determine whether prostate cancer is "current" prostate cancer or "history of" prostate cancer.)

a. What is the main term for compression fracture?

_____

b. Using "Fracture" as the main term and "compression" as the subterm, what are you directed to do?

_____

Before you continue to look up other possible subterms, you need to consider why the patient has severe low back pain. You may need to query the physician or review the record to determine whether the compression fracture was or was not due to trauma. The term idiopathic means of unknown cause; the term pathologic means due to a disease or accompanying a disease. Let us assume that the patient record substantiates a diagnosis of a fracture due to a disease (pathologic). Under Fracture, locate pathologic and then the subterm "vertebrae." You are then forwarded to 733.13. Is that the correct code according to the Tabular?

c. The second diagnosis in the differential diagnoses is metastasis from prostate cancer. Locating cancer in the Index, you find: "*see also* Neoplasm, by site, malignant." The potential neoplasm is of the bone. "Neoplasm" is the main term and "bone" is a subterm. Secondary is the type of malignancy because the record states that this patient has prostate cancer (primary) and now has the potential to have bone (secondary) cancer. Under the "Secondary" column, what is the correct code for "Neoplasm, bone" for this patient?

Code: _____

An additional code would be assigned for the prostate cancer.

 STOP *The difference between Guidelines Section II, D (Two or More Comparative or Contrasting Conditions), and Section II, E (Symptom[s] Followed by Contrasting/Comparative Diagnosis) is the way the physician states the final diagnosis. In the Guideline Section II, D, examples, symptoms are documented but the physician states "X versus Y" instead of listing the symptoms. In Guideline Section II, E, the physician states the diagnosis as "symptoms due to X versus Y."*

Symptom(s) Followed by Contrasting/Comparative Diagnoses

OFFICIAL GUIDELINES FOR CODING AND REPORTING

SECTION II. E. A symptom(s) followed by contrasting/comparative diagnoses

When a symptom(s) is followed by contrasting/comparative diagnoses, the symptom code is sequenced first. All the contrasting/comparative diagnoses should be coded as additional diagnoses.

inpatient

EXERCISE 15–10 *Symptom(s) Followed by Contrasting/ Comparative Diagnoses*

1 The patient presents with knee pain of 3 months' duration, with no known trauma, either bucket-handle tear of medial meniscus or loose body in the knee joint. The final diagnosis is knee pain due to buckethandle tear of medial meniscus versus loose body in the knee joint.

There will be three codes for this case: one for the **pain** in the knee joint, one for the **tear** in the meniscus, and one for the **loose body** in the knee joint.

a. Using "Pain, joint, knee" for the first condition, what is the correct code?

Code: _____

b. Using "Tear, meniscus, bucket handle, old," what is the correct second code?

Code: _____

c. Using "Loose, body, joint, knee," what is the correct third code?

Code: _____

Observation for Suspected Conditions

OFFICIAL GUIDELINES FOR CODING AND REPORTING

SECTION I. C. 18. Classification of Factors Influencing Health Status and Contact with Health Service (Supplemental V01-V89)

Note: The chaper specific guidelines provide additional information about the use of V codes for specified encounters.

a. Introduction
ICD-9-CM provides codes to deal with encounters for circumstances other than a disease or injury. The Supplementary Classification of Factors Influencing Health Status and Contact with Health Services (V01.0-V89) is provided to deal with occasions when circumstances other than a disease or injury (codes 001-999) are recorded as a diagnosis or problem.

There are four primary circumstances for the use of V codes:

1) A person who is not currently sick encounters the health services for some specific reason, such as to act as an organ donor, to receive prophylactic care, such as inoculations or health screenings, or to receive counseling on health related issues.

2) A person with a resolving disease or injury, or a chronic, long-term condition requiring continuous care, encounters the health care system for specific aftercare of that disease or injury (e.g., dialysis for renal disease; chemotherapy for malignancy; cast change). A diagnosis/symptom code should be used whenever a current, acute, diagnosis is being treated or a sign or symptom is being studied.

3) Circumstances or problems influence a person's health status but are not in themselves a current illness or injury.

4) Newborns, to indicate birth status

b. V codes used in any healthcare setting.
V codes are for use in any healthcare setting. V codes may be used as either a first listed (principal diagnosis code in the inpatient setting) or secondary code, depending on the circumstances of the encounter. Certain V codes may only be used as first listed, others only as secondary codes. *See Section I.C.18.e, V Code Table.*

inpatient/outpatient

Codes from the V71.0-V71.9 series, Observation and evaluation for suspected conditions, are assigned as principal or first-listed diagnoses for encounters or admissions to evaluate the patient's condition when there is some evidence to suggest the existence of an abnormal condition or following an accident or other incident that ordinarily results in a health problem, and where no supporting evidence for the suspected condition is found and no treatment is currently required. The fact that the patient may be scheduled for continuing observation in the office/clinic setting following discharge does not limit the use of this category.

EXERCISE 15-11 *Observation for Suspected Conditions*

1 The patient fell off his motorcycle when turning too sharply and hit his head on the sidewalk. The patient was wearing a helmet. The examination reveals no outwardly apparent head injury. The only injury noted on examination is abrasion of the elbow. The patient is admitted overnight to the observation unit to rule out head injury.

There will be three codes on this case: one for the **observation** of the injury (a V code), one for the **abrasion**, and one for the **cause** (an E code).

a. Hospital observation is located in the Index under the main term "Observation." Listed under the main term are the reasons for observation. The subterm is "accident NEC." Check the code in the Tabular. What is the V code?

Code: _____

b. The second code is for the abrasion to the elbow. When you locate the term "abrasion" in the Index, you are referred to "*see also* Injury, superficial, by site." Locate "Injury, superficial, arm." What is the code for the abrasion?

Code: _____

(See the cross-reference in the Tabular, and discover whether a fourth digit is needed for specificity.)

c. The E code would be E816.2.

2 A patient is admitted for observation and further evaluation following an alleged rape.

a. There is only one code for this case. What is that V code?

Code: _____

Original Treatment Plan Not Carried Out

OFFICIAL GUIDELINES FOR CODING AND REPORTING

SECTION II. F. Original treatment plan not carried out

Sequence as the principal diagnosis the condition, which after study occasioned the admission to the hospital, even though treatment may not have been carried out due to unforeseen circumstances.

EXERCISE 15-12 *Original Treatment Plan Not Carried Out*

1 A patient is admitted to the hospital for an elective cholecystectomy. The patient has chronic cholecystitis, and gallstones were visualized on x-ray films. After admission, it is noticed that the patient has a fever, is coughing, and shows some patchy infiltrates on the chest x-ray film. Surgery is canceled because the patient may have pneumonia.

This case will have three codes: the cholecystitis with gallstones (cholelithiasis), pneumonia, and surgery not done.

a. Cholelithiasis with cholecystitis, without mention of obstruction. What is the code?

Code: _____

b. What is the pneumonia code?

Code: _____

c. The surgery that was not done is located in the Index under "Surgery, not done because of." Why was the surgery not done?

_____

d. What is the code for the surgery not done?

Code: _____

No procedure code is submitted because no procedure was done.

2 A patient is admitted for elective sterilization by tubal ligation. The patient and her husband decide not to go through with the surgery, and the surgery is canceled.

a. How many codes will there be for this case and what are the main terms for each?

_____

b. What is the V code for the sterilization?

Code: _____

c. What is the code for the surgery not done?

Code: _____

No ICD-9-CM procedure code is submitted because no procedure was performed.

V CODES AND LATE EFFECTS

There are 17 chapters in Volume 1, Tabular List, of the ICD-9-CM. Each of the chapters represents a different organ system or type of disease. You will review each of the chapters, but first, there are some special codes that you need to know about—V codes and late effects.

V Codes

Let's begin with the V codes. In the Tabular, the V codes follow code 999.9. If you have an ICD-9-CM manual available, locate the V codes now. Notice that V codes have only two digits before the decimal point, and a V precedes the number. V codes can be located in the Index like any other code. Often, the most difficult thing about the V code is locating the V code term in the Index. To help you become familiar with how to locate V codes in the Index, review the following, the most common Index terms for locating V codes:

Admission	Examination	Prophylactic
Aftercare	Fitting of	Replacement
Attention to	Follow-up	Screening
Boarder	Health, Healthy	Status
Care (of)	History	Supervision (of)
Carrier	Maintenance	Test
Checking	Maladjustment	Transplant
Contraception	Observation	Unavailability of medical facilities
Counseling	Problem	
Dialysis	Procedure (surgical)	Vaccination
Donor		

V codes are most often used in outpatient settings, that is, ambulatory care centers, physicians' offices, and outpatient departments of hospitals. There are four circumstances in which V codes are used:

1. A patient is not currently sick but receives health care services.

> ### Example
> An elderly patient comes to the clinic for an influenza vaccination. The patient is not currently sick but receives the health care service of a vaccination.
>
> Index: **Vaccination**, prophylactic, influenza V04.81
>
> Tabular: **V04 Need for prophylactic vaccination and inoculation against certain diseases**
>
> **V04.8 Other viral diseases**
>
> **V04.81 Influenza**
>
> Code: V04.81 Influenza vaccination

2. A patient with a known disease or injury receives health services for specific treatment of the disease or injury.

> ### Example
> A patient with breast cancer reports to the outpatient department of the hospital for a chemotherapy session. The patient is not currently ill but receives health care services for specific treatment of cancer.
>
> Index: **Chemotherapy**, encounter (for) V58.11
>
> Tabular: **V58 Encounter for other and unspecified procedures and aftercare**
>
> **V58.11 Encounter for antineoplastic chemotherapy**
>
> Code: V58.11 Chemotherapy treatment
>
> The breast cancer (174.9) would also be coded, but you will learn about the details of that later in the chapter; for now, concentrate on the use of the V codes. V codes should not be mistaken for procedure codes. There is an ICD-9-CM procedure code to identify chemotherapy (99.25). Facility policy and the setting will determine the assignment of the procedure code.

3. A circumstance or problem is present and influences a patient's health status but is not in itself a current illness or injury. (In these situations the V code should be used only as a supplementary or secondary code.)

> ### Example
> A patient who is allergic to penicillin is admitted to the hospital for treatment of pneumonia using intravenous antibiotic. The patient receives treatment for the pneumonia, but the patient's allergy to penicillin is a special consideration in the treatment received.
>
> Index: **History** (personal) of, allergy to, antibiotic agent NEC V14.1, penicillin V14.0
>
> Tabular: **V14 Personal history of allergy to penicillin**
>
> **V14.0 Penicillin**
>
> Code: V14.0 History of allergy to penicillin
>
> Additionally, the pneumonia (486) would be coded as the first-listed or principal diagnosis, but you are focusing only on the use of V codes right now.

4. To indicate the birth status and outcome of the delivery of a newborn.

Example

A live, healthy newborn infant is the result of a vaginal delivery in the hospital.

Index: **Newborn**, single, born in hospital V30.00

Tabular: **V30 Single live born**

The third digit "0" means born in hospital, and the fourth digit "0" means delivery without mention of cesarean delivery.

Code: V30.00 Vaginal delivery of a single, live-born newborn

EXERCISE 15–13 *V Codes*

Fill in the V code(s) for the following:

1 Admission for cardiac pacemaker adjustment

 Code(s): _____

2 Insertion of subdermal implantable contraceptive

Code(s): _____

3 Personal history of cancer of the prostate

Code(s): _____

4 Baby in for MMR (measles, mumps, rubella) vaccination

Code(s): _____

5 Screening mammogram

Code(s): _____

6 Clinic visit for pre-employment physical examination

Code(s): _____

CAUTION *Often, the patient record states that there is a "history of" a disease: for example, "history of diabetes mellitus." This does not mean that the patient no longer has diabetes mellitus, but that the patient's medical history includes diabetes mellitus. You would not assign a V code to indicate a previous history of diabetes mellitus, but instead would assign the code for the current disease of diabetes mellitus (250.0X). If there is any question regarding the current status of the disease, check with the physician. You may also want to offer some physician education regarding the documentation of past history of diseases.*

Late Effects Late effects codes are not assigned to a separate chapter in the Tabular. Instead, you must first identify a case as a late effect and then code it as such. You use late effects codes when the acute phase of the illness or injury has passed but a residual remains. Sometimes an acute illness or injury leaves a patient with a residual health problem that remains after the illness or injury has resolved. The **residual** is coded **first** and **then** the **late effects** code is assigned to indicate the cause of the residual. An example would be scars (residual) that remain after a severe burn (cause). The late effects code is accessed in the Index under the main term "Late."

In most instances, two codes will be assigned—one code for the residual that is being treated and one code that indicates the late effect. There is no time limit for the development of a residual. It may be evident at the time of the acute illness or it may occur months after an injury. It is also possible that a patient may develop more than one residual. For example, a patient who has had a stroke may develop right-sided hemiparesis (paralysis of one side) and aphasia (loss of ability to communicate).

A person cannot have a current hip fracture (820.8) and a late effect of hip fracture (905.3). The code is either a current injury or a condition caused by a prior injury. It cannot be both at the same time. (The only exception to this rule is in category 438, Late effects of cerebrovascular disease; this is explained below.)

OFFICIAL GUIDELINES FOR CODING AND REPORTING

SECTION I. B. 12. Late Effects

A late effect is the residual effect (condition produced) after the acute phase of an illness or injury has terminated. There is no time limit on when a late effect code can be used. The residual may be apparent early, such as in cerebrovascular accident cases, or it may occur months or years later, such as that due to a previous injury. Coding of late effects generally requires two codes sequenced in the following order: The condition or nature of the late effect is sequenced first. The late effect code is sequenced second.

An exception to the above guidelines are those instances where the code for late effect is followed by a manifestation code identified in the Tabular List and title, or the late effect code has been expanded (at the fourth and fifth-digit levels) to include the manifestation(s). The code for the acute phase of an illness or injury that led to the late effect is never used with a code for the late effect.

inpatient/outpatient

OFFICIAL GUIDELINES FOR CODING AND REPORTING

SECTION I. C. 7. d. Late Effects of Cerebrovascular Disease

1) Category 438, Late Effects of Cerebrovascular disease

Category 438 is used to indicate conditions classifiable to categories 430-437 as the causes of late effects (neurologic deficits), themselves classified elsewhere. These "late effects" include neurologic deficits that persist after initial onset of conditions classifiable to 430-437. The neurologic deficits caused by cerebrovascular disease may be present from the onset or may arise at any time after the onset of the condition classifiable to 430-437.

2) Codes from category 438 with codes from 430-437

Codes from category 438 may be assigned on a health care record with codes from 430-437, if the patient has a current cerebrovascular accident (CVA) and deficits from an old CVA.

3) Code V12.54

Assign code V12.54, Transient ischemic attack (TIA), and cerebral infarction without residual deficits (and not a code from category 438) as an additional code for history of cerebrovascular disease when no neurologic deficits are present.

inpatient/outpatient

Example

Diagnosis:	Dysphagia due to a previous cerebrovascular accident
Residual:	Dysphagia

The dysphagia is a problem that remains following the acute illness of the cerebrovascular accident.

Cause:	Cerebrovascular accident

(This patient had a previous cerebrovascular accident.)

Terms to code:	Dysphagia [residual]
	Cerebrovascular accident [cause]

The late effect of cerebrovascular accident is reported with a combination code. Locate the terms "Late, effect, cerebrovascular disease, with dysphagia" and you will be directed to 438.82, which includes both the residual and the cause in one code.

EXERCISE 15–14 *Residual and Cause*

Write the term(s) that represent the residual and the cause of the following cases on the lines provided:

1 Scars of the face resulting from third-degree burns suffered 1 year ago

Residual _____

Cause _____

2 Constrictive pericarditis due to old tuberculosis infection

Residual _____

Cause _____

3 Residual foreign body in femur due to gunshot injury years ago

Residual _____

Cause _____

4 Mental retardation due to previous poliomyelitis

Residual _____

Cause _____

5 Leg pain resulting from old fracture of femur

Residual _____

Cause _____

To locate the late effects codes in the ICD-9-CM, use the entry "Late, effects" in the Index. There are numerous subterms that describe the various late effects. Review and become familiar with the late effects subterms.

Assign the code for the acute injury or disease first; then refer to the Index "Late, effects" for that injury or disease. Next, reference the Tabular to ensure the codes are correct and assign any further digits indicated.

EXERCISE 15-15   *Residual and Cause Codes*

Now you identify the residual and cause terms and code the following diagnoses:

1 Traumatic arthritis following fracture of the left ankle 3 years ago

Residual _____

Code: _____

Cause: _____

Code: _____

2 Aphasia due to cerebrovascular accident 6 months ago (requires one combination code)

Residual: _____

Cause: _____

Code: _____

3 Sensorineural deafness due to previous meningitis

Residual: _____

Code: _____

Cause: _____

Code: _____

CHAPTER-SPECIFIC GUIDELINES

Chapter 1 in the Tabular is Infectious and Parasitic Diseases, which classifies diseases according to the etiology, or cause, of the disease. Because infectious or parasitic conditions can affect various parts of the body, the chapter contains a wide variety of codes.

Infectious and Parasitic Diseases

In this chapter there are many instances of combination coding and multiple coding. Remember: **Combination coding** applies when one code fully describes the condition. **Multiple coding** is acceptable when it takes more than one code to fully describe the condition, so the sequencing of multiple codes may have to be considered.

From the Trenches

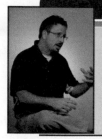

"I try to always keep people aware that we're not just translating an ICD-9 narrative into a code—that's a patient we're dealing with. It's not just a piece of paper, it's not just words we're handling—it's still a patient."

JOHN

Example

Combination Coding

Diagnosis:	Candidiasis infection of the mouth
Index:	**Candidiasis**, candidal, mouth 112.0
Tabular:	**112.0 Candidiasis of mouth**
Code:	112.0 Candidiasis infection of the mouth

The code 112.0 fully describes the diagnosis.

Multiple Coding

Diagnosis:	Urinary tract infection due to *Escherichia coli (E. coli)*
Index:	**Infection**, infected, infective, urinary (tract) NEC 599.0
Tabular:	**599.0 Urinary tract infection, site not specified**

Use additional code to identify organism, such as *Escherichia coli [E. coli]* (041.4)

Code 599.0 does not fully describe the condition. The instructions in the Tabular for code 599.0 state that you are to also code the organism causing the urinary tract infection. To locate a causative organism, you locate the main term "Infection" in the Index and then the subterm of the specific organism, which in the example is *Escherichia coli*. The urinary tract infection is sequenced first and the bacterial organism follows.

Example

Index:	**Infection**, infected, infective, Escherichia coli NEC 041.4
Tabular:	**041 Bacterial infection in conditions classified elsewhere and of unspecified site**
	041.4 Escherichia coli [E. coli]
Codes:	599.0, 041.4 Urinary tract infection due to *Escherichia coli (E. coli)*

Multiple coding is necessary to fully describe the infection of the urinary tract and the causative organism, *E. coli*.

Human Immunodeficiency. Another important category in Chapter 1 is 042 Human Immunodeficiency Virus (HIV) Disease. Review the guidelines for HIV codes.

OFFICIAL GUIDELINES FOR CODING AND REPORTING

SECTION I. C. C1. a. Infectious and Parasitic Diseases (001-139)

a. Human Immunodeficiency Virus (HIV) Infections

1) Code only confirmed cases

Code only confirmed cases of HIV infection/illness. This is an exception to the hospital inpatient guideline Section II, H.

In this context, "confirmation" does not require documentation of positive serology or culture for HIV; the provider's diagnostic statement that the patient is HIV positive, or has an HIV-related illness is sufficient.

2) Selection and sequencing of HIV codes

(a) Patient admitted for HIV-related condition

inpatient/outpatient

inpatient

inpatient

If a patient is admitted for an HIV-related condition, the principal diagnosis should be 042, followed by additional diagnosis codes for all reported HIV-related conditions.

(b) Patient with HIV disease admitted for unrelated condition

If a patient with HIV disease is admitted for an unrelated condition (such as a traumatic injury), the code for the unrelated condition (e.g., the nature of injury code) should be the principal diagnosis. Other diagnoses would be 042 followed by additional diagnosis codes for all reported HIV-related conditions.

(c) Whether the patient is newly diagnosed

Whether the patient is newly diagnosed or has had previous admissions/encounters for HIV conditions is irrelevant to the sequencing decision.

inpatient/outpatient

(d) Asymptomatic human immunodeficiency virus

V08 Asymptomatic human immunodeficiency virus [HIV] infection, is to be applied when the patient without any documentation of symptoms is listed as being "HIV positive," "known HIV," "HIV test positive," or similar terminology. Do not use this code if the term "AIDS" is used or if the patient is treated for any HIV-related illness or is described as having any condition(s) resulting from his/her HIV positive status; use 042 in these cases.

(e) Patients with inconclusive HIV serology

Patients with inconclusive HIV serology, but no definitive diagnosis or manifestations of the illness, may be assigned code 795.71, Inconclusive serologic test for Human Immunodeficiency Virus [HIV].

(f) Previously diagnosed HIV-related illness.

Patients with any known prior diagnosis of an HIV-related illness should be coded to 042. Once a patient has developed an HIV-related illness, the patient should always be assigned code 042 on every subsequent admission/encounter. Patients previously diagnosed with any HIV illness (042) should never be assigned to 795.71 or V08.

(g) HIV Infection in Pregnancy, Childbirth and the Puerperium

During pregnancy, childbirth or the puerperium, a patient admitted (or presenting for a health care encounter) because of an HIV-related illness should receive a principal diagnosis of 647.6X, Other specified infectious and parasitic diseases in the mother classifiable elsewhere, but complicating the pregnancy, childbirth or the puerperium, followed by 042 and the code(s) for the HIV-related illness(es). Codes from Chapter 15 always take sequencing priority.

Patients with asymptomatic HIV infection status admitted (or presenting for a health care encounter) during pregnancy, childbirth, or the puerperium should receive codes of 647.6X and V08.

(h) Encounters for testing for HIV

If a patient is being seen to determine his/her HIV status, use code V73.89, Screening for other specified viral disease. Use code V69.8, Other problems related to lifestyle, as a secondary code if an asymptomatic patient is in a known high risk group for HIV. Should a patient with signs or symptoms or illness, or a confirmed HIV related diagnosis be tested for HIV, code the signs and symptoms or the diagnosis. An additional counseling code V65.44 may be used if counseling is provided during the encounter for the test.

When a patient returns to be informed of his/her HIV test results use code V65.44, HIV counseling, if the results of the test are negative.

If the results are positive but the patient is asymptomatic use code V08, Asymptomatic HIV infection. If the results are positive and the patient is symptomatic use code 042, HIV infection, with codes for the HIV related symptoms or diagnosis. The HIV counseling code may also be used if counseling is provided for patients with positive test results.

SECTION IV. A. Selection of first-listed condition

In the outpatient setting, the term first-listed diagnosis is used in lieu of principal diagnosis.

In determining the first-listed diagnosis the coding conventions of ICD-9-CM, as well as the general and disease specific guidelines take precedence over the outpatient guidelines.

Diagnoses often are not established at the time of the initial encounter/visit. It may take two or more visits before the diagnosis is confirmed.

The most critical rule involves beginning the search for the correct code assignment through the Alphabetic Index. Never begin searching initially in the Tabular List as this will lead to coding errors.

As stated in Guideline Section I. C. 1. you do not assign 042 to a patient's record or insurance claim unless the diagnosis of HIV is a confirmed diagnosis. The assignment of the code prior to confirmation may cause the patient many unwarranted problems if the patient does not have HIV. Use extreme caution when assigning 042.

Note: This statement is **very** important. You are **never** to code HIV unless you are certain of the diagnosis. This diagnosis stays in the patient's record forever.

Infectious and Parasitic Diseases

OFFICIAL GUIDELINES FOR CODING AND REPORTING

SECTION I. C. 1. b.

b. Septicemia, Systematic Inflammatory Response Syndrome (SIRS), Sepsis, Severe Sepsis, and Septic Shock

(1) SIRS, Septicemia, and Sepsis

(a) The terms *septicemia* and *sepsis* are often used interchangeably by providers, however they are not considered synonymous terms. The following descriptions are provided for reference but do not preclude querying the provider for clarification about terms used in the documentation:

(i) Septicemia generally refers to a systemic disease associated with the presence of pathological microorganisms or toxins in the blood, which can include bacteria, viruses, fungi or other organisms.

(ii) Systemic inflammatory response syndrome (SIRS) generally refers to the systemic response to infection, trauma/burns, or other insult (such as cancer) with symptoms including fever, tachycardia, tachypnea, and leukocytosis.

(iii) Sepsis generally refers to SIRS due to infection.

(iv) Severe sepsis generally refers to sepsis with associated acute organ dysfunction.

(b) The Coding of SIRS, sepsis and severe sepsis

The coding of SIRS, sepsis, and severe sepsis requires a minimum of 2 codes: a code for the underlying cause (such as infection or trauma) and a code from subcategory 995.9 Systemic inflammatory response syndrome (SIRS).

(i) The code for the underlying cause (such as infection or trauma) must be sequenced before the code from subcategory 995.9 Systemic inflammatory response syndrome (SIRS).

(ii) Sepsis and severe sepsis require a code for the systemic infection (038.xx, 112.5, etc.) and either code 995.91, Sepsis, or 995.92,

inpatient

Severe sepsis. If the causal organism is not documented, assign code 038.9, Unspecified septicemia.

(iii) Severe sepsis requires additional code(s) for the associated acute organ dysfunction(s).

(iv) If a patient has sepsis with multiple organ dysfunctions, follow the instructions for coding severe sepsis.

(v) Either the term sepsis or SIRS must be documented to assign a code from subcategory 995.9.

(vi) *See Section I.C.17.g), Injury and poisoning, for information regarding systemic inflammatory response syndrome (SIRS) due to trauma/burns and other non-infectious processes.*

(c) Due to the complex nature of sepsis and severe sepsis, some cases may require querying the provider prior to assignment of the codes.

2) Sequencing sepsis and severe sepsis

(a) Sepsis and severe sepsis as principal diagnosis

If sepsis or severe sepsis is present on admission, and meets the definition of principal diagnosis, the systemic infection code (e.g., 038.xx, 112.5, etc.) should be assigned as the principal diagnosis, followed by code 995.91, Sepsis, or 995.92, Severe sepsis, as required by the sequencing rules in the Tabular List. Codes from subcategory 995.9 can never be assigned as a principal diagnosis. A code should also be assigned for any localized infection, if present.

If the sepsis or severe sepsis is due to a postprocedual infection, see Section I.C.10 for guidelines related to sepsis due to postprocedural infection.

(b) Sepsis and severe sepsis as secondary diagnoses

When sepsis or severe sepsis develops during the encounter (it was not present on admission), the systemic infection code and code 995.91 or 995.92 should be assigned as secondary diagnoses.

(c) Documentation unclear as to whether sepsis or severe sepsis is present on admission

Sepsis or severe sepsis may be present on admission but the diagnosis may not be confirmed until sometime after admission. If the documentation is not clear whether the sepsis or severe sepsis was present on admission, the provider should be queried.

3) Sepsis/SIRS with Localized Infection

If the reason for admission is both sepsis, severe sepsis, or SIRS and a localized infection, such as pneumonia or cellulitis, a code for the systemic infection (038.xx, 112.5, etc) should be assigned first, then code 995.91 or 995.92, followed by the code for the localized infection. If the patient is admitted with a localized infection, such as pneumonia, and sepsis/SIRS doesn't develop until after admission, see guideline I.C.1.b.2.b.

If the localized infection is postprocedural, see Section I.C.10 for guidelines related to sepsis due to postprocedural infection.

Note: The term urosepsis is a nonspecific term. If that is the only term documented then only code 599.0 should be assigned based on the default for the term in the ICD-9-CM index, in addition to the code for the causal organism if known.

4) Bacterial Sepsis and Septicemia

In most cases, it will be a code from category 038, Septicemia, that will be used in conjunction with a code from subcategory 995.9 such as the following:

(a) Streptococcal sepsis

If the documentation in the record states streptococcal sepsis, codes 038.0, Streptococcal septicemia, and code 995.91 should be used, in that sequence.

(b) Streptococcal septicemia

If the documentation states streptococcal septicemia, only code 038.0 should be assigned, however, the provider should be queried whether the patient has sepsis, an infection with SIRS.

5) Acute organ dysfunction that is not clearly associated with the sepsis

If a patient has sepsis and an acute organ dysfunction, but the medical record documentation indicates that the acute organ dysfunction is related to a medical condition other than the sepsis, do not assign code 995.92, Severe sepsis. An acute organ dysfunction must be associated with the sepsis in order to assign the severe sepsis code. If the documentation is not clear as to whether an acute organ dysfunction is related to the sepsis or another medical condition, query the provider.

6) Septic shock

(a) Sequencing of septic shock

Septic shock generally refers to circulatory failure associated with severe sepsis, and, therefore, it represents a type of acute organ dysfunction.

For all cases of septic shock, the code for the systemic infection should be sequenced first, followed by codes 995.92 and 785.52. Any additional codes for other acute organ dysfunctions should also be assigned. As noted in the sequencing instructions in the Tabular List, the code for septic shock cannot be assigned as a principal diagnosis.

(b) Septic Shock without documentation of severe sepsis

Septic shock indicates the presence of severe sepsis.

Code 995.92, Severe sepsis, must be assigned with code 785.52, Septic shock, even if the term severe sepsis is not documented in the record. The "use additional code" note and the "code first" note in the tabular support this guideline.

7) Sepsis and septic shock complicating abortion and pregnancy

Sepsis and septic shock complicating abortion, ectopic pregnancy, and molar pregnancy are classified to category codes in Chapter 11 (630-639).

See section I.C.11.

8) Negative or inconclusive blood cultures

Negative or inconclusive blood cultures do not preclude a diagnosis of septicemia or sepsis in patients with clinical evidence of the condition, however, the provider should be queried.

9) Newborn sepsis

See section I.C.15.j for information on the coding of newborn sepsis.

10) Sepsis due to a Postprocedural Infection

(a) Documentation of causal relationship

As with all postprocedural complications, code assignment is based on the provider's documentation of the relationship between the infection and the procedure.

(b) Sepsis due to postprocedural infection

In cases of postprocedural sepsis, the complication code, such as code 998.59, Other postoperative infection, or 674.3x, Other complications of obstetrical surgical wounds should be coded first followed by the appropriate sepsis codes (systemic infection dose and either code 995.91 or 995.92). An additional code(s) for any acute organ dysfunction should also be assigned for cases of severe sepsis.

11) External cause of injury codes with SIRS

Refer to Section I.C.19.a.7 for instruction on the use of external cause of injury codes with codes for SIRS resulting from trauma.

inpatient

12) Sepsis and Severe Sepsis Associated with Non-infectious Process

(a) Sequencing <u>of sepsis/severe sepsis associated with non-infectious processes</u>

In some cases, a non-infectious process, such as trauma, may lead to an infection which can result in sepsis or severe sepsis. If sepsis or severe sepsis is documented as associated with a non-infectious condition, such as a burn or serious injury, and this condition meets the definition for principal diagnosis, the code for the non-infectious condition should be sequenced first, followed by the code for the systemic infection and either code 995.91, Sepsis, or 995.92, Severe sepsis. Additional codes for any associated acute organ dysfunction(s) should also be assigned for cases of severe sepsis. If the sepsis or severe sepsis meets the definition of principal diagnosis, the systemic infection and sepsis codes should be sequenced before the non-infectious condition. When both the associated non-infectious condition and the sepsis or severe sepsis meet the definition of principal diagnosis, either may be assigned as principal diagnosis.

See Section I.C.1.b.2)(a) for guidelines pertaining to sepsis or severe sepsis as the principal diagnosis.

(b) Only one SIRS (subcategory 995.9) code should be assigned

Only one code from subcategory 995.9 should be assigned for SIRS associated with trauma or other non-infectious condition. Assign the SIRS code (subcategory 995.9) that corresponds to the principal diagnosis. That is, if trauma or a non-infectious condition is the underlying cause, assign code 995.93 or 995.94. If an infection is the underlying cause, assign code 995.91 or 995.92.

See Section I.C.17.g for information on the coding of SIRS due to trauma/ burns or other non-infectious disease processes.

Point 8 means that if the patient has the signs and symptoms (clinical evidence) of septicemia, but the laboratory tests (blood cultures) do not confirm the diagnosis, the physician may still list the diagnosis of septicemia.

EXERCISE 15–16 *Infectious and Parasitic Diseases*

Code the following infectious diseases:

1 Viral gastroenteritis

♻ Code(s): _____

2 Septicemia due to *Pseudomonas* species with septic shock

♻ Code(s): _____

3 Acute poliomyelitis

♻ Code(s): _____

4 Candidal vaginal infection

♻ Code(s): _____

Neoplasms   Chapter 2 in the Tabular is similar to Chapter 1, Infectious and Parasitic Diseases, in that it classifies diseases according to the etiology, or cause, of the disease. Neoplastic conditions can affect all parts of the body. Before you learn more about what is in Chapter 2, we will quickly review some of the specific terminology.

EXERCISE 15–17 *Neoplasms Terminology*

Match the following terms to the correct definitions:

1 neoplasm ——
2 malignant ——
3 primary ——
4 secondary ——
5 benign ——
6 in situ ——
7 uncertain behavior ——
8 unspecified nature ——
9 morphology ——

a. not usually progressive

b. malignancy that is located within the original site of development

c. used to describe a cancerous tumor that grows worse over time

d. study of neoplasms

e. refers to the behavior of a neoplasm as neither malignant nor benign but having characteristics of both malignant and benign neoplasms

f. when the behavior or histology of a neoplasm is not known or not specified

g. site to which a malignant tumor has spread

h. site of origin or where the tumor originated

i. new tumor growth that can be benign or malignant

Neoplasm Codes. Locating a code for a neoplasm is a two-step process:

1. First, locate the morphology or histologic type of the neoplasm in the Index. Examples of histology types are carcinoma, adenocarcinoma, sarcoma, melanoma, lymphoma, lipoma, adenoma.
2. Once you have located the morphology, review all modifiers and subterms, and then follow the instructions or verify the code listed. Most often you will be instructed to turn to the Neoplasm Table in the Index to find the code.

When you locate the morphology of the neoplasm, you can identify the "M," or morphology code. The M codes are in parentheses following the morphology. M codes are used in some inpatient settings and are optional, so facility policy would determine their usage. Mostly, M codes are used by the tumor registrar (the person who records morphology information). M codes are not required on insurance forms.

M codes are alphanumeric codes and are listed in Appendix A of the ICD-9-CM code book. The alphanumeric structure of the morphology codes starts with the letter M, followed by four digits that indicate the histologic type of neoplasm, and a slash, followed by a fifth digit that indicates the behavior.

Behavior

/0 = Benign

/1 = Uncertain whether benign or malignant
　　　Borderline malignancy

/2 = Carcinoma in situ
　　　Intraepithelial
　　　Noninfiltrating
　　　Noninvasive

/3 = Malignant, primary site

/6 = Malignant, metastatic site
　　　Secondary site

/9 = Malignant, uncertain whether primary or metastatic site

The following example shows how the morphology codes are used. This information is provided not because you will use the M codes when coding diagnoses, but rather so you will understand what M codes are and how M codes are used by those who gather morphology information.

Example

ICD-9-CM Codes and Morphology Codes

Diagnosis:	Adenocarcinoma of the upper-outer quadrant right breast with metastasis to the axillary lymph nodes
Index:	**Adenocarcinoma** (M8140/3)—*see also* Neoplasm, by site, malignant
Neoplasm Table:	Breast, upper-outer quadrant 174.4 (primary column)
	Lymph, lymphatic, gland (secondary column), axilla, axillary 196.3
Tabular:	**174 Malignant neoplasm of female breast**
	174.4 Upper-outer quadrant
	196 Secondary and unspecified malignant neoplasm of lymph nodes
	196.3 Lymph nodes of axilla and upper limb
Codes:	174.4, 196.3 Adenocarcinoma of the upper-outer quadrant right breast with metastasis to the axillary lymph nodes

But wait, you're not finished yet. You have two M codes to assign to this diagnosis before you are finished—one for the primary adenocarcinoma and one for a secondary adenocarcinoma. Both M codes will have the same histologic type of adenocarcinoma, but the fifth digit will be different to indicate the primary and secondary behaviors.

Index:	**Adenocarcinoma** (M8140/3)—*see also* Neoplasm, by site, malignant
M code:	**primary** adenocarcinoma of the breast, M8140/3 (3 indicates primary site)
M code:	**secondary** adenocarcinoma of the axillary lymph nodes, M8140/6 (6 indicates secondary site)
ICD-9-CM and M Codes:	174.4, M8140/3, 196.3, M8140/6 Adenocarcinoma of the upper-outer quadrant right breast with metastasis to the axillary lymph nodes

Note that the M codes are sequenced after the ICD-9-CM diagnosis code to which they refer.

OFFICIAL GUIDELINES FOR CODING AND REPORTING

SECTION I. C. 2. Neoplasms (140-239)

<u>General guidelines</u>

Chapter 2 of the ICD-9-CM contains the codes for most benign and all malignant neoplasms. Certain benign neoplasms, such as prostatic adenomas, may be found in the specific body system chapters. To properly code a neoplasm it is necessary to determine from the record if the neoplasm is benign, in situ, malignant, or of uncertain histologic behavior. If malignant, any secondary (metastatic) sites should also be determined.

The neoplasm table in the Alphabetic Index should be referenced first. However, if the histological term is documented, that term should be referenced first, rather than going immediately to the Neoplasm Table, in order to determine which column in the Neoplasm Table is appropriate. For example, if the documentation indicates "adenoma," refer to the term in the Alphabetic Index to review the entries under this term and the instructional note to "see also neoplasm, by site, benign." The table provides the proper code based on the type of neoplasm and the site. It is important to select the proper column in the table that corresponds to the type of neoplasm. The tabular should then be referenced to verify that the correct code has been selected from the table and that a more specific site code does not exist.

See Section I.C.18.d.4. for information regarding V codes for genetic susceptibility to cancer.

a. Treatment directed at the malignancy

If the treatment is directed at the malignancy, designate the malignancy as the principal diagnosis.

b. Treatment of secondary site

When a patient is admitted because of a primary neoplasm with metastasis and treatment is directed toward the secondary site only, the secondary neoplasm is designated as the principal diagnosis even though the primary malignancy is still present.

c. Coding and sequencing of complications

Coding and sequencing of complications associated with the malignancies or with the therapy thereof are subject to the following guidelines:

1) Anemia associated with malignancy

When admission/encounter is for management of an anemia associated with the malignancy, and the treatment is only for anemia, the appropriate anemia code (such as code 285.22, Anemia in neoplastic disease) is designated as the principal diagnosis and is followed by the appropriate code(s) for the malignancy.

Code 285.22 may also be used as a secondary code if the patient suffers from anemia and is being treated for the malignancy.

2) Anemia associated with chemotherapy, immunotherapy and radiation therapy

When the admission/encounter is for management of an anemia associated with chemotherapy, immunotherapy or radiotherapy and the only treatment is for the anemia, the anemia is sequenced first followed by code E933.1. The appropriate neoplasm code should be assigned as an additional code.

3) Management of dehydration due to the malignancy

When the admission/encounter is for management of dehydration due to the malignancy or the therapy, or a combination of both, and only the dehydration is being treated (intravenous rehydration), the dehydration is sequenced first, followed by the code(s) for the malignancy.

4) Treatment of a complication resulting from a surgical procedure

When the admission/encounter is for treatment of a complication resulting from a surgical procedure, designate the complication as the principal or first-listed diagnosis if treatment is directed at resolving the complication.

d. Primary malignancy previously excised

When a primary malignancy has been previously excised or eradicated from its site and there is no further treatment directed to that site and there is no evidence of any existing primary malignancy, a code from category V10, Personal history of malignant neoplasm, should be used to indicate the former site of the malignancy. Any mention of extension, invasion, or metastasis to another site is coded as a secondary malignant neoplasm to that site. The secondary site may be the principal or first-listed with the V10 code used as a secondary code.

e. Admission/Encounters involving chemotherapy, immunotherapy and radiation therapy

1) Episode of care involves surgical removal of neoplasm

When an episode of care involves the surgical removal of a neoplasm, primary or secondary site, followed by adjunct chemotherapy or radiation treatment during the same episode of care, the neoplasm code should be assigned as principal or first-listed diagnosis, using codes in the 140-198 series or where appropriate in the 200-203 series.

2) Patient admission/encounter solely for administration of chemotherapy, immunotherapy and radiation therapy

If a patient admission/encounter is solely for the administration of chemotherapy, immunotherapy or radiation therapy assign code V58.0, Encounter for radiation therapy, or V58.11, Encounter for antineoplastic chemotherapy, or V58.12, Encounter for antineoplastic immunotherapy as the first-listed or principal diagnosis. If a patient receives more than one of these therapies during the same admission more than one of these codes may be assigned, in any sequence.

3) Patient admitted for radiotherapy/chemotherapy and immunotherapy and develops complications

When a patient is admitted for the purpose of radiotherapy, immunotherapy or chemotherapy and develops complications such as uncontrolled nausea and vomiting or dehydration, the principal or first-listed diagnosis is V58.0, Encounter for radiotherapy, or V58.11, Encounter for antineoplastic chemotherapy, or V58.12, Encounter for antineoplastic immunotherapy, followed by any codes for the complications.

f. Admission/encounter to determine extent of malignancy

When the reason for admission/encounter is to determine the extent of the malignancy, or for a procedure such as paracentesis or thoracentesis, the primary malignancy or appropriate metastatic site is designated as the principal or first-listed diagnosis, even though chemotherapy or radiotherapy is administered.

g. Symptoms, signs, and ill-defined conditions listed in Chapter 16 associated with neoplasms

Symptoms, signs, and ill-defined conditions listed in Chapter 16 characteristic of, or associated with, an existing primary or secondary site malignancy cannot be used to replace the malignancy as principal or first-listed diagnosis, regardless of the number of admissions or encounters for treatment and care of the neoplasm.

See Section I.C.18.d.14, Encounter for prophylactic organ removal.

h. Admission/encounter for pain control/management

See Section I.C.6.a.5 for information on coding admission/encounter for pain control/management.

V codes are also frequently used when coding neoplasms. There are V codes present in the ICD-9-CM to indicate the history of a malignant neoplasm (V10.00-V10.9). These history codes are used to indicate a primary malignant neoplasm that is no longer present. Remember that in the V code section, you were presented with information about documenting a "history of" a disease. Be careful in determining whether the physician is indicating a past and current history of a condition or a true past history. With neoplasms there is often a true "history of" whereby the condition previously existed but is no longer present.

There are also encounter codes for chemotherapy (V58.11) and radiotherapy (V58.0). When coding an encounter for chemotherapy, immunotherapy (V58.12), or radiotherapy, code the V code first, followed by the active code for the malignant neoplasm, even if that neoplasm has already been removed. As long as the neoplasm is being treated with adjunctive therapy following a surgical removal of the cancer, you can code that neoplasm as if it still exists. You would not assign a "history of" V code because the neoplasm is the reason for the treatment. Instead, the neoplasm is coded as a current or active disease.

EXERCISE 15-18 *Neoplasm Codes*

1 A patient is admitted for chemotherapy for ovarian cancer.

Two codes are needed for this case: one for the encounter for chemotherapy and the other for the malignant, primary, ovarian neoplasm.
   Locate in the Index and verify in the Tabular the two codes necessary to code this case.

   Code(s): _____ _____

2 A patient is admitted for radiation therapy for metastatic bone cancer. The patient had a mastectomy for breast cancer 3 years earlier.

There is a code for the admission for radiation management, which will be a V code; a code for the secondary, malignant, bone neoplasm; and a V code for the history of malignant neoplasm of the breast. What are these three codes?

   Code(s): _____ _____ _____

3 A patient is admitted with chest pain, shortness of breath, and a history of bloody sputum. Diagnostic x-ray film shows a mass in the bronchial tube. A diagnostic bronchoscopy is performed and is positive for cancer. The pathology report states "metastatic carcinoma of bronchus, primary unknown." The patient chooses to undergo chemotherapy.

   a. What is the description of the principal diagnosis? _____

   b. What is the subsequent diagnosis description? _____

   c. Is metastatic carcinoma of the bronchus considered a primary or secondary malignant

      neoplasm? _____

   d. What are the diagnosis codes for this case?

      Code(s): _____ _____

4 A patient is admitted with uncontrolled nausea and vomiting after chemotherapy treatment for lung cancer.

   a. How many codes would be needed to accurately report this case? _____

   b. What is the principal diagnosis? _____

c. What is the secondary diagnosis? _____

d. What is the code for the principal diagnosis?

    Code: _____

e. What is the code for the secondary diagnosis and the E code?

    Code(s): _____ _____

Unknown Site or Unspecified. There is an entry on the Neoplasm Table that states "unknown site or unspecified." This code, 199.1, is used to indicate either an unknown or an unspecified primary or secondary malignancy. If there is a known secondary site, a code must be assigned to the primary site or the history of a primary site. It is possible for a primary site to be unknown.

QUICK CHECK 15-3

Where in the Neoplasm Table in the Index are the codes for "unknown or unspecified site" located?

_____

Example

Diagnosis:	Metastatic bone cancer.

This statement indicates that the bone cancer is a secondary neoplasm, but there is no indication of the location of the primary site.

Index:	**Cancer** (M8000/3)—*see also* Neoplasm, by site, malignant
Neoplasm Table:	Bone 198.5 (secondary)
	Unknown site or unspecified 199.1 (primary)
Tabular:	**198 Secondary malignant neoplasm of other specified site**
	198.5 Bone and bone marrow
Tabular:	**199 Malignant neoplasm without specification of site**
	199.1 Other
Codes:	198.5, 199.1 Metastatic bone cancer (if the treatment is for the secondary site)
	199.1, 198.5 Metastatic bone cancer (if the treatment or diagnostic workup is for the primary site)

The sequencing of the primary and secondary neoplasms is dependent on the treatment circumstances documented in the health record. If treatment was directed toward the secondary malignancy, that code would be sequenced first. If treatment was focused on determining the site of the unknown primary malignancy, that code would be sequenced first.

EXERCISE 15-19   *More Neoplasms*

Practice assigning ICD-9-CM codes as well as the appropriate M codes for the following neoplasms:

1 Multiple myeloma

    Code(s): ——————————— ———————————

2 Carcinoma in situ, cervix

    Code(s): ——————————— ———————————

3 Cancer of the sigmoid colon with spread to the peritoneum

    Code(s): ——————————— ——————————— ———————————

4 Adenocarcinoma of the prostate with metastasis to the bone

    ⊛ Code(s): ———————————

5 Metastatic cancer to the brain; primary unknown (treatment directed to metastatic site)

    ⊛ Code(s): ———————————

6 Metastatic carcinoma of the breast to the lungs; the breast carcinoma has been removed by mastectomy

    ⊛ Code(s): ———————————

Endocrine, Nutritional, and Metabolic Diseases and Immunity Disorders

Chapter 3 in the Tabular describes diseases or conditions affecting the endocrine system. The endocrine system involves glands that are located throughout the body and are responsible for secreting hormones into the bloodstream. Also included in Chapter 3 are diseases or conditions that affect nutritional and metabolic status as well as disorders of the immune system.

One of the frequently used category codes in Chapter 3 is 250 Diabetes Mellitus. When you locate diabetes in the Index, you will note that for many of the subterms, two codes are listed. The 250.X code is followed by an italicized code in brackets. This is because multiple coding is common for diabetes inasmuch as both the manifestation (symptom) and the etiology (cause—diabetes) are coded.

> **Example**
>
> Index: **Diabetes**, retinopathy, background, 250.5X *[362.01]*

There are four five-digit subclassifications for use with category 250. It is essential that you read these before assigning codes for diagnosis of diabetes mellitus (DM). The fifth digits identify the type of diabetes: 2 is type II or unspecified type, uncontrolled; and 3 is type I [juvenile type], uncontrolled. It is best if the health care providers document the type of diabetes mellitus. You should not assume that because a patient is receiving insulin that he or she is a type I diabetic because a type II diabetic may be receiving insulin. If there is any question regarding the type of diabetes, query the physician. In order to appropriately assign the fifth digits 2 or 3, uncontrolled diabetes, the physician must document that the patient's DM is uncontrolled or out of control. If a complication is specified (250.1-250.8), assign the appropriate fourth and fifth digits; do not use the .9 (unspecified).

Example

Diagnosis: Diabetic iritis

Index: **Diabetes, diabetic**, iritis 250.5 *[364.42]*

The first code (250.5) indicates the etiology (diabetes) and the second code *[364.42]* indicates the manifestation (iritis). You need two codes to describe diagnoses. You will always list first the etiology and then the manifestation.

Tabular: **250.5 Diabetes with ophthalmic manifestations**

Use additional code to identify manifestation, as. . . . :

364.4 Vascular disorders of iris and ciliary body

The Tabular also indicates that a fifth digit should be added for greater specificity.

Tabular: **364.4 Vascular disorders of iris and ciliary body**

364.42 Rubeosis iridis

Even though the 364.42 entry above does not specifically indicate iritis, you trust the code that is listed in the Index. You could also look up the main term "Iritis" in the Index and be directed to the same codes.

Index: **Iritis** 364.3, diabetic 250.5 *[364.42]*

You are directed to the same codes.

Code(s):   250.50, 364.42 Diabetic iritis

The codes must be sequenced in this order to indicate that the iritis is a manifestation of the diabetes.

To code a disease or condition as a manifestation of DM, it must be stated that the disease or condition is diabetic or due to the diabetes. A cause-and-effect relationship must be stated or evident. If you are unsure of the relationship, you must clarify this relationship with the physician.

If a cause-and-effect relationship is not evident or stated and no further indication of the relationship can be obtained, the following codes would be assigned. An exception would be gangrene or osteomyelitis because of the index entry "with."

Example

Diagnosis: Diabetes mellitus and iritis

Index: **Diabetes, diabetic** 250.0

Note—Use the following fifth-digit subclassification with category 250:

The Note in the Index directs you to use a fifth digit for greater specificity.

Tabular: **250.0 Diabetes mellitus without mention of complication**

Index: **Iritis 364.3**

Tabular: **364.3 Unspecified iridocyclitis**

Code(s):   250.00 Diabetes and 364.3 Iritis

Note that codes (250.00 and 364.3) are different because a cause-and-effect relationship was not established—the iritis is not reported as a manifestation of the diabetes in this case.

EXERCISE 15–20 *Endocrine, Nutritional, and Metabolic Diseases and Immunity Disorders*

Fill in the codes for the following:

1 Addison's disease

   Code: _____

2 Dehydration

   Code: _____

3 Diabetes mellitus with hypoglycemic coma

   Code: _____

4 Graves' disease with thyrotoxic crisis

   Code: _____

Diseases of the Blood and Blood-Forming Organs

Chapter 4, Diseases of the Blood and Blood-Forming Organs, is a short chapter with only 10 categories. The **anemia** category is often used because anemia is the most common blood disease. Anemia is the main term under which you will find the many subterms that relate to anemia. In addition to there being numerous subterms for anemia, many of those subterms have lengthy additional subterms listed under them.

There are two anemias that are easy to confuse—anemia of chronic disease and chronic anemia. These two diagnostic statements do not have the same meaning. In anemia of chronic disease, the word "chronic" describes the nature of the disease that is the cause of the anemia, for example, Anemia due to neoplastic disease. The neoplasm is the chronic disease causing the anemia. Code anemia (285.22) and then assign the appropriate code to identify the neoplastic process. In the diagnostic statement chronic, simple anemia, the word "chronic" describes the anemia. Let's see what difference these diagnostic statements make in code assignment.

Example

Diagnosis: Anemia of chronic disease

In this diagnosis statement, you do not know what the chronic disease is.

Index: **Anemia**

The Index has a subterm (in, chronic illness, 285.29) that further directs you in the choice of the correct code.

Tabular: **285.2 Anemia of chronic disease**
Code: **285.29 Anemia of other chronic disease**

Diagnosis: Chronic simple anemia
Index: **Anemia 285.9, chronic simple 281.9**

In this example, the Index does indicate a subterm that further directs you to chronic simple 281.9.

Tabular: **281.9 Unspecified deficiency anemia**
Code: 281.9 Chronic simple anemia

If there is any question about the classification of the anemia, check with the physician.

EXERCISE 15–21 *Diseases of the Blood and Blood-Forming Organs*

Fill in the codes for the following:

1 Pernicious anemia

Code: _____

2 Disseminated intravascular coagulation (DIC)

Code: _____

3 Hemophilia

Code: _____

4 Acute blood-loss anemia

Code: _____

5 Familial polycythemia

Code: _____

Mental Disorders

Chapter 5 in the Tabular is Mental Disorders. The chapter includes four sections: organic psychotic conditions; other psychoses; neurotic, personality, and other nonpsychotic mental disorders; and mental retardation.

Your understanding of the definitions of these mental disorders is necessary to enable you to code the diagnoses accurately. When assigning codes from Chapter 5, you need to take extra care to select the appropriate code(s) and code only diagnoses that are documented in the medical record. Mental disorders can be difficult to code because physicians are not always as specific in their diagnostic statements as might be required by the codes in this chapter. When in doubt, always check with the physician. Just one term in the medical record can make a big difference in the code(s) you use.

You should be aware that there is a V code for history of alcoholism (V11.3). Instead of using that code you use the **alcoholism** code (303.9x) with the fifth digit 3, which specifies in remission. It is rare to assign code V11.3 because the disease of alcoholism cannot be cured.

Five-Digit Subclassification. A five-digit subclassification is provided for categories 303-305 to indicate the patient's pattern of use of alcohol or drugs:

-0:	unspecified	
-1:	continuous:	Alcohol: refers to daily intake of large amounts of alcohol or regular heavy drinking on weekends or days off from work
		Drugs: daily or almost daily use of drugs
-2:	episodic:	Alcohol: refers to alcoholic binges lasting weeks or months, followed by long periods of sobriety
		Drugs: indicates short periods between drug use or use on weekends
-3:	remission:	Refers either to a complete cessation of alcohol or drug intake or to the period during which decreasing intake leading toward cessation is taking place

Another commonly encountered instance is the instruction to Use additional code to identify the associated neurological condition or Use additional code to identify cerebral atherosclerosis (437.0). Pay close attention to the instructions given in the Tabular when you see these words.

Example

Diagnosis:	Arteriosclerotic dementia with delirium
Index:	**Dementia 294.8, arteriosclerotic (simple type) (uncomplicated) 290.40, with, delirium 290.41**
Tabular:	**290 Senile and presenile organic psychotic conditions**
	290.4 Vascular dementia
	Use additional code to identify cerebral atherosclerosis (437.0)
	290.41 Vascular dementia with delirium
Tabular:	**437 Other and ill-defined cerebrovascular disease**
	437.0 Cerebral atherosclerosis
Codes:	290.41, 437.0 Arteriosclerotic dementia with delirium

EXERCISE 15–22 *Mental Disorders*

Now you have a chance to show your skill by coding the following:

1 Alzheimer's dementia with aggressive behavior

Code(s): _____ _____

2 Depression with anxiety

Code: _____

3 Profound mental retardation

🌐 Code(s): _____

4 Anorexia nervosa

🌐 Code(s): _____

5 Delirium tremens due to chronic alcoholism, continuous

🌐 Code(s): _____

Diseases of the Nervous System and Sense Organs

Chapter 6, Diseases of the Nervous System and Sense Organs, in the Tabular describes diseases or conditions affecting the central nervous system and the peripheral nervous system. It also includes disorders and diseases of the eyes and ears.

The chapter uses some combination codes in which one code identifies both the manifestation and the etiology.

Example

Diagnosis:	Pneumococcal meningitis

This diagnostic statement means the meningitis is due to pneumococcal bacteria.

Index:	**Meningitis**, pneumococcal 320.1

Tabular:	**320 Bacterial meningitis**
	320.1 Pneumococcal meningitis
Code:	320.1 Pneumococcal meningitis

Code 320.1 includes the manifestation of meningitis and also the etiology of pneumococcal organism. No separate code is required for the organism in this case.

In Chapter 6, you will also find conditions that are manifestations of other diseases. These categories appear in italics in the Tabular and provide instructions to code the underlying disease process first.

Example

| Diagnosis: | Chronic iridocyclitis due to sarcoidosis |
| Index: | **Iridocyclitis** NEC 364.3, chronic, in, sarcoidosis 135 *[364.11]* |

Entries such as 135 *[364.11]* instruct you to code the sarcoidosis (135) first, followed by the chronic iridocyclitis (364.11). Both codes need to be verified in the Tabular.

Tabular:	**135 Sarcoidosis**
Tabular:	**364 Disorders of iris and ciliary body**
	364.11 Chronic iridocyclitis in diseases classified elsewhere
	Code first underlying disease, as:
	sarcoidosis (135)
	tuberculosis (017.3)
Codes:	135, 364.11 Chronic iridocyclitis due to sarcoidosis

EXERCISE 15–23 *Diseases of the Nervous System and Sense Organs*

Fill in the codes for the following:

1 Meningitis due to *Proteus morganii*

 Code(s): _____

2 Multiple sclerosis

 Code(s): _____

3 Acute otitis media

 Code(s): _____

4 Primary open-angle glaucoma

 Code(s): _____

5 Bell's palsy

 Code(s): _____

Diseases of the Circulatory System

Chapter 7, Diseases of the Circulatory System, in the Tabular contains diseases of heart and blood vessels.

Hypertension is probably one of the most common conditions coded in this chapter. The Hypertension Table is located in the Index, as shown in Fig. 15–2. This table provides a complete listing of all conditions due to or associated with hypertension. The first column identifies the hypertensive

INDEX TO DISEASES		Hypertension	
	Malignant	Benign	Unspecified
Hypertension, hypertensive (arterial) (arteriolar) (crisis) (degeneration) (disease) (essential) (fluctuating) (idiopathic) (intermittent) (labile) (low renin) (orthostatic) (paroxysmal) (primary) (systemic) (uncontrolled) (vascular)	401.0	(#1) 401.1	(#3) 401.9
with			
chronic kidney disease	—	—	—
stage I through stage IV, or unspecified	403.00	403.10	403.90
stage V or end stage renal disease	403.01	403.11	403.91
heart involvement (conditions classifiable to 425.8, 428, 429.0-429.3, 429.8, 429.9 due to hypertension) (see also Hypertension, heart)	402.00	402.10	402.90
with kidney involvement — see Hypertension, cardiorenal			
renal involvement (only conditions classifiable to 585, 586, 587) (excludes conditions classifiable to 584) (see also Hypertension, kidney)	403.00	403.10	403.90
with heart involvement — see Hypertension, cardiorenal			
failure (and sclerosis) (see also Hypertension, kidney).......................	403.01	403.11	(#4) 403.91
sclerosis without failure (see also Hypertension, kidney)	403.00	403.10	403.90
accelerated (see also Hypertension, by type, malignant)	401.0	—	—
antepartum — see Hypertension, complicating pregnancy, childbirth, or the puerperium			
cardiorenal (disease)	404.00	404.10	404.90
with			
chronic kidney disease	—	—	—
stage I through stage IV or unspecified	404.00	404.10	404.90
and heart failure	404.01	404.11	404.91
stage V or end stage renal disease	404.02	404.12	404.92
and heart failure	404.03	404.13	404.93
heart failure	404.01	404.11	404.91
and chronic kidney disease	404.02	404.12	404.92
stage I through stage IV or unspecified	404.02	404.12	404.92
stage V or end stage renal disease	404.03	404.13	404.93
cardiovascular disease (arteriosclerotic) (sclerotic).....................................	(#2) 402.00	402.10	402.90
with			
heart failure	402.01	402.11	402.91
renal involvement (conditions classifiable to 403) (see also Hypertension, cardiorenal).............	404.00	404.10	404.90
cardiovascular renal (disease) (sclerosis) (see also Hypertension, cardiorenal)................	404.00	404.10	404.90

Condition →

FIGURE 15–2 Hypertension Table, Index to Diseases. (From International Classification of Diseases, 9th Revision. U.S. Department of Health and Human Services, Public Health Service, Centers for Medicare and Medicaid Services.)

condition, such as accelerated, antepartum, cardiovascular disease, cardiorenal, and cerebrovascular disease. The remaining three columns, entitled malignant, benign, and unspecified, constitute the subcategories of hypertensive disease.

Malignant hypertension is an accelerated, severe form of hypertension, manifested by headaches, blurred vision, dyspnea, and uremia. This type of hypertension usually causes permanent organ damage and has a poor prognosis. **Benign hypertension** is a continuous, mild blood pressure elevation that can usually be controlled by medication. **Unspecified hypertension** has not been specified in the medical record as either benign or malignant.

There is no defined threshold of blood pressure above which an individual is considered hypertensive. Commonly, a sustained diastolic pressure of above 90 mm Hg and a sustained systolic pressure of above 140 mm Hg constitutes hypertension.

Benign hypertension remains fairly stable over the years and is compatible with a long life, but if untreated it is an important risk factor in coronary heart disease and cerebrovascular disease.

Malignant hypertension is commonly associated with abrupt onset and runs a course measured in months. It causes irreversible organ damage and often ends with renal failure or cerebral hemorrhage. Usually a person with malignant hypertension complains of headaches and vision difficulties. Blood pressure of 200/140 mm Hg is not uncommon.

Hypertensive heart disease refers to the secondary effects on the heart of prolonged, sustained, systemic hypertension. The heart has to work against greatly increased resistance, and that results in high blood pressure. The primary effect is the thickening of the left ventricle, which finally results in heart failure.

There are two sections in this chapter that have instructions to Use additional code to identify presence of hypertension (401-405). The sections are Ischemic Heart Disease (410-414) and Cerebrovascular Disease (430-438). There are also a number of guidelines that pertain to hypertension or other hypertensive disease processes.

OFFICIAL GUIDELINES FOR CODING AND REPORTING

SECTION I. C. 7. a Diseases of Circulatory System (390-459)

a. Hypertension

Hypertension Table

The Hypertension Table, found under the main term, "Hypertension", in the Alphabetic Index, contains a complete listing of all conditions due to or associated with hypertension and classifies them according to malignant, benign, and unspecified.

1) Hypertension, Essential, or NOS

Assign hypertension (arterial) (essential) (primary) (systemic) (NOS) to category code 401 with the appropriate fourth digit to indicate malignant (.0), benign (.1), or unspecified (.9). Do not use either .0 malignant or .1 benign unless medical record documentation supports such a designation.

2) Hypertension with Heart Disease

Heart conditions (425.8, 429.0-429.3, 429.8, 429.9) are assigned to a code from category 402 when a causal relationship is stated (due to hypertension) or implied (hypertensive). Use an additional code from category 428 to identify the type of heart failure in those patients with heart failure. More than one code from category 428 may be assigned if the patient has systolic or diastolic failure and congestive heart failure.

The same heart conditions (425.8, 429.0-429.3, 429.8, 429.9) with hypertension, but without a stated causal relationship, are coded separately. Sequence according to the circumstances of the admission/encounter.

3) Hypertensive Chronic Kidney Disease

Assign codes from category 403, Hypertensive chronic kidney disease, when conditions classified to categories 585-587 are present. Unlike hypertension with heart disease, ICD-9-CM presumes a cause-and-effect relationship and classifies chronic kidney disease (CKD) with hypertension as hypertensive chronic kidney disease.

Fifth digits for category 403 should be assigned as follows:
- 0 with CKD stage I through stage IV, or unspecified
- 1 with CKD stage V or end stage renal disease

The appropriate code from category 585, Chronic kidney disease, should be used as a secondary code with a code from category 403 to identify the stage of chronic kidney disease.

See Section I.C.10.a for information on the coding of chronic kidney disease.

4) Hypertensive Heart and Chronic Kidney Disease

Assign codes from combination category 404, Hypertensive heart and chronic kidney disease, when both hypertensive kidney disease and hypertensive heart disease are stated in the diagnosis. Assume a relationship between the hypertension and the chronic kidney disease,

inpatient/outpatient

whether or not the condition is so designated. Assign an additional code from category 428, to identify the type of heart failure. More than one code from category 428 may be assigned if the patient has systolic or diastolic failure and congestive heart failure.

Fifth digits for category 404 should be assigned as follows:
- 0 without heart failure and with chronic kidney disease (CKD) stage I through stage IV, or unspecified
- 1 with heart failure and with CKD stage I through stage IV, or unspecified
- 2 without heart failure and with CKD stage V or end stage renal disease
- 3 with heart failure and with CKD stage V or end stage renal disease

The appropriate code from category 585, Chronic kidney disease, should be used as a secondary code with a code from category 404 to identify the stage of kidney disease.

See Section I.C.10.a for information on the coding of chronic kidney disease.

5) Hypertensive Cerebrovascular Disease

First assign codes from 430-438, Cerebrovascular disease, then the appropriate hypertension code from categories 401-405.

6) Hypertensive Retinopathy

Two codes are necessary to identify the condition. First assign the code from subcategory 362.11, Hypertensive retinopathy, then the appropriate code from categories 401-405 to indicate the type of hypertension.

7) Hypertension, Secondary

Two codes are required: one to identify the underlying etiology and one from category 405 to identify the hypertension. Sequencing of codes is determined by the reason for admission/encounter.

8) Hypertension, Transient

Assign codes 796.2, Elevated blood pressure reading without diagnosis of hypertension, unless patient has an established diagnosis of hypertension. Assign code 642.3X for transient hypertension of pregnancy.

9) Hypertension, Controlled

Assign appropriate code from categories 401-405. This diagnostic statement usually refers to an existing state of hypertension under control by therapy.

10) Hypertension, Uncontrolled

Uncontrolled hypertension may refer to untreated hypertension or hypertension not responding to current therapeutic regimen. In either case, assign the appropriate code from categories 401-405 to designate the stage and type of hypertension. Code to the type of hypertension.

Guideline Section I. C. 7. a. 3. instructs you to assume that there is a cause-and-effect relationship between hypertension and renal diseases that are categorized in the range of codes 585-587. The physician might not indicate that they are related, but the coder must assume this relationship.

Chronic renal failure (CRF), chronic kidney disease (CKD), and chronic renal insufficiency (CRI) when reported with hypertension are reported as follows:

CRF/CKD/CRI + hypertension	403.90 + 585.9
CKD stage 1 + hypertension	403.90 + 585.1
CKD stage 2 + hypertension	403.90 + 585.2
CKD stage 3 + hypertension	403.90 + 585.3
CKD stage 4 + hypertension	403.90 + 585.4
CKD stage 5 + hypertension	403.91 + 585.5
CKD stage 6 or ESRD or on dialysis + hypertension	403.91 + 585.6
Patient with CKD on any type of dialysis	403.91 + 585.6 + V45.1

Code *410* Acute myocardial infarction (MI) requires a fifth digit assignment and includes specific instructions that must be carefully read.

A fifth digit of 1 indicates an initial episode of care for an MI and can be assigned to the same patient for a different admission providing treatment for the initial episode of care for the MI. A patient could be diagnosed with acute MI and be transferred to a larger facility for further investigation and care. The diagnoses at both facilities would sequence the acute MI first with the fifth-digit 1 at both facilities.

A fifth digit of 2 indicates subsequent care and is used when a patient is readmitted for testing or further care within 8 weeks of the initial episode. For example, a patient had an acute myocardial infarction and was discharged from the hospital. Four weeks later, that same patient was admitted for a cardiovascular procedure. The myocardial infarction would be coded 410.92 to indicate a subsequent episode of care with fifth digit 2. Note that code 412 is assigned for a healed (old) myocardial infarction that is not showing any symptoms (asymptomatic). You would not assign a V code history of MI in this situation.

As you review the following examples, refer to Fig. 15–2 for the codes highlighted in each example.

Examples

Hypertension

Diagnosis:	Congestive heart failure **with** benign hypertension
Tabular:	**428.0 Congestive heart failure**
	401.1 Hypertension, benign (indicated as 1 in Fig. 15–2)

The key word in the above diagnosis statement is "with," which indicates two conditions. Both the congestive heart failure and the benign hypertension are coded because each is a separate condition.

Diagnosis:	Dilated cardiomyopathy **due to** malignant hypertension
Index:	**Hypertension,** cardiovascular disease, 402.00 (indicated as 2 in Fig. 15–2)
Tabular:	**402 Hypertensive heart disease**
	402.0 Malignant
	402.00 Without heart failure

In this example, the hypertension caused the cardiomyopathy. The key words here are "due to," which indicates that one condition caused the other condition.

Diagnosis:	Acute renal failure **with** hypertension
Tabular:	**584.9 Acute renal failure,** unspecified
Tabular:	**401.9 Hypertension,** unspecified (indicated as 3 in Fig. 15–2)

You would code the hypertension separately because the word "with" is included in the diagnostic statement. Under Hypertension, renal involvement, in Fig. 15–2, you will see an Excludes note. The note indicates that conditions classifiable to 584 (acute renal failure) are excluded from the codes for hypertension with renal involvement. The condition in this example is acute renal failure (584); so, you cannot assign a renal involvement hypertension codes. Thus, the code for the hypertension in this example is 401.9, Hypertension, unspecified, with no code for the acute renal failure. The key term included in this diagnosis is "acute" renal failure. See how the coding changes when the term chronic is stated within the diagnosis statement.

INDEX TO DISEASES **Hypertension**

	Malignant	Benign	Unspecified
Hypertension—*continued*			
pulmonary (artery) (idiopathic) (primary) (solitary)—*continued*			
with cor pulmonale (chronic)	—	—	416.0
acute	—	—	416.8
secondary	—	—	416.8
renal (disease) (*see also* Hypertension, kidney)	403.00	403.10	403.90
renovascular NEC	405.01	405.11	405.91
secondary NEC	405.09	405.19	405.99
due to			
aldosteronism, primary	405.09	405.19	405.99
brain tumor	405.09	405.19	405.99
bulbar poliomyelitis	405.09	405.19	405.99
calculus			
kidney	405.09	405.19	405.99
ureter	405.09	405.19	405.99
coarctation, aorta	405.09	405.19	405.99
Cushing's disease	405.09	405.19	405.99
glomerulosclerosis (*see also* Hypertension, kidney)	403.00	403.10	403.90
periarteritis nodosa	405.09	405.19	405.99
pheochromocytoma	405.09	405.19	405.99
polycystic kidney(s)	405.09	405.19	405.99
polycythemia	405.09	405.19	405.99
porphyria	405.09	405.19	405.99
pyelonephritis	405.09	405.19	405.99
renal (artery)			
aneurysm	405.01	405.11	405.91
anomaly	405.01	405.11	405.91
embolism	405.01	405.11	405.91
fibromuscular hyperplasia	405.01	405.11	405.91
occlusion	405.01	405.11 #5	405.91
stenosis	405.01	405.11	405.91
thrombosis	405.01	405.11	405.91
transient	—	—	796.2
of pregnancy	—	—	642.3

Secondary hypertension → *secondary NEC*

FIGURE 15–3 Secondary hypertension. (From International Classification of Diseases, 9th Revision. U.S. Department of Health and Human Services, Public Health Service, Centers for Medicare and Medicaid Services.)

Fig. 15–3 shows the portion of the Hypertension Table that includes the secondary hypertension codes. **Secondary hypertension** means that the hypertension is caused by another condition.

Example

Diagnosis: Secondary, benign hypertension, due to renal artery occlusion

Tabular: **405.11 Hypertension**, secondary, due to renal (artery), occlusion, benign (indicated as 5 in Fig. 15–3)

In the previous example, the renal artery occlusion caused the hypertension and so is correctly coded to category 405. You would also assign a code to the renal artery occlusion (593.81) because the renal artery occlusion is causing the secondary hypertension.

Example

Code: 593.81, 405.11 Secondary, benign hypertension, due to renal
             artery occlusion

The renal artery occlusion is causing the hypertension and when treated may result in the disappearance of the hypertension.

According to Guideline Section I. C. 7. a. 7. the sequencing is determined by the reason for admission/encounter.

OFFICIAL GUIDELINES FOR CODING AND REPORTING

SECTION I. C. 7. a. 11. Elevated Blood Pressure

For a statement of elevated blood pressure without further specificity, assign code 796.2, Elevated blood pressure reading without diagnosis of hypertension, rather than a code from category 401.

EXERCISE 15–24 *Diseases of the Circulatory System*

Fill in the codes for the following:

1 Congestive heart failure

 ✿ Code(s): _____

2 Acute subendocardial infarction, initial episode

 ✿ Code(s): _____

3 Secondary hypertension due to periarteritis nodosa

 ✿ Code(s): _____

4 Cerebral infarction due to thrombosis, brain

 ✿ Code(s): _____

5 Subarachnoid hemorrhage

 ✿ Codes(s): _____

Diseases of the Respiratory System

Chapter 8, Diseases of the Respiratory System, in the Tabular includes diseases and disorders of the respiratory tract; it starts with the nasal passages and follows a path to the lungs. Note that at the beginning of Chapter 8 there is an instructional note that covers the entire chapter. The note states, "Use additional code to identify infectious organism." You should be aware that in this chapter the organism is already identified in some codes, and you would not assign an additional code to identify the specific infectious organism.

Examples

Diagnosis:	Pneumonia due to *Klebsiella pneumoniae*
Index:	**Pneumonia**, *Klebsiella pneumoniae*, 482.0
Tabular:	**482 Other bacterial pneumonia**
	482.0 Pneumonia due to Klebsiella pneumoniae
Code:	482.0 Pneumonia due to *Klebsiella pneumoniae*

The code 482.0 is a combination code that includes the disease process (pneumonia) with the causative organism *(Klebsiella pneumoniae)*. In this instance, you would not need to assign an additional code because the organism is identified in the code 482.0.

In the following example, two codes are necessary, one to describe the disease process (manifestation) and one to indicate the causative organism (etiology).

Diagnosis:	Acute maxillary sinusitis due to *Hemophilus influenzae*
Index:	**Sinusitis** (accessory) (nasal) (hyperplastic) (nonpurulent) (purulent) (chronic) 473.9
	acute 461.9
	maxillary 461.0
Tabular:	**461 Acute sinusitis**
	461.0 Maxillary
Index:	**Infection, infected, infective** (opportunistic), *Hemophilus influenzae* NEC 041.5
Tabular:	**041 Bacterial infection in conditions classified elsewhere and of unspecified site**
	041.5 Hemophilus influenzae [H. influenzae]
Codes:	461.0, 041.5 Acute maxillary sinusitis due to *Hemophilus influenzae*

The manifestation is listed first and the etiology is listed second.

Now, let's learn how to code the respiratory condition of chronic obstructive pulmonary disease (COPD), which falls within the category 496 Chronic airway obstruction NEC. The note under code 496 indicates that this code cannot be assigned with any code from categories 491-493 (491 is chronic bronchitis, 492 is emphysema, and 493 is asthma). The Excludes note under code 496 indicates that COPD specified "(as) (with) asthma (493.2)" cannot be assigned to code 496; rather, reference 493.2.

Example

Diagnosis:	COPD with asthma
Index:	**Asthma, asthmatic** (bronchial) (catarrh) (spasmodic) 493.9, with, chronic obstructive pulmonary disease (COPD) 493.2
Tabular:	**493 Asthma**
	493.2 Chronic obstructive asthma

This code is not complete yet because it needs a fifth digit. You have three fifth-digit choices:

0 unspecified

1 with status asthmaticus*

2 with (acute) exacerbation

*Note: Status asthmaticus is the most severe form of asthma attack and can last for days or weeks.

To code the asthma with status asthmaticus, the physician provides specific documentation of the condition. If the clinical condition is severe enough that you suspect that the patient has status asthmaticus, clarification by the physician should be sought.

Code: 493.20 COPD with asthma

EXERCISE 15-25   *Diseases of the Respiratory System*

Fill in the codes for the following:

1 Croup

  ✪ Code(s): _____

2 Respiratory failure due to congestive heart failure

  ✪ Code(s): _____

3 COPD with chronic bronchitis (without exacerbation)

  ✪ Code(s): _____

4 Influenza with acute bronchitis

  ✪ Code(s): _____

5 Pneumonia due to *Hemophilus influenzae*

  ✪ Code(s): _____

Diseases of the Digestive System

Chapter 9, Diseases of the Digestive System, in the Tabular describes diseases or conditions affecting the digestive system. Digestion starts when food is taken into the mouth and follows the gastrointestinal tract until it leaves the body through the anus. The categories are sequenced in a manner that follows that path, starting with disorders of the teeth.

Throughout the chapter, as in other chapters, you must pay close attention to fifth-digit assignment and carefully read the *Excludes* notes and any other instructions. Also important in the chapter is the presence of **hemorrhage** (bleeding) associated with the diseases. The physician may not always indicate the presence of hemorrhage, and the coder must review the record and then clarify with the physician the appropriate code assignment.

Example	
Diagnosis:	Diverticulitis of the colon with hemorrhage
Index:	**Diverticulitis** (acute), colon (perforated) 562.11, with hemorrhage 562.13

Note that the presence of hemorrhage makes a difference in the code assignment: without, 562.11; with, 562.13.

Tabular:	**562 Diverticula of intestine**
	562.13 Diverticulitis of colon with hemorrhage
Code:	562.13 Diverticulitis of the colon with hemorrhage

If you begin your search for the above diagnosis of "Diverticulitis of the colon with hemorrhage" using the main term "Hemorrhage, gastrointestinal," you will find 578.9. When you reference 578.9 in the Tabular, you will find a long list of *Excludes*. Note that in the list of *Excludes* is "diverticulitis, intestine: large (562.13)." This means that you cannot assign 578.9, gastrointestinal hemorrhage, when there is a mention of diverticulitis of the intestine, as in the above example.

578 Gastrointestinal hemorrhage

EXCLUDES *that with mention of:*
angiodysplasia of stomach and duodenum (537.83)
angiodysplasia of intestine (569.85)
diverticulitis, intestine:
large (562.13)
small (562.03)
diverticulosis, intestine:
large (562.12)
small (562.02)
gastritis and duodenitis (535.0-535.6)
ulcer:
duodenum, gastric, gastrojejunal, or peptic (531.00-534.91)

If you are coding a diagnosis of gastrointestinal (GI) hemorrhage with any of the listed Excludes diagnoses, and if the GI hemorrhage is due to the GI condition, only the combination code should be assigned.

Example

Diagnosis: Gastrointestinal hemorrhage due to acute antral ulcer

Index: **Ulcer, ulcerated, ulcerating, ulceration, ulcerative** 707.9,
antral—*see* ulcer, stomach, stomach (eroded) (peptic) (round) 531.9, acute 531.3, with hemorrhage 531.0

Tabular: **531 Gastric ulcer**

531.0 Acute with hemorrhage

Code 531.0 is not a complete code. You must assign a fifth digit. There is no mention of obstruction in the diagnosis, so the fifth digit assigned would be 0, without mention of obstruction, 531.00.

Referencing hemorrhage in the Index, you are directed to 578 again and you note that the Excludes notes indicate not to code gastrointestinal hemorrhage with mention of gastric ulcer. So no further code is needed, as the hemorrhage is included in the code for the ulcer (531.00).

Index: **Hemorrhage, hemorrhagic** (nontraumatic) 459.0

gastrointestinal (tract) 578.9

Tabular: **578 Gastrointestinal hemorrhage**

EXCLUDES *that with mention of:*
Ulcer:
duodenal, gastric, gastrojejunal, or peptic (531.00-534.91)

Code: 531.00 Gastrointestinal hemorrhage due to acute antral ulcer

---

CODING SHOT For a hemorrhage to be coded, there does not have to be active bleeding; however, there must be documentation in the medical record that supports the fact that active bleeding has occurred and the physician must identify the source of bleeding for the combination code to be assigned.

From the Trenches

"If you enjoy working with numbers and solving mysteries—and you have that fundamental need to do what is right for the patient, then coding could be an option for you. Those things are inherent, no matter where you go in the profession."

JOHN

It is so important to verify code assignment in the Tabular. It is only when you check the Tabular that you can know for certain about the Includes and *Excludes*, which are not listed anywhere else. So be certain to always, always check the Tabular before assigning a code.

EXERCISE 15-26 *Diseases of the Digestive System*

Fill in the codes for the following:

1 Appendicitis with peritonitis

Code(s): _____

2 Gastrointestinal bleeding due to acute duodenal ulcer

Code(s): _____

3 Acute and chronic cholecystitis with cholelithiasis

Code(s): _____

4 Gastroenteritis

Code(s): _____

5 Gastroesophageal reflux

Code(s): _____

Diseases of the Genitourinary System

Chapter 10, Diseases of the Genitourinary System, in the Tabular includes conditions and diseases of the male and female genital organs and urinary tract. Disorders of the breast (categories 610-611) are also included in the chapter.

Once again, when you are dealing with infections of the urinary tract or the genital organs, you are instructed to use an additional code to identify the organism.

Example

Diagnosis: Acute prostatitis due to *Streptococcus*

Index: **Prostatitis** (congestive) (suppurative) 601.9

acute 601.0

Tabular: **601 Inflammatory diseases of prostate**

601.0 Acute prostatitis

Index:	**Infection, infected, infective** (opportunistic)
	streptococcal NEC 041.00
Tabular:	**041 Bacterial infection in conditions classified elsewhere and of unspecified site**
	041.0 Streptococcus
	041.00 Streptococcus, unspecified
Codes:	601.0, 041.00 Acute prostatitis due to *Streptococcus*

EXERCISE 15–27 *Diseases of the Genitourinary System*

Fill in the codes for the following diagnostic statements:

1 Pelvic inflammatory disease (PID)

    Code(s): _____

2 Hematuria

    Code(s): _____

3 Acute and chronic pyelonephritis

    Code(s): _____

4 Benign prostatic hypertrophy (BPH)

    Code(s): _____

5 Fibrocystic breast disease

    Code(s): _____

Complications of Pregnancy, Childbirth, and the Puerperium

Chapter 11, Complications of Pregnancy, Childbirth, and the Puerperium, of the Tabular is probably the most difficult chapter from which to code. One reason is that pregnancy and childbirth are natural functions, and physicians often overlook documentation of diagnoses that should be coded. Another reason is that there is extensive use of multiple coding in the chapter. Also, fifth-digit assignment for pregnancy is often difficult to determine. There are instructions throughout this chapter that must be read thoroughly. Obstetric coding can also be difficult because you may not use this chapter as frequently as some of the other chapters, so you won't be as familiar with the special notes and coding instructions.

CODING SHOT An ectopic pregnancy is one in which the fertilized ovum implants outside the uterus, usually in the fallopian tube. Ectopic and Molar Pregnancy (630-633) contains instructions to use an additional code from category 639 to identify any complication(s).

Category 639, Complications following abortion and ectopic and molar pregnancies, are used to report genital tract and pelvic infection (639.0), delayed or excessive hemorrhage (639.1), damage to pelvic organ and tissue (639.2), renal failure (639.3), metabolic disorder (639.4), shock (639.5), embolism (639.6), and other specified complications (639.8), or unspecified complications (639.9). You cannot use 639, Complications, with any code from categories 634-638 (abortion) because the complications for the abortion are classified according to the fourth-digit subcategory codes. Examples are 635 Legally induced abortion, 635.1 Complicated by delayed or excessive hemorrhage. As stated previously, you use 639, Complications, to identify any complications related to codes 630-633. You also use 639, Complications, when the complication is the reason for the medical care, and the abortion, ectopic, or molar pregnancy was taken care of during a previous episode.

Complications related mainly to pregnancy (640-649) designate fifth-digit subclassifications that are of special note:

0 unspecified as to episode of care or not applicable
1 delivered, with or without mention of antepartum condition
2 delivered, with mention of postpartum complication
3 antepartum condition or complication
4 postpartum condition or complication

The fifth digit 0 is used when an abortion is due to or associated with a complication included in the chapter. To use the fifth digits 1 and 2, a delivery must have occurred during that stay. The 1 is assigned to cases in which an antepartum condition has or has not been noted. The fifth digits 3 and 4 are used when no delivery has occurred during that stay or visit. The 3 is used for antepartum conditions, and the 4 for postpartum conditions. When you review the categories and subcategories throughout the chapter, you will note that many subcategories may indicate that you can use only certain fifth digits with a particular code. For example, with code 641.1, Hemorrhage from placenta previa, the only fifth digits that can be used are 0, 1, or 3. Neither 2 nor 4 can be used because placenta previa occurs **before** a baby is delivered and 2 and 4 are assigned **after** delivery.

When coding multiple diagnoses from one inpatient stay, certain combinations of fifth digits are used to classify that stay or visit. These fifth-digit combinations are:

1 only, or with 2; NOT with 0, 3, or 4
2 only, or with 1; NOT with 0, 3, or 4
3 only, NOT with 0, 1, 2, or 4
4 only, NOT with 0, 1, 2, or 4

Category 650, Normal delivery, cannot be used with any other code that falls within the range 630-676 because these codes refer to other than normal delivery. Code 650 is used only when all of the following are documented:

▪ A full-term, single liveborn infant is delivered.
▪ There are no antepartum or postpartum conditions classifiable to 630-676 (other than normal delivery).
▪ The presentation is cephalic, requiring minimal assistance and without fetal manipulation or the use of instrumentation.
▪ An episiotomy can be performed.

Most deliveries do not fit the above criteria for a 650 Normal Delivery code assignment.

Category V27 Outcome of delivery can be assigned as an additional code to the mother's record. This is indexed under the term "Outcome."

CODING SHOT It may be helpful to code the mother's and baby's records at the same time. Conditions documented on the birth certificate may appear on the newborn's record but may not appear on the mother's record. As always, the individual record must support the codes assigned, so additional documentation may have to be obtained from the physician.

OFFICIAL GUIDELINES FOR CODING AND REPORTING

SECTION I. C. 11. b. Selection of OB Principal or First-listed Diagnosis

3) Episodes when no delivery occurs

In episodes when no delivery occurs, the principal diagnosis should correspond to the principal complication of the pregnancy, which necessitated the encounter. Should more than one complication exist, all of which are treated or monitored, any of the complication codes may be sequenced first.

Example

Diagnosis:	Iron deficiency anemia complicating pregnancy, antepartum
Index:	**Pregnancy** (single) (uterine) (without sickness) V22.2
	complicated (by) 646.9
	anemia (conditions classifiable to 280-285) 648.2
Tabular:	**648.2 Anemia**

This code is not complete because it lacks fifth digit assignment and there are instructions to Use additional code(s) to identify the **condition**, which means to identify the type of anemia. The ICD-9-CM information indicates that you can assign fifth digits 0-4. No delivery has occurred and the condition is stated as being antepartum; therefore, the fifth digit 3 is assigned, 648.23. The next step is to locate the additional code to identify the type of anemia.

Index:	**Anemia** 285.9, deficiency 281.9, iron (Fe) 280.9
Tabular:	**280.9 Iron deficiency anemia, unspecified**
Codes:	648.23, 280.9 Iron deficiency anemia complicating pregnancy, antepartum

The first code, 648.23, indicates that the anemia is a complication of the pregnancy, and the second code, 280.9, provides greater specificity as to the type of anemia as being iron deficiency anemia.

Chapter 4 can be somewhat confusing at the beginning because there is an *Excludes* note that states, "anemia complicating pregnancy or the puerperium (648.2)." In Chapter 11 you are directed to "Also code the condition." This means that anemias are assumed to be complications of pregnancy and you should follow the instructions given for code 648.2. The code from the obstetric chapter would be sequenced first, followed by the anemia code.

OFFICIAL GUIDELINES FOR CODING AND REPORTING

SECTION I. C. 11. Complications of Pregnancy, Childbirth, and the Puerperium (630-677)

a. General Rules for Obstetric Cases

1) Codes from Chapter 11 and sequencing priority

Obstetric cases require codes from Chapter 11, codes in the range 630-677, Complications of Pregnancy, Childbirth, and the Puerperium. Chapter 11 codes have sequencing priority over codes from other chapters. Additional codes from other chapters may be used in conjunction with chapter 11 codes to further specify conditions. Should the provider document that the pregnancy is incidental to the encounter, then code V22.2 should be used in place of any chapter 11 codes. It is the provider's responsibility to state that the condition being treated is not affecting the pregnancy.

2) Chapter 11 codes used only on the maternal record

Chapter 11 codes are to be used only on the maternal record, never on the record of the newborn.

3) Chapter 11 fifth-digits

Categories 640-648, 651-676 have required fifth-digits, which indicate whether the encounter is antepartum, postpartum and whether a delivery has also occurred.

4) Fifth-digits, appropriate for each code

The fifth-digits, which are appropriate for each code number, are listed in brackets under each code. The fifth-digits on each code should all be consistent with each other. That is, should a delivery occur all of the fifth-digits should indicate the delivery.

b. Selection of OB Principal or First-Listed Diagnosis

1) Routine oupatient prenatal visits

For routine outpatient prenatal visits when no complications are present codes V22.0, Supervision of normal first pregnancy, and V22.1, Supervision of other normal pregnancy, should be used as the first-listed diagnoses. These codes should not be used in conjunction with chapter 11 codes.

2) Prenatal outpatient visits for high-risk patients

For prenatal outpatient visits for patients with high-risk pregnancies, a code from category V23, Supervision of high-risk pregnancy, should be used as the first-listed diagnosis. Secondary chapter 11 codes may be used in conjunction with these codes if appropriate.

3) Episodes when no delivery occurs

In episodes when no delivery occurs, the principal diagnosis should correspond to the principal complication of the pregnancy, which necessitated the encounter. Should more than one complication exist, all of which are treated or monitored, any of the complications codes may be sequenced first.

4) When a delivery occurs

When a delivery occurs, the principal diagnosis should correspond to the main circumstances or complication of the delivery. In cases of cesarean delivery, the selection of the principal diagnosis should correspond to the reason the cesarean delivery was performed unless the reason for admission/encounter was unrelated to the condition resulting in the cesarean delivery.

5) Outcome of delivery

An outcome of delivery code, V27.0-V27.9, should be included on every maternal record when a delivery has occurred. These codes are not to be used on subsequent records or on the newborn record.

c. Fetal Conditions Affecting the Management of the Mother

1) Codes from category 655

Known or suspected fetal abnormality affecting management of the mother, and category 656, Other fetal and placental problems affecting the management of the mother, are assigned only when the fetal condition is actually responsible for modifying the management of the mother, i.e., by requiring diagnostic studies, additional observation, special care, or termination of pregnancy. The fact that the fetal condition exists does not justify assigning a code from this series to the mother's record.

inpatient/outpatient

2) In utero surgery

In cases when surgery is performed on the fetus, a diagnosis code from category 655, Known or suspected fetal abnormalities affecting management of the mother, should be assigned identifying the fetal condition. Procedure code 75.36, Correction of fetal defect, should be assigned on the hospital inpatient record.

No code from Chapter 15, the perinatal codes, should be used on the mother's record to identify fetal conditions. Surgery performed in utero on a fetus is still to be coded as an obstetric encounter.

d. HIV Infection in Pregnancy, Childbirth and the Puerperium

During pregnancy, childbirth or the puerperium, a patient admitted because of an HIV-related illness should receive a principal diagnosis of 647.6X, Other specified infectious and parasitic diseases in the mother classifiable elsewhere, but complicating the pregnancy, childbirth or the puerperium, followed by 042 and the code(s) for the HIV-related illness(es). Patients with asymptomatic HIV infection status admitted during pregnancy, childbirth, or the puerperium should receive codes of 647.6X and V08.

inpatient

e. Current Conditions Complicating Pregnancy

Assign a code from subcategory 648.x for patients that have current conditions when the condition affects the management of the pregnancy, childbirth, or the puerperium. Use additional secondary codes from other chapters to identify the conditions, as appropriate.

inpatient/outpatient

f. Diabetes mellitus in pregnancy

Diabetes mellitus is a significant complicating factor in pregnancy. Pregnant women who are diabetic should be assigned code 648.0x, Diabetes mellitus complicating pregnancy, and a secondary code from category 250, Diabetes mellitus, to identify the type of diabetes. Code V58.67, Long-term (current) use of insulin, should also be assigned if the diabetes mellitus is being treated with insulin.

g. Gestational diabetes

Gestational diabetes can occur during the second and third trimester of pregnancy in women who were not diabetic prior to pregnancy. Gestational diabetes can cause complications in the pregnancy similar to those of preexisting diabetes mellitus. It also puts the woman at greater risk of developing diabetes after the pregnancy. Gestational diabetes is coded to 648.8x, Abnormal glucose tolerance. Codes 648.0x and 648.8x should never be used together on the same record.

Code V58.67, Long-term (current) use of insulin, should also be assigned if the gestational diabetes is being treated with insulin.

h. Normal Delivery, Code 650

1) Normal delivery

Code 650 is for use in cases when a woman is admitted for a full-term normal delivery and delivers a single, healthy infant without any complications antepartum, during the delivery, or postpartum during the delivery episode. Code 650 is always a principal diagnosis. It is not to be used if any other code from chapter 11 is needed to describe a current complication of the antenatal, delivery, or perinatal period. Additional

inpatient

inpatient

codes from other chapters may be used with code 650 if they are not related to or are in any way complicating the pregnancy.

2) Normal delivery with resolved antepartum complication
Code 650 may be used if the patient had a complication at some point during her pregnancy, but the complication is not present at the time of the admission for delivery.

3) V27.0, Single liveborn, outcome of delivery
V27.0, Single liveborn, is the only outcome of delivery code appropriate for use with 650.

inpatient/outpatient

i. The Postpartum and Peripartum Periods

1) Postpartum and peripartum periods
The postpartum period begins immediately after delivery and continues for six weeks following delivery. The peripartum period is defined as the last month of pregnancy to five months postpartum.

2) Postpartum complication
A postpartum complication is any complication occurring within the six-week period.

3) Pregnancy-related complications after 6-week period
Chapter 11 codes may also be used to describe pregnancy-related complications after the six-week period should the provider document that a condition is pregnancy related.

4) Postpartum complications occurring during the same admission as delivery
Postpartum complications that occur during the same admission as the delivery are identified with a fifth digit of "2." Subsequent admissions/encounters for postpartum complications should be identified with a fifth digit of "4."

5) Admission for routine postpartum care following delivery outside hospital
When the mother delivers outside the hospital prior to admission and is admitted for routine postpartum care and no complications are noted, code V24.0, Postpartum care and examination immediately after delivery, should be assigned as the principal diagnosis.

6) Admission following delivery outside hospital with postpartum conditions
A delivery diagnosis code should not be used for a woman who has delivered prior to admission to the hospital. Any postpartum conditions and/or postpartum procedures should be coded.

inpatient/outpatient

j. Code 677, Late effect of complication of pregnancy

1) Code 677
Code 677, Late effect of complication of pregnancy, childbirth, and the puerperium is for use in those cases when an initial complication of a pregnancy develops a sequelae requiring care or treatment at a future date.

2) After the initial postpartum period
This code may be used at any time after the initial postpartum period.

3) Sequencing of Code 677
This code, like all late effect codes, is to be sequenced following the code describing the sequelae of the complication.

inpatient/outpatient

k. Abortions

1) Fifth-digits required for abortion categories
Fifth-digits are required for abortion categories 634-637. Fifth-digit 1, incomplete, indicates that all of the products of conception have not been expelled from the uterus. Fifth-digit 2, complete, indicates that all products of conception have been expelled from the uterus prior to the episode of care.

2) Code from categories 640-648 and 651-659

A code from categories 640-648 and 651-659 may be used as additional codes with an abortion code to indicate the complication leading to the abortion.

Fifth digit 3 is assigned with codes from these categories when used with an abortion code because the other fifth digits will not apply. Codes from the 660-669 series are not to be used for complications of abortion.

3) Code 639 for complications

Code 639 is to be used for all complications following abortion. Code 639 cannot be assigned with codes from categories 634-638.

4) Abortion with Liveborn Fetus

When an attempted termination of pregnancy results in a liveborn fetus assign code 644.21, Early onset of delivery, with an appropriate code from category V27, Outcome of Delivery. The procedure code for the attempted termination of pregnancy should also be assigned.

5) Retained Products of Conception following an abortion

Subsequent admissions for retained products of conception following a spontaneous or legally induced abortion are assigned the appropriate code from category 634, Spontaneous abortion, or 635 Legally induced abortion, with a fifth digit of "1" (incomplete). This advice is appropriate even when the patient was discharged previously with a discharge diagnosis of complete abortion.

EXERCISE 15–28 *Complications of Pregnancy, Childbirth, and the Puerperium*

Fill in the codes for the following:

1 Blighted ovum

🌐 Code(s): _____

2 Incomplete spontaneous abortion; dilation and curettage (D&C) performed

🌐 Code(s): _____

3 False labor of 38-week pregnancy, undelivered

🌐 Code(s): _____

4 Vaginal delivery of liveborn single infant with fourth-degree perineal laceration; obstetric laceration repaired (include appropriate V code for outcome of delivery)

🌐 Code(s): _____

5 Obstructed labor due to cephalopelvic disproportion; liveborn single infant delivered by lower segment cesarean section

🌐 Code(s): _____

Diseases of the Skin and Subcutaneous Tissue

Chapter 12, Diseases of the Skin and Subcutaneous Tissue, in the Tabular describes diseases or conditions of the integumentary system. This chapter is one of the shorter chapters in the ICD-9-CM manual. When reviewing the first categories listed, such as 681, 682, and 683, you will note that multiple coding may be necessary for some conditions.

Example

Diagnosis: Cellulitis right small finger due to *Staphylococcus aureus*

Index: **Cellulitis** (diffuse) (with lymphangitis) (*see also* abscess) 682.9, finger (intrathecal) (periosteal) (subcutaneous) (subcuticular) 681.00

Tabular: **681 Cellulitis and abscess of finger and toe**

         681.0 Finger

         681.00 Cellulitis and abscess, unspecified

There is an instructional note that directs you to identify the organism when assigning code 681.00. To locate the code for the causative organism you look up the main term "Infection" in the Index.

Index: **Infection, infected, infective** (opportunistic) 136.9, staphylococcal, NEC 041.10, aureus 041.11

Tabular: **041 Bacterial infection in conditions classified elsewhere and of unspecified site**

         041.1 Staphylococcus

         041.11 Staphylococcus aureus

The Tabular states, "Use additional code, if desired, to identify organism, such as *Staphylococcus* (041.1)." Code 041.1 must have a fifth-digit assignment before it can be assigned, and you would know this only if you verified the code in the Tabular and found that the five-digit code 041.11 specifies *Staphylococcus aureus*.

Code(s):   681.00, 041.11 Cellulitis right small finger due to *Staphylococcus aureus*

The code for the organism is used as an additional code and is sequenced after the disease or condition.

EXERCISE 15–29   *Diseases of the Skin and Subcutaneous Tissue*

Fill in the codes for the following:

1 Pruritus

   Code(s): _____

2 Heat rash

   Code(s): _____

3 Psoriasis

   Code(s): _____

4 Decubitus ulcer buttock

   Code(s): _____

5 Dermatitis due to poison ivy

   Code(s): _____

Diseases of the Musculoskeletal System and Connective Tissue

Chapter 13, Diseases of the Musculoskeletal System and Connective Tissue, in the Tabular describes diseases or conditions of the bone, joints, and muscles. It is important to refer to the note at the beginning of the chapter because that is where you will find the information on the fifth-digit subclassifications that are used for categories 711-712, 715-716, 718-719, and 730. If you turn to category 711, you will see the fifth-digit subclassifications again, but not in the same detail as is found at the beginning of the chapter.

Example

Diagnosis:	Pyogenic arthritis of the wrist
Index:	**Arthritis**, arthritic (acute) (chronic) (subacute), 716.9 pyogenic or pyemic 711.0
Tabular:	**711 Arthropathy associated with infections**
	711.0 Pyogenic arthritis

Code 711.0 is not a valid code until you assign a fifth digit to indicate the site. When reviewing the subclassifications, you must identify whether the wrist is part of the forearm or part of the hand. You need to refer to that note at the beginning of the chapter, where you will note that fifth digit "3 forearm includes the radius, ulna and wrist joint."

Code:	711.03 Pyogenic arthritis of the wrist

Pathologic, or spontaneous, fractures are also coded in Chapter 13. A pathologic, or spontaneous, fracture is a break in a bone that occurs because of a bone disease or a change surrounding the bone tissue that makes the bone weak. For a pathologic fracture, you code the fracture and the disease process responsible for the fracture, such as osteoporosis or metastatic cancer of the bone. It is possible to have a small trauma associated with a pathologic fracture. Suppose, for example, an elderly woman with severe osteoporosis bumps her hip against the doorway and sustains a fractured hip. This would be classifiable as a pathologic fracture because a person with healthy bones would not fracture a hip as the result of a small trauma such as bumping the hip on a doorway. If there is any question about whether a fracture is pathologic or due to trauma, ask the physician what caused the fracture.

A pathologic fracture is serious because healing may be delayed by the underlying bone disease. Also, if a pathologic fracture is documented and no other disease process is indicated, review the record or clarify with the physician the underlying cause of the fracture.

Example

Diagnosis:	Pathologic fracture of the hip due to severe osteoporosis
Index:	**Fracture** (abduction) (adduction) (avulsion) (compression) (crush) (dislocation) (oblique) (separation) (closed) 829.0, pathologic (cause unknown) 733.10, hip 733.14
Tabular:	**733.1 Pathologic fracture**
	733.14 Pathologic fracture of neck of femur

Now, a second code will identify the underlying disease.

Index:	**Osteoporosis** (generalized) 733.00
Tabular:	**733.0 Osteoporosis**
	733.00 Osteoporosis, unspecified
Codes:	733.14, 733.00 Pathologic fracture of the hip due to severe osteoporosis

---

The instructions for category 730, Osteomyelitis, periostitis, and other infections involving bone, direct you to identify any organism as an additional code. It is easy to miss the instructions when they are stuck between an *Excludes* note and the list of fifth-digit subclassifications. Highlight these instructions in your ICD-9-CM until you become familiar with their use when coding in this area. Any additional information you can add to your code book to make you a better coder—add it.

EXERCISE 15–30 *Diseases of the Musculoskeletal System and Connective Tissue*

Fill in the codes for the following:

1 Rheumatoid arthritis

Code: _____

2 Pain in the neck

Code: _____

3 Recurrent dislocation, right shoulder

Code: _____

4 Spontaneous fracture left humerus due to metastatic bone cancer; history of cancer of the breast previously excised

Code(s): _____ _____ _____

Congenital Anomalies and Certain Conditions Originating in the Perinatal Period

Chapters 14 and 15, Congenital Anomalies and Certain Conditions Originating in the Perinatal Period, in the Tabular describe congenital anomalies and conditions that originate in the perinatal period. An **anomaly** is an abnormality of a structure or organ. **Congenital** means that it is an abnormality that one was born with. Some anomalies are noticeable and so are discovered at birth. In cases of other anomalies, it may be a number of months or even years before they are discovered. If there is any question about whether a condition is acquired or congenital, you can review the record or clarify the case with the physician.

The perinatal period extends through the 28 days following birth. The term perinatal applies only to the baby and **postpartum** applies to the mother. Codes from this chapter can still be used beyond that time frame, but as the chapter title indicates, the condition must have originated during the perinatal period.

OFFICIAL GUIDELINES FOR CODING AND REPORTING

SECTION I. C. 15. Newborn (Perinatal) Guidelines (760-779)

For coding and reporting purposes the perinatal period is defined as before birth through the 28th day following birth. The following guidelines are provided for reporting purposes. Hospitals may record other diagnoses as needed for internal data use.

a. General Perinatal Rule
1) Chapter 15 Codes
They are <u>never</u> for use on the maternal record. Codes from Chapter 11, the obstetric chapter, are never permitted on the newborn record. Chapter 15 codes may be used throughout the life of the patient if the condition is still present.

inpatient

2) Sequencing of perinatal codes

Generally, codes from Chapter 15 should be sequenced as the principal/first-listed diagnosis on the newborn record, with the exception of the appropriate V30 code for the birth episode, followed by codes from any other chapter that provide additional detail. The "use additional code" note at the beginning of the chapter supports this guideline. If the index does not provide a specific code for a perinatal condition, assign code 779.89, Other specified conditions originating in the perinatal period, followed by the code from another chapter that specifies the condition. Codes for signs and symptoms may be assigned when a definitive diagnosis has not been established.

3) Birth process or community acquired conditions

If a newborn has a condition that may be either due to the birth process or community acquired and the documentation does not indicate which it is, the default is due to the birth process and the code from Chapter 15 should be used. If the condition is community-acquired, a code from Chapter 15 should not be assigned.

4) Code all clinically significant conditions

All clinically significant conditions noted on routine newborn examination should be coded. A condition is clinically significant if it requires:

- clinical evaluation; or
- therapeutic treatment; or
- diagnostic procedures; or
- extended length of hospital stay; or
- increased nursing care and/or monitoring; or
- has implications for future health care needs

Note: The perinatal guidelines listed above are the same as the general coding guidelines for "additional diagnoses", except for the final point regarding implications for future health care needs. Codes should be assigned for conditions that have been specified by the provider as having implications for future health care needs. Codes from the perinatal chapter should not be assigned unless the provider has established a definitive diagnosis.

b. Use of Codes V30-V39

When coding the birth of an infant, assign a code from categories V30-V39, according to the type of birth. A code from this series is assigned as a principal diagnosis, and assigned only once to a newborn at the time of birth.

c. Newborn Transfers

If the newborn is transferred to another institution, the V30 series is not used at the receiving hospital.

d. Use of Category V29

1) Assigning a code from category V29

Assign a code from category V29, Observation and evaluation of newborns and infants for suspected conditions not found, to identify those instances when a healthy newborn is evaluated for a suspected condition that is determined after study not to be present. Do not use a code from category V29 when the patient has identified signs and symptoms of a suspected problem; in such cases, code the sign or symptom.

A code from category V29 may also be assigned as a principal code for readmissions or encounters when the V30 code no longer applies. Codes from category V29 are for use only for healthy newborns and infants for which no condition after study is found to be present.

2) V29 code on a birth record

A V29 code is to be used as a secondary code after the V30, Outcome of delivery, code.

e. Use of other V codes on perinatal records

V codes other than V30 and V29 may be assigned on a perinatal or newborn record code. The codes may be used as a principal or first-listed diagnosis for specific types of encounters or for readmissions or encounters when the V30 code no longer applies.

See Section I.C.18 for information regarding the assignment of V codes.

f. Maternal Causes of Perinatal Morbidity

Codes from categories 760-763, Maternal causes of perinatal morbidity and mortality, are assigned only when the maternal condition has actually affected the fetus or newborn. The fact that the mother has an associated medical condition or experiences some complication of pregnancy, labor or delivery does not justify the routine assignment of codes from these categories to the newborn record.

g. Congenital Anomalies in Newborns

For the birth admission, the appropriate code from category V30, Liveborn infants according to type of birth, should be used, followed by any congenital anomaly codes, categories 740-759. Use additional secondary codes from other chapters to specify conditions associated with the anomaly, if applicable.

Also, see Section I.C.14 for information on the coding of congenital anomalies.

h. Coding of Additional Perinatal Diagnoses

1) Assigning codes for conditions that require treatment

Assign codes for conditions that require treatment or further investigation, prolong the length of stay, or require resource utilization.

2) Codes for conditions specfied as having implications for future health care needs

Assign codes for conditions that have been specified by the provider as having implications for future health care needs.

Note: This guideline should not be used for adult patients.

3) Codes for newborn conditions originating in the perinatal period

Assign a code for newborn conditions originating in the perinatal period (categories 760-779), as well as complications arising during the current episode of care classified in other chapters, only if the diagnoses have been documented by the responsible provider at the time of transfer or discharge as having affected the fetus or newborn.

i. Prematurity and Fetal Growth Retardation

Providers utilize different criteria in determining prematurity. A code for prematurity should not be assigned unless it is documented. The 5th digit assignment for codes from category 764 and subcategories 765.0 and 765.1 should be based on the recorded birth weight and estimated gestational age.

A code from subcategory 765.2, Weeks of gestation, should be assigned as an additional code with category 764 and codes from 765.0 and 765.1 to specify weeks of gestation as documented by the provider in the record.

j. Newborn sepsis

Code 771.81, Septicemia [sepsis] of newborn, should be assigned with a secondary code from category 041, Bacterial infections in conditions classified elsewhere and of unspecified site, to identify the organism. It is not necessary to use a code from subcategory 995.9, Systemic inflammatory response syndrome (SIRS), on a newborn record. A code from category 038, Septicemia, should not be used on a newborn record. Code 771.81 describes the sepsis.

As Guideline Section I. C. 15. b. states, code the birth from categories V30-V39, Liveborn infant according to type of birth. This code is used only once on the birth record because it indicates the type of birth.

On the baby's birth record the appropriate V code is sequenced first as the principal diagnosis. If any other conditions or congenital anomalies are documented, they are coded as secondary diagnoses.

Example

Diagnosis: Newborn male delivered in the hospital by cesarean section and with Down's syndrome

Index: **Newborn** (infant) (liveborn), single, born in hospital (without mention of cesarean delivery or section) V30.00; with cesarean delivery or section V30.01

Tabular: **V30 Single liveborn**

The code is not complete until you have coded it to the fourth and fifth digit subclassifications. The fourth digit is "0" for born in the hospital and the fifth digit is "1" for delivered by cesarean delivery. The code would be V30.01. Now you need to code the Down's syndrome.

Index: **Syndrome**—*see also* disease, Down's (mongolism) 758.0

Tabular: **758 Chromosomal anomalies**

758.0 Down's syndrome

Codes: V30.01, 758.0 Newborn male delivered by cesarean section in the hospital; Down's syndrome.

In the preceding example, if that baby was transferred to a second facility for treatment of the Down's syndrome, no V code would be used by the second facility to identify delivery. The V code can be used only once, as the principal diagnosis at the birthing facility. The principal diagnosis code would be Down's syndrome (758.0) at the second facility.

You have to be careful about assigning codes from the 760-763 categories, Maternal Causes of Perinatal Morbidity and Mortality. Many times the mother has a condition, but that condition has no untoward (negative) effect on the baby or fetus. Codes from these categories are to be used only when the maternal condition has **affected** the health of the newborn.

EXERCISE 15–31 *Congenital Anomalies and Certain Conditions Originating in the Perinatal Period*

Fill in the codes for the following:

1 Congenital absence of the earlobe

Code: _____

2 Newborn male delivered in the hospital via vaginal delivery; undescended left testicle (will reevaluate in 6 weeks)

Code(s): _____ _____

3 Three-year-old diagnosed with fragile X syndrome

⊛ Code(s): _____

4 Newborn transferred to a facility because of congenital dislocation of right hip (code as the facility transferred to)

⊛ Code(s): _____

Symptoms, Signs, and Ill-Defined Conditions

Chapter 16, Symptoms, Signs, and Ill-Defined Conditions, in the Tabular includes symptoms, signs, abnormal results of investigations and other ill-defined conditions. Signs and symptoms codes are used for encounters until a definitive diagnosis can be made.

You use the codes from Chapter 16 when

- no more specific diagnosis can be made after investigation
- signs and symptoms existing at the time of the initial encounter prove to be transient, or a cause cannot be determined
- a patient fails to return and all you have is a provisional diagnosis
- a case is referred elsewhere before a definitive diagnosis can be made
- a more precise diagnosis is not available for any other reason
- certain symptoms that represent important problems in medical care exist and it might be desirable to classify them in addition to the known cause

You do not code from Chapter 16 when a definitive diagnosis is available. Consider, for example, this diagnostic statement: "Right lower quadrant abdominal pain due to acute appendicitis." The code for right lower quadrant abdominal pain is 789.03, which is located in Chapter 16. But because the reason for the pain is the acute appendicitis, you would not include the code for the symptom of abdominal pain, rather you would assign 540.9 for the acute appendicitis, which is the definitive diagnosis.

You do not code from Chapter 16 when the symptom is considered to be routinely associated with the disease process. Consider, for example, this diagnostic statement: "Cough and fever with pneumonia." Both cough and fever are symptoms of the pneumonia; therefore, you would not assign codes for either symptom. The only code you would assign is 486 for the pneumonia.

A disease reference book comes in handy until you become more familiar with disease symptoms. If you do not know which symptoms are associated with a given disease, look them up in a reference or ask a colleague.

Finding the codes for **abnormal investigations** in the Index is a little tricky. The codes are found under the main term "Findings, abnormal, without diagnosis (examination) (laboratory test)." Some entries may also be found under the main term "Elevation," such as blood pressure and body temperature.

Example

Diagnosis: Abnormal liver scan

Index: **Findings, abnormal, without diagnosis** (examination) (laboratory test) 796.4, scan NEC 794.9, liver 794.8

Tabular: **794 Nonspecific abnormal results of function studies**
794.8 Liver

Code: 794.8 Abnormal liver scan

EXERCISE 15–32 *Symptoms, Signs, and Ill-Defined Conditions*

Fill in the codes for the following:

1 Fussy infant

Code: _____

2 Pleuritic-type chest pain

Code: _____

3 Abnormal mammogram

Code: _____

4 Seizure

Code: _____

5 Elevated blood pressure reading

Code: _____

Injury and Poisoning

OFFICIAL GUIDELINES FOR CODING AND REPORTING

inpatient/outpatient

SECTION I. C. 19. Supplemental Classification of External Causes of Injury and Poisoning (E-codes, E800-E999)

Introduction: These guidelines are provided for those who are currently collecting E codes in order that there will be standardization in the process. If your institution plans to begin collecting E codes, these guidelines are to be applied. The use of E codes is supplemental to the application of ICD-9-CM diagnosis codes. E codes are never to be recorded as principal diagnoses (first-listed in the non-inpatient setting) and are not required for reporting to CMS.

External causes of injury and poisoning codes (E codes) are intended to provide data for injury research and evaluation of injury prevention strategies. E codes capture how the injury or poisoning happened (cause), the intent (unintentional or accidental; or intentional, such as suicide or assault), and the place where the event occurred.

Some major categories of E codes include:

transport accidents

poisoning and adverse effects of drugs, medicinal substances and biologicals

accidental falls

accidents caused by fire and flames

accidents due to natural and environmental factors

late effects of accidents, assaults or self-injury

assaults or purposely inflicted injury

suicide or self inflicted injury

These guidelines apply for the coding and collection of E codes from records in hospitals, outpatient clinics, emergency departments, other ambulatory care settings and provider offices, and nonacute care settings, except when other specific guidelines apply.

a. General E Code Coding Guidelines

1) Used with any code in the range of 001-V84.8
An E code may be used with any code in the range of 001-V84.8 which indicates an injury, poisoning, or adverse effect due to an external cause.

2) Assign the appropriate E code for all initial treatments
Assign the appropriate E code for the initial encounter of an injury, poisoning, or adverse effect of drugs, not for subsequent treatment.
External cause of injury codes (E-codes) may be assigned while the acute fracture codes are still applicable.
See Section I.C.17.b.1 for coding of acute fractures.

3) Use the full range of E codes

Use the full range of E codes to completely describe the cause, the intent, and the place of the occurrence, if applicable, for all injuries, poisonings, and adverse effects of drugs.

4) Assign as many E codes as necessary

Assign as many E codes as necessary to fully explain each cause. If only one E code can be recorded, assign the E code most related to the principal diagnosis.

5) The selection of the appropriate E code

The selection of the appropriate E code is guided by the Index to External Causes, which is located after the alphabetical index to diseases and by Inclusion and Exclusion notes in the Tabular List.

6) E code can never be a principal diagnosis

An E code can never be a principal (first listed) diagnosis.

7) External cause code(s) with systemic inflammatory response syndrome (SIRS)

An external cause code is not appropriate with a code from subcategory 995.9, unless the patient also has an injury, poisoning, or adverse effect of drugs.

b. Place of Occurrence Guideline

Use an additional code from category E849 to indicate the Place of Occurrence for injuries and poisonings. The Place of Occurrence describes the place where the event occurred and not the patient's activity at the time of the event.

Do not use E849.9 if the place of occurrence is not stated.

c. Adverse Effects of Drugs, Medicinal, and Biological Substances Guidelines

1) Do not code directly from the Table of Drugs

Do not code directly from the Table of Drugs and Chemicals. Always refer back to the Tabular List.

2) Use as many codes as necessary to describe

Use as many codes as necessary to describe completely all drugs, medicinal or biological substances.

3) If the same E code would describe the causative agent

If the same E code would describe the causative agent for more than one adverse reaction, assign the code only once.

4) If two or more drugs, medicinal or biological substances

If two or more drugs, medicinal or biological substances are reported, code each individually unless the combination code is listed in the Table of Drugs and Chemicals. In that case, assign the E code for the combination.

5) When a reaction results from the interaction of a drug(s)

When a reaction results from the interaction of a drug(s) and alcohol, use poisoning codes and E codes for both.

6) If the reporting format limits the number of E codes

If the reporting format limits the number of E codes that can be used in reporting clinical data, code the one most related to the principal diagnosis. Include at least one from each category (cause, intent, place) if possible.

If there are different fourth digit codes in the same three digit category, use the code for "Other specified" of that category. If there is no "Other specified" code in that category, use the appropriate "Unspecified" code in that category.

If the codes are in different three-digit categories, assign the appropriate E code for other multiple drugs and medicinal substances.

7) Codes from the E930-E949 series

Codes from the E930-E949 series must be used to identify the causative substance for an adverse effect of drug, medical and biological substances, correctly prescribed and properly administered. The effect, such as tachycardia, delirium, gastrointestinal hemorrhaging, vomiting, hypokalemia, hepatitis, renal failure, or respiratory failure, is coded and followed by the appropriate code from the E930-E949 series.

d. Multiple Cause E Code Coding Guidelines

If two or more events cause separate injuries, an E code should be assigned for each cause. The first listed E code will be selected in the following order:

E codes for child and adult abuse take priority over all other E codes. *See Section I.C.19.e. Child and Adult Abuse Guidelines*

E codes for terrorism events take priority over all other E codes except child and adult abuse

E codes for cataclysmic events take priority over all other E codes except child and adult abuse and terrorism.

E codes for transport accidents take priority over all other E codes except cataclysmic events and child and adult abuse and terrorism.

The first-listed E code should correspond to the cause of the most serious diagnosis due to an assault, accident, or self-harm, following the order of hierarchy listed above.

e. Child and Adult Abuse Guidelines

1) Intentional injury

When the cause of an injury or neglect is intentional child or adult abuse, the first listed E code should be assigned from categories E960-E968, Homicide and injury purposely inflicted by other persons (except category E967). An E code from category E967, Child and adult battering and other maltreatment, should be added as an additional code to identify the perpetrator, if known.

2) Accidental intent

In cases of neglect when the intent is determined to be accidental, E code E904.0, Abandonment or neglect of infant and helpless person, should be the first listed E code.

f. Unknown or Suspected Intent Guidelines

1) If the intent (accident, self-harm, assault) of the cause of an injury or poisoning is unknown

If the intent (accident, self-harm, assault) of the cause of an injury or poisoning is unknown or unspecified, code the intent as undetermined E980-E989.

2) If the intent (accident, self-harm, assault) of the cause of an injury or poisoning is questionable

If the intent (accident, self-harm, assault) of the cause of an injury or poisoning is questionable, probable or suspected, code the intent as undetermined E980-E989.

g. Undetermined Cause

When the intent of an injury or poisoning is known, but the cause is unknown, use codes E928.9, Unspecified accident, E958.9, Suicide and self-inflicted injury by unspecified means, and E968.9, Assault by unspecified means.

These E codes should rarely be used, as the documentation in the medical record, in both the inpatient outpatient, and other settings, should normally provide sufficient detail to determine the cause of the injury.

h. Late Effects of External Cause Guidelines

1) Late effect E codes

Late effect E codes exist for injuries and poisonings but not for adverse effects of drugs, misadventures, and surgical complications.

   2) Late effect E codes (E929, E959, E969, E977, E989, or E999.1)

     A late effect E code (E929, E959, E969, E977, E989, or E999.1) should be used with any report of a late effect or sequela resulting from a previous injury or poisoning (905-909).

   3) Late effect E code with a related current injury

     A late effect E code should never be used with a related current nature of injury code.

   4) Use of late effect E codes for subsequent visits

     Use a late effect E code for subsequent visits when a late effect of the initial injury or poisoning is being treated. There is no late effect E code for adverse effects of drugs.

     Do not use a late effect E code for subsequent visits for follow-up care (e.g., to assess healing, to receive rehabilitative therapy) of the injury or poisoning when no late effect of the injury has been documented.

i. Misadventures and Complications of Care Guidelines

   1) Code range E870-E876

     Assign a code in the range of E870-E876 if misadventures are stated by the provider.

   2) Code range E878-E879

     Assign a code in the range of E878-E879 if the provider attributes an abnormal reaction or later complication to a surgical or medical procedure, but does not mention misadventure at the time of the procedure as the cause of the reaction.

j. Terrorism Guidelines

   1) Cause of injury identified by the Federal Government (FBI) as terrorism

     When the cause of an injury is identified by the Federal Government (FBI) as terrorism, the first-listed E-code should be a code from category E979, Terrorism. The definition of terrorism employed by the FBI is found at the inclusion note at E979. The terrorism E-code is the only E-code that should be assigned. Additional E codes from the assault categories should not be assigned.

   2) Cause of an injury is suspected to be the result of terrorism

     When the cause of an injury is suspected to be the result of terrorism a code from category E979 should not be assigned. Assign a code in the range of E codes based circumstances on the documentation of intent and mechanism.

   3) Code E979.9, Terrorism, secondary effects

     Assign code E979.9, Terrorism, secondary effects, for conditions occurring subsequent to the terrorist event. This code should not be assigned for conditions that are due to the initial terrorist act.

   4) Statistical tabulation of terrorism codes

     For statistical purposes these codes will be tabulated within the category for assault, expanding the current category from E960-E969 to include E979 and E999.1.

Chapter 17, Injury and Poisoning, in the Tabular is a very long chapter that includes the codes that range from 800 to 999. At the beginning of this chapter there are notes that provide you with specific instructions for the entire chapter. A recent addition to this chapter is the statement that coders should "Use E code(s) to identify the cause and intent of the injury or poisoning (E800-E999)." You learned how to assign E codes in Chapter 14.

There are numerous guidelines that pertain to injuries and poisonings. See Figs. 15–4 through 15–6.

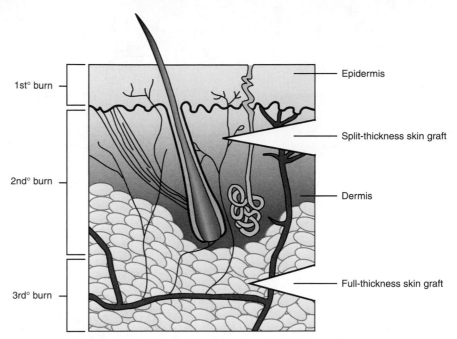

FIGURE 15–4 First-, second-, and third-degree burns.

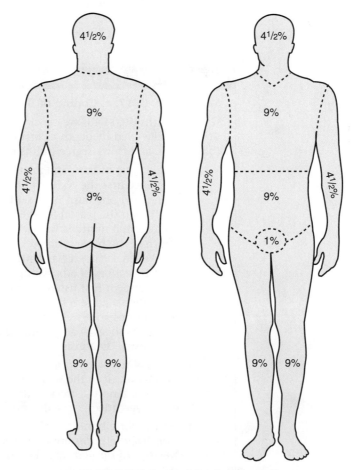

FIGURE 15–5 Rule of nines, adult.

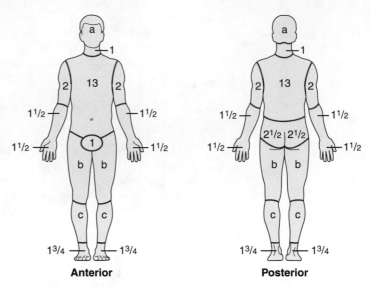

Anterior   **Posterior**

Relative percentage of body surface areas (% BSA) affected by growth

	0 yr	1 yr	5 yr	10 yr	15 yr
a – 1/2 of head	9 1/2	8 1/2	6 1/2	5 1/2	4 1/2
b – 1/2 of 1 thigh	2 3/4	3 1/4	4	4 1/4	4 1/2
c – 1/2 of lower leg	2 1/2	2 1/2	2 3/4	3	3 1/4

FIGURE 15–6 Lund-Browder chart for estimating the extent of burns on children.

OFFICIAL GUIDELINES FOR CODING AND REPORTING

SECTION I. C. 17. c. Coding of Burns

Current burns (940-948) are classified by depth, extent and by agent (E code). Burns are classified by depth as first degree (erythema), second degree (blistering), and third-degree (full-thickness involvement).

1) Sequencing of burn and related condition codes
   Sequence first the code that reflects the highest degree of burn when more than one burn is present.
   a. When the reason for the admission or encounter is for treatment of external multiple burns, sequence first the code that reflects the burn of the highest degree.
   b. When a patient has both internal and external burns, the circumstances of admission govern the selection of the principal diagnosis or first-listed diagnosis.
   c. When a patient is admitted for burn injuries and other related conditions such as smoke inhalation and/or respiratory failure, the circumstances of admission govern the selection of the principal or first-listed diagnosis.

2) Burns of the same local site
   Classify burns of the same local site (three-digit category level, 940-947) but of different degrees to the subcategory identifying the highest degree recorded in the diagnosis *[as is illustrated in Fig. 15–4].*

3) Non-healing burns
   Non-healing burns are coded as acute burns.
   Necrosis of burned skin should be coded as a non-healed burn.

4) Code 958.3, Posttraumatic wound infection
   Assign code 958.3, Posttraumatic wound infection, not elsewhere classified, as an additional code for any documented infected burn site.

inpatient/outpatient

inpatient/outpatient

5) Assign separate codes for each burn site

When coding burns, assign separate codes for each burn site. Category 946 Burns of Multiple specified sites, should only be used if the locations of the burns are not documented.

Category 949, Burn, unspecified, is extremely vague and should rarely be used.

6) Assign codes from category 948, Burns

Burns classified according to extent of body surface involved, when the site of the burn is not specified or when there is a need for additional data. It is advisable to use category 948 as additional coding when needed to provide data for evaluating burn mortality, such as that needed by burn units. It is also advisable to use category 948 as an additional code for reporting purposes when there is mention of third-degree burn involving 20 percent or more of the body surface.

In assigning a code from category 948:

Fourth-digit codes are used to identify the percentage of total body surface involved in a burn (all degree).

Fifth-digits are assigned to identify the percentage of body surface involved in third-degree burn.

Fifth-digit zero (0) is assigned when less than 10 percent or when no body surface is involved in a third-degree burn.

Category 948 is based on the classic "rule of nines" *[as illustrated in Figs. 15–5 and 15–6]* in estimating body surface involved: head and neck are assigned nine percent, each arm nine percent, each leg 18 percent, the anterior trunk 18 percent, posterior trunk 18 percent, and genitalia one percent. Providers may change these percentage assignments when necessary to accommodate infants and children who have proportionately larger heads than adults and patients who have large buttocks, thighs, or abdomen that involve burns.

7) Encounters for treatment of late effects of burns

Encounters for the treatment of the late effects of burns (i.e., scars or joint contractures) should be coded to the residual condition (sequelae) followed by the appropriate late effect code (906.5-906.9). A late effect E code may also be used, if desired.

8) Sequelae with a late effect code and current burn

When appropriate, both a sequela with a late effect code, and a current burn code may be assigned on the same record (when both a current burn and sequelae of an old burn exist).

d. Coding of Debridement of Wounds, Infection, or Burn

Excisional debridement involves surgical removal or cutting away, as opposed to a mechanical (brushing, scrubbing, washing) debridement.

For coding purposes, excisional debridement is assigned to code 86.22. Nonexcisional debridement is assigned to code 86.28.

C. 17. Injury and Poisoning (800-999)

a. Coding of Injuries

When coding injuries, assign separate codes for each injury unless a combination code is provided, in which case the combination code is assigned. Multiple injury codes are provided in ICD-9-CM, but should not be assigned unless information for a more specific code is not available. These codes are not to be used for normal, healing surgical wounds or to identify complications of surgical wounds.

The code for the most serious injury, as determined by the provider, and the focus of treatment, is sequenced first.

1) Superficial injuries

Superficial injuries such as abrasions or contusions are not coded when associated with more severe injuries of the same site.

inpatient/outpatient

2) Primary injury with damage to nerves/blood vessels
When a primary injury results in minor damage to peripheral nerves or blood vessels, the primary injury is sequenced first with additional code(s) from categories 950-957, Injury to nerves and spinal cord, and/or 900-904, Injury to blood vessels. When the primary injury is to the blood vessels or nerves, that injury should be sequenced first.

b. Coding of Traumatic Fractures
The principle of multiple coding of injuries should be followed in coding fractures. Fractures of specified sites are coded individually by site in accordance with both the provisions within categories 800-829 and the level of detail furnished by medical record content. Combination categories for multiple fractures are provided for use when there is insufficient detail in the medical record (such as trauma cases transferred to another hospital), when the reporting form limits the number of codes that can be used in reporting pertinent clinical data, or when there is insufficient specificity at the fourth-digit or fifth-digit level. More specific guidelines are as follows:

1) Acute Fractures vs. Aftercare
Traumatic fractures are coded using the acute fracture codes (800-829) while the patient is receiving active treatment for the fracture. Examples of active treatment are: surgical treatment, emergency department encounter, and evaluation and treatment by a new physician.

Fractures are coded using the aftercare codes (subcategories V54.0, V54.1, V54.8, or V54.9) for encounters after the patient has completed active treatment of the fracture and is receiving routing care for the fracture during the healing or recovery phase. Examples of fracture aftercare are: cast change or removal, removal of external or internal fixation device, medication adjustment, and follow up visits following fracture treatment.

Care for complications of surgical treatment for fracture repairs during the healing or recovery phase should be coded with the appropriate complication codes.

Care of complications of fractures, such as malunion and nonunion, should be reported with the appropriate codes.

Pathologic fractures are not coded in the 800-829 range, but instead are assigned to subcategory 733.1. *See Section I.C.13.a for additional information.*

2) Multiple fractures of same limb
Multiple fractures of same limb classifiable to the same three-digit or four-digit category are coded to that category.

3) Multiple unilateral or bilateral fractures of same bone
Multiple unilateral or bilateral fractures of same bone(s) but classified to different fourth-digit subdivisions (bone part) within the same three-digit category are coded individually by site.

4) Multiple fracture categories 819 and 828
Multiple fracture categories 819 and 828 classify bilateral fractures of both upper limbs (819) and both lower limbs (828), but without any detail at the fourth-digit level other than open and closed type of fracture.

5) Multiple fractures sequencing
Multiple fractures are sequenced in accordance with the severity of the fracture. The provider should be asked to list the fracture diagnoses in the order of severity.

Fracture is the first section in the chapter and it contains the codes assigned for fractures caused by trauma. A fracture not indicated as closed or open should be classified as closed. If you have any doubt, check with the physician as to the nature of the fracture. A dislocation and fracture of the same bone would be coded to the fracture site because that is the highest level of specificity and fracture is more severe than dislocation. You are also instructed in the Index to see fracture by site. The cross-reference "see" is a mandatory instruction that tells you to go to Fracture and not to code the dislocation separately. When you locate the main term "dislocation" in the Index, you are directed to "see Fracture, by site." You locate Fracture in the Index on the basis of the anatomic location of the fracture.

Examples

Diagnosis: Fracture, right patella with abrasions of the site

Index: **Fracture**, patella (closed) 822.0

Tabular: **822 Fracture of patella**

 822.0 Closed

Code(s): 822.0 Fracture, right patella with abrasions of the site

When a fracture is not specified as open or closed, assign a code that indicates a closed fracture. You would not assign a code for the abrasions when there is a more severe injury (the fracture) at the same site, as in the following example.

Diagnosis: Fractured hip with dislocation

Index: **Dislocation**, with fracture—*see* Fracture by site.

The "*see* Fracture by site" means the dislocation is included with the fracture code.

Index: **Fracture**, hip (closed) 820.8

Tabular: **820 Fracture of neck of femur**

 820.8 Unspecified part of neck of femur, closed

Code(s): 820.8 Fractured hip with dislocation

The guidelines for **burns** direct you to sequence the highest degree of burn first. If you are coding a third-degree burn of the hand and a second-degree burn of the chest wall, you would sequence the code for the third-degree burn of the hand first, followed by the second-degree burn of the chest.

If different degrees of burns are documented at the same site, assign a code to the highest degree only. If, for example, the patient has first- and second-degree burns to the hand, you would code only the second-degree burn to the hand because that is the highest level of specificity and the most severe.

Facilities may choose to capture data regarding the extent of body area burned. In this case, the rule of nines is applied (refer to Figs. 15–5 and 15–6). The Index entry is "Burn . . . 949.0" with a note indicating that the fifth digit is added to indicate the extent of body surface involved (in percentage).

Burns are located in the Index by referring to the main term "Burn," subterms according to the site (abdomen or thigh), and finally to the degree of burn (second or third).

Codes from the 948 category can be used alone or in combination with other specific burn codes. The inclusion of codes from 948 are important for statistical purposes and may affect reimbursement. The use of the three-digit code 948 indicates a burn condition. The **fourth** digit indicates the **total percentage** of the body that has been burnt—including all first-, second-, and third-degree burns. The **fifth** digit (0-9) indicates the percentage of the body that has received **third-degree** burns. It is not the coder's job to calculate the percentages, but you should seek clarification from the physician if documentation is missing or unclear.

Examples

Diagnosis: First- and second-degree burn to the back

Index: **Burn,** back, second degree 942.24

Tabular: **942 Burn of trunk**

               942.2 Blisters, epidermal [second degree]

A fifth digit is used to indicate the specific location of the burn to the trunk. In this case, the fifth digit 4 is used to indicate the location, back, 942.24.

Code(s):   942.24 First- and second-degree burn to the back

Note that the diagnosis includes first- and second-degree burns and the code assigned indicates second-degree burns: You code only the highest degree when the burns are at the same site.

Diagnosis: Second-degree burn, 1%, chin, and third-degree burn, 3%, scapular region, for a total of 4% of the body

Index: **Burn,** chin, second 941.24

Tabular: **941 Burn of face, head, and neck**

               941.2 Blisters, epidermal loss [second degree]

A fifth digit is used to indicate the specific location of the burn to the face, head, or neck. In this case, the fifth digit 4 is used to indicate the location, chin, 941.24. Now, to code the burn to the scapular region:

Index: **Burn,** scapular region, third degree 943.36

Tabular: **943 Burn of upper limb, except wrist and hand**

               943.3 Full thickness skin loss [third degree NOS]

A fifth digit is used to indicate the specific location of the burn. In this case, the fifth digit 6 is used to indicate the location, scapular region, 943.36.

But wait! You need one more code to finish coding this example—one to indicate the body surface involved.

Index: **Burn,** extent, less than 10%, 948.0

Tabular: **948.0 Burn [any degree] involving less than 10% of body surface**

The fifth digit "0" is required to indicate less than 10% total body surface was involved, 948.00.

Code(s):   943.36, 941.24, 948.00 Third-degree burn, scapular region, and second-degree burn, chin; with the 948.00 indicating that there is less than 10% third-degree burn on less than 10% of the body surface.

E codes for burns are assigned, as per facility policy, for all initial treatments.

EXERCISE 15–33 *Burns*

Code the burn, extent of the body surface involved, and percentage of body surface burned using the rule of nines.

1 A 3-year-old receives third-degree burns of the abdomen, 10%, and second-degree burns of the thigh, 5%, after pulling a pot of hot water on herself

   Third-degree Code: _____ Second-degree Code: _____

   E Code: _____ Degree and Percentage Code:_____

2 Infected third-degree burn, left thigh, 4½%, subsequent treatment

   Code(s): _____ _____ _____

3 First- and second-degree burn, right foot, 2¼%, due to bonfire

 🌀 Code(s): _____

4 Non-healing third-degree burn, right hand, 2¼%; excisional debridement performed by physician; patient seen 10 days ago for initial treatment

 🌀 Code(s): _____

5 Second-degree burn, right forearm, 2%; first-degree burn, right little finger, 4%; and third-degree burn, right chest wall, 5%, subsequent treatment

 🌀 Code(s): _____

Wounds (lacerations) are found under the main term "Wound." There are three subcategories in some of the wound codes. These injuries can be classified as

1. Without mention of complication
2. Complicated
3. With tendon involvement

A **complicated wound** is one that includes documentation of delayed healing, delayed treatment, foreign body, or primary infection.

QUICK CHECK 15-4

In the Index under Wound, there is information included for coding:
a. Penetrating wounds of internal organs
b. Insect bites
c. Crush injuries
d. All of the above

Example

Diagnosis:	Infected wound of the right knee
Index:	**Wound**, knee 891.0, complicated 891.1
Tabular:	**891 Open wound of knee, leg [except thigh], and ankle**
	891.1 Complicated
Codes:	891.1 Infected wound of the right knee

The coding of adverse effects and poisonings is probably the most difficult part of this chapter. It takes some practice to distinguish between an adverse effect and a poisoning. Because the physician is probably not going to use those specific terms in the diagnostic statement, you must question the physician if you are uncertain whether the diagnosis is an adverse effect or a poisoning.

OFFICIAL GUIDELINES FOR CODING AND REPORTING

SECTION I. C. 17. E. Adverse Effects, Poisoning, and Toxic Effects

The properties of certain drugs, medicinal and biological substances, or combinations of such substances, may cause toxic reactions. The occurrence of drug toxicity is classified in ICD-9-CM as follows:

inpatient/outpatient

1) Adverse Effect

When the drug was correctly prescribed and properly administered, code the reaction plus the appropriate code from the E930-E949 series. Codes from E930-E949 series must be used to identify the causative substance for adverse effect of drug, medicinal and biological substances correctly prescribed and properly administered. The effect, such as tachycardia, delirium, gastrointestinal hemorrhaging, vomiting, hypokalemia, hepatitis, renal failure, or respiratory failure, is coded and followed by the appropriate code from E930-E949 series.

Adverse effects of therapeutic substances correctly prescribed and properly administered (toxicity, synergistic reaction, side effect, and idiosyncratic reaction) may be due to (1) differences among patients, such as age, sex, disease, and genetic factors, and (2) drug-related factors, such as type of drug, route of administration, duration of therapy, dosage, and bioavailability.

An **adverse effect** occurs when a drug has been correctly prescribed and properly administered and the patient develops a reaction. Everything has been done correctly by the physician and the patient, but a reaction or adverse effect has occurred because of the drug.

When coding adverse effects, you code the **effect** first, followed by the E code from the **therapeutic** column in the Table of Drugs and Chemicals. (You use the therapeutic column because the medication was prescribed by the physician as a therapy for a condition.)

Example

Diagnosis:	Urticaria due to penicillin (properly taken and prescribed)
Index:	**Urticaria** 708.9, due to, drugs 708.0
Tabular:	**708 Urticaria**
	708.0 Allergic urticaria

You now need to code the drug using the Table of Drugs and Chemicals.

Table of Drugs:	Penicillin (any type) E930.0
Tabular:	**E930 Antibiotics**
	E930.0 Penicillins
Codes:	708.0, E930.0 Urticaria due to penicillin

The code for the effect (urticaria, 708.0) is listed first and the cause (penicillin, E930.0) next.

The E codes from this section (E930-E949) are considered required E codes. Thus, therapeutic E codes for adverse effects must be assigned. E codes are never assigned as a principal diagnosis but are always considered an additional code.

There is a code available for an **unknown adverse effect.** For example, if the physician has documented a reaction due to penicillin and you cannot determine from the record what the exact adverse effect has been, you would code unknown adverse effect. Adverse effects can be found in the Index under the main term "Effect, adverse," and the subterm "drugs and medicinals correct substance properly taken 995." The correct codes for an unknown adverse effect due to penicillin are 995.20 and E930.0.

A **poisoning** occurs when drugs or other chemical substances are taken not according to a physician's instruction. Poisonings occur in a variety of ways:

■ The wrong dosage is given in error, either during medical treatment or by nonmedical personnel such as the mother or the patient herself or himself.

■ The medication is given to the wrong person.

■ The medication is taken by the wrong person.

■ A medication overdose has occurred.

■ Medications (prescription or over-the-counter) have been taken in combination with alcohol or other recreational drugs.

■ Over-the-counter medications have been taken in combination with prescription medications without physician approval.

OFFICIAL GUIDELINES FOR CODING AND REPORTING

SECTION I. C. 17. E. 2. Poisoning

(a) Error was made in drug prescription
Error made in drug prescription or in the administration of the drug by provider, nurse, patient, or other person, use the appropriate poisoning code from the 960-979 series.

(b) Overdose of a drug intentionally taken
If an overdose of a drug was intentionally taken or administered and resulted in drug toxicity, it would be coded as a poisoning (960-979 series).

(c) Nonprescribed drug taken with corectly prescribed and properly administered drug
If a nonprescribed drug or medicinal agent was taken in combination with a correctly prescribed and properly administered drug, any drug toxicity or other reaction resulting from the interaction of the two drugs would be classified as a poisoning.

(d) Sequencing of poisoning
When coding a poisoning or reaction to the improper use of a medication (e.g., wrong dose, wrong substance, wrong route of administration) the poisoning code is sequenced first, followed by a code for the manifestation. If there is also a diagnosis of drug abuse or dependence to the substance, the abuse or dependence is coded as an additional code.
See Section I.C.3.a.6.b. if poisoning is the result of insulin pump malfunctions and Section I.C.19 for general use of E-codes.

inpatient/outpatient

Poisoning codes are found in the Table of Drugs and Chemicals. You must always sequence the poisoning code first, then code any manifestation of the poisoning, such as coma, second. You also assign the corresponding E code from the Table of Drugs and Chemicals. If there is no documentation to indicate otherwise, you use the E code from the accidental column.

 CAUTION *You CANNOT use an E code from the therapeutic column (E930-E940) with a poisoning code because they are mutually exclusive. Something that is therapeutic (intended for treatment) could not be a poisoning (harmful).*

Example

Diagnosis: Coma due to accidental overdose of Valium (Valium is the brand name for benzodiazepine)

When you look up the main term "Overdose" in the Index, you are referred to the Table of Drugs and Chemicals.

Table of Drugs:	Valium 969.4 (poisoning)
	E853.2 (accidental)
Tabular:	**969 Poisoning by psychotropic agents**
	969.4 Benzodiazepine-based tranquilizers
Tabular:	**E853 Accidental poisoning by tranquilizers**
	E853.2 Benzodiazepine-based tranquilizers
Index:	**Coma 780.01**
Tabular:	**780 General symptoms**
	780.01 Coma
Codes:	969.4, 780.01, E853.2 Coma due to accidental overdose of Valium. Note that the poisoning code (969.4) is sequenced first, followed by the manifestation (780.01) and then the E code.

If there has been no manifestation (coma, in the above case) of the poisoning, you would assign only the poisoning code (969.4) with the appropriate E code. When a patient undergoes a poisoning that involves more than one drug or chemical, there could be a different poisoning code and E code for each drug or chemical.

OFFICIAL GUIDELINES FOR CODING AND REPORTING

SECTION II. G. Complications of surgery and other medical care

When the admission is for treatment of a complication resulting from surgery or other medical care, the complication code is sequenced as the principal diagnosis. If the complication is classified to the 996-999 series and the code lacks the necessary specificity in describing the complication, an additional code for the specific complication should be assigned.

inpatient/outpatient

EXERCISE 15–34 *Injury/Poisoning and Complications*

In the Index, you will find complications of medical and surgical procedures under the main term "Complications." Locate "Complications" in the Index.

What code does the Index direct you to for the following complications?

1 Breast implants, infection

Code: _____

2 Bone marrow graft, rejection

Code: _____

3 Surgical procedures, stitch abscess

Code: _____

4 Cardiac pacemaker, (device) mechanical complication

Code: _____

When coding complications of surgical or medical care, you must be careful to be sure that actual complications are present. A surgical complication is one that takes place as a result of the procedure. Just because a complication occurs following a procedure does not mean the complication is a surgical complication. Do not assume a cause-and-effect relationship. Clarify any doubt or questions with the physician.

MORE GENERAL GUIDELINES

You have now reviewed all of the chapter-specific guidelines. However, there are a few more guidelines to consider.

OFFICIAL GUIDELINES FOR CODING AND REPORTING

SECTION III. Reporting Additional Diagnoses

The UHDDS item #11-b defines Other Diagnoses as "all conditions that coexist at the time of admission, that develop subsequently, or that affect the treatment received and/or the length of stay. Diagnoses that relate to an earlier episode which have no bearing on the current hospital stay are to be excluded." UHDDS definitions apply to inpatients in acute care, short-term, long term care and psychiatric hospital setting. The UHDDS definitions are used by acute care short-term hospitals to report inpatient data elements in a standardized manner. These data elements and their definitions can be found in the July 31, 1985, Federal Register (Vol. 50, No. 147), pp. 31038-40.

Since that time the application of the UHDDS definitions has been expanded to include all non-outpatient settings (acute care, short term, long term care and psychiatric hospitals; home health agencies; rehab facilities; nursing homes, etc).

inpatient

Reporting Other (Additional) Diagnoses

The general rule is that for reporting purposes, the term "other diagnoses" is interpreted to refer to additional conditions that affect patient care in terms of requiring:

- clinical evaluation
- therapeutic treatment
- diagnostic procedures
- extended length of hospital stay, or
- increased nursing care and/or monitoring

The listing of the diagnoses in the medical record is the responsibility of the attending physician.

OFFICIAL GUIDELINES FOR CODING AND REPORTING

SECTION III. INTRODUCTION (PARAGRAPH 3)

The following guidelines are to be applied in designating "other diagnoses" when neither the Alphabetic Index nor the Tabular List in ICD-9-CM provide direction. The listing of the diagnoses in the patient record is the responsibility of the attending provider.

A. Previous conditions

If the provider has included a diagnosis in the final diagnostic statement, such as the discharge summary or the face sheet, it should ordinarily be coded. Some providers include in the diagnostic statement resolved conditions or diagnoses and status-post procedures from previous admission that have no bearing on the current stay. Such conditions are not to be reported and are coded only if required by hospital policy.

However, history codes (V10-V19) may be used as secondary codes if the historical condition or family history has an impact on current care or influences treatment.

inpatient/outpatient

EXERCISE 15–35 *Previous Conditions*

Circle the conditions in the following diagnostic lists that would NOT be coded:

1 Herpes zoster

   History of hysterectomy

   Diabetes

2 Influenza

   Hypertension (currently controlled by medication)

   History of peptic ulcer disease

OFFICIAL GUIDELINES FOR CODING AND REPORTING

SECTION I. B. 7. Conditions that are an integral part of a disease process

Signs and symptoms that are associated routinely with a disease process should not be assigned as additional codes, unless otherwise instructed by the classification.

SECTION I. B. 8. Conditions that are not an integral part of a disease process

Additional signs and symptoms that may not be associated routinely with a disease process should be coded when present.

SECTION III. B. Abnormal findings

Abnormal findings (laboratory, x-ray, pathologic, and other diagnostic results) are not coded and reported unless the provider indicates their clinical significance. If the findings are outside the normal range and the attending provider has ordered other tests to evaluate the condition or prescribed treatment, it is appropriate to ask the provider whether the abnormal finding should be added.

   Please note: This differs from the coding practices in the outpatient setting for coding encounters for diagnostic tests that have been interpreted by a provider.

inpatient/outpatient

EXERCISE 15–36 *Other Diagnoses*

Circle the diagnoses that should NOT be coded:

1 Acute myocardial infarction

   Chest pain

   Shortness of breath

   Congestive heart failure

2 Fractured hip

   Hip pain

   Contusion of hip

In the following cases, would anemia be coded?

3 A patient is admitted with a fractured femur and undergoes an open reduction. Laboratory values following surgery show a hemoglobin level of 8 mg/dL. No additional workup is done or treatment provided.

_____

4 A patient is admitted for reduction of a hip fracture but receives two units of blood following two reports of hemoglobin volumes of 7 and 8 mg/dL.

_____

In the following case, would the potassium level be coded?

5 A patient with gastroenteritis has a blood sample drawn that shows low levels of potassium. The physician initials the test result but does not order potassium supplements or additional laboratory studies.

_____

DIAGNOSTIC CODING AND REPORTING GUIDELINES FOR OUTPATIENT SERVICES

The outpatient guidelines do not address specific sequencing or diseases as the inpatient guidelines do. Although it is not stated in the Guidelines, you will follow the inpatient coding guidelines in situations in which there are no clear outpatient coding guidelines. For example, in an outpatient setting, you would follow the hypertension guidelines and the sequencing of injuries according to severity as is done when following the inpatient guidelines.

OFFICIAL GUIDELINES FOR CODING AND REPORTING

Note: Any green text signifies edits for accuracy and is not included in the Official Guidelines for Coding and Reporting.

SECTION IV. Diagnostic Coding and Reporting Guidelines for Outpatient Services

These coding guidelines for outpatient diagnoses have been approved for use by hospitals/providers in coding and reporting hospital-based outpatient services and provider-based office visits.

Information about the use of certain abbreviations, punctuation, symbols, and other conventions used in the ICD-9-CM Tabular List (code numbers and titles) can be found Section IA of these guidelines, under "Conventions Used in the Tabular List." Information about the correct sequence to use in finding a code is described in Section I.

The terms encounter and visit are often used interchangeably in describing outpatient service contacts and, therefore, appear together in these guidelines without distinguishing one from the other.

Though the conventions and general guidelines apply to all settings, coding guidelines for outpatient and provider reporting of diagnoses will vary in a number of instances from those for inpatient diagnoses, recognizing that:

The Uniform Hospital Discharge Data Set (UHDDS) definition of principal diagnosis applies only to inpatients in acute, short-term, long-term care and psychiatric hospitals.

Coding guidelines for inconclusive diagnoses (probable, suspected, rule out, etc.) were developed for inpatient reporting and do not apply to outpatients.

A. Selection of first-listed condition

In the outpatient setting, the term first-listed diagnosis is used in lieu of principal diagnosis.

In determining the first-listed diagnosis the coding conventions of ICD-9-CM, as well as the general and disease specific guidelines take precedence over the outpatient guidelines.

Diagnoses often are not established at the time of the initial encounter/visit. It may take two or more visits before the diagnosis is confirmed.

The most critical rule involves beginning the search for the correct code assignment through the Alphabetic Index. Never begin searching initially in the Tabular List as this will lead to coding errors.

1. Outpatient Surgery
   When a patient presents for outpatient surgery, code the reason for the surgery as the first-listed diagnosis (reason for the encounter), even if the surgery is not performed due to a contraindication.

2. Observation Stay
   When a patient is admitted for observation for a medical condition, assign a code for the medical condition as the first-listed diagnosis. When a patient presents for outpatient surgery and develops complications requiring admission to observation, code the reason for the surgery as the first reported diagnosis (reason for the encounter), followed by codes for the complications as secondary diagnoses.

B. Codes from 001.0 through V84.8 (V86.1)
   The appropriate code or codes from 001.0 through V84.8 must be used to identify diagnoses, symptoms, conditions, problems, complaints, or other reason(s) for the encounter/visit.

C. Accurate reporting of ICD-9-CM diagnosis codes
   For accurate reporting of ICD-9-CM diagnosis codes, the documentation should describe the patient's condition, using terminology which includes specific diagnoses as well as symptoms, problems, or reasons for the encounter. There are ICD-9-CM codes to describe all of these.

D. Selection of codes 001.0 through 999.9
   The selection of codes 001.0 through 999.9 will frequently be used to describe the reason for the encounter. These codes are from the section of ICD-9-CM for the classification of diseases and injuries (e.g., infectious and parasitic diseases; neoplasms; symptoms, signs, and ill-defined conditions, etc.)

E. Codes that describe symptoms and signs
   Codes that describe symptoms and signs, as opposed to diagnoses, are acceptable for reporting purposes when a diagnosis has not been established (confirmed) by the provider. Chapter 16 of ICD-9-CM, Symptoms, Signs, and Ill-defined conditions (Conditions) (codes 780.0-799.9), contains many, but not all codes for symptoms.

F. Encounters for circumstances other than a disease or injury
   ICD-9-CM provides codes to deal with encounters for circumstances other than a disease or injury. The Supplementary Classification of factors (Factors) Influencing Health Status and Contact with Health Services (V01.0-V84.8) is provided to deal with occasions when circumstances other than a disease or injury are recorded as diagnosis or problems. *See Section I.C.18 for information on V-codes.*

G. Level of Detail in Coding

1. ICD-9-CM codes with 3, 4, or 5 digits
   ICD-9-CM is composed of codes with either 3, 4, or 5 digits. Codes with three digits are included in ICD-9-CM as the heading of a category of codes that may be further subdivided by the use of fourth and/or fifth digits, which provide greater specificity.

2. Use of full number of digits required for a code
   A three-digit code is to be used only if it is not further subdivided. Where fourth-digit subcategories and/or fifth-digit subclassifications are provided, they must be assigned. A code is invalid if it has not been coded to the full number of digits required for that code. *See also*

discussion under Section I.b.3., General Coding Guidelines, Level of Detail in Coding.

H. ICD-9-CM code for the diagnosis, condition, problem, or other reason for encounter/visit

List first the ICD-9-CM code for the diagnosis, condition, problem, or other reason for encounter/visit shown in the medical record to be chiefly responsible for the services provided. List additional codes that describe any coexisting conditions. In some cases the first-listed diagnosis may be a symptom when a diagnosis has not been established (confirmed) by the physician.

I. Uncertain Diagnosis

Do not code diagnoses documented as "probable", "suspected," "questionable," "rule out," or "working diagnosis" or other similar terms indicating uncertainty. Rather, code the condition(s) to the highest degree of certainty for that encounter/visit, such as symptoms, signs, abnormal test results, or other reason for the visit.

Please note: This differs from the coding practices used by short-term, acute care, long-term care, and psychiatric hospitals.

J. Chronic diseases

Chronic diseases treated on an ongoing basis may be coded and reported as many times as the patient receives treatment and care for the condition(s).

K. Code all documented conditions that coexist

Code all documented conditions that coexist at the time of the encounter/visit, and require or affect patient care treatment or management. Do not code conditions that were previously treated and no longer exist. However, history codes (V10-V19) may be used as secondary codes if the historical condition or family history has an impact on current care or influences treatment.

L. Patients receiving diagnostic services only

For patients receiving diagnostic services only during an encounter/visit, sequence first the diagnosis, condition, problem, or other reason for encounter/visit shown in the medical record to be chiefly responsible for the outpatient services provided during the encounter/visit. Codes for other diagnoses (e.g., chronic conditions) may be sequenced as additional diagnoses.

For encounters for routine laboratory/radiology testing in the absence of any signs, symptoms, or associated diagnosis, assign V72.5 to V72.6. If routine testing is performed during the same encounter as a test to evaluate a sign, symptom, or diagnosis, it is appropriate to assign both the V code and the code describing the reason for the non-routine test.

For outpatient encounters for diagnostic tests that have been interpreted by a physician, and the final report is available at the time of coding, code any confirmed or definitive diagnosis(es) documented in the interpretation. Do not code related signs and symptoms as additional diagnoses.

Please note: This differs from the coding practice in the hospital inpatient setting regarding abnormal findings on test results.

M. Patients receiving therapeutic services only

For patients receiving therapeutic services only during an encounter/visit, sequence first the diagnosis, condition, problem, or other reason for encounter/visit shown in the medical record to be chiefly responsible for the outpatient services provided during the encounter/visit. Codes for other diagnoses (e.g., chronic conditions) may be sequenced as additional diagnoses.

The only exception to this rule is that when the primary reason for the admission/encounter is chemotherapy, radiation therapy, or rehabilitation, the appropriate V code for the service is listed first, and the diagnosis or problem for which the service is being performed listed second.

N. Patients receiving preoperative evaluations only

For patients receiving preoperative evaluations only, sequence first a code from category V72.8, Other specified examinations, to describe the pre-op consultations. Assign a code for the condition to describe the reason for the outpatient

surgery as an additional diagnosis. Code also any findings related to the pre-op evaluation.

O. Ambulatory surgery

For ambulatory surgery, code the diagnosis for which the surgery was performed. If the postoperative diagnosis is known to be different from the preoperative diagnosis at the time the diagnosis is confirmed, select the postoperative diagnosis for coding, since it is the most definitive.

P. Routine outpatient prenatal visits

For routine outpatient prenatal visits when no complications are present, codes V22.0, Supervision of normal first pregnancy, or V22.1, Supervision of other normal pregnancy, should be used as the principal diagnosis. These codes should not be used in conjunction with chapter 11 codes.

Preoperative Clearance

Often a surgeon will want a preoperative clearance done by the patient's primary care provider, often due to a chronic or pre-existing condition. When the primary care provider is coding the diagnosis for this visit the first-listed code/primary diagnosis must be the appropriate V code to show the encounter is a preop clearance, then the condition code/diagnosis for the condition requiring surgery, followed by the condition requiring the clearance. The V code will be one of the following:

V72.81 Preoperative cardiovascular examination

V72.82 Preoperative respiratory examination

V72.83 Other specified preoperative examination

V72.84 Preoperative examination, unspecified

OVERVIEW OF ICD-10-CM AND ICD-10-PCS

Development of the ICD-10

The tenth edition of the *International Classification of Diseases* (ICD-10) was issued in 1993 by the World Health Organization (WHO), and WHO is responsible for maintaining it. The ICD-10 does not include a procedure classification (Volume 3). Each world government is responsible for adapting the ICD-10 to suit its own country's needs. For example, Australia uses the ICD-10-AM, that is, the ICD-10-Australian Modification. Each government is responsible for ensuring that its modifications conform with the WHO's conventions in the ICD-10. In the United States, the Centers for Medicare and Medicaid Services is responsible for developing the procedure classification entitled the ICD-10-PCS (PCS stands for Procedure Coding System). The National Center for Health Statistics (NCHS) is responsible for the disease classification system (Volumes 1 and 2) entitled ICD-10-CM (CM stands for Clinical Modification). The ICD-10-CM and ICD-10-PCS are scheduled for introduction sometime after the year 2010.

The ICD-10 is already widely used in Europe, but conversion to the new edition in the United States has taken a great deal of time to implement. One reason for the additional time needed for conversion is that the ICD-9-CM is the basis for the hospital billing system in the United States. In addition, Medicare Severity Diagnosis Related Groups (MS-DRG) is the prospective payment system in place for reimbursement of Medicare hospital inpatient stays, and the MS-DRG system is based on the ICD-9-CM.

At the time of publication of this textbook, the final versions of the ICD-10-CM and ICD-10-PCS had not been released. Therefore, all information presented here is based on the draft version of the ICD-10-CM.

Development of the ICD-10-CM to Replace the ICD-9-CM, Volumes 1 and 2

The ICD-10-CM will replace ICD-9-CM, Volumes 1 and 2. Prior to the implementation of the new edition, extensive consultation and review must take place with physician groups, clinical coders, and others. The NCHS has established a 20-member Technical Advisory Panel made up of representatives of the health care and coding communities to provide input during the development of the 10th edition.

Improvements in the ICD-10-CM. Notable improvements in the content and format of the ICD-10-CM include:

- the addition of information relevant to ambulatory and managed care encounters
- the expansion of injury codes

   Extensive expansion of the injury codes allows for greater specificity. For example, S50.351 is the new code for Superficial foreign body of right elbow.

- the creation of combination diagnosis/symptom codes to reduce the number of codes needed to fully describe a condition

   For example, I25.12 is the new code for Atherosclerotic heart disease with unstable angina. Under the ICD-9-CM, two codes are required to classify both diagnoses.

- the addition of a sixth character

   For example, S06.336 is the new code for Contusion and laceration of brainstem with prolonged [<24 hrs.] loss of consciousness . . .

- the incorporation of common fourth and fifth digit subclassifications

   For example, F10.04 is the new code for Alcohol abuse with alcohol-induced mood disorder.

- the updating and greater specificity of diabetes mellitus codes

   For example, E11.21 is the new code for Type 2 diabetes mellitus with nephropathy.

- the facilitation of providing greater specificity when assigning codes

Structure of the System. ICD-10-CM contains 21 chapters and excludes the supplementary classifications found in ICD-9-CM. The E and V codes of ICD-9-CM have been incorporated throughout the ICD-10-CM. Chapter titles in the ICD-10-CM remain the same except for the presence of two new chapters: Chapter VII, Diseases of the Eye and Adnexa, and Chapter VIII, Diseases of the Ear and Mastoid Process.

Crosswalk. As a part of the conversion, a **crosswalk** has been developed. This crosswalk converts ICD-9-CM codes to ICD-10-CM codes. Fig. 15–7 illustrates a section of the crosswalk. Sometimes, more than one ICD-10-CM code crosswalks from the ICD-9-CM code. In these instances, the possible matches are noted in a Best Match column. For example, in Fig. 15–7 the ICD-9-CM code 281.1, Vitamin B_{12} deficiency anemia NEC, has five possible matches with ICD-10-CM codes. In the Best Match column, the symbol "#a" indicates that the best match for 281.1 is ICD-10-CM code D51.9. Every ICD-9-CM code is crosswalked to ICD-10-CM code(s) in this way.

Index. The Index for the ICD-10-CM is alphabetic, as illustrated in Fig. 15–8. As in the ICD-9-CM, the ICD-10-CM index presents the main terms in bold type, and subterms indented under the main term. After the index entry, a code is provided. Sometimes, only the first four digits of the code are given. To ensure that you have chosen the correct code and/or to obtain the remaining digits, you must refer to the Tabular.

Tabular. The 21 chapters of the Tabular are arranged in numeric order after the first letter assigned to the chapter. For example, the letter R is assigned to the chapter regarding symptoms. Fig. 15–9 illustrates a portion of the chapter concerning symptoms. Note that in the index (see Fig. 15–8) the main entry is Abdomen, abdominal, and the first subterm is "acute," directing the coder to the Tabular location, R10.0. Now, note in the Tabular (Fig. 15–9) the location of R10.0 as Acute abdomen.

ICD-9-CM to ICD-10-CM Conversion
Diseases of the Blood and Blood-forming Organs
(pound sign (#) following ICD-10-CM code indicates the best match of one to many matches)

ICD-9-CM Code	ICD-9-CM Abbreviated Title	ICD-10-CM Code	Best Match	ICD-10-CM Abbreviated Title
280	IRON DEFICIENCY ANEMIAS			
280.0	IRON DEF ANEM DT BL LOSS	D50.0		CHRONIC BLOOD LOSS ANEMIA
280.1	IRON DEF ANEM DT DIET	D50.8		FE DEFICIENCY ANEMIA NEC
280.8	IRON DEFICIT ANEMIAS NEC	D50.1		SIDEROPENIC DYSPHAGIA
280.8	IRON DEFICIT ANEMIAS NEC	D50.8	#b	FE DEFICIENCY ANEMIA NEC
280.9	IRON DEFICIT ANEMIA NOS	D50.9		FE DEFICIENCY ANEMIA NOS
281	OTHER DEFICIENCY ANEMIAS			
281.0	PERNICIOUS ANEMIA	D51.0		PERNICIOUS ANEMIA
281.1	VIT B12 DEFIC ANEMIA NEC	D51.1		HEREDIT MEGALOBLAST ANEM
281.1	VIT B12 DEFIC ANEMIA NEC	D51.2		TRANSCOBALAMIN DEF ANEM
281.1	VIT B12 DEFIC ANEMIA NEC	D51.3		DIETARY B12 DEF ANEM NEC
281.1	VIT B12 DEFIC ANEMIA NEC	D51.8		B12 DEFICIENC ANEM NEC
281.1	VIT B12 DEFIC ANEMIA NEC	D51.9	#a	B12 DEFICIENC ANEM NOS

ICD-10-CM Best Match for 281.1

Best Match Designation

FIGURE 15–7 ICD-9-CM to ICD-10-CM Conversion (crosswalk). (Courtesy U.S. Department of Health and Human Services, Centers for Medicare and Medicaid Services.)

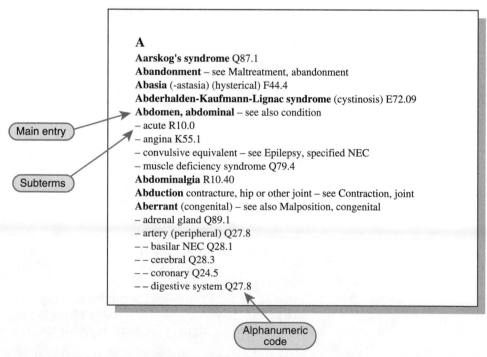

A

Aarskog's syndrome Q87.1
Abandonment – see Maltreatment, abandonment
Abasia (-astasia) (hysterical) F44.4
Abderhalden-Kaufmann-Lignac syndrome (cystinosis) E72.09
Abdomen, abdominal – see also condition
– acute R10.0
– angina K55.1
– convulsive equivalent – see Epilepsy, specified NEC
– muscle deficiency syndrome Q79.4
Abdominalgia R10.40
Abduction contracture, hip or other joint – see Contraction, joint
Aberrant (congenital) – see also Malposition, congenital
– adrenal gland Q89.1
– artery (peripheral) Q27.8
– – basilar NEC Q28.1
– – cerebral Q28.3
– – coronary Q24.5
– – digestive system Q27.8

Main entry

Subterms

Alphanumeric code

FIGURE 15–8 ICD-10-CM Index. (Courtesy U.S. Department of Health and Human Services, Centers for Medicare and Medicaid Services.)

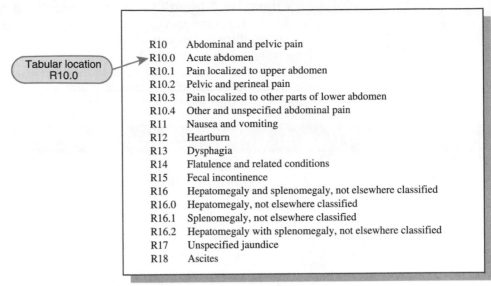

R10	Abdominal and pelvic pain
R10.0	Acute abdomen
R10.1	Pain localized to upper abdomen
R10.2	Pelvic and perineal pain
R10.3	Pain localized to other parts of lower abdomen
R10.4	Other and unspecified abdominal pain
R11	Nausea and vomiting
R12	Heartburn
R13	Dysphagia
R14	Flatulence and related conditions
R15	Fecal incontinence
R16	Hepatomegaly and splenomegaly, not elsewhere classified
R16.0	Hepatomegaly, not elsewhere classified
R16.1	Splenomegaly, not elsewhere classified
R16.2	Hepatomegaly with splenomegaly, not elsewhere classified
R17	Unspecified jaundice
R18	Ascites

Tabular location R10.0

FIGURE 15–9 ICD-10-CM Tabular. (Courtesy U.S. Department of Health and Human Services, Centers for Medicare and Medicaid Services.)

Development of the ICD-10-PCS to Replace the ICD-9-CM, Volume 3

The new structure will allow more expansion than was possible with the ICD-9-CM. Because the ICD-9-CM lacks specificity (exactness) and does not provide for sufficient expansion to support government payment systems and data needs, CMS contracted with 3M Health Information Systems to develop the ICD-10-PCS to replace the ICD-9-CM procedure codes for reporting inpatient procedures.

Four major objectives guided the development of ICD-10-PCS:

1. **Completeness.** There should be a unique code for all substantially different procedures. Currently, procedures performed on different body parts, using different approaches or of different types, are sometimes assigned the same code.

2. **Expandability.** As new procedures are developed, the structure of the ICD-10-PCS should allow for their incorporation as unique codes.

3. **Multiaxial.** ICD-10-PCS should have a structure such that each code character has, as much as possible, the same meaning, both within the specific procedure section and across procedure sections.

4. **Standardized terminology.** Although the meaning of a specific word can vary in common usage, ICD-10-PCS should not include multiple meanings for the same term; each term should be assigned a specific meaning, and ICD-10-PCS should include definitions of the terminology.

A complete, expandable, multiaxial ICD-10-PCS with standardized terminology will allow coding specialists to determine accurate codes with minimal effort.

The Seven Characters of the ICD-10-PCS

The ICD-10-PCS has a seven-character alphanumeric code structure. Each character has as many as 34 different values: 10 digits (0-9) and 24 letters (A-H, J-N, and P-Z) may be assigned to each character. The letters O and I are not used in order to avoid confusion with the digits 0 and 1. In the ICD-10-PCS, the term "procedure" is used to refer to the complete designation of the seven characters. Procedures are divided into sections according to the type of procedure.

Character 1 Identifies the Section. The first character of the procedure code identifies the section. To assign an ICD-10-PCS code, the section where the procedure is coded must be identified. For example, a chest x-ray is in the Imaging section, a breast biopsy is in the Medical and Surgical section, and crisis intervention is in the Mental Health section. Each section is identified by a specific character—number or letter. Section titles and numbers/letters are shown in Fig. 15–10.

EXERCISE 15–37 *ICD-10-PCS First Character*

Using Fig. 15–10, identify the first character that would be assigned to the following procedures:

1 _____ Gait training (Rehabilitation)

2 _____ Cesarean section (Obstetrics)

3 _____ Computerized tomography, spine (Imaging)

4 _____ Cholecystectomy (Medical/Surgical)

5 _____ Insertion of radium into cervix (brachytherapy) (Radiation Oncology)

6 _____ Cranioplasty (Medical/Surgical)

Changing Characters. Characters 2 through 7 have a standard meaning within each section but may have different meanings across sections. The meanings for each character are described in each section. For example, Fig. 15–11 shows the meanings of the seven characters for the Medical and Surgical sections, and Fig. 15–12 shows the meanings for the Imaging section. Notice that several characters have different meanings across these sections. For instance, the third character in medical and surgical procedures (Fig. 15–11) is used to define the root *operation* (extraction, insertion, removal, etc.), whereas the third character in imaging procedures (Fig. 15–12) is used to define the root *type* (fluoroscopy, MRI, CT, ultrasonography, etc.).

Sections

0	Medical and Surgical
1	Obstetrics
2	Placement
3	Administration
4	Measurement and Monitoring
5	Imaging
6	Nuclear Medicine
7	Radiation Oncology
8	Osteopathic
9	Rehabilitation and Diagnostic Audiology
B	Extracorporeal Assistance and Performance
C	Extracorporeal Therapies
D	Laboratory
F	Mental Health
G	Chiropractic
H	Miscellaneous

FIGURE 15–10 Sections of ICD-10-PCS. (Courtesy U.S. Department of Health and Human Services, Centers for Medicare and Medicaid Services.)

FIGURE 15-11 Medical and surgical procedures. (Courtesy U.S. Department of Health and Human Services, Centers for Medicare and Medicaid Services.)

1	2	3	4	5	6	7
Section	Body system	Root operation	Body part	Approach	Device	Qualifier

FIGURE 15-12 Imaging procedures. (Courtesy U.S. Department of Health and Human Services, Centers for Medicare and Medicaid Services.)

1	2	3	4	5	6	7
Section	Body system	Root type	Body part	Contrast	Contrast/Qualifier	Qualifier

 STOP *Each code must include seven characters. If a character is not applicable to a specific procedure, the letter Z is used.*

Character 2 Is the Body System. The second character identifies the body system in all sections except Rehabilitation and Mental Health. In these two sections, the second character identifies the type of procedure performed.

Character 3 Is the Root Operation. The third character identifies the root operation in all sections except Radiation Oncology, Rehabilitation, and Mental Health. In many sections, only a few root operations are performed, and these operations are defined for use in that section. The Medical and Surgical section uses an extensive list of root operations. The Obstetrics and Placement sections use some of these same root operations as well as section-specific root operations. See Table 15–1 for a list of the Medical and Surgical root operations definitions, explanations, and examples.

TABLE 15-1

MEDICAL AND SURGICAL ROOT OPERATIONS

0	Alteration	**Definition:** Modifying the natural anatomic structure of a body part without affecting the function of the body part
		Explanation: Principal purpose is to improve appearance.
		Examples: Face lift Breast augmentation
1	Bypass	**Definition:** Altering the route of passage of the contents of a tubular body part
		Explanation: Rerouting contents around an area of a body part to another distal (downstream) area in the normal route; to another different but similar route and body part; or to an abnormal route and another dissimilar body part.
		Encompasses: Diversion, reroute, shunt
		Examples: Gastrojejunal bypass Coronary artery bypass
2	Change	**Definition:** Taking out or off a device from a body part and putting back an identical or similar device in or on the same body part without cutting or puncturing the skin or a mucous membrane
		Explanation: Requires no invasive intervention
		Example: Change of a drainage tube
3	Control	**Definition:** Stopping, or attempting to stop, postprocedural bleeding
		Explanation: Confined to postprocedural bleeding and limited to the Anatomic Regions, Upper Extremities, and Lower Extremities Body Systems

Table continued on following page

TABLE 15–1

MEDICAL AND SURGICAL ROOT OPERATIONS (Continued)

		Examples: Control of postprostatectomy bleeding Control of postpneumonectomy bleeding
4	**Creation**	**Definition:** Making a new structure that does not physically take the place of a body part
		Explanation: Confined to sex change operations in which genitalia are made
		Encompasses: Formation
		Examples: Creation of an artificial vagina in a male Creation of an artificial penis in a female
5	**Destruction**	**Definition:** Eradicating all or a portion of a body part
		Explanation: The actual physical destruction of all or a portion of a body part by the direct use of energy, force, or a destructive agent. No tissue is taken out.
		Encompasses: Ablation, cauterization, coagulation, crushing, electrocoagulation, fulguration, mashing, obliteration
		Examples: Fulguration of a rectal polyp Crushing of a fallopian tube
6	**Detachment**	**Definition:** Cutting off all or a portion of an extremity
		Explanation: Pertains only to extremities. The body part determines the level of the detachment. All of the body parts distal to the detachment level are detached.
		Encompasses: Amputation
		Examples: Shoulder disarticulation Below-knee amputation
7	**Dilation**	**Definition:** Expanding the orifice or the lumen of a tubular body part
		Explanation: Stretching by pressure using intraluminal instrumentation
		Examples: Dilation of the trachea Dilation of the anal sphincter
8	**Division**	**Definition:** Separating, without taking out, all or a portion of a body part
		Explanation: Separating into two or more portions by sharp or blunt dissection
		Encompasses: Bisection
		Examples: Bisection of an ovary Spinal cordotomy Division of a patent ductus
9	**Drainage**	**Definition:** Taking into or letting out of fluids and/or gases in a body part
		Explanation: The fluids or gases may be normal or abnormal.
		Encompasses: Aspiration, evacuation, marsupialization, needle puncture, rupture, stabbing, suction, taping, unbridling, undercutting, window formation
		Examples: I & D of an abscess Thoracentesis
B	**Excision**	**Definition:** Cutting out or off, without replacement, a portion of a body part
		Explanation: Involves the act of cutting using a sharp instrument or other method such as a hot knife or laser
		Encompasses: Biopsy, core needle biopsy, debridement, debulk, fine needle aspiration, punch, shuck, trim, wedge
		Examples: Partial nephrectomy Wedge ostectomy Pulmonary segmentectomy
C	**Extirpation**	**Definition:** Taking or cutting out solid matter from a body part
		Explanation: Taking out solid matter (which may or may not have been broken up) by cutting with either a sharp instrument or other method such as a hot knife or laser, by blunt dissection, by pulling, by stripping, or by suctioning, with the intent not to take out any appreciable amount of the body part. The solid matter may be imbedded in the tissue of the body part or in the lumen of a tubular body part.
		Examples: Sequestrectomy Cholelithotomy
D	**Extraction**	**Definition:** Taking out or off all or a portion of a body part
		Explanation: The body part is not completely dissected free but is pulled or stripped by the use of force (manual, suction, etc.) from its location.
		Encompasses: Abrasion, avulsion, strip

TABLE 15–1

MEDICAL AND SURGICAL ROOT OPERATIONS (Continued)

		Examples: Tooth extraction Vein stripping Dermabrasion
F	**Fragmentation**	**Definition:** Breaking down solid matter in a body part
		Explanation: Physically breaking up solid matter not normally present in a body part, such as stones and foreign bodies. The breakup may be accomplished by direct physical force or by shock waves that are applied directly or indirectly through intervening layers. The resulting debris is not taken out but is passed from the body or absorbed by the body. The solid matter may be in the lumen of a tubular body part or in a body cavity.
		Encompasses: Pulverization
		Examples: Lithotripsy, urinary stones Lithotripsy, gallstones
G	**Fusion**	**Definition:** Joining together portions of an articular body part, rendering the articular body part immobile
		Explanation: Confined to joints
		Examples: Spinal fusion Ankle arthrodesis
H	**Insertion**	**Definition:** Putting into a body a nonbiologic appliance that monitors, assists, performs, or prevents a physiologic function, but does not physically take the place of a body part
		Encompasses: Cutdown, implantation, passage
		Examples: Implantation of a radioactive element Insertion of a diaphragmatic pacemaker
J	**Inspection**	**Definition:** Visually and/or manually exploring a body part
		Explanation: Looking at a body part directly or with an optical instrument or feeling the body part directly or through intervening body layers
		Encompasses: Checking, entering, examining, exploring, exposing, opening, probing
		Examples: Diagnostic arthroscopy Exploratory laparotomy
K	**Map**	**Definition:** Locating the route of passage of electrical impulses and/or locating functional areas in a body part
		Explanation: Confined to the cardiac conduction mechanism and the central nervous system
		Encompasses: Localization
		Examples: Mapping of cardiac conduction pathways Location of cortical areas
L	**Occlusion**	**Definition:** Completely closing the orifice or lumen of a tubular body part
		Explanation: Can be accomplished intraluminally or extraluminally
		Encompasses: Clamping, clipping, embolizing, interrupting, ligating, stopping, suturing
		Examples: Ligation of the vas deferens Fallopian tube ligation
M	**Reattachment**	**Definition:** Putting back into or onto a body all or a portion of a body part
		Explanation: Pertains only to body parts and appendages that have been severed; may or may not involve the reestablishment of vascular and nervous supplies
		Encompasses: Replantation
		Examples: Reattachment of penis Reattachment of a hand Replantation of parathyroids
N	**Release**	**Definition:** Freeing a body part
		Explanation: Eliminating abnormal compression or restraint by force or by sharp or blunt dissection. Some of the restraining tissue may be taken out, but none of the body part itself is taken out.
		Encompasses: Decompressing, freeing, lysing, mobilizing, relaxing, relieving, sectioning, taking down
		Examples: Lysing of peritoneal adhesions Freeing of median nerve
P	**Removal**	**Definition:** Taking out or off a device from a body part
		Explanation: May or may not involve invasive penetration
		Examples: Removal of a drainage tube Removal of a cardiac pacemaker

Table continued on following page

TABLE 15-1

MEDICAL AND SURGICAL ROOT OPERATIONS (Continued)

Q Repair

Definition: Restoring, to the extent possible, a body part to its natural anatomic structure

Explanation: An operation of exclusion. Most of the other operations are some type of repair, but if the objective of the procedure is one of the other operations, then that operation is coded. If none of the other operations is performed to accomplish the repair, then the operation "repair" is coded.

Encompasses: Closure, correction, fixation, reconstruction, reduction, reformation, reinforcement, restoration, stitching, suturing

Examples: Tracheoplasty
Suture laceration
Herniorrhaphy

R Replacement

Definition: Putting into or onto a body biologic or synthetic material that physically takes the place of all or a portion of a body part

Explanation: The biologic material may be living similar or dissimilar tissue from the same individual or nonliving similar or dissimilar tissue from the same individual, another individual, or an animal. The body part replaced may have been taken out previously or replaced previously or may be taken out concurrently with the replacement.

Examples: Replacement of external ear with synthetic prosthesis
Total hip replacement
Replacement of part of the aorta
Free skin graft
Pedicle skin graft

S Reposition

Definition: Moving to its normal location or other suitable location all or a portion of a body part

Explanation: The body part repositioned is aberrant, compromised, or has been detached. If attached, it may or may not be detached to accomplish the repositioning.

Examples: Repositioning of an undescended testicle
Repositioning of an aberrant kidney

T Resection

Definition: Cutting out or off, without replacement, all of a body part

Explanation: Involves the act of cutting with a sharp instrument or other method such as a hot knife or laser

Examples: Total gastrectomy
Pneumonectomy
Total nephrectomy

V Restriction

Definition: Partially closing the orifice or lumen of a tubular body part

Explanation: Can be accomplished intraluminally or extraluminally

Encompasses: Banding, cerclage, collapse, compression, packing, tamponade

Examples: Fundoplication
Cervical cerclage

W Revision

Definition: Correcting a portion of a previously performed procedure

Explanation: Redoing a portion of a previously performed procedure that has failed to function as intended. Revisions exclude the complete redo of the procedure and procedures to correct complications that do not require the redoing of a portion of the original procedure, such as the control of bleeding.

Examples: Revision of hip replacement
Revision of gastroenterostomy

X Transfer

Definition: Moving, without taking out, all or a portion of a body part to another location to take over the function of all or a portion of a body part

Explanation: The body part transferred is not detached from the body. Its vascular and nerve supply remain intact. The body part whose function is taken over may or may not be similar.

Encompasses: Transposition

Examples: Nerve transfer
Tendon transfer

Y Transplantation

Definition: Putting in or on all or a portion of a living body part taken from another individual or animal to physically take the place and/or function of all or a portion of a similar body part

Explanation: The native body part may or may not be taken out. The transplanted body part may physically take the place of the native body part or may simply take over all or a portion of its function.

Examples: Lung transplant
Kidney transplant

EXERCISE 15-38 *Root Operation*

Place the character for the root operation term before its definition:

1 ＿＿ Taking or letting out fluids and/or gases from a body part

2 ＿＿ Freeing a body part

3 ＿＿ Taking out or off a device from a body part

4 ＿＿ Visually and/or manually exploring a body part

5 ＿＿ Restoring to the extent possible a body part to its natural anatomic structure

6 ＿＿ Altering the route of passage of the contents of a tubular body part

7 ＿＿ Cutting out or off, without replacement, all of a body part

8 ＿＿ Eradicating all or a portion of a body part

9 ＿＿ Correcting a portion of a previously performed procedure

10 ＿＿ Cutting out or off, without replacement, a portion of a body part

1 Bypass
4 Destruction
7 Drainage
8 Excision
L Release
M Removal
N Repair
R Resection
G Inspection
T Revision

A Closer Look at Root Operations. The root operation is described by one of the main terms, as outlined in Table 15–1 (e.g., alteration, destruction, transfer). These root operations can be grouped into types of operations, such as operations that always involve devices: insertion, replacement, removal, change. Table 15–2 shows the root operations grouped by types.

EXERCISE 15-39 *Root Operation Terms*

Using Table 15–2, identify the root operation term for each example:

1 ＿＿＿＿ Tendon transfer

2 ＿＿＿＿ Appendectomy

3 ＿＿＿＿ Diagnostic bronchoscopy

4 ＿＿＿＿ Kidney transplant

5 ＿＿＿＿ Cardioverter-defibrillator implantation

6 ＿＿＿＿ Removal of pulse generator for pacemaker

7 ＿＿＿＿ Lithotripsy, bladder stone

8 ＿＿＿＿ Fallopian tube ligation

9 ＿＿＿＿ Elbow replacement revision

10 ＿＿＿＿ Lysis peritoneal adhesions

TABLE 15-2

ROOT OPERATIONS BY TYPE

Operation	Action	Object	Modification	Example
Operations that take out or eliminate all or a portion of a body part				
Excision	Cutting out or off	Portion of a body part	Without replacing the body part	Sigmoid polypectomy
Resection	Cutting out or off	All of a body part	Without replacing the body part	Total nephrectomy
Extraction	Taking out or off	All or a portion of a body part	Without replacing the body part	Tooth extraction
Destruction	Eradicating	All or a portion of a body part	Without taking out any of the body part	Fulguration of rectal polyp
			Without replacing the body part	
Detachment	Cutting off	All or a portion of an extremity	Without replacing the extremity	Below-knee amputation
Operations that involve putting in or on, putting back, or moving living body parts				
Transplantation	Putting in or on	All or a portion of a living body part	Taking from other individual or animal; physically takes the place and/or function of all or a portion of a body part	Heart transplant
Reattachment	Putting back in or on	All or a portion of a body part	Attaching a body part that was detached	Reattachment of finger
Reposition	Moving	All or a portion of a body part	Putting into its normal or another suitable location; body part may or may not be detached	Repositioning of undescended testicle
Transfer	Moving	All or a portion of a body part	Without taking out the body part; takes over function of similar body part	Tendon transfer
Operations that take out or eliminate solid matter, fluids, or gases from a body part				
Drainage	Taking in or letting out	Fluid and/or gases of a body part	Without taking out any of the body part	I & D of an abscess
Extirpation	Taking in or cutting out	Solid matter in a body part	Without taking out any of the body part	Sequestrectomy
Fragmentation	Breaking down	Solid matter in a body part	Without taking out any of the body part or any of the solid matter	Lithotripsy, gallstones
Operations that involve only examination of body parts and regions				
Inspection	Visually and/or manually exploring	A body part		Diagnostic arthroscopy
Map	Locating	Route of passage of electrical impulses		Cardiac conduction pathways
		Functional areas in a body part		Location of cortical areas
Operations that can be performed only on tubular body parts				
Bypass	Altering the route of passage	Contents of tubular body part	May include use of living tissue, nonliving biologic material or synthetic material that does not take the place of the body part	Gastrojejunal bypass
Dilation	Expanding	Orifice or lumen of a tubular body part	By applying pressure	Dilation of anal sphincter
Occlusion	Completely closing	Orifice or lumen of a tubular body part		Fallopian tube ligation
Restriction	Partially closing	Orifice or lumen of a tubular body part		Cervical cerclage

TABLE 15-2

ROOT OPERATIONS BY TYPE (Continued)

Operation	Action	Object	Modification	Example
Operations that always involve devices				
Insertion	Putting in	Nonbiologic appliance	Does not physically take the place of body part	Pacemaker insertion
Replacement	Putting in or on	Biologic or synthetic material; living tissue taken from same individual	Physically takes the place of all or a portion of a body part	Total hip replacement
Removal	Taking out or off	Device		Removal of cardiac pacemaker
Change	Taking out or off and putting back	Identical or similar device	Without cutting or puncturing the skin or mucous membrane	Change of a drainage tube
Miscellaneous operations				
Alteration	Modifying	Natural anatomic structures of a body part	Without affecting function of a body part	Face lift
Creation	Making	New structure	Does not physically take the place of a body part	Creation of an artificial vagina
Control	Stopping or attempting to stop	Postprocedural bleeding		Postprostatectomy bleeding
Division	Separating	A body part	Without taking out any of the body part	Bisection of ovary
Fusion	Joining together	An articular body part	Rendering a body part immobile	Spinal fusion
Release	Freeing	A body part	By eliminating compression or restriction; without taking out any of the body part	Lysing of peritoneal adhesions
Repair	Restoring	To the extent possible, a body part and its natural anatomic structure	May include use of living tissue, nonliving biologic material, or synthetic material that does not take the place of or take over the function of the body part	Hernia repair
Revision	Correcting	Portion of a previously performed procedure	Procedure failing to function as intended	Revision hip replacement

The Index

ICD-10-PCS codes are described in both the Index and the Tabular List. The Index, which allows codes to be located by means of an alphabetic lookup, is divided into two parts. The first part of the Index includes the following sections:

- Medical and Surgical
- Obstetrics
- Placement
- Measurement and Monitoring
- Administration
- Extracorporeal Assistance and Performance
- Extracorporeal Therapies
- Miscellaneous Sections

The first part of the Index is arranged according to root operation terms and has subentries based on:

- Body System
- Body Part

- Operation (for Revision)
- Device (for Change)

The Index may also be consulted for a specific operation term such as "Hysterectomy," where a cross-reference directs you to see "Resection, Female Reproductive System, OVT." Although you need to become very familiar with the root operations, you may be able to locate a code for a specific operation such as an appendectomy more rapidly by looking under the term "Appendectomy" than by consulting the root operation term "Resection," subterms "by Body Part," and "Appendix." See Fig. 15–13 for an example of the Index of the ICD-10-PCS.

The second part of the Index covers the remaining sections. This part is also arranged by root operations. For example:

- Imaging—Fluoroscopy by Body System, by Body Part
- Nuclear Medicine—Nonimaging Assay by Body System, by Body Part
- Osteopathic—Treatment by Region

Codes may also be located in the second part of the Index by specific procedures such as Chest x-ray—see Plain Radiography, Anatomical Regions. The Index refers you to a specific entry in the Tabular List by providing the first three or four digits of the procedure code. It is always necessary to refer to the Tabular List to obtain the complete code because the Index contains only the first few numbers and letters.

Fasciotomy – see Resection, Bursa, Ligaments, Fascia 0MB....
Fasciectomy – see Excision, Bursa, Ligaments, Fascia 0MT....
Fascioplasty – see Repair, Bursa, Ligaments, Fascia 0MG....
Fine Needle Aspiration – see Excision
Fix – see Repair
Flushing – see Irrigation
Formation – see Creation
Fragmentation
   by Body System
      Anatomical Regions 0XF....
      Central Nervous System 00F...
      Eye 08F...
      Female Reproduction System 0VF....
      Gastrointestinal System 0DF...
      Heart & Great Vessels 02F....
      Hepatobiliary System & Pancreas 0FF....
      Mouth & Throat 0CF....
      Respiratory System 0BF....
      Urinary System 0TF....
   by Body Part
      Ampulla of Vater 0FFB....
      Anus 0DFQ....
      Appendix 0DFJ....
      Bladder 0TF8....
      Bladder Neck 0TF9....
      Bronchus
         Lingula 0BF9....
         Lower Lobe 0BF....
         Main 0BF....
         Middle Lobe, Right 0BF5....
         Segmental, Lingula 0BF9....
         Upper Lobe 0BF....

FIGURE 15–13 ICD-10-PCS Index. (Courtesy U.S. Department of Health and Human Services, Centers for Medicare and Medicaid Services.)

The Tabular List Completes the Code

The Tabular List provides the remaining characters needed to complete the code given in the Index. The Tabular List is arranged by sections, and most sections are subdivided by body systems. For each body system, the Tabular List begins with a listing of the operations performed, that is, the root operations. When a procedure involves distinct parts, multiple codes are provided. For example, a section of the listing of operations performed in respect to the central nervous system is as follows:

- Bypass
- Change
- Destruction
- Division
- Drainage
- Excision

The Tabular List for each body system also includes a listing of the body parts, approaches, devices, and qualifiers for that system. These listings are followed by separate tables for each root operation in the body system. At the top of each of the tables is the name of the section, body system, and root operation as well as the definition of the root operation. The list is formatted as a grid, with rows and columns. The four columns in the grid represent the last four characters of the code (which are labeled Body Part, Approach, Device, and Qualifier in the Obstetrics and Medical and Surgical sections). Each row in the grid specifies the allowable combinations of the last four characters. For example, looking at the grid in Fig. 15–14, you can see that the code for delivery of retained products of conception is 10Y1BZZ:

1 Obstetrics

0 Pregnancy

Y Delivery

1 Products of Conception, Retained

B Transorifice Intraluminal

Z None

Z None

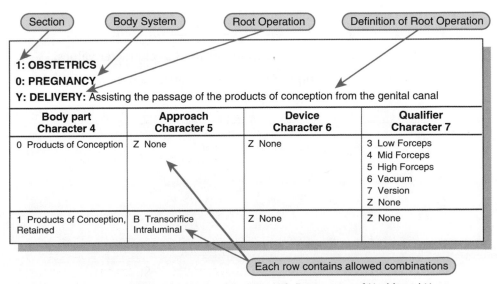

FIGURE 15–14 ICD-10-PCS Tabular. (Courtesy U.S. Department of Health and Human Services, Centers for Medicare and Medicaid Services.)

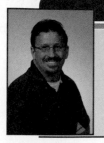

From the Trenches

"You have to look internally and find out what drives you . . . It really is being aware of your own interests, what motivates you, what stimulates you to get up in the morning and go to work . . . You have to really know yourself—and what motivates you."

JOHN

Code 10Y1BZZ would be the only allowable code for Products of Conception, Retained, because you may not complete a code by choosing entries from different rows (a row may consist of multiple entries in a box). Thus the code 10Y1B<u>Z6</u> is not permitted because the qualifier 6 can be used only with the body part 0; it cannot be used with body part 1. If you begin the code with 0, Products of Conception, you must continue to choose from the available numbers or letters in that same line. So, with the qualifier 6, the code would have to be 10Y0ZZ6.

EXERCISE 15–40   *ICD-10-PCS Format*

Complete the following:

Achievement of the four major objectives guiding the development of the ICD-10-PCS will result in a classification system that is

1 _____

2 _____

3 _____

4 _____

Provide the requested information about the ICD-10-PCS code structure:

5 The ICD-10-PCS has a _____ character code structure.

6 The characters in ICD-10-PCS are _____.

7 Each character has up to _____ different values.

8 The letters _____ are not used as character values.

9 The complete specification of seven characters describes a(n) _____

_____ in the ICD-10-PCS.

CHAPTER REVIEW

CHAPTER 15, PART I, THEORY

List, define, or describe the following, as directed:

1 The UHDDS definition of a Principal Diagnosis is

_____

_____

_____

_____

2 List two of the four cooperating parties that agree on coding principles: _____

_____

CHAPTER 15, PART II, PRACTICAL

Using the ICD-9-CM and coding guidelines, fill in the codes for the following:

3 Combined spinal cord degeneration due to pernicious anemia

Code(s): _____

_____

4 Carcinoma, in situ, of the lip, vermilion border

Code: _____

5 Bilateral occlusion of carotid arteries

Code: _____ _____

6 Subacute bacterial endocarditis

Code: _____ _____

7 Nephrogenic diabetes insipidus

Code: _____

8 Ovarian cyst

Code: _____

9 Uterine fibroids complicating pregnancy, 23 weeks' gestation

Code: _____

10 Acute bronchitis with chronic obstructive bronchitis

Code(s): _____

11 Group B streptococcal pneumonia

Code(s): _____

12 Obstructed labor caused by cephalopelvic disproportion, delivered liveborn male

Code(s): _____

13 Term birth, 2268 grams, delivered by cesarean section, with intrauterine growth retardation

Code(s): _____

14 Alzheimer's disease

Code(s): _____

15 Hypertension with end-stage renal disease

Code(s): _____

16 Anal fistula

Code(s): _____

Fill in the ICD-9-CM codes for the following cases:

17 Mr. Jones presents to the emergency department with acute abdominal pain. After a thorough examination and diagnostic x-ray film, Mr. Jones is diagnosed with acute small bowel obstruction and taken immediately to surgery.

Code: _____

18 Mrs. Smith is at 32 weeks' gestation and is admitted with severe bleeding with abdominal cramping. An emergency ultrasound is done and fetal monitors are applied. She is diagnosed with total placenta previa with indications of fetal distress. An emergency cesarean section is done, with delivery of a viable male infant.

Codes: _____

_____ _____

_____ _____

19 Mr. Jensen is status post colon resection 3 months ago for sigmoid colon cancer and is now admitted for adjunct chemotherapy.

Code(s): _____

20 Miss Halliday is an 80-year-old woman who presents to the emergency department with a history of abdominal pain, fever, and burning with urination. Urine culture is obtained, and Miss Halliday is admitted for workup to rule out urosepsis.

Code(s): _____

21 Mr. Johnson is admitted to the hospital with chest and epigastric pain. He is evaluated by the emergency department physician with a diagnosis of rule out myocardial infarction. Mr. Johnson is then transferred to a larger facility for further workup.

Code(s): _____

In the following cases, identify the principal diagnosis and all other diagnoses. Assign the appropriate ICD-9-CM codes.

CASE STUDY 1

History of Present Illness

The patient is a 68-year-old female, status post motor vehicle accident 3 months ago. The patient had an open fracture that was treated initially with traction for 6 to 8 weeks. After initial treatment with traction, the patient was placed in a cast brace. She presents with a complaint of pain in the left femur and inability to bear weight on her leg. The patient was referred from an orthopedic surgeon. The past medical history was significant for no history of myocardial infarction or renal disease and no asthma. The patient had undergone no previous procedures with the exception of debridement of the open fracture. Otherwise the patient's history was unremarkable. The patient was taking no medications and had no known allergies. She underwent a preoperative workup that included a gallium scan.

Physical Examination

The heart, lungs, and abdomen were benign. The left knee had a 30-degree extension lag. There was motion with the knee approximately 30 degrees from horizontal axis to 90 degrees of flexion. The patella was difficult to palpate, and it was very difficult to tell at the time of examination whether motion was occurring at the fracture or whether it was occurring at the knee joint. The vascular examination was unremarkable.

Laboratory Data and Course in Hospital

The x-ray film showed nonunion of the left femur. The gallium scan obtained preoperatively was unremarkable, and there was no evidence of infection.

Treatment

On May 14, the patient underwent open reduction and internal fixation of the left femur fracture with a 90-degree dynamic condylar screw and side plate. The patient tolerated the procedure well. She received two units of her own autologous blood at the time of surgery. Postoperatively she was quite anemic, with hemoglobin of 6 to 7 mg/dL. The patient was asymptomatic clinically, and her vascular examination was intact. On postoperative day 2, she had motion in the left knee from 0 to 30 degrees of flexion. She was placed in continuous

passive motion and was up with physical therapy but non-weight-bearing on the left leg. Physical therapy was tolerated well. The hospital course was benign. The wound was clean and dry, and the neurovascular examination was unchanged. The x-ray films obtained before discharge showed maintenance of alignment of the left femur. The patient's staples were removed on postoperative day 7. She was placed in a cast brace and was discharged home after being independent in physical therapy.

Final Diagnosis

Nonunion of the left femur

Procedure

Open reduction and internal fixation of the left femur with 90-degree screw and site plate.

22 🌐 Code(s): _____

CASE STUDY 2

History of Present Illness

This 50-year-old disabled male is a resident of a nursing home who has been admitted because of marked congestion and respiratory distress. He is known to have mental retardation and frequent urinary tract and pulmonary infections. He has a recurrent epileptic disorder that is well controlled on Dilantin.

Physical Examination

On admission, vital signs include a temperature of 101° F, respiratory rate of 32 breaths per minute, heart rate of 82 beats per minute, and blood pressure of 120/70 mm Hg. Examination of the chest reveals bilateral crepitations. There is moderate redness and edema of the scrotal skin.

Laboratory Data and Course in Hospital

His white blood cell count is 8.5; hemoglobin, 12.9 g/dL; polymorphonuclear leukocytes, 64; bands, 19; lymphocytes, 10; monocytes, 6; and eosinophils, 1. Urinalysis shows moderate bacterial and 11 white blood cell count. Urine culture shows mixed flora. The repeat urine culture shows *Providencia stuartii* sensitive to Fortaz. Sputum culture reveals the presence of methicillin-resistant *Staphylococcus aureus,* sensitive to vancomycin. Chest x-ray film shows bilateral pulmonary infiltrates. Arterial blood gases on room air show a P_{O_2} of 48, P_{CO_2} of 30, and pH of 7.50. When repeated with the patient on oxygen, P_{O_2} is 66,

P_{CO_2} is 36, and pH is 7.45. The patient is treated with intravenous vancomycin and intravenous Fortaz. His pulmonary infiltrate decreases. His oral intake has been somewhat poor, and he has been given intravenous fluids off and on. The nursing staff at the nursing home note that his intake, in terms of eating and taking fluids, is much better. His medications at the nursing home include Dilantin, 200 mg twice a day; Tegretol, 400 mg at 8 am and 4 pm, and 200 mg at 8 pm; and Cipro, 500 mg twice a day; and his maintenance medications are continued. This patient is being discharged today.

Final Diagnosis

Acute respiratory insufficiency

Bilateral pneumonia due to staphauerus

Mental retardation

Epilepsy; UTI due to *Provincia stuartii*

23 ⊛ Code(s): _____

CASE STUDY 3

History of Present Illness

The patient is an 80-year-old female with a known history of advanced metastatic carcinoma of the breast, which was the primary site. (The breast cancer is no longer present but has metastasized to other unspecified areas.) The patient has been admitted because of increased shortness of breath and severe pain. The pain is worse in her left chest, and this is associated with increased shortness of breath. At the time of admission, the patient is in so much pain that she is unable to remember her history. The patient initially presented for congestive heart failure more than a year earlier. This was subsequently found to be secondary to metastatic breast cancer, after left mastectomy, 3 years ago. The patient had previously been on chemotherapy.

Course in Hospital

The patient is treated initially with intravenous pain medication to control her pain, and subsequently her condition becomes stable on oral medication. By the time of discharge, the patient is stable on oral Vicodin. She is able to eat. Admission blood urea nitrogen (BUN) was 38 mg/dL with creatinine of 1.3 mg/dL secondary to dehydration. By the time of discharge, these levels have improved. Admission glucose of 225 mg/dL is down to 110 mg/dL at discharge.

Discharge Diagnoses

Uncontrolled pain, secondary to widely metastatic breast carcinoma

Dehydration

Type II diabetes mellitus, uncontrolled

24 What is the principal diagnosis and the code for the principal diagnosis for this patient?

Diagnosis and code: _____

25 What are the other diagnoses for this patient and what are the codes for these other diagnoses?

⊛ Diagnosis and code(s): _____

_____

QUICK CHECK ANSWERS

QUICK CHECK 15-1
Various, depending upon publisher

QUICK CHECK 15-2
"Use additional code to identify organism, such as Staphylococcus (041.1)"

QUICK CHECK 15-3
Above the "notes" on the first page of the Neoplasm Table in the Index

Listed alphabetically within the table under "unknown" or "unspecified"

QUICK CHECK 15-4
d. All of the above

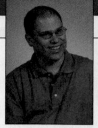

"Coding is a diverse field, so there are a lot of opportunities in many areas...Find an area of interest and become an expert in it; make yourself valuable."

Keith Russell, CPC, CPC-H
Senior Compliance Analyst
Baylor College of Medicine
Houston, Texas

Third-Party Reimbursement Issues

Chapter Topics

Introduction

The Basic Structure of the Medicare Program

The Importance of the *Federal Register*

Inpatient Prospective Payment System (IPPS)

The Quality Improvement Organizations (QIOs)

What Is the Outpatient Resource-Based Relative Value Scale (RBRVS)?

The Prospective Payment System for the Skilled Nursing Facility

Outpatient Medicare Reimbursement System— APC

Medicare Fraud and Abuse

The Managed Health Care Concept

Chapter Review

Quick Check Answers

Learning Objectives

After completing this chapter you should be able to

1. Distinguish between Medicare Part A and Part B.
2. Define "QIO."
3. Locate information in the Federal Register.
4. Identify major elements of the IPPS.
5. Explain the purpose of QIOs.
6. Explain the RBRVS system.
7. State the structure of the APC system.
8. Understand the framework of Medicare Fraud and Abuse.
9. Identify the major components of Managed Health Care.

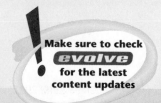

Make sure to check **evolve** for the latest content updates

INTRODUCTION

You now have an understanding of the coding systems used in the outpatient and inpatient health care settings. Each of the coding systems plays a key role in the reimbursement of providers of patient health care services. In your role as a medical coder, it is your responsibility to ensure that you code accurately and completely to optimize reimbursement for services provided.

Today, the elderly compose the fastest growing segment of our population. Medical advances allow people to live longer and healthier lives than ever before. Consider that in 1949 there were four persons age 19 and younger for every one person age 65 and older; in 2030 there will be one person age 19 and younger for every one person older than age 65.[1]

RATIO OF CHILDREN 19 AND YOUNGER TO PERSONS 65 AND OLDER[1,2]

- 4 : 1 1949
- 2 : 1 1988
- 1 : 1 2030

Persons enrolled in Medicare coverage increased from 19 million in 1967 to 43 million in 2008.[3] Medicare is big business, with Outlays for Mandatory Medicare spending at $207.9 billion in 1997 and $373.7 billion in 2006.[4] The program is expected to grow to $862 billion in 2016 and provide for 77 million beneficiaries.[5]

Increasing numbers of elderly people, technologic advances, and improved access to health care have increased consumer use of health care services. As more people use health care services, coding becomes even more important to appropriate reimbursement and cost control.

You must understand that your responsibility is to ensure that the data reported are as accurate as possible, not only for classification and study purposes but also to obtain appropriate reimbursement. Ethical issues surface and must be dealt with by coding personnel. Guidelines must always be followed in the assignment of codes. Instruction from internal and external sources (e.g., administration, review organizations, third-party payers) that may increase reimbursement but conflict with coding guidelines must be discussed and resolved. The principal diagnosis must match the documentation. The sequencing in Medicare Severity Diagnosis Related Group (MS-DRG) payment must always be substantiated by the medical records. Upcoding (maximizing), assigning comorbidity/complications based only on laboratory values, and using nonphysician impressions/assessments without physician agreement are all clearly fraudulent, prompting ethical concerns when coding for reimbursement.

Reimbursement usually comes from third-party payers. By far, the largest third-party payer is the government through the Medicare program. Because the Medicare program plays such an important role in reimbursement, the rules and regulations that govern Medicare reimbursement will be your first topic of study.

THE BASIC STRUCTURE OF THE MEDICARE PROGRAM

The Medicare program was established in 1965 with the passage of the Social Security Act. The Medicare Program dramatically increased the involvement of the government in health care. The program consists of Part A (Hospital Insurance) and Part B (Supplemental Medical Insurance). Part A pays for the cost of hospital/facility care, and Part B pays for physician services and durable medical equipment that are not paid for under Part A.

Medicare was originally designed for people 65 and over, but later, people who were eligible for disability benefits from Social Security were also covered under the Medicare program, along with those experiencing permanent kidney failure. Individuals covered under Medicare are called **beneficiaries.**

The Secretary of the Department of Health and Human Services (DHHS) is responsible for the administration of the federal Medicare program. Within the Department, the operation of Medicare is delegated to the Centers for Medicare and Medicaid Services (CMS), formerly the Health Care Financing Administration (HCFA). The funds to run Medicare are generated from payroll taxes paid by employers and employees. The Social Security Administration is responsible for collecting and handling the funds. CMS's function is to promote the general welfare of the public.

CMS's mission and vision are:

CMS's Mission:	To ensure effective, up-to-date health care coverage and to promote quality care for beneficiaries.
CMS's Vision:	To achieve a transformed and modernized health care system.
CMS will accomplish our mission by continuing to transform and modernize America's health care system.[6]	

CMS handles the daily operation of the Medicare program through the use of Medicare Administrative Contractors (MACs) (was Fiscal Intermediaries, FIs). The **MACs** do the paperwork for Medicare and are usually insurance companies that bid for a contract with CMS to handle the Medicare program in a specific area. The monies for Medicare flow from the Social Security Administration through the CMS to the MACs and, finally, are paid to beneficiaries and providers.

In 2003, the Medicare Prescription Drug Improvement and Modernization Act passed and allows CMS to reduce the administrative structure from 48 FIs to 19 MACs. There are 15 Part A & B MACs (Fig. 16–1), and 4 Durable Medical Equipment (DME) MACs (Fig. 16–2). The full implementation will be approximately 2011.

Physicians, hospitals, and other suppliers that furnish care or supplies to Medicare patients are called **providers.** Providers must be licensed by local and state health agencies to be eligible to provide Medicare patients' services or supplies. Providers must also meet various additional Medicare requirements before payment can be made for their services.

Medicare pays for 80% of covered charges, and the beneficiary pays the remaining 20%. The beneficiary pays deductibles, premiums, and coinsurance payments. (The 2009 deductible for Part A is $1,068[7] and for Part B, $135.[7]) **Coinsurance** is the 20% that Medicare does not pay. Often, beneficiaries have additional insurance to cover out-of-pocket expenses.

Beneficiary Pays: Deductible, premiums, coinsurance (20%), non-covered services

Medicare Pays: Covered services (80%)

The maximum out-of-pocket amounts are set each year according to formulas established by Congress and published in the *Federal Register.* New amounts usually take effect each January 1.

What Is QIO?

Claims sent in by the providers of services are processed by MACs according to Medicare guidelines. Providers can sign a **Quality Improvement Organization (QIO) agreement** with a MAC to accept assignment on all claims submitted to Medicare. QIO providers were previously termed PROs (Participating Provider Organizations). Under the direction of CMS, the Quality Improvement Organization program consists of a national network of QIOs, responsible for each U.S. state, territory, and the District of Columbia. QIOs work with consumers and physicians, hospitals, and other caregivers to refine care delivery systems to make sure patients get the right

Part A and B MAC Jurisdictions

Jurisdiction	States Included in Jurisdiction
1	American Samoa, California, Guam, Hawaii, Nevada, and Northern Mariana Islands
2	Alaska, Idaho, Oregon, and Washington
3	Arizona, Montana, North Dakota, South Dakota, Utah, and Wyoming
4	Colorado, New Mexico, Oklahoma, and Texas
5	Iowa, Kansas, Missouri, and Nebraska
6	Illinois, Minnesota, and Wisconsin
7	Arkansas, Louisiana, and Mississippi
8	Indiana and Michigan
9	Florida, Puerto Rico, and U.S. Virgin Islands
10	Alabama, Georgia, and Tennessee
11	North Carolina, South Carolina, Virginia, and West Virginia
12	Delaware, District of Columbia, Maryland, New Jersey, and Pennsylvania
13	Connecticut and New York
14	Maine, Massachusetts, New Hampshire, Rhode Island, and Vermont
15	Kentucky and Ohio

FIGURE 16–1   Part A and B MAC jurisdictions.[8]

Durable Medical Equipment (DME) MAC Jurisdictions

Jurisdiction	States Included in Jurisdiction
A	Connecticut, Delaware, District of Columbia, Maine, Maryland, Massachusetts, New Hampshire, New Jersey, New York, Pennsylvania, Rhode Island, and Vermont
B	Illinois, Indiana, Kentucky, Michigan, Minnesota, Ohio, and Wisconsin
C	Alabama, Arkansas, Colorado, Florida, Georgia, Louisiana, Mississippi, New Mexico, North Carolina, Oklahoma, Puerto Rico, South Carolina, Tennessee, Texas, U.S. Virgin Islands, Virginia, and West Virginia
D	Alaska, American Samoa, Arizona, California, Guam, Hawaii, Idaho, Iowa, Kansas, Missouri, Montana, Nebraska, Nevada, North Dakota, Northern Mariana Islands, Oregon, South Dakota, Utah, Washington, and Wyoming

FIGURE 16–2   Durable Medical Equipment jurisdictions.[9]

care at the right time, particularly patients from underserved populations.[10] **Accepting assignment** means that the provider will accept what Medicare allows and not bill the patient for the difference between what the service costs and what Medicare allows. For example, a QIO provider renders a service that costs $100 and bills Medicare for the service; Medicare allows $58, and the provider accepts the Medicare payment as payment in full. Now, you are probably asking yourself why anyone would agree to this. The patient does not pay the $42 difference, nor does Medicare. The amount is written off by the provider as if the service really cost only $58 to provide. This is a good deal for Medicare and the patient, but what about the provider? Why would he or she agree to decreased payments?

Incentives have been established to encourage providers to become QIO providers. Congress has mandated the following incentives:

FOR QIO PROVIDERS:

- Direct payment is made on all claims.
- A 5% higher fee schedule than that for non-QIO providers.
- Faster processing of claims.
- The provider's name is listed in the QIO directory, which is made available to each Medicare patient, along with identification as a QIO provider who accepts assignment on all claims.
- Hospital referrals for outpatient care must provide the patient with the name and address of at least one QIO provider.

FOR NON-QIO PROVIDERS:

- Payment goes to the patient on all claims.
- A 5% lower fee schedule than that for QIO providers.
- Slower processing of claims is the norm.
- A statement on the Explanation of Benefits (EOB) sent to the patient reminds the patient that the use of a participating physician will lower out-of-pocket expenses.

FOR QIO:

- A bonus is offered for each recruited and enrolled QIO provider.

There are incentives for providers to participate in the Medicare program! Incentives backed by Congress. Currently, more than half of all physicians in the nation are participating providers. (More on QIOs later in this chapter.)

Part A: Hospital Insurance

Hospitals report services for Part A services by using ICD-9-CM codes and Medicare Severity Diagnosis Related Groups (MS-DRGs) assignment. MS-DRGs are discussed later in this chapter. Beneficiaries are automatically eligible for Part A, hospital insurance, when they are eligible for Medicare benefits.

During a hospital inpatient stay, Part A pays for a semiprivate room (two to four beds), meals and special diet, plus all other medically necessary services except personal-convenience items and private-duty nurses. Part A can also help pay for inpatient care in a Medicare-certified skilled nursing facility if the patient's condition requires daily skilled nursing or rehabilitation services that can be provided only in a skilled nursing facility. Skilled nursing care means care that can be performed only by or under the supervision of licensed nursing personnel. Skilled rehabilitation services may include such services as physical therapy performed by or under the supervision of a professional therapist. The skilled nursing care and skilled rehabilitation services received must be based on a physician's orders. Part A pays for a semiprivate room in the skilled nursing facility, plus meals, nursing services, and drugs. Personal-convenience items, private-duty nurses, and custodial nursing home services are provided to covered beneficiaries who have chronic long-term illnesses or disabilities.

Part A can pay for covered home health care visits from a participating home health agency. The visits can include part-time skilled nursing care and physical therapy or speech therapy when the services are approved by a physician.

Hospice provides relief (palliative) care and support care to terminally ill patients. Part A also pays for hospice care for terminally ill patients when a physician has certified that the patient is terminally ill, the patient has elected to receive care from a hospice rather than the standard Medicare benefits, and the hospice is Medicare-certified. Items covered include nursing services, physician services, and certain other medically necessary services.[7]

Part B: Supplementary Insurance

Part B is not automatically provided to beneficiaries when they become eligible for Medicare. Instead, beneficiaries must purchase the benefits with a monthly premium.[7] Part B helps to pay for medically necessary physicians' services, outpatient hospital services, home health care, and a number of other medical services and supplies that are not covered by Part A. These Part B services are reported using ICD-9-CM codes for the diagnosis, CPT codes for the procedure (service), and HCPCS codes (national codes) for the additional supplies and services.

Part C: Medicare Advantage

Medicare Part C is also known as Medicare Advantage (formerly Medicare + Choice) and is a set of health care options from which Medicare beneficiaries can choose their health care providers. The options available under Part C are:

- Health Maintenance Organization (HMO)
- Point of Service plans (POS)
- Provider-Sponsored Organizations (PSO)
- Preferred Provider Organization (PPO)
- Medical Savings Account (MSA)
- Private plans (fee-for-service)
- Religious fraternal benefit society plans

The managed plan, such as an HMO, has a contract to deliver Medicare services under the plan and provides the same services to all beneficiaries enrolled under Part C. The beneficiary is still under the coverage of Medicare, but has opted to utilize a different way of receiving services.

Part D: Prescription Drugs

The Medicare Prescription Drug, Improvement, and Modernization Act of 2003 (MMA) (Pub. L. 108–173, enacted December 8, 2003) established a prescription drug benefit under Part D of the Medicare Program. On January 1, 2006, Medicare beneficiaries could enroll in the Medicare prescription drug plan (Part D) and could choose between several plans that offered drug coverage. Medicare beneficiaries are charged a premium each month to be a member of these plans and receive the Medicare Part D drug benefit.

QUICK CHECK 16-1

Match the Medicare Part or Parts with the correct phrase(s) below.

a. Part A   b. Part B   c. Part C   d. Part D

1. Automatic coverage under social security _____
2. Optional coverage under social security _____
3. Hospice care coverage _____
4. Prescription drug coverage _____
5. Physician visit coverage _____
6. Beneficiary pays premium for coverage _____
7. Codes assigned for payment using ICD-9-CM, Vol 1, 2; CPT, HCPCS _____

EXERCISE 16–1 *Medicare*

Using the information presented in this chapter, complete the following:

1 The major third-party reimburser in the United States is _____.

2 The Medicare program was established in what year? _____

3 Hospital Insurance is Medicare, Part _____.

4 Supplemental Medical Insurance is Medicare, Part _____.

CHECK THIS OUT ☞ The CMS website is located at http://www.cms.hhs.gov. It contains information about the Medicare program, and through it, you can link to useful information concerning Medicare providers.

THE IMPORTANCE OF THE *FEDERAL REGISTER*

The *Federal Register* is the official publication for all "Presidential Documents," "Rules and Regulations," "Proposed Rules," and "Notices." When the government institutes national changes, those changes are published in the *Federal Register*. You must be aware of the changes listed in the *Federal Register* that relate to reimbursement of Medicare so as to submit Medicare charges correctly.

Most of the information in this chapter is about rules that the government has developed and introduced through the *Federal Register*. You might wonder why so much time is to be spent on learning how to follow the guidelines set by the government for reimbursement when it is only one third-party payer. The answer is simple: Because the government is the largest third-party payer in the nation, even a slight change in the rules governing reimbursement to providers can have a major consequence. For example, there was a 45% decrease in the number of inpatient hospital beds between 1975 and 1996.[2] Many of the reasons for this decrease are directly related to the government-implemented inpatient reimbursement system

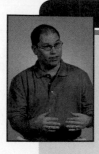

From the Trenches

Why should a coder consider getting certified?

"Certification indicates a level of competence and many employers now require applicants to be certified. Plus, salary surveys have shown that certified coders command higher salaries than non-certified coders."

KEITH

that you will learn about in this chapter—MS-DRGs. Often, more than 33% of the patients in a hospital are Medicare patients. Because the government is such an important payer in the health care system, you must know how to interpret the government's directives published in the *Federal Register*. In addition, many commercial insurers are adopting Medicare payment philosophies for their own reimbursement policies. The government has changed health care reimbursement through the Medicare program, and even more changes are promised.

If you have the *Federal Register* available to you through a library or via the internet, locating and reviewing some of the issues would be an excellent educational activity for you.

CHECK THIS OUT 🖝 You can access the *Federal Register* on the website for the National Archives and Records Administration at www.gpoaccess.gov/fr/index.html. This site houses issues of the *Federal Register* from 1994 to the present.

The October editions of the *Federal Register* are of special interest to **hospital** facilities because the hospital updates are released in that edition. **Outpatient** facilities are especially interested in the November or December edition of the *Federal Register* because Medicare reimbursements for outpatient services are usually published in one of those editions. Each year, when changes to the various payment systems are proposed, those proposed changes are published early in the year, and a period of several months is offered to interested parties to comment and make suggestions on the proposed changes. The final rules are usually published in the fall editions. The changes presented in fall editions of the *Federal Register* are implemented in the following calendar year.

Fig. 16–3 shows a copy of a portion of a *Federal Register;* it is marked to indicate the location of the following details[11]:

1. The regulation's issuing office
2. The subject of the notice
3. The agency
4. The action
5. A summary
6. The dates
7. The address
8. Contacts for further information
9. Supplementary information

Items 1 through 9 are always placed before the Final Rule, which is the official statement of the entire rule.

9. Supplementary information

5342   Federal Register / Vol. 73, No. 19 / Tuesday, January 29, 2008 / Proposed Rules

1. Issuing office →

DEPARTMENT OF HEALTH AND HUMAN SERVICES

Centers for Medicare & Medicaid Services

42 CFR Part 412

[CMS–1393–P]

RIN 0938–AO94

2. Subject →

Medicare Program; Prospective Payment System for Long-Term Care Hospitals RY 2009: Proposed Annual Payment Rate Updates, Policy Changes, and Clarification

3. Agency →

AGENCY: Centers for Medicare & Medicaid Services (CMS), HHS.

4. Action →

ACTION: Proposed rule.

5. Summary →

SUMMARY: This proposed rule would update the annual payment rates for the Medicare prospective payment system (PPS) for inpatient hospital services provided by long-term care hospitals (LTCHs). In addition, we are proposing to consolidate the annual July 1 update for payment rates and the October 1 update for Medicare severity long-term care diagnosis related group (MS–LTC–DRG) weights to a single fiscal year (FY) update.

In this proposed rule, we are also clarifying various policy issues.

This proposed rule would also describe our evaluation of the possible one-time adjustment to the Federal payment rate.

6. Dates →

DATES: To be assured consideration, comments must be received at one of the addresses provided below, no later than 5 p.m. on March 24, 2008.

7. Address →

ADDRESSES: In commenting, please refer to file code CMS–1393–P. Because of staff and resource limitations, we cannot accept comments by facsimile (FAX) transmission.

You may submit comments in one of four ways (please choose only one of the ways listed):

8. Further information →

1. *Electronically.* You may submit electronic comments on specific issues in this regulation to *http:// www.regulations.gov/.* Follow the instructions for "Comment or Submission" and enter the filecode to find the document accepting comment.

2. *By regular mail.* You may mail written comments (one original and two copies) to the following address ONLY:

Centers for Medicare & Medicaid Services, Department of Health and Human Services, *Attention:* CMS–1393–P, P.O. Box 8013, Baltimore, MD 21244–8013.

Please allow sufficient time for mailed comments to be received before the close of the comment period.

3. *By express or overnight mail.* You may send written comments (one original and two copies) to the following address ONLY:

Centers for Medicare & Medicaid Services, Department of Health and Human Services, Attention: CMS–1393–P, Mail Stop C4–26–05, 7500 Security Boulevard, Baltimore, MD 21244–1850.

4. *By hand or courier.* If you prefer, you may deliver (by hand or courier) your written comments (one original and two copies) before the close of the comment period to one of the following addresses. If you intend to deliver your comments to the Baltimore address, please call telephone number (410) 786–7195 in advance to schedule your arrival with one of our staff members.

Room 445–G, Hubert H. Humphrey Building, 200 Independence Avenue, SW., Washington, DC 20201; or 7500 Security Boulevard, Baltimore, MD 21244–1850.

(Because access to the interior of the HHH Building is not readily available to persons without Federal Government identification, commenters are encouraged to leave their comments in the CMS drop slots located in the main lobby of the building. A stamp-in clock is available for persons wishing to retain a proof of filing by stamping in and retaining an extra copy of the comments being filed.)

Comments mailed to the addresses indicated as appropriate for hand or courier delivery may be delayed and received after the comment period.

Submission of comments on paperwork requirements. You may submit comments on this document's paperwork requirements by mailing your comments to the addresses provided at the end of the "Collection of Information Requirements" section in this document.

For information on viewing public comments, see the beginning of the **SUPPLEMENTARYINFORMATION** section.

→ **FOR FURTHER INFORMATION CONTACT:**

Tzvi Hefter, (410) 786–4487 (General information).

Judy Richter, (410) 786–2590 (General information, payment adjustments for special cases, onsite discharges and readmissions, interrupted stays, co-located providers, and short-stay outliers).

Michele Hudson, (410) 786–5490 (Calculation of the payment rates, MS–LTC–DRGs, relative weights and case-mix index, market basket, wage index, budget neutrality, and other payment adjustments).

Ann Fagan, (410) 786–5662 (Patient classification system).

Linda McKenna, (410) 786–4537 (Payment adjustments and interrupted stay).

Elizabeth Truong, (410) 786–6005 (Federal rate update, budget neutrality, other adjustments, and calculation of the payment rates).

Michael Treitel, (410) 786–4552 (High cost outliers and cost-to-charge ratios).

Table of Contents

FIGURE 16–3 Example of page from the *Federal Register.* (From *Federal Register,* January 29, 2008, Vol. 73, No. 19, Proposed Rules.)

EXERCISE 16–2 *Federal Register*

Answer the following questions:

1 Which edition of the *Federal Register* is of special interest to hospital facilities?

_____

2 Which edition of the *Federal Register* is of special interest to outpatient facilities?

_____

Using Fig. 16–3, answer the following questions:

3 What is the issuing office? _____

4 What is the last date for comment to be received on this proposal? _____

5 According to the Summary section in Figure 16–3, what does LTCH mean?

_____

_____

6 According to the "For Further Information Contact" section in Figure 16–3, who could give you

further information related to the issue addressed in this *Federal Register*? _____

INPATIENT PROSPECTIVE PAYMENT SYSTEM (IPPS)

The design and development of the DRGs began in the late 1960s at Yale University. The initial motivation for developing the DRGs was to create a framework for monitoring the quality of care and the utilization of services in a hospital setting. The first large-scale application of the DRGs was in the late 1970s in New Jersey. The New Jersey State Department of Health used DRGs as the basis of a prospective payment system in which hospitals were reimbursed a fixed DRG-specific amount for each patient treated. In 1982, the Tax Equity and Fiscal Responsibility Act (TEFRA) modified the Medicare hospital reimbursement limits to include a system based on DRGs. In 1983, Congress amended the Social Security Act to include a national DRG-based hospital prospective payment system for all Medicare patients.

Facilities contract with Medicare to furnish acute inpatient care. These facilities agreed to accept a predetermined amount under the Inpatient Prospective Payment System (IPPS). The discharge is the basis of payment and the discharge is based on the diagnosis(es) and procedure(s) furnished during the hospital stay. The discharge diagnosis(es) and procedure(s) are assigned to a Medicare Severity Diagnosis Related Group (MS-DRG). Groups of MS-DRGs have similar clinical problems that are expected to require similar amounts of hospital resources. Each MS-DRG has a relative weight assigned that reflects the expected costliness of the inpatient treatment for that group of patients.

The payment rate is adjusted based on several factors, such as, if the facility has a resident teaching program for medical students or if the facility serves a disproportionate large share of low-income patients. The IPPS payment rate is to cover the average costs the provider incurred when furnishing care to that type of case. To arrive at the IPPS payment rate, a dollar figure (standardized amount) is divided into labor and non-labor related portions. The labor portion is adjusted by a wage index that reflects the labor costs for various geographic areas. For example, the average salary for a registered nurse in New York is higher than the average salary for a registered nurse in Montana. The adjusted labor amount is added to the non-labor amount. This total adjusted amount was multiplied by the relative weight for the specific MS-DRG. Any adjusted payment factors, such as the medical resident teaching program or treatment of a disproportionate large share of low income patients, is calculated to arrive at the facilities payment for the specific MS-DRG.

The patient's principal diagnosis and up to 8 secondary diagnoses indicate comorbidities (the presence of disease/disorder in addition to the principal diagnosis) or complications and determines the final MS-DRG payment. Assignment of the MS-DRG may be affected by up to 6 procedures that may have been furnished during the hospital stay.

The MS-DRG system became fully transitioned from the predecessor, DRG system, in 2008. At that time, the system underwent several major revisions that significantly reduce the payment rate. Under the new MS-DRG system there are three levels of severity based on the secondary diagnosis codes:

1. MCC (Major Complication/Comorbidity) reflects the highest level of severity

2. CC (Complication/Comorbidity) is the next level of severity

3. Non-CC (Non-Complication/Comorbidity) does not significantly affect the severity of the illness or resources used by the facility during the patient stay

Another significant change was that all related outpatient department services delivered on the day of or 3 days prior to admission are now included in the payment for the inpatient stay and are not reported separately. Payment is also reduced when a patient has a short length of stay (LOS) and then transfers to another acute care hospital or, in some instances, to a post-acute care setting. These types of transfers used to be factored into the payment to be more beneficial to the hospitals, but these factors have been removed from the MS-DRG system.

Setting Payment Rates

The IPPS payments are developed and annually updated by CMS through a series of adjustments. The discharge base rate standardized payment amount is now a set amount. CMS states that the payment was designed to cover all costs incurred by the facility, but as in the establishment of the original DRG program, decreases in payment will require the facilities to become even more efficient. Some costs are excluded from the IPPS, such as organ acquisition.

A national IPPS rate is established each year for the operating and capital costs. In 2008, the amount of the operating base rate was $4,990.60 and the capital base rate was $426.14. The rates are the basis of payment for the year. The operating payments include labor and supply costs. The capital payment includes depreciation, interest, rent, property-related insurance, and taxes.

Relative Weights and Adjustments

A relative weight is assigned to each MS-DRG and recalculated each year based on mathematical averages of 15 typical hospital departments. Cost-of-living adjustments (COLA) are made for increases in the operating and capital base rates. For example, in Alaska and Hawaii the cost of living is significantly greater than other states.

There is also a 70% allowance for bad debts that result from beneficiaries not paying their co-payments or deductibles. The facility must demonstrate that a reasonable effort was made to collect the unpaid amounts.

There are additional adjustments (5.5%) available for teaching hospitals, those who serve a disproportionate share of low-income patients (based on facility size and number of patients served in the low-income bracket), and rural hospitals (based on a separate formula). Rural hospitals that are in areas determined to be Critical Access Hospitals (CAH) are paid on a cost basis and not under the IPPS.

There are some cases that are so costly that the facility cannot offset the loss to other MS-DRG categories. Under the IPPS, a fixed amount of loss is established each year. For 2008, the amount was $22,185. Hospitals are paid 80% of their costs once they have exceeded the fixed loss amount. For burn cases, hospitals are paid 90% over the fixed loss amount. To fund these amounts, all MS-DRGs were decreased a predetermined amount to ensure that the overall CMS spending did not exceed the fixed budget amount.

Under the MS-DRG system, payments for patients transferred to other facilities were significantly reduced when the patient's length of stay (LOS) is at least 1 day less than the geometric mean LOS (mathematical average of all lengths of stay for that MS-DRG) or is transferred to another acute care hospital covered under the IPPS.

Major Diagnostic Categories

There are 25 Major Diagnostic Categories (MDC) of the Medicare Severity Diagnosis Related Groups (MS-DRGs) as illustrated in Figure 16–4. Some of these categories are based on body systems, such as nervous, circulatory, and digestive systems, and some on injuries, burns, trauma, etc. After the initial grouping, the MDCs are further divided into either surgical or medical as illustrated in Figure 16–5. Note that the first decision in the MDC flow chart is based on if a operating room procedure was or was not performed. If the patient did have an operating room procedure, the next choice is if the surgery was major, minor, other, or unrelated. Each of the choices has a number of MS-DRGs attached. If the patient did not have surgery, the next choice is the type of principal diagnosis of neoplasm, a condition related or not related to the organ system, symptoms, or other diagnosis. Each type of principal diagnosis has a number of MS-DRGs attached.

Let us code a discharge diagnosis of major chest trauma. The index of the MS-DRG manual indicates that major chest trauma is coded to MDC 4 as illustrated in Figure 16–6. The main portion of the manual is then referenced and MDC 4 is located, as illustrated in Figure 16–7. The choices for a major chest trauma are:

1. with Major Complication or Comorbidity (MCC), MS-DRG 183,
2. with no MCC but with a Complication or Comorbidity (CC), 184,
3. or with no MCC and no CC, 185

Based on the documentation of a discharge diagnosis of major chest trauma, the coder assigns one of the three MS-DRGs. The ICD-9-CM codes are listed after the MS-DRGs; refer to Figure 16–7. Upon referencing the medical documentation, the major chest trauma was stated to be "three fractured ribs (closed)." The decimal points are removed from the code, so 80703 is ICD-9-CM code 807.03 for a three fractures, closed. The coder inputs the diagnoses codes, with or without MCC/CC, into the grouper and the MS-DRG is identified.

Complications and comorbidities are displayed in Appendix C of the MS-DRG manual.

Major Diagnostic Categories

1 - Diseases and Disorders of the Nervous System
2 - Diseases and Disorders of the Eye
3 - Diseases and Disorders of the Ear, Nose, Mouth and Throat
4 - Diseases and Disorders of the Respiratory System
5 - Diseases and Disorders of the Circulatory System
6 - Diseases and Disorders of the Digestive System
7 - Diseases and Disorders of the Hepatobiliary System and Pancreas
8 - Diseases and Disorders of the Musculoskeletal System and Connective Tissue
9 - Diseases and Disorders of the Skin, Subcutaneous Tissue and Breast
10 - Endocrine, Nutritional and Metabolic Diseases and Disorders
11 - Diseases and Disorders of the Kidney and Urinary Tract
12 - Diseases and Disorders of the Male Reproductive System
13 - Diseases and Disorders of the Female Reproductive System
14 - Pregnancy, Childbirth and the Puerperium
15 - Newborns and Other Neonates with Conditions Originating in the Perinatal Period
16 - Diseases and Disorders of the Blood and Blood Forming Organs and Immunological Disorders
17 - Myeloproliferative Diseases and Disorders, and Poorly Differentiated Neoplasms
18 - Infectious and Parasitic Diseases (Systemic or Unspecified Sites)
19 - Mental Diseases and Disorders
20 - Alcohol/Drug Use and Alcohol/Drug Induced Organic Mental Disorders
21 - Injuries, Poisonings and Toxic Effects of Drugs
22 - Burns
23 - Factors Influencing Health Status and Other Contacts with Health Services
24 - Multiple Significant Trauma
25 - Human Immunodeficiency Virus Infections

FIGURE 16–4 Major Diagnostic Categories of the Medicare Severity Diagnosis Related Groups. (From Medicare Severity Diagnosis Related Groups, Version 25.0, Definitions Manual, 3M Health Information Systems.)

Grouper and ICD-9-CM Diagnosis Codes

A computer program, called a grouper, is used to input the principal diagnosis and other critical information about a patient (diagnosis, procedures, and discharge status). The grouper then provides the correct MS-DRG assignment for the case on the basis of the information the coder inputs. Did you know that even today's sophisticated computers do not come close to your capabilities! You have tremendous potential! The computer is only as smart as the operator. You will be the operator of the grouper, and the quality of the information you input will determine the quality of the information that is output.

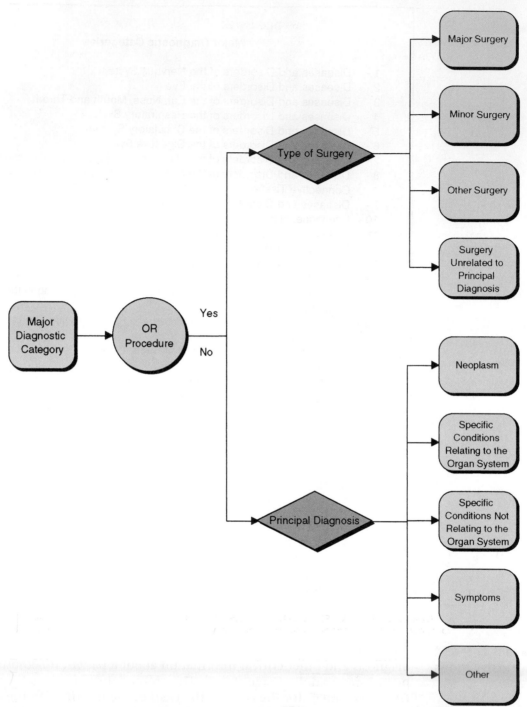

FIGURE 16–5 Typical MS-DRG structure for a Major Diagnostic Category. The Medical and Surgical Classes are further divided based on the presence of complications or comorbidities. (From Medicare Severity Diagnosis Related Groups, Version 25.0, Definitions Manual, 3M Health Information Systems.)

MS-DRG INDEX

MS-DRG	MS-DRG description	MDC	Page
134	OTHER EAR, NOSE, MOUTH & THROAT O.R. PROCEDURES W/O CC/MCC	3	117
135	SINUS & MASTOID PROCEDURES W CC/MCC	3	119
136	SINUS & MASTOID PROCEDURES W/O CC/MCC	3	119
137	MOUTH PROCEDURES W CC/MCC	3	119
138	MOUTH PROCEDURES W/O CC/MCC	3	119
139	SALIVARY GLAND PROCEDURES	3	120
146	EAR, NOSE, MOUTH & THROAT MALIGNANCY W MCC	3	120
147	EAR, NOSE, MOUTH & THROAT MALIGNANCY W CC	3	120
148	EAR, NOSE, MOUTH & THROAT MALIGNANCY W/O CC/MCC	3	120
149	DYSEQUILIBRIUM	3	121
150	EPISTAXIS W MCC	3	121
151	EPISTAXIS W/O MCC	3	121
152	OTITIS MEDIA & URI W MCC	3	122
153	OTITIS MEDIA & URI W/O MCC	3	122
154	NASAL TRAUMA & DEFORMITY W MCC	3	123
155	NASAL TRAUMA & DEFORMITY W CC	3	123
156	NASAL TRAUMA & DEFORMITY W/O CC/MCC	3	123
157	DENTAL & ORAL DISEASES W MCC	3	125
158	DENTAL & ORAL DISEASES W CC	3	125
159	DENTAL & ORAL DISEASES W/O CC/MCC	3	125
163	MAJOR CHEST PROCEDURES W MCC	4	137
164	MAJOR CHEST PROCEDURES W CC	4	137
165	MAJOR CHEST PROCEDURES W/O CC/MCC	4	137
166	OTHER RESP SYSTEM O.R. PROCEDURES W MCC	4	138
167	OTHER RESP SYSTEM O.R. PROCEDURES W CC	4	138
168	OTHER RESP SYSTEM O.R. PROCEDURES W/O CC/MCC	4	138
175	PULMONARY EMBOLISM W MCC	4	139
176	PULMONARY EMBOLISM W/O MCC	4	139
177	RESPIRATORY INFECTIONS & INFLAMMATIONS W MCC	4	139
178	RESPIRATORY INFECTIONS & INFLAMMATIONS W CC	4	139
179	RESPIRATORY INFECTIONS & INFLAMMATIONS W/O CC/MCC	4	139
180	RESPIRATORY NEOPLASMS W MCC	4	141
181	RESPIRATORY NEOPLASMS W CC	4	141
182	RESPIRATORY NEOPLASMS W/O CC/MCC	4	141
183	MAJOR CHEST TRAUMA W MCC	4	141
184	MAJOR CHEST TRAUMA W CC	4	141
185	MAJOR CHEST TRAUMA W/O CC/MCC	4	141
186	PLEURAL EFFUSION W MCC	4	142
187	PLEURAL EFFUSION W CC	4	142
188	PLEURAL EFFUSION W/O CC/MCC	4	142
189	PULMONARY EDEMA & RESPIRATORY FAILURE	4	142
190	CHRONIC OBSTRUCTIVE PULMONARY DISEASE W MCC	4	142
191	CHRONIC OBSTRUCTIVE PULMONARY DISEASE W CC	4	142
192	CHRONIC OBSTRUCTIVE PULMONARY DISEASE W/O CC/MCC	4	142
193	SIMPLE PNEUMONIA & PLEURISY W MCC	4	143
194	SIMPLE PNEUMONIA & PLEURISY W CC	4	143
195	SIMPLE PNEUMONIA & PLEURISY W/O CC/MCC	4	143
196	INTERSTITIAL LUNG DISEASE W MCC	4	143
197	INTERSTITIAL LUNG DISEASE W CC	4	143
198	INTERSTITIAL LUNG DISEASE W/O CC/MCC	4	143
199	PNEUMOTHORAX W MCC	4	144
200	PNEUMOTHORAX W CC	4	144
201	PNEUMOTHORAX W/O CC/MCC	4	144
202	BRONCHITIS & ASTHMA W CC/MCC	4	144
203	BRONCHITIS & ASTHMA W/O CC/MCC	4	144
204	RESPIRATORY SIGNS & SYMPTOMS	4	145
205	OTHER RESPIRATORY SYSTEM DIAGNOSES W MCC	4	145
206	OTHER RESPIRATORY SYSTEM DIAGNOSES W/O MCC	4	145

Major chest trauma MS-DRGs →

MDC

← Page number in manual

FIGURE 16-6 MS-DRG Index. (From Medicare Severity Diagnosis Related Groups, Version 25.0, Definitions Manual, 3M Health Information Systems.)

MDC 4 DEFINITION OF MS-DRGs

Major Complication or Comorbidity

Complication or Comorbidity

Major Chest Trauma

MCC	CC		MS-DRG
Yes			183
No	Yes		184
No	No		185

MS-DRGs

MS-DRG 183 MAJOR CHEST TRAUMA W MCC
MS-DRG 184 MAJOR CHEST TRAUMA W CC
MS-DRG 185 MAJOR CHEST TRAUMA W/O CC/MCC

Principle Diagnosis ICD-9-CM Codes

PRINCIPAL DIAGNOSIS

80703	Fracture three ribs-clos	80711	Fracture one rib-open
80704	Fracture four ribs-close	80712	Fracture two ribs-open
80705	Fracture five ribs-close	80713	Fracture three ribs-open
80706	Fracture six ribs-closed	80714	Fracture four ribs-open
80707	Fracture seven ribs-clos	80715	Fracture five ribs-open
80708	Fx eight/more rib-closed	80716	Fracture six ribs-open
80709	Fx mult ribs NOS-closed	80717	Fracture seven ribs-open
80710	Fracture rib NOS-open	80718	Fx eight/more ribs-open

FIGURE 16-7 Definitions of MS-DRGs. (From Medicare Severity Diagnosis Related Groups, Version 25.0, Definitions Manual, 3M Health Information Systems.)

EXERCISE 16-3 MS-DRG Information

After locating the principal diagnosis in your ICD-9-CM, use Fig. 16–8 to answer the following questions:

1 Can a complication/comorbidity of a concussion with a brief (29 minutes) coma (850.11) be used with a principal diagnosis of a cerebral laceration with open intracranial wound (851.32)?

NO, because 850.11 has 851.32 listed as a C/C.

2 Can a complication/comorbidity of a dislocation of the third cervical vertebra (closed) be used as a complication/comorbidity with the principal diagnosis of whiplash?

NO

3 Can the complication/comorbidity of dislocation of the sixth cervical vertebra (open) be used as a complication/comorbidity with the principal diagnosis of injury to the external carotid artery?

Yes

Fill in the blanks with the correct word(s):

4 The design and development of the DRGs began in the late 1960s at which university?

Yale

5 The first large-scale application of the DRGs was in the late 1970s in which state?

New Jersey

APPENDIX C - DIAGNOSES DEFINED AS COMPLICATIONS OR COMORBIDITIES

83901   Disloc 1st cerv vert-cl
80500-80518,80600-80619,
8068-8069,83900-83918,8470,
8488-8489,8798-8799,9290-9299,
95200-95209,9588,9598-9599

83902   Disloc 2nd cerv vert-cl
80500-80518,80600-80619,
8068-8069,83900-83918,8470,
8488-8489,8798-8799,9290-9299,
95200-95209,9588,9598-9599

83903   Disloc 3rd cerv vert-cl
80500-80518,80600-80619,
8068-8069,83900-83918,8470,
8488-8489,8798-8799,9290-9299,
95200-95209,9588,9598-9599

83904   Disloc 4th cerv vert-cl
80500-80518,80600-80619,
8068-8069,83900-83918,8470,
8488-8489,8798-8799,9290-9299,
95200-95209,9588,9598-9599

83905   Disloc 5th cerv vert-cl
80500-80518,80600-80619,
8068-8069,83900-83918,8470,
8488-8489,8798-8799,9290-9299,
95200-95209,9588,9598-9599

83906   Disloc 6th cerv vert-cl
80500-80518,80600-80619,
8068-8069,83900-83918,8470,
8488-8489,8798-8799,9290-9299,
95200-95209,9588,9598-9599

83907   Disloc 7th cerv vert-cl
80500-80518,80600-80619,
8068-8069,83900-83918,8470,
8488-8489,8798-8799,9290-9299,
95200-95209,9588,9598-9599

83908   Disloc mult cerv vert-cl
80500-80518,80600-80619,
8068-8069,83900-83918,8470,
8488-8489,8798-8799,9290-9299,
95200-95209,9588,9598-9599

83910   Disloc cerv vert NOS-opn
80500-80518,80600-80619,
8068-8069,83900-83918,8470,
8488-8489,8798-8799,9290-9299,
95200-95209,9588,9598-9599

83911   Disloc lst cerv vert-opn
80500-80518,80600-80619,
8068-8069,83900-83918,8470,
8488-8489,8798-8799,9290-9299,
95200-95209,9588,9598-9599

83912   Disloc 2nd cerv vert-opn
80500-80518,80600-80619,

8068-8069,83900-83918,8470,
8488-8489,8798-8799,9290-9299,
95200-95209,9588,9598-9599

83913   Disloc 3rd cerv vert-opn
80500-80518,80600-80619,
8068-8069,83900-83918,8470,
8488-8489,8798-8799,9290-9299,
95200-95209,9588,9598-9599

83914   Disloc 4th cerv vert-opn
80500-80518,80600-80619,
8068-8069,83900-83918,8470,
8488-8489,8798-8799,9290-9299,
95200-95209,9588,9598-9599

83915   Disloc 5th cerv vert-opn
80500-80518,80600-80619,
8068-8069,83900-83918,8470,
8488-8489,8798-8799,9290-9299,
95200-95209,9588,9598-9599

83916   Disloc 6th cerv vert-opn
80500-80518,80600-80619,
8068-8069,83900-83918,8470,
8488-8489,8798-8799,9290-9299,
95200-95209,9588,9598-9599

83917   Disloc 7th cerv vert-opn
80500-80518,80600-80619,
8068-8069,83900-83918,8470,
8488-8489,8798-8799,9290-9299,
95200-95209,9588,9598-9599

83918   Disloc mlt cerv vert-opn
80500-80518,80600-80619,
8068-8069,83900-83918,8470,
8488-8489,8798-8799,9290-9299,
95200-95209,9588,9598-9599

8500   Concussion w/o coma
80000-80199,80300-80499,
8500-85219,85221-85419,
8738-8739,8798-8799,9050,
9251-9252,9290-9299,9588-9590,
9598-9599

8501   Concussion-brief coma
80000-80199,80300-80499,
8500-85219,85221-85419,
8738-8739,8798-8799,9050,
9251-9252,9290-9299,9588-9590,
9598-9599

8502   Concussion-moderate coma
80000-80199,80300-80499,
8500-85219,85221-85419,
8738-8739,8798-8799,9050,
9251-9252,9290-9299,9588-9590,
9598-9599

C
C

FIGURE 16–8   Appendix C, Diagnoses Defined as Complications or Comorbidities. (From Medicare Severity Diagnosis Related Groups, Version 25.0, Definitions Manual, 3M Health Information Systems.)

THE PURPOSE OF QUALITY IMPROVEMENT ORGANIZATIONS (QIOs)

An attempt to monitor payment and ensure quality care for hospital services came about when Congress amended the Social Security Act of 1972 and established the Professional Standards Review Organization (PSRO). The PSRO was a voluntary group of physicians who monitored the necessity of hospital admissions and reviewed the treatment costs and medical records of hospitals. But the cost of operating the PSRO was more than the amount the program saved each year. Congress wanted a program that had stricter controls over Medicare reimbursement for inpatient costs. Congress was concerned that within the prospective payment system there was an incentive for hospitals to increase admissions, increase readmissions, and code hospital stays into higher-priced diagnostic categories so as to receive higher payments. So Congress created control peer review organizations (PROs). The creation of the PROs was made possible under the provision of the Tax Equity and Fiscal Responsibility Act (TEFRA), which gave the CMS the right to contract with private organizations for review purposes.

Quality Improvement Organizations (QIOs), formerly known as Peer Review Organization (PRO), is a group of doctors and other health care experts that are paid by CMS to do reviews. QIOs review complaints about the quality of health care services given to Medicare beneficiaries in hospitals, skilled nursing facilities, Comprehensive Outpatient Rehabilitation Facilities (CORFs), and home health agencies. QIOs also review cases from hospitals to make sure the care is medically necessary, provided in the appropriate setting, and coded correctly. In addition, QIOs provide assistance to hospitals, nursing homes, physician offices, and home health agencies in measuring and improving quality.[12]

MACs (Medicare Administrative Contractors) make the appropriate referrals to the QIO for medical necessity determination and accept referrals from the QIO. MACs also process payment adjustments submitted by the QIO based on medical necessity determinations and MS-DRG validations. MACs also receive notification of billing errors from the QIO and resolve the error.[12]

EXERCISE 16–4 *Quality Improvement Organizations*

Fill in the blanks with the correct word(s):

1 The creation of Peer Review Organizations was made possible under the provision of what act?

    TEFRA

2 QIO is a group of doctors and other health care professionals that reviews the care given to

    _____.

3 The QIOs also review cases from hospitals to make sure the care was _medically_

    necessary, provided in the appropriate _setting_, and _coded_ correctly.

4 This organization receives notification of billing errors from the QIO.

    MAC's

From the Trenches

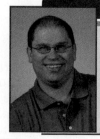

"Being certified opens many doors, but it also gives a level of credibility and confidence to your work, which makes a difference when dealing with other professions."

KEITH

WHAT IS THE OUTPATIENT RESOURCE-BASED RELATIVE VALUE SCALE (RBRVS)?

Physician payment reform was implemented to:

1. Decrease Medicare expenditures

2. Redistribute physicians' payments more equitably

3. Ensure quality health care at a reasonable rate

Before January 1, 1992, payment under Medicare Part B for physicians' services was based on a reasonable charge that, under the Social Security Act, could not exceed the lowest of (1) the physician's actual charge for the service, (2) the physician's customary charge for the service, or (3) the prevailing charges of physicians for similar services in the locality.

The act also required that the local prevailing charge for a physician's service not exceed the level in effect for that service in the locality for the fiscal year ending on June 30, 1973. Some provision was made for changes in the level on the basis of economic changes. When there were economic changes in the country, the Medicare Economic Index (MEI) reflected these changes. Until 1992, the MEI tied increases in the Medicare prevailing charges to increases in the costs of physicians' practice and general wage rates throughout the economy as compared with the index base year. The MEI was first published in the *Federal Register* on June 16, 1975, and has been recalculated annually since then.

Congress mandated the MEI as part of the 1972 Amendments to the Social Security Act. The 1972 Amendment to the Act did not specify the particular type of index to be used; however, the present form of the MEI follows the recommendations outlined by the Senate Finance Committee in its report accompanying the legislation. The MEI attempts to present an equitable measure for changes in the costs of physicians' time and operating expenses.

A major change took place in Medicare in 1989 with the enactment of the Omnibus Budget Reconciliation Act of 1989 (OBRA), Public Law 101-239. Section 6102 of PL 101-239 amended Title XVIII of the Social Security Act by adding Section 1848, Payment for Physician Services. The new section contained three major elements:

1. Establishment of standard rates of increase of expenditures for physicians' services

2. Replacement of the reasonable charge payment mechanism by a fee schedule for physicians' services

3. Replacement of the maximum actual allowable charge (MAAC), which limits the total amount non-QIO physicians could charge

Revisions were made and a new Omnibus Budget Reconciliation Act of 1990 was passed. OBRA 1990 contained several modifications and clarifications of the provisions establishing the physician fee schedule. This final rule required that before January 1 of each year, beginning with 1992, the Secretary establish, by regulation, fee schedules that determine payment amounts for all physicians' services furnished in all fee schedule areas for the year.

The physician fee schedule is updated each April 15 and is composed of three basic elements:

1. The relative value units for each service

2. A geographic adjustment factor to adjust for regional variations in the cost of operating a health care facility

3. A national conversion factor

CHECK THIS OUT ☞ The CMS Physician Fee Schedule Search can be accessed at http://www.cms.hhs.gov/pfslookup/02_PFSsearch.asp to locate the current pricing by code.

Medicare volume performance standards have been developed to be used as a tool to monitor annual increases in Part B expenditures for physicians' services and, when appropriate, to adjust payment levels to reflect the success or failure in meeting the performance standards. Various financial protections have been designed and instituted on behalf of the Medicare beneficiary. Uniformity of administration and standardization of procedures, policies, and coding have been implemented so that all Medicare MACs communicate on the same level and use the same language.

National Fee Schedule

Beginning January 1, 1992, the Medicare Fee Schedule (MFS) replaced the reasonable-charge payment system. All physicians' services are paid on the basis of the amounts indicated in the new MFS. Reimbursement is made at 80% of the fee schedule amount, subject to the annual Part B Medicare deductible. The fee schedule applies to Medicare payment for physicians' services and supplies furnished "incidental to" physicians' services, outpatient physical and occupational therapy services, diagnostic tests, and radiology services. The fee schedule applies when payment is made to either physicians or suppliers.

Relative Value Unit

Nationally, unit values have been assigned for each service, and they are determined on the basis of the resources necessary to the physician's performance of the service. By analyzing a service, a Harvard team was able to identify its separate parts and assign each part a relative value unit (RVU). These parts or components are as follows:

1. Work. The work component is identified as the amount of time, the intensity of effort, and the technical expertise required for the physician to provide the service.

2. Overhead. The overhead component is identified as the allocation of costs associated with the physician's practice (e.g., rent, staffing, supplies) that must be expended in order to provide a service.

3. Malpractice. The malpractice component is identified as the cost of the medical malpractice insurance coverage associated with providing service.

The sum of the units established for each component of the service equals the total RVUs of a service.

A relative value of 1 has been established for a midlevel, established-patient office visit (99213). All other services are valued at, above, or below this service relative to the work, overhead, and malpractice expenses associated with the service.

Geographic Practice Cost Index

The Urban Institute developed scales that measure cost differences in various areas. The Geographic Practice Cost Indices (GPCIs) have been established for each of the prevailing charge localities. An entire state may be considered a locality for purposes of physician payment reform. The GPCIs reflect the relative costs of practice in a given locality compared with the national average. The national average is 1. A separate GPCI has been established and is applied to each component of a service.

Conversion Factor

The conversion factor (CF) is a national dollar amount that is applied to all services paid on the basis of the Medicare Fee Schedule. Congress provided a CF to be used to convert RVUs to dollars. The CF is updated annually on the basis of the data sources, which indicate

- Percent changes to the Medicare Economic Index (MEI)
- Percent changes in physician expenditures

- The relationship of expenditures to volume performance standards
- Change in access and quality

The CF varies according to the type of service provided (e.g., medical, surgical, nonsurgical).

The Transition

To prevent extreme fluctuation in Medicare reimbursement amounts, some of the fee schedule amounts were subject to a 5-year transitional phase-in. A historical payment base charge (HPBC) was established for all services so it could be used in a comparison with the fee schedule allowance. Simply put, this means that Medicare allowed 5 years to bring the prices for services to the fee schedule amounts. Those prices that were higher than the fee schedule slowly dropped during this period, and those that were lower were slowly raised. By 1996, all prices for services reflected the fee schedule amount.

CHECK THIS OUT ☞ The Physician Fee Schedule (PFS) is located at http://www.cms.hhs.gov/PhysicianFeeSched/PFSRVF/list.asp#TopOfPage

Medicare Volume Performance Standards

The Medicare Volume Performance Standards (MVPS) are best thought of as an object. "It" represents the government's estimate of how much growth is appropriate for nationwide physician expenditures paid by the Part B Medicare program. The purpose of MVPS is to guide Congress in its consideration of the appropriate annual payment update.

The Secretary of Health and Human Services must make MVPS recommendations to Congress by April 15 for the upcoming fiscal year, and by May 15, the Physician Payment Review Commission (PPRC) must make its recommendations for the fiscal year. Congress has until October 15 to establish the MVPS by either accepting or modifying the two proposed MVPS recommendations.

If Congress does not react by October 15, the MVPS rate is established by using a default mechanism. If the default mechanism is used, the Secretary is then required to publish a notice in the *Federal Register* that provides the formula for deriving the MVPS.

Variations in health care usage by Medicare patients occur every year. Because Medicare strives for balanced billing, if CMS agrees to pay for additional services not previously paid for or increases the weights of CPT codes, thus increasing reimbursement, then discounts are taken across the board so that more money than authorized is not spent and the budget is balanced.

Beneficiary Protection

Several provisions in the Physician Payment Reform were designed to protect Medicare beneficiaries.

1. As of September 1, 1990, all providers must file claims for their Medicare patients (free of charge). In addition, claims must be submitted within 15 ~~to 27~~ months from the date of service or they will be subject to a 10% reduction in payment.
2. The Omnibus Budget Reconciliation Act of 1989 requires the physician to accept the amount paid for eligible Medicaid services (mandatory assignment).
3. Effective January 1, 1991, the Maximum Actual Allowable Charge (MAAC) limitations that applied to unassigned physician charges were replaced by new billing limits called limiting charges. The provisions of the new limitations state that nonparticipating physicians and suppliers cannot charge more than the stated limiting charge on unassigned claims.

Limiting Charge

In 1991 and 1992, the limiting charge was specific to each physician. Beginning in 1993, the limiting charge for a service has been the same for all physicians within a locality, regardless of specialty. The limiting charge for each service also appears on the beneficiary's Explanation of Medicare Benefits.

The limiting charge applies to every service listed in the Medicare Physicians' Fee Schedule that is performed by a nonparticipating physician. This includes global, professional, and technical services performed by a physician. When a nonphysician provider (e.g., portable x-ray supplier, laboratory technician) provides the technical component of a service that is on the fee schedule, the limiting charge does not apply. CPT codes are assigned many different prices. The amount determined by multiplying the RVU weight by the geographic index and the conversion factor is called the fee schedule amount. If a physician is participating, he or she receives the fee schedule amount. If the physician is not participating, the fee schedule amount or the allowable payment is slightly less than the participating physician's payment. The limiting amount is a percentage over the allowable (e.g., 115% times the allowable amount). The limiting charge is important because that is the maximum amount a Medicare patient can be billed for a service. For covered services, Medicare usually pays 80% of the allowable amount. The beneficiary is then balance-billed, which means that the patient is billed the difference between what Medicare pays and the limiting charge.

Example

Limiting charge is	$115	(Maximum charge)
Allowable is	$100	
Medicare pays	$80	(Medicare pays 80%)
Patient is billed	$35	($20, 20% of $100, and $15, the remainder of the limiting charge maximum)

Physicians may round the limiting charge to the nearest dollar if they do this consistently for all services.

Uniformity Provision

Equitable use of the Medicare fee schedule requires a payment system with a uniform policy and uniform procedures. Because the relative value of the work component of a service is the same nationwide (except for a geographic practice cost adjustment), it is important that when physicians across the country are paid for a service they be paid for the same amount, or "package," of work. For example, the preoperative and postoperative periods included in the payment must be the same. To prevent variation in interpretation, standard definitions of services are required.

Adjustments

Whenever an adjustment of the full fee schedule amount is made to a service, the limiting charge for that service must be adjusted. Medicare has provided adjusted limiting charges to providers for services to which the site-of-service limitation applies, the assistant-at-surgery limitation applies, and multiple surgery limitations apply, and when only a portion of the global surgical package is being provided. These adjustments are identified on the physician disclosure, which is provided to all physicians during the participating enrollment period each year.

Adjustments to the limiting charge must be manually calculated before submitting unassigned claims for all services in which a fee schedule limitation applies.

Payments to nonparticipating physicians will not exceed 95% of the physician fee schedule for a service.

Site-of-Service Limitations

Services that are performed primarily in office settings are subject to a payment discount if they are performed in outpatient hospital departments. There is a national list of procedures that are performed 50% of the time in the office setting. These procedures are subject to site-of-service limitations, which means that a discount is taken on any service that is performed in a setting other than a clinic setting. For instance, an arthrocentesis is normally performed in the office. If a physician provides this service in a hospital outpatient setting, the limiting charge will be less than that for the office setting. This is because the hospital will also be billing Medicare for the use of the room and the supplies. Medicare has a built-in practice expense, or overhead, for the clinic setting (the RVU weight for practice expense), and Medicare doesn't want to pay twice for the overhead. So part of the overhead is reduced from the physician's payment to make up for the hospital payment. For these procedures, the practice expense RVU is reduced by 50%. Payment is the lower of the actual charge or the reduced fee schedule amount. Physicians who bill an emergency department visit are not subject to the outpatient limit on these services.

Surgical Modifier Circumstances

Multiple Surgery

General. If a surgeon performs more than one procedure on the same patient on the same day, discounts are made on all subsequent procedures. Medicare will pay 100% of the fee for the highest value procedure, 50% for the second most expensive procedure, and 25% for the third, fourth, and fifth procedures. Discounting is why the service (CPT code) that you place the modifier on is so important! Each procedure after the fifth procedure requires documentation and special carrier review to determine the payment amount. These discount amounts are subject to review every year by the CMS.

Commercial insurers often follow discount limits different from those of Medicare, as established by their own individual reimbursement policies.

Endoscopic Procedures. In the case of multiple endoscopic procedures, Medicare allows the full value of the highest valued endoscopy, plus the difference between the next highest endoscopy and the base endoscopy. As in all other reimbursement issues, some non-Medicare carriers follow this pricing method, whereas others follow their own multiple-procedure discounting policies.

Dermatologic Surgery. For certain dermatology services, there are CPT codes that indicate that multiple surgical procedures have been performed. When the CPT code description states "additional," the general multiple-procedure rules do not apply.

Providers Furnishing Part of the Global Fee Package.

Under the fee schedule, Medicare pays the same amount for surgical services furnished by several physicians as it pays if only one physician furnished all of the services in the global package.

Medicare pays each physician directly for his or her part of the global surgical services. The policy is written with the assumption that the surgeon always furnishes the usual and necessary preoperative and intraoperative services and also, with a few exceptions, in-hospital postoperative services. In most cases, the surgeon also furnishes the postoperative office services necessary to ensure normal recovery from the surgery. Recognizing that there are cases in which the surgeon turns over the out-of-hospital recovery care to another physician, Medicare has determined percentages for families of procedures for paying usual out-of-hospital postoperative care if furnished by someone other than the surgeon. These are weighted percentages based on the percentage of total global surgical work.

Again, become familiar with individual third-party payer policies, because some may not split their global payments in this manner.

Physicians Who Assist at Surgery. Physicians assisting the primary physician in a procedure receive a set percentage of the total fee for the service. Medicare sets the payment level for assistants-at-surgery at 16% of the fee schedule amount for the global surgical service. Non-Medicare payers may set this percentage at 20% or more. CPT modifiers -80 (Assistant Surgeon), -81 (Minimum Assistant Surgeon), and -82 (Assistant Surgeon, when qualified resident surgeon not available) would be appended to the code to indicate the type of assistant.

Two Surgeons and Surgical Team. When two surgeons of different specialties perform a procedure, each is paid an equal percentage of the global fee. For co-surgeons, Medicare pays 125% of the global fee, dividing the payment equally between the two surgeons (or each will receive 62.5% of the global fee). No payment is made for an assistant-at-surgery in these cases.

For team surgery, a medical director determines the payment amounts on an individual basis. Modifiers -62 (Two Surgeons) or -66 (Surgical Team) would be appended to the code.

QUICK CHECK 16-2

Match the modifier or modifiers with the correct definition.

	Modifiers
1. Multiple Surgery _____	a. -56
2. Part of Global Fee Package ____ ____ ____	b. -80
3. Assistant Physicians ____ ____ ____	c. -54
4. Two Surgeons _____	d. -51
5. Surgical Team _____	e. -55
	f. -62
	g. -82
	h. -66
	i. -81

Purchased Diagnostic Services. For physicians who bill for a diagnostic test performed by an outside supplier, the fee schedule amount is limited to the lower of the billing physician's fee schedule amount or the price he or she paid for the service.

Reoperations. The amount paid by Medicare for a return trip to the operating room for treatment of a complication is limited to the intraoperative portion of the code that best describes the treatment of the complications.

When an unlisted procedure is billed because no other code exists to describe the treatment, payment is based on a maximum of 50% of the value of the intraoperative services originally performed.

Commercial insurance companies again have their own guidelines. Many do not take discounts for these subsequent surgical procedures. Modifiers -78 (Return to Operating Room for a Related Procedure During the Postoperative Period) or -79 (Unrelated Procedure or Service by the Same Physician During the Postoperative Period) would be appended to the code to more specifically identify that the service was a reoperation.

EXERCISE 16–5 *RBRVS*

Fill in the blanks with the correct words:

1 What does RBRVS stand for? *Resource Based Relative Value Scale*

2 The Medicare Economic Index is published in what publication? *Fed Register*

3 In 1989, a major change took place in Medicare with the enactment of *OBRA*

THE PROSPECTIVE PAYMENT SYSTEM FOR THE SKILLED NURSING FACILITY

Effective July 1, 1998, a per diem prospective payment system (PPS) for skilled nursing facilities (SNFs) was implemented to cover all costs (routine, ancillary, and capital) related to services provided to Medicare Part A beneficiaries. Federal rates were established using fiscal year (FY) 1995 cost reports, and per diem payments are case-mix-adjusted according to a classification system entitled Resource Utilization Groups III (RUGS III).

Information collected by completing the Minimum Data Set 2.0 (MDS 2.0) resident assessment instrument (RAI) determines the amount of per diem payments for each SNF admission. Payments are case-mix-adjusted on the basis of data from the MDS 2.0 and relative weights determined by SNF staff time. The per diem rate is adjusted for geographic variation in wages, using the hospital wage index, and rates are expected to increase each federal fiscal year using an SNF market-basket index.

OUTPATIENT MEDICARE REIMBURSEMENT SYSTEM—APC

Medicare payments for hospital services, both inpatient and outpatient, were historically based on the customary and reasonable cost of a service. In 1983, the law that governs Medicare was revised to move from this cost-based payment to a prospective payment system (PPS) for hospital inpatients. Outpatient hospital services continued to operate on the cost-based system. Advances in medical technology and changes in practices (such as more outpatient surgery) brought a shift in the site of medical care from the inpatient to the outpatient setting. In the years that followed, Congress enacted many laws to try to curb this shift to outpatient-based services, but to no avail. OBRA 1986 (the Omnibus Budget Reconciliation Act of 1986) contained a requirement to replace the existing outpatient hospital cost-based system with a PPS. Also with OBRA 1986 came the ability to require hospitals to report claims for services under the CMS Healthcare Common Procedural Coding System (HCPCS). This coding requirement provided data to CMS about the specific services being provided on an outpatient basis. These data were used to develop the outpatient PPS.

CMS conducted research into ways to classify outpatient services for the purposes of developing the outpatient PPS. The resulting report cited the Ambulatory Patient Groups (APGs), developed by 3M Health Information Systems under a cooperative grant with CMS, as the most promising classification system for grouping outpatient services, and recommended that APG-like groups be used in the hospital PPS. The APG-like groups were named Ambulatory Patient Classifications (APCs) and were scheduled for implementation on January 1, 1999. Implementation was final on August 1, 2000.

Introduction to Ambulatory Payment Classifications

APCs are a system for reimbursing facilities for Medicare outpatient health care. They are mandatory for all hospital outpatient services. They include inpatient services covered under Part B for beneficiaries who are entitled to Part A benefits but who have exhausted their Part A benefits or otherwise are not involved in a hospital stay covered by Part A. Patients who receive partial hospitalization services furnished by community mental health centers also qualify to have their services paid for under the PPS of APCs. In general, the definition of a hospital outpatient is an individual who is not an inpatient of the hospital but who is registered as an outpatient.

A coinsurance amount is calculated for each APC based on 20% of the national median charge for services in the APC. The coinsurance amount for an APC will not change until such time as the amount becomes 20% of the total APC payment.

Fig. 16–9 shows the broad range of categories of services provided under the Medicare program and which categories are paid according to the APC rate. The APC system consists of groups of services that are covered under this hospital outpatient prospective payment system (OPPS). Each procedure is then assigned into a group of APCs, and the payment rate and beneficiary payment portion are identified (Fig. 16–10). The services are identified by HCPCS codes and descriptions. The APCs identify the packaged services that are included in each APC. Packaged services are those that are recognized as contributing to the cost of the services in the APC, but that Medicare does not pay for separately. Under the APC system, packaged services include the operating room, recovery room, anesthesia, medical/surgical supplies, pharmaceuticals, observation, blood, intraocular lenses, casts and splints, donor tissue, and various incidental services such as venipuncture. Also bundled into the APC is any medical visit that takes place on the same date of service as a scheduled outpatient surgery. Registration of the patient, taking of vital signs, insertion of an IV, preparation for surgery, and so forth, are packaged into and paid for as a part of the APC group to which the surgical procedure or service is classified.

APC packaging includes certain items such as anesthesia, supplies, certain drugs, and the use of the recovery and observation rooms. Multiple APC surgical procedures furnished during the same operative session will be discounted. Discounting operates on the same principle as the surgical package. The first surgical procedure is paid at 100% and the second surgical procedure is paid at 50%. Another discounting situation occurs when the surgical procedure is terminated after the patient has been prepared for surgery but before the induction of the anesthesia. In this case, the payment would be 50% of the usual APC payment.

ADDENDUM D1. — OPPS PAYMENT STATUS INDICATORS

Indicator	Item/Code/Service	OPPS Payment Status
A	Services furnished to a hospital outpatient that are paid under a fee schedule or payment system other than OPPS, for example: • Ambulance Services. • Clinical Diagnostic Laboratory Services .... • Non-Implantable Prosthetic and Orthotic Devices. • EPO for ESRD Patients. • Physical, Occupational, and Speech Therapy. • Routine Dialysis Services for ESRD Patients Provided in a Certified Dialysis Unit of a Hospital. • Diagnostic Mammography. • Screening Mammography	Not paid under OPPS. Paid by fiscal intermediaries/MACs under a fee schedule or payment system other than OPPS. Not subject to deductible or coinsurance. Not subject to deductible.
B	Codes that are not recognized by OPPS when submitted on an outpatient hospital Part B bill type (12x and 13x).	Not paid under OPPS. • May be paid by fiscal intermediaries/MACs when submitted on a different bill type, for example, 75x (CORF), but not paid under OPPS. • An alternate code that is recognized by OPPS when submitted on an outpatient hospital Part B bill type (12x and 13x) may be available.
C	Inpatient Procedures	Not paid under OPPS. Admit patient. Bill as inpatient.
D	Discontinued Codes	Not paid under OPPS or any other Medicare payment system.
E	Items, Codes, and Services: • That are not covered by Medicare based on statutory exclusion. • That are not covered by Medicare for reasons other than statutory exclusion. • That are not recognized by Medicare but for which an alternate code for the same item or service may be available. • For which separate payment is not provided by Medicare.	Not paid under OPPS or any other Medicare payment system.
F	Corneal Tissue Acquisition; Certain CRNA Services and Hepatitis B Vaccines.	Not paid under OPPS. Paid at reasonable cost.
G	Pass-Through Drugs and Biologicals	Paid under OPPS; separate APC payment includes pass-through amount.
H	Pass-Through Device Categories	Separate cost-based pass-through payment; not subject to copayment.
K	(1) Nonpass-Through Drugs and Biologicals .... (2) Therapeutic Radiopharmaceuticals .... (3) Brachytherapy Sources .... (4) Blood and Blood Products	(1) Paid under OPPS; separate APC payment. (2) Paid under OPPS; separate APC payment. (3) Paid under OPPS; separate APC payment. (4) Paid under OPPS; separate APC payment.
L	Influenza Vaccine; Pneumococcal Pneumonia Vaccine	Not paid under OPPS. Paid at reasonable cost; not subject to deductible or coinsurance.
M	Items and Services Not Billable to the Fiscal Intermediary/MAC.	Not paid under OPPS.
N	Items and Services Packaged into APC Rates	Paid under OPPS; payment is packaged into payment for other services, including outliers. Therefore, there is no separate APC payment.
P	Partial Hospitalization	Not paid under OPPS; per diem APC payment.
Q	Packaged Services Subject to Separate Payment under OPPS Payment Criteria.	Paid under OPPS; Addendum B displays APC assignments when services are separately payable. (1) Separate APC payment based on OPPS payment criteria. (2) If criteria are not met, payment is packaged into payment for other services, including outliers. Therefore, there is no separate APC payment.
S	Significant Procedure, Not Discounted when Multiple	Paid under OPPS; separate APC payment.
T	Significant Procedure, Multiple Reduction Applies	Paid under OPPS; separate APC payment.
V	Clinic or Emergency Department Visit	Paid under OPPS; separate APC payment.
X	Ancillary Services	Paid under OPPS; separate APC payment.
Y	Non-Implantable Durable Medical Equipment	Not paid under OPPS. All institutional providers other than home health agencies bill to DMERC.

FIGURE 16–9 A listing of groups of services and the payment status for each group.[13]

APC	HCPCS Code	Group Title	Short Descriptor	SI	Relative Weight	Payment Rate	National Unadjusted Copayment	Minimum Unadjusted Copayment
0001		Level I Photochemotherapy		S	0.5204	33.15	7.00	6.63
0001	96900		Ultraviolet light therapy					
0001	96910		Photochemotherapy with UV-B					
0001	96912		Photochemotherapy with UV-A					
0002		Level I Fine Needle Biopsy/Aspiration		T	1.1915	75.89		15.18
0002	10021		Fna w/o image					
0002	19001		Drain breast lesion add-on					
0002	36680		Insert needle, bone cavity					
0002	G0364		Bone marrow aspirate & biopsy					
0003		Bone Marrow Biopsy/Aspiration		T	3.239	206.30		41.26
0003	38220		Bone marrow aspiration					
0003	38221		Bone marrow biopsy					
0004		Level I Needle Biopsy/Aspiration Except Bone Marrow		T	4.5062	287.01		57.40
0004	10022		Fna w/ image					
0004	19000		Drainage of breast lesion					
0004	19100		Bx breast percut w/o image					
0004	20615		Treatment of bone cyst					
0004	47399		Liver surgery procedure					
0004	48999		Pancreas surgery procedure					
0004	54800		Biopsy of epididymis					
0004	55000		Drainage of hydrocele					
0004	60001		Aspirate/inject thyroid cyst					
0004	60100		Biopsy of thyroid					
0005		Level II Needle Biopsy/Aspiration Except Bone Marrow		T	7.3012	465.04		93.01

Labels: APC number, HCPCS code, Group title, Description, Status indicator, Payment rate, Copayment, Copayment

FIGURE 16–10 APCs with group titles and payment rates.[14]

EXERCISE 16–6 *APCs*

Fill in the blanks:

1 APC stands for

_____

_____.

2 The final implemented of APCs was August 1 of this year. _____

3 The coinsurance amount for the beneficiaries under the APC system is _____ percent.

4 According to Figure 16–9, status indicator D indicates a code that has been _____.

MEDICARE FRAUD AND ABUSE

What Are Fraud and Abuse?

The Medicare program is subject to fraud and abuse, as is any third-party payer program. But because Medicare is the largest third-party payer, it has the most comprehensive anti-fraud and -abuse program. You must understand the specifics of this program because you will be filing Medicare claims. CMS is responsible for establishing the regulations that monitor the Medicare program for fraud and abuse.

CHECK THIS OUT ☞ Check out free Web-based training course on fraud and abuse available at the CMS website http://cms.meridianksi.com/kc/main/kc_frame.asp?kc_ident=kc0001&loc=1

Fraud is the intentional deception or misrepresentation that an individual knows to be false or does not believe to be true and makes it knowing that the deception could result in some unauthorized benefit to himself/herself or some other person. Fraud involves both deliberate intention to deceive and an expectation of an unauthorized benefit. By this definition, it is fraud if a claim is filed for a service rendered to a Medicare patient when that service was not actually provided. How could this type of fraud happen? The fact is that most Medicare patients sign a standing approval, which is kept on file in the medical office. Having a standing approval is convenient for the patient and for the coding staff. After the patient has received a service, the Medicare claim is filed automatically, without the patient's having to sign the form. But a standing approval also makes it easy for unscrupulous persons to submit charges for services never provided. This circumstance also makes it possible for extra services to be submitted in addition to services that were provided (upcoding). Suppose, for example, a patient came in for an office visit and a claim was submitted for an in-office surgical procedure. That's also fraud.

🖐 **CAUTION** *The most common kind of fraud arises from a false statement or misrepresentation made, or caused to be made, that results in additional payment by the Medicare program.*

Who Are the Violators? The violator may be a physician or other practitioner, a hospital or other institutional provider, a clinical laboratory or other supplier, an employee of any provider, a billing service, a beneficiary, a Medicare carrier employee, or any person in a position to file a claim for Medicare benefits. You will be the person filing Medicare claims so you have to be careful about the claims you submit—it's important to validate that the service was provided by consulting the medical record or the physician.

Fraud schemes range from those committed by individuals acting alone to broad-based activities perpetrated by institutions or groups of individuals, sometimes employing sophisticated telemarketing and other promotional techniques to lure consumers into serving as unwitting tools in the schemes. Seldom do such perpetrators target just one insurer; nor do they focus exclusively on either the public or the private sector. Rather, most are found to be defrauding several private- and public-sector victims such as Medicare simultaneously.

What Forms Does Fraud Take? The most common forms of Medicare fraud are:

- Billing for services not furnished
- Misrepresenting a diagnosis to justify a payment
- Soliciting, offering, or receiving a kickback
- Unbundling, or "exploding," charges
- Falsifying certificates of medical necessity, plans of treatment, and medical records to justify payment
- Billing for additional services not furnished as billed—that is, upcoding
- Routine waiver of copayment

Who Says What Is Fraudulent? CMS administers the Medicare program. CMS's responsibilities include managing contractor claims payment, overseeing fiscal audit and/or overpayment prevention and recovery, and developing and monitoring the payment safeguards necessary to detect and respond to payment errors or abusive patterns of service delivery. Within CMS's Bureau of Program Operations is the Office of Benefits Integrity (OBI), which oversees Medicare's payment safeguard program, including carrier and intermediary operations related to fraud, audit, medical review, the collection of overpayments, and the imposition of civil monetary penalties (CMPs) for certain violations of Medicare law.

The Office of the Inspector General (OIG), Department of Health and Human Services, is responsible for developing an annual work plan that outlines the ways in which the Medicare program is monitored to identify fraud and abuse. The plan is a published public document that provides the evaluation methods and approaches that will be taken the following year to monitor the Medicare program. For example, in the 2008 Work Plan, the following is listed as the review of "Incident to" services:

MEDICARE "INCIDENT TO" SERVICES

We will review Medicare claims for services furnished "incident to" the professional services of selected physicians. Medicare Part B generally pays for services "incident to" a physician's professional service; such services are typically performed by a nonphysician staff member in the physician's office. Federal regulations at 42 CFR § 410.26(b) specify criteria for "incident to" services. We will examine the Medicare services that selected physicians bill "incident to" their professional services and the qualifications and appropriateness of the staff who perform them. This study will review medical necessity, documentation, and quality of care for "incident to" services.[15]

This excerpt from the OIG Work Plan identifies a specific area to be monitored in that year. The OIG charges the MACs with doing the actual monitoring. (Recall that insurance companies bid for the opportunity to be the MAC for Medicare and handle the payments to providers for Medicare services.) The OIG Work Plan sets the broad boundaries for monitoring the Medicare program for fraud and abuse.

CHECK THIS OUT ☞ The site http://www.oig.doc.gov/oig/reports/other_publications/ contains the OIG work plan for the current year and previous years.

The Specific Regulations Are in the IOMs

CMS establishes the specific regulations in the Internet-Only Manuals (IOMs) for the providers and carriers to follow. You will deal with regulations as you code Medicare claims in order to know what is allowable.

CHECK THIS OUT ☞ The IOMs are located at http://www.cms.hhs.gov/Manuals/IOM/list.asp and 100-08, Medicare Program Integrity Manual, with many directions on fraud and abuse.

Attempts to defraud the Medicare program may take a variety of forms. The following are some examples of how fraud may be perpetrated in the Medicare medical insurance program:

- Billing for services or supplies that were not provided. This includes billings for "no shows," i.e., billing Medicare for services that were not actually furnished because patients failed to keep their appointments;
- Misrepresenting the diagnosis for the patient to justify the services or equipment furnished;

- Altering claim forms to obtain a higher payment amount;
- Deliberately applying for duplicate payment, e.g., billing both Medicare and the beneficiary for the same service or billing both Medicare and another insurer in an attempt to get paid twice;
- Soliciting, offering, or receiving a kickback, bribe, or rebate, e.g., paying for a referral of patients in exchange for the ordering of diagnostic tests and other services or medical equipment;
- Unbundling or "exploding" charges, e.g., the billing of a multichannel set of lab tests to appear as if the individual tests had been performed.
- Completing Certificates of Medical Necessity (CMN) for patients not personally and professionally known by the provider;
- Misrepresenting the services rendered (upcoding or the use of procedure codes not appropriate for the item or service actually furnished), amounts charged for services rendered, identity of the person receiving the services, dates of services, etc;
- Billing for noncovered services, e.g., routine foot care billed as a more involved form of foot care to obtain payment;
- Participating in schemes that involve collusion between a provider and a beneficiary, or between a supplier and a provider, and result in higher costs or charges to the Medicare program;
- Using another person's Medicare card to obtain medical care;
- Utilizing split billing schemes (e.g., billing procedures over a period of days when all treatment occurred during one visit);
- Participating in schemes that involve collusion between a provider and a carrier employee where the claim is assigned, e.g., the provider deliberately overbills for services, and the carrier employee then generates adjustments with little or no awareness on the part of the beneficiary;
- Manipulating claims data on unassigned claims for one's own benefit, e.g., through manipulation of beneficiary address or the claims history record, a carrier employee could generate adjustment payments against many beneficiary records and cause payments to be mailed to an address known only to him/her; and
- Billing based on "gang visits," e.g., a physician visits a nursing home and bills for 20 nursing home visits without furnishing any specific service to, or on behalf of, individual patients.

How to Protect Yourself. As you can see from the preceding information about Medicare fraud and abuse, CMS is very serious about identifying those who try to take advantage of the program. As the person submitting the Medicare claims, you are one of those whom the CMS holds responsible for submitting truthful and accurate claims. If you are unsure about a charge or a request, check with the physician or other supervisory personnel to ensure that you are submitting the correct charges for each patient. In this way, you protect the Medicare program, your facility, and yourself.

CHECK THIS OUT ☞ CMS fraud and abuse guidelines at http://www.cms. hhs.gov/MDFraudAbuseGenInfo/

THE MANAGED HEALTH CARE CONCEPT

Health care in the United States is the best in the world, and people come from all over the world to access the health care that U.S. residents take for granted. Physicians and health care have traditionally been held in high esteem by U.S. citizens. Whatever it took to provide access to high-quality health care is what these citizens demanded. Historically, the government responded to these demands by funding the research, facilities, and services necessary to keep the U.S. health system on the cutting edge of medical advances. But the research, facilities, and services are extremely expensive, and many U.S. citizens are also demanding a balanced federal budget.

Health care services in the United States are undergoing rapid change. The U.S. health care system has been financed through traditional health insurance systems, which paid providers on a fee-for-service basis and allowed beneficiaries relative freedom in their selection of health care providers. Health insurance has become an important benefit of employment. Employers became the primary purchasers of health insurance, and the rising cost of health care is reflected in the premiums employers pay and the subsequent decrease in employer-sponsored coverage. Private purchasers of health insurance have also seen a steady increase in their health insurance premiums, until many are forced to go "bare," forgoing health insurance due to the high costs. Fewer people now have health insurance coverage as a benefit of their employment. The number of uninsured people increased to 47 million in 2008,[16] and the number of uninsured continues to rise as employers and individuals find health care insurance out of their reach. One way of containing health care costs that has widespread popularity is managed health care.

The term "managed health care" refers to the concept of establishing networks of health care providers that offer an array of health care services under the umbrella of a single organization. A managed health care organization may be a group of physicians, hospitals, and health plans responsible for the health services for an enrolled individual or group. The organization coordinates the total health care services required by its enrollees. The purpose of managed health care is to provide cost-effectiveness of services and theoretically to improve the health care services provided to the enrollee by ensuring access to all required health services.

Many models are used to deliver managed health care: Health Maintenance Organizations (HMOs), Individual Practice Associations (IPAs), Group Practice, Multiple Option Plan, Medicare Risk HMOs, Preferred Provider Organizations (PPOs), and the Staff model. Each of these models delivers managed health care using a different structure.

Currently, 80 million persons are enrolled in HMOs.[17] HMO and PPO enrollees make up 41% of the U.S. population. The use of the managed health care approach varies widely with geography. There continues to be a rise in the percentage of employers opting for a managed care health plan for their employees; this indicates the employers' search for cost containment while offering the benefit of health coverage to employees.

The managed care industry has evolved from small, regional nonprofit plans to large, national, for-profit companies. Eleven national managed care companies now account for half of all HMO enrollment.

The pressure on the government to cut expenses and balance the budget guarantees the continued increases in market share for managed care. The government mandated the use of managed care within the Medicaid program, and the number of Medicaid beneficiaries enrolled in managed care continues to increase.

In the early stages of development, the managed care market included networks that allowed the enrollees a broad choice of providers. As the market segments for managed care expanded, choice for the enrollees decreased.

Types of HMOs

A **Managed Care Organization (MCO)** is a group that is responsible for the health care services offered to an enrolled group or person. The organization coordinates or manages the care of the enrollee. The MCO contains costs by negotiating with various health care entities—hospitals, clinics, laboratories, and so forth—for a discounted rate for services provided to its enrollees. Providers of the health care services must receive prior approval from the MCO before services are rendered. For example, a physician may want to conduct a certain high-cost diagnostic test, but before the test can be conducted, the MCO must give the physician approval. The MCO uses a gatekeeper, usually the primary care physician of the patient, who can authorize the patient's need to seek health care services outside of the established organization. For example, a certain specialist may not be available within the MCO, and the primary care physician can recommend that the enrollee be referred to such a specialist. If the enrollee were to see the specialist without the recommendation of the primary care physician and the approval of the MCO, the enrollee would be responsible for charges incurred. MCOs develop practice guidelines that evaluate the appropriateness and medical necessity of medical care provided to the enrollee by the physicians, which gives the MCO control over what care is provided to the enrollee.

A **Preferred Provider Organization (PPO)** is a group of providers who form a network and who have agreed to provide services to enrollees at a discounted rate. Enrollees are usually responsible for paying a portion of the costs (cost sharing) when using a PPO provider. Enrollees who seek health care outside of the PPO providers pay an additional out-of-pocket cost. The out-of-pocket costs are established by the PPO to discourage the use of outside providers. The PPOs do not use a gatekeeper, but they do have strict guidelines that denote approved expenses and how much the enrollee will pay.

A **Health Maintenance Organization (HMO)** is a delivery system that allows the enrollee access to all health care services. The HMO is the "total package" approach to health care organizations, and the out-of-pocket expenses are minimal. However, the enrollee is assigned a primary care physician who manages all the health care needs of the enrollee and acts as the gatekeeper for the enrollee. Services are prepaid by the HMO. For example, the HMO pays a laboratory to provide services at a negotiated price and the services are prepaid by the HMO. The gatekeeper has authority to allow the enrollee access to the services available or authorize services outside of those the HMO has available. The gatekeeper has strong incentives to contain costs for the HMO by controlling and managing the health care services provided to the enrollee. The HMO can directly employ the physician in the **Staff Model** HMO or contract the physician through the **Individual Practice Associations (IPA)** model in which the physician provides services for a set fee. Either way, the physician has an incentive to service the cost containment needs of the HMO.

An **Exclusive Provider Organization (EPO)** has many of the same features as an HMO except that the providers of the services are not prepaid. Instead, the providers are paid on a fee-for-service basis. The **Group Practice Model (GPM)** is a form of HMO in which an organization of physicians contracts with the HMO to provide services to the enrollees of the HMO. A payment is negotiated, the HMO pays the group, and then the group pays the individual physicians.

Medicare Advantage (formerly **Medicare + Choice**) is a Medicare-funded alternative to the standard Medicare supplemental coverage. Medicare Advantage is a standard HMO; however, it is provided to Medicare beneficiaries rather than the traditional fee-for-service model historically used by Medicare. The enrollees pay out of pocket if they choose to go outside the network of providers. **Point-of-Service (POS)** benefits allow enrollees to receive services outside of the HMO's health care network, but at increased cost in copayments, in coinsurance, or in a deductible. The POS benefit is one that the HMO may choose to offer, but it is not required, and the CMS does not provide any additional funding for this benefit. However, the HMO that offers this option is more attractive to a potential enrollee, because the lack of access to providers outside of a predefined network is the one reason people do not join a managed health care organization. The POS benefit option is also referred to as an **open-ended HMO** or a **self-referral option**. The POS benefit is attractive not only to Medicare enrollees who wish to be treated by providers not available in their plan's network but also to those who travel and would like access to routine medical care while temporarily (for fewer than 90 days) out of their plan's service area.

Program for All-Inclusive Care for the Elderly (PACE) is a program developed to address the needs of long-term care clients, providers, and payers. The program provides a comprehensive package of services that permits the clients to continue to live in their homes while receiving services rather than being placed in an institution.

Managed health care is now part of the fabric of the U.S. health care system. The "richer" plans of traditional insurance companies are often no longer an option to a great segment of the population.

Drawbacks of the HMO. There are some significant drawbacks to the HMO concept in terms of access to health care. Consider that providers (physicians in particular) have an incentive to keep treatment costs to a minimum. Traditionally, a physician's primary concern was what was in the best interest of the patient, not what was in the best interest of containment of cost. This fundamental change transformed physicians into gatekeepers for third-party payers and transformed third-party payers into developers of guidelines that ultimately control the services patients can and do receive. The patient-physician relationship has shifted to a physician/third-party-payer relationship, which leaves the patient at the mercy of the third-party payer. Many lawsuits have been brought by patients who allege that lack of treatment caused harm and sometimes death. Cost-containment issues, and hence HMOs, raise many ethical and legal issues that will continue to involve patients, providers, and third-party payers.

CHAPTER REVIEW

CHAPTER 16, PART I, THEORY

Complete the following:

1 What two insurance programs were established in 1965 by amendments to the Social Security Act?

_____

_____

2 The Secretary of DHHS has delegated responsibility for Medicare to which department?

_____

_____

3 Who administers funds for Medicare?

4 Who is eligible for Medicare?

_____

_____

5 QIO stands for

_____

6 A CORF stands for

_____ _____

_____ _____

7 List the three components of the relative value unit:

_____

_____

_____

8 What does RBRVS stand for?

_____

9 What is the fastest growing segment of our population today?

_____

10 What is the name given to the groups that handle the daily operations of the Medicare program?

_____

QUICK CHECK ANSWERS

QUICK CHECK 16-1
1. a
2. b, c, d
3. a
4. d
5. b
6. b, c, d
7. b, c

QUICK CHECK 16-2
1. d
2. a, c, e
3. b, g, i
4. f
5. h

References

1. Resident Population of the United States: Middle Series Projections, by Age and Sex, US Bureau of the Census, March 1996, p. 2015-2030.
2. 1996 HCFA Statistics. Bureau of Data Management, HCFA Pub. No. 03394, Sept. 1996.
3. Medicare 2000, 35 Years of Improving Americans' Health and Security, http://www.cms.hhs.gov/TheChartSeries/downloads/35chartbk.pdf
4. http://www.cbo.gov/ftpdocs/77xx/doc7731/01-24-BudgetOutlook.pdf
5. http://www.nchc.org/facts/Economy/effects_on_the_federal_budget.pdf
6. http://www.cms.hhs.gov/MissionVisionGoals/downloads/CMSStrategicActionPlan06-09_061023a.pdf
7. http://www.cms.hhs.gov/apps/media/press/factsheet.asp?Counter=2488&intNumPerPage=10&checkDate=&checkKey=&srchType=1&numDays=3500&srchOpt=0&srchData=&srchOpt=0&srchData=&keywordType=All&chkNewsType=6&intPage=&showAll=&pYear=&year=&desc=&cboOrder=date
8. http://www.cms.hhs.gov/MedicareContractingReform/Downloads/PrimaryABMACJurisdictionFactSheets.pdf
9. http://www.cms.hhs.gov/MedicareContractingReform/Downloads/DMEMACJurisdictionFactSheets.pdf
10. http://www.cms.hhs.gov/QualityImprovementOrgs/01_overview.asp
11. Federal Register, 73(19), January 29, 2008, p. 5342.
12. http://www.cms.hhs.gov/MedicareContractingReform/downloads/MACImplementationHandbook.pdf
13. http://www.cms.hhs.gov/HospitalOutpatientPPS/Downloads/CMS1392P_Addendum_D1.pdf
14. http://www.cms.hhs.gov/ASCPayment
15. http://oig.hhs.gov/publications/docs/workplan/2008/Work_Plan_FY_2008.pdf
16. US Department of Labor: http://www.bls.gov/cex
17. National Committee for Quality Assurance (NCQA) website at http://www.ncqa.org/tabid/566/Default.aspx

ICD-9-CM Official Guidelines for Coding and Reporting

Reprinted as released by the Centers for Medicare and Medicaid Services and the National Center for Health Statistics. See http://www.cdc.gov/nchs/datawh/ ftpserv/ftpicd9/ftpicd9.htm#guidelines. You can also check the Evolve website for the latest updates at http://evolve.elsevier.com/Buck/step/.

Effective October 1, 2008
Narrative changes appear in bold text
Items underlined have been moved within the guidelines since
October 1, 2007
The guidelines include the updated V Code Table

The Centers for Medicare and Medicaid Services (CMS) and the National Center for Health Statistics (NCHS), two departments within the U. S. Federal Government's Department of Health and Human Services (DHHS) provide the following guidelines for coding and reporting using the International Classification of Diseases, 9th Revision, Clinical Modification (ICD-9-CM). These guidelines should be used as a companion document to the official version of the ICD-9-CM as published on CD-ROM by the U.S. Government Printing Office (GPO).

These guidelines have been approved by the four organizations that make up the Cooperating Parties for the ICD-9-CM: the American Hospital Association (AHA), the American Health Information Management Association (AHIMA), CMS, and NCHS. These guidelines are included on the official government version of the ICD-9-CM, and also appear in *"Coding Clinic for ICD-9-CM"* published by the AHA.

These guidelines are a set of rules that have been developed to accompany and complement the official conventions and instructions provided within the ICD-9-CM itself. These guidelines are based on the coding and sequencing instructions in Volumes I, II and III of ICD-9-CM, but provide additional instruction. Adherence to these guidelines when assigning ICD-9-CM diagnosis and procedure codes is required under the Health Insurance Portability and Accountability Act (HIPAA). The diagnosis codes (Volumes 1-2) have been adopted under HIPAA for all healthcare settings. Volume 3 procedure codes have been adopted for inpatient procedures reported by hospitals. A joint effort between the healthcare provider and the coder is essential to achieve complete and accurate documentation, code assignment, and reporting of diagnoses and procedures. These guidelines have been developed to assist both the healthcare provider and the coder in identifying those diagnoses and procedures that are to be reported. The importance of consistent, complete documentation in the medical record cannot be overemphasized. Without such documentation accurate coding cannot be achieved. The entire record should be reviewed to determine the specific reason for the encounter and the conditions treated.

The term encounter is used for all settings, including hospital admissions. In the context of these guidelines, the term provider is used throughout the guidelines to mean physician or any qualified health care practitioner who is legally accountable for establishing the patient's diagnosis. Only this set of guidelines, approved by the Cooperating Parties, is official.

The guidelines are organized into sections. Section I includes the structure and conventions of the classification and general guidelines that apply to the entire classification, and chapter-specific guidelines that correspond to the chapters as they are arranged in the classification. Section II includes guidelines for selection of principal diagnosis for non-outpatient settings. Section III includes guidelines for reporting additional diagnoses in non-outpatient settings. Section IV is for outpatient coding and reporting.

ICD-9-CM Official Guidelines for Coding and Reporting

Section I.   Conventions, general coding guidelines and chapter specific guidelines

 A. Conventions for the ICD-9-CM

  1. Format:

  2. Abbreviations

   a. Index abbreviations

   b. Tabular abbreviations

  3. Punctuation

  4. Includes and Excludes Notes and Inclusion terms

  5. Other and Unspecified codes

   a. "Other" codes

   b. "Unspecified" codes

  6. Etiology/manifestation convention ("code first", "use additional code" and "in diseases classified elsewhere" notes)

  7. "And"

  8. "With"

  9. "See" and "See Also"

 B. General Coding Guidelines

  1. Use of Both Alphabetic Index and Tabular List

  2. Locate each term in the Alphabetic Index

  3. Level of Detail in Coding

  4. Code or codes from 001.0 through V84.8

  5. Selection of codes 001.0 through 999.9

  6. Signs and symptoms

  7. Conditions that are an integral part of a disease process

  8. Conditions that are not an integral part of a disease process

  9. Multiple coding for a single condition

8. Chapter 8: Diseases of Respiratory System (460-519)
   a. Chronic Obstructive Pulmonary Disease [COPD] and Asthma
   b. Chronic Obstructive Pulmonary Disease [COPD] and Bronchitis
   c. Acute Respiratory Failure
   d. Influenza due to identified avian influenza virus (avian influenza)
9. Chapter 9: Diseases of Digestive System (520-579)
   Reserved for future guideline expansion
10. Chapter 10: Diseases of Genitourinary System (580-629)
    a. Chronic kidney disease
11. Chapter 11: Complications of Pregnancy, Childbirth, and the Puerperium (630-679)
    a. General Rules for Obstetric Cases
    b. Selection of OB Principal or First-listed Diagnosis
    c. Fetal Conditions Affecting the Management of the Mother
    d. HIV Infection in Pregnancy, Childbirth and the Puerperium
    e. Current Conditions Complicating Pregnancy
    f. Diabetes mellitus in pregnancy
    g. Gestational diabetes
    h. Normal Delivery, Code 650
    i. The Postpartum and Peripartum Periods
    j. Code 677, Late effect of complication of pregnancy
    k. Abortions
12. Chapter 12: Diseases Skin and Subcutaneous Tissue (680-709)
    a. **Pressure ulcer stage codes**
    Reserved for future guideline expansion
13. Chapter 13: Diseases of Musculoskeletal and Connective Tissue (710-739)
    a. Coding of Pathologic Fractures
14. Chapter 14: Congenital Anomalies (740-759)
    a. Codes in categories 740-759, Congenital Anomalies
15. Chapter 15: Newborn (Perinatal) Guidelines (760-779)
    a. General Perinatal Rules
    b. Use of codes V30-V39
    c. Newborn transfers
    d. Use of category V29
    e. Use of other V codes on perinatal records
    f. Maternal Causes of Perinatal Morbidity
    g. Congenital Anomalies in Newborns
    h. Coding Additional Perinatal Diagnoses

SECTION I. ▪ *Conventions, general coding guidelines and chapter specific guidelines*

The conventions, general guidelines and chapter-specific guidelines are applicable to all health care settings unless otherwise indicated.

  A. **Conventions for the ICD-9-CM**
     The conventions for the ICD-9-CM are the general rules for use of the classification independent of the guidelines. These conventions are incorporated within the index and tabular of the ICD-9-CM as instructional notes. The conventions are as follows:

1. **Format:**
   The ICD-9-CM uses an indented format for ease in reference

2. **Abbreviations**
   a. **Index abbreviations**
      NEC   "Not elsewhere classifiable"
      This abbreviation in the index represents "other specified" when a specific code is not available for a condition the index directs the coder to the "other specified" code in the tabular.

   b. **Tabular abbreviations**
      NEC   "Not elsewhere classifiable"
      This abbreviation in the tabular represents "other specified". When a specific code is not available for a condition the tabular includes an NEC entry under a code to identify the code as the "other specified" code.
      (See Section I.A.5.a. "Other" codes").

      NOS   "Not otherwise specified" This abbreviation is the equivalent of unspecified.
      (See Section I.A.5.b., "Unspecified" codes)

3. **Punctuation**
   [ ]   Brackets are used in the tabular list to enclose synonyms, alternative wording or explanatory phrases. Brackets are used in the index to identify manifestation codes.
   (See Section I.A.6. "Etiology/manifestations")

   ( )   Parentheses are used in both the index and tabular to enclose supplementary words that may be present or absent in the statement of a disease or procedure without affecting the code number to which it is assigned. The terms within the parentheses are referred to as nonessential modifiers.

   :   Colons are used in the Tabular list after an incomplete term which needs one or more of the modifiers following the colon to make it assignable to a given category.

4. **Includes and Excludes Notes and Inclusion terms**
   Includes: This note appears immediately under a three-digit code title to further define, or give examples of, the content of the category.

   Excludes: An excludes note under a code indicates that the terms excluded from the code are to be coded elsewhere. In some cases the codes for the excluded terms should not be used in conjunction with the code from which it is excluded. An example of this is a congenital condition excluded from an acquired form of the same condition. The congenital and acquired codes should not be used together. In other cases, the excluded terms may be used together with an excluded code. An example of this is when fractures of different bones are coded to different codes. Both codes may be used together if both types of fractures are present.

Inclusion terms: List of terms is included under certain four and five digit codes. These terms are the conditions for which that code number is to be used. The terms may be synonyms of the code title, or, in the case of "other specified" codes, the terms are a list of the various conditions assigned to that code. The inclusion terms are not necessarily exhaustive. Additional terms found only in the index may also be assigned to a code.

5. **Other and Unspecified codes**

   a. **"Other" codes**

   Codes titled "other" or "other specified" (usually a code with a 4th digit 8 or fifth-digit 9 for diagnosis codes) are for use when the information in the medical record provides detail for which a specific code does not exist. Index entries with NEC in the line designate "other" codes in the tabular. These index entries represent specific disease entities for which no specific code exists so the term is included within an "other" code.

   b. **"Unspecified" codes**

   Codes (usually a code with a 4th digit 9 or 5th digit 0 for diagnosis codes) titled "unspecified" are for use when the information in the medical record is insufficient to assign a more specific code.

6. **Etiology/manifestation convention ("code first", "use additional code" and "in diseases classified elsewhere" notes)**

   Certain conditions have both an underlying etiology and multiple body system manifestations due to the underlying etiology. For such conditions, the ICD-9-CM has a coding convention that requires the underlying condition be sequenced first followed by the manifestation. Wherever such a combination exists, there is a "use additional code" note at the etiology code, and a "code first" note at the manifestation code. These instructional notes indicate the proper sequencing order of the codes, etiology followed by manifestation.

   In most cases the manifestation codes will have in the code title, "in diseases classified elsewhere." Codes with this title are a component of the etiology/manifestation convention. The code title indicates that it is a manifestation code. "In diseases classified elsewhere" codes are never permitted to be used as first listed or principal diagnosis codes. They must be used in conjunction with an underlying condition code and they must be listed following the underlying condition.

There are manifestation codes that do not have "in diseases classified elsewhere" in the title. For such codes a "use additional code" note will still be present and the rules for sequencing apply.

In addition to the notes in the tabular, these conditions also have a specific index entry structure. In the index both conditions are listed together with the etiology code first followed by the manifestation codes in brackets. The code in brackets is always to be sequenced second.

The most commonly used etiology/manifestation combinations are the codes for Diabetes mellitus, category 250. For each code under category 250 there is a use additional code note for the manifestation that is specific for that particular diabetic manifestation. Should a patient have more than one manifestation of diabetes, more than one code from category 250 may be used with as many manifestation codes as are needed to fully describe the patient's complete diabetic condition. The category 250 diabetes codes should be sequenced first, followed by the manifestation codes.

"Code first" and "Use additional code" notes are also used as sequencing rules in the classification for certain codes that are not part of an etiology/manifestation combination.

See - Section I.B.9. "Multiple coding for a single condition".

7. **"And"**

    The word "and" should be interpreted to mean either "and" or "or" when it appears in a title.

8. **"With"**

    The word "with" in the alphabetic index is sequenced immediately following the main term, not in alphabetical order.

9. **"See" and "See Also"**

    The "see" instruction following a main term in the index indicates that another term should be referenced. It is necessary to go to the main term referenced with the "see" note to locate the correct code.

    A "see also" instruction following a main term in the index instructs that there is another main term that may also be referenced that may provide additional index entries that may be useful. It is not necessary to follow the "see also" note when the original main term provides the necessary code.

B. **General Coding Guidelines**

1. **Use of Both Alphabetic Index and Tabular List**

    Use both the Alphabetic Index and the Tabular List when locating and assigning a code. Reliance on only the Alphabetic Index or the Tabular List leads to errors in code assignments and less specificity in code selection.

2. **Locate each term in the Alphabetic Index**

    Locate each term in the Alphabetic Index and verify the code selected in the Tabular List. Read and be guided by instructional notations that appear in both the Alphabetic Index and the Tabular List.

3. **Level of Detail in Coding**

Diagnosis and procedure codes are to be used at their highest number of digits available.

ICD-9-CM diagnosis codes are composed of codes with 3, 4, or 5 digits. Codes with three digits are included in ICD-9-CM as the heading of a category of codes that may be further subdivided by the use of fourth and/or fifth digits, which provide greater detail.

A three-digit code is to be used only if it is not further subdivided. Where fourth-digit subcategories and/or fifth-digit subclassifications are provided, they must be assigned. A code is invalid if it has not been coded to the full number of digits required for that code. For example, Acute myocardial infarction, code 410, has fourth digits that describe the location of the infarction (e.g., 410.2, Of inferolateral wall), and fifth digits that identify the episode of care. It would be incorrect to report a code in category 410 without a fourth and fifth digit.

ICD-9-CM Volume 3 procedure codes are composed of codes with either 3 or 4 digits. Codes with two digits are included in ICD-9-CM as the heading of a category of codes that may be further subdivided by the use of third and/or fourth digits, which provide greater detail.

4. **Code or codes from 001.0 through V89.09**

The appropriate code or codes from 001.0 through **V89.09** must be used to identify diagnoses, symptoms, conditions, problems, complaints or other reason(s) for the encounter/visit.

5. **Selection of codes 001.0 through 999.9**

The selection of codes 001.0 through 999.9 will frequently be used to describe the reason for the admission/encounter. These codes are from the section of ICD-9-CM for the classification of diseases and injuries (e.g., infectious and parasitic diseases; neoplasms; symptoms, signs, and ill-defined conditions, etc.).

6. **Signs and symptoms**

Codes that describe symptoms and signs, as opposed to diagnoses, are acceptable for reporting purposes when a related definitive diagnosis has not been established (confirmed) by the provider. Chapter 16 of ICD-9-CM, Symptoms, Signs, and Ill-defined conditions (codes 780.0 - 799.9) contain many, but not all codes for symptoms.

7. **Conditions that are an integral part of a disease process**

Signs and symptoms that are **associated routinely with a disease process** should not be assigned as additional codes, unless otherwise instructed by the classification.

8. **Conditions that are not an integral part of a disease process**

Additional signs and symptoms that may not be associated routinely with a disease process should be coded when present.

9. Multiple coding for a single condition

In addition to the etiology/manifestation convention that requires two codes to fully describe a single condition that affects multiple body systems, there are other single conditions that also require more than one code. "Use additional code" notes are found in the tabular at codes that are not part of an etiology/manifestation pair where a secondary code is useful to fully describe a condition. The sequencing rule is the same as the etiology/manifestation pair - , "use additional code" indicates that a secondary code should be added.

For example, for infections that are not included in chapter 1, a secondary code from category 041, Bacterial infection in conditions classified elsewhere and of unspecified site, may be required to identify the bacterial organism causing the infection. A "use additional code" note will normally be found at the infectious disease code, indicating a need for the organism code to be added as a secondary code.

"Code first" notes are also under certain codes that are not specifically manifestation codes but may be due to an underlying cause. When a "code first" note is present and an underlying condition is present the underlying condition should be sequenced first.

"Code, if applicable, any causal condition first", notes indicate that this code may be assigned as a principal diagnosis when the causal condition is unknown or not applicable. If a causal condition is known, then the code for that condition should be sequenced as the principal or first-listed diagnosis.

Multiple codes may be needed for late effects, complication codes and obstetric codes to more fully describe a condition. See the specific guidelines for these conditions for further instruction.

10. Acute and Chronic Conditions

If the same condition is described as both acute (subacute) and chronic, and separate subentries exist in the Alphabetic Index at the same indentation level, code both and sequence the acute (subacute) code first.

11. Combination Code

A combination code is a single code used to classify:
Two diagnoses, or
A diagnosis with an associated secondary process (manifestation)
A diagnosis with an associated complication
Combination codes are identified by referring to subterm entries in the Alphabetic Index and by reading the inclusion and exclusion notes in the Tabular List.

Assign only the combination code when that code fully identifies the diagnostic conditions involved or when the Alphabetic Index so directs. Multiple coding should not be used when the classification provides a combination code that clearly identifies all of the elements documented in the diagnosis. When the combination code lacks necessary specificity in describing the manifestation or complication, an additional code should be used as a secondary code.

12. **Late Effects**

A late effect is the residual effect (condition produced) after the acute phase of an illness or injury has terminated. There is no time limit on when a late effect code can be used. The residual may be apparent early, such as in cerebrovascular accident cases, or it may occur months or years later, such as that due to a previous injury. Coding of late effects generally requires two codes sequenced in the following order: The condition or nature of the late effect is sequenced first. The late effect code is sequenced second.

An exception to the above guidelines are those instances where the code for late effect is followed by a manifestation code identified in the Tabular List and title, or the late effect code has been expanded (at the fourth and fifth-digit levels) to include the manifestation(s). The code for the acute phase of an illness or injury that led to the late effect is never used with a code for the late effect.

13. **Impending or Threatened Condition**

Code any condition described at the time of discharge as "impending" or "threatened" as follows:

If it did occur, code as confirmed diagnosis.

If it did not occur, reference the Alphabetic Index to determine if the condition has a subentry term for "impending" or "threatened" and also reference main term entries for "Impending" and for "Threatened."

If the subterms are listed, assign the given code.

If the subterms are not listed, code the existing underlying condition(s) and not the condition described as impending or threatened.

14. **Reporting Same Diagnosis Code More than Once**
Each unique ICD-9-CM diagnosis code may be reported only once for an encounter. This applies to bilateral conditions or two different conditions classified to the same ICD-9-CM diagnosis code.

15. **Admissions/Encounters for Rehabilitation**
When the purpose for the admission/encounter is rehabilitation, sequence the appropriate V code from category V57, Care involving use of rehabilitation procedures, as the principal/first-listed diagnosis. The code for the condition for which the service is being performed should be reported as an additional diagnosis.

Only one code from category V57 is required. Code V57.89, Other specified rehabilitation procedures, should be assigned if more than one type of rehabilitation is performed during a single encounter. A procedure code should be reported to identify each type of rehabilitation therapy actually performed.

16. **Documentation for BMI and Pressure Ulcer Stages**

For the Body Mass Index (BMI) and pressure ulcer stage codes, code assignment may be based on medical record documentation from clinicians who are not the patient's provider (i.e., physician or other qualified healthcare practitioner legally accountable for establishing the patient's diagnosis), since this information is typically documented by other clinicians involved in the care of the patient (e.g., a dietitian often documents the BMI and nurses often documents the pressure ulcer stages). However, the associated diagnosis (such as overweight, obesity, or pressure ulcer) must be documented by the patient's provider. If there is conflicting medical record documentation, either from the same clinician or different clinicians, the patient's attending provider should be queried for clarification.

The BMI and pressure ulcer stage codes should only be reported as secondary diagnoses. As with all other secondary diagnosis codes, the BMI and pressure ulcer stage codes should only be assigned when they meet the definition of a reportable additional diagnosis (see Section III, Reporting Additional Diagnoses).

C. **Chapter-Specific Coding Guidelines**

In addition to general coding guidelines, there are guidelines for specific diagnoses and/or conditions in the classification. Unless otherwise indicated, these guidelines apply to all health care settings. Please refer to Section II for guidelines on the selection of principal diagnosis.

1. **Chapter 1: Infectious and Parasitic Diseases (001-139)**

   a. **Human Immunodeficiency Virus (HIV) Infections**

      1) **Code only confirmed cases**

         Code only confirmed cases of HIV infection/illness. This is an exception to the hospital inpatient guideline Section II, H.

         In this context, "confirmation" does not require documentation of positive serology or culture for HIV; the provider's diagnostic statement that the patient is HIV positive, or has an HIV-related illness is sufficient.

      2) **Selection and sequencing of HIV codes**

         (a) **Patient admitted for HIV-related condition**

            If a patient is admitted for an HIV-related condition, the principal diagnosis should be 042, followed by additional diagnosis codes for all reported HIV-related conditions.

         (b) **Patient with HIV disease admitted for unrelated condition**

            If a patient with HIV disease is admitted for an unrelated condition (such as a traumatic injury), the code for the unrelated condition (e.g., the nature of injury code) should be the principal diagnosis. Other diagnoses would be 042 followed by additional diagnosis codes for all reported HIV-related conditions.

(c) **Whether the patient is newly diagnosed**
Whether the patient is newly diagnosed or has had previous admissions/encounters for HIV conditions is irrelevant to the sequencing decision.

(d) **Asymptomatic human immunodeficiency virus**
V08 Asymptomatic human immunodeficiency virus [HIV] infection, is to be applied when the patient without any documentation of symptoms is listed as being "HIV positive," "known HIV," "HIV test positive," or similar terminology. Do not use this code if the term "AIDS" is used or if the patient is treated for any HIV-related illness or is described as having any condition(s) resulting from his/her HIV positive status; use 042 in these cases.

(e) **Patients with inconclusive HIV serology**
Patients with inconclusive HIV serology, but no definitive diagnosis or manifestations of the illness, may be assigned code 795.71, Inconclusive serologic test for Human Immunodeficiency Virus [HIV].

(f) **Previously diagnosed HIV-related illness**
Patients with any known prior diagnosis of an HIV-related illness should be coded to 042. Once a patient has developed an HIV-related illness, the patient should always be assigned code 042 on every subsequent admission/encounter. Patients previously diagnosed with any HIV illness (042) should never be assigned to 795.71 or V08.

(g) **HIV Infection in Pregnancy, Childbirth and the Puerperium**
During pregnancy, childbirth or the puerperium, a patient admitted (or presenting for a health care encounter) because of an HIV-related illness should receive a principal diagnosis code of 647.6X, Other specified infectious and parasitic diseases in the mother classifiable elsewhere, but complicating the pregnancy, childbirth or the puerperium, followed by 042 and the code(s) for the HIV-related illness(es). Codes from Chapter 15 always take sequencing priority.

Patients with asymptomatic HIV infection status admitted (or presenting for a health care encounter) during pregnancy, childbirth, or the puerperium should receive codes of 647.6X and V08.

(h) Encounters for testing for HIV

If a patient is being seen to determine his/her HIV status, use code V73.89, Screening for other specified viral disease. Use code V69.8, Other problems related to lifestyle, as a secondary code if an asymptomatic patient is in a known high risk group for HIV. Should a patient with signs or symptoms or illness, or a confirmed HIV related diagnosis be tested for HIV, code the signs and symptoms or the diagnosis. An additional counseling code V65.44 may be used if counseling is provided during the encounter for the test.

When a patient returns to be informed of his/her HIV test results use code V65.44, HIV counseling, if the results of the test are negative.

If the results are positive but the patient is asymptomatic use code V08, Asymptomatic HIV infection. If the results are positive and the patient is symptomatic use code 042, HIV infection, with codes for the HIV related symptoms or diagnosis. The HIV counseling code may also be used if counseling is provided for patients with positive test results.

b. Septicemia, Systemic Inflammatory Response Syndrome (SIRS), Sepsis, Severe Sepsis, and Septic Shock

1) SIRS, Septicemia, and Sepsis

(a) The terms *septicemia* and *sepsis* are often used interchangeably by providers, however they are not considered synonymous terms. The following descriptions are provided for reference but do not preclude querying the provider for clarification about terms used in the documentation:

(i) Septicemia generally refers to a systemic disease associated with the presence of pathological microorganisms or toxins in the blood, which can include bacteria, viruses, fungi or other organisms.

(ii) Systemic inflammatory response syndrome (SIRS) generally refers to the systemic response to infection, trauma/ burns, or other insult (such as cancer) with symptoms including fever, tachycardia, tachypnea, and leukocytosis.

(iii) Sepsis generally refers to SIRS due to infection.

(iv) Severe sepsis generally refers to sepsis with associated acute organ dysfunction.

(b) The Coding of SIRS, sepsis and severe sepsis

The coding of SIRS, sepsis and severe sepsis requires a minimum of 2 codes: a code for the underlying cause (such as infection or trauma) and a code from subcategory 995.9 Systemic inflammatory response syndrome (SIRS).

  (i) The code for the underlying cause (such as infection or trauma) must be sequenced before the code from subcategory 995.9 Systemic inflammatory response syndrome (SIRS).

  (ii) Sepsis and severe sepsis require a code for the systemic infection (038.xx, 112.5, etc.) and either code 995.91, Sepsis, or 995.92, Severe sepsis. If the causal organism is not documented, assign code 038.9, Unspecified septicemia.

  (iii) Severe sepsis requires additional code(s) for the associated acute organ dysfunction(s).

  (iv) If a patient has sepsis with multiple organ dysfunctions, follow the instructions for coding severe sepsis.

  (v) Either the term sepsis or SIRS must be documented to assign a code from subcategory 995.9.

  (vi) See Section I.C.17.g), Injury and poisoning, for information regarding systemic inflammatory response syndrome (SIRS) due to trauma/burns and other non-infectious processes.

(c) Due to the complex nature of sepsis and severe sepsis, some cases may require querying the provider prior to assignment of the codes.

2) Sequencing sepsis and severe sepsis

(a) Sepsis and severe sepsis as principal diagnosis

If sepsis or severe sepsis is present on admission, and meets the definition of principal diagnosis, the systemic infection code (e.g., 038.xx, 112.5, etc) should be assigned as the principal diagnosis, followed by code 995.91, Sepsis, or 995.92, Severe sepsis, as required by the sequencing rules in the Tabular List. Codes from subcategory 995.9 can never be assigned as a principal diagnosis. A code should also be assigned for any localized infection, if present.

If the sepsis or severe sepsis is due to a postprocedural infection, see Section

I.C.1.b.10 for guidelines related to sepsis due to postprocedural infection.

(b) **Sepsis and severe sepsis as secondary diagnoses**

When sepsis or severe sepsis develops during the encounter (it was not present on admission), the systemic infection code and code 995.91 or 995.92 should be assigned as secondary diagnoses.

(c) **Documentation unclear as to whether sepsis or severe sepsis is present on admission**

Sepsis or severe sepsis may be present on admission but the diagnosis may not be confirmed until sometime after admission. If the documentation is not clear whether the sepsis or severe sepsis was present on admission, the provider should be queried.

3) **Sepsis/SIRS with Localized Infection**

If the reason for admission is both sepsis, severe sepsis, or SIRS and a localized infection, such as pneumonia or cellulitis, a code for the systemic infection (038.xx, 112.5, etc) should be assigned first, then code 995.91 or 995.92, followed by the code for the localized infection. If the patient is admitted with a localized infection, such as pneumonia, and sepsis/SIRS doesn't develop until after admission, see guideline I.C.1.b.2.b). If the localized infection is postprocedural, *see Section I.C.1.b.10 for guidelines related to sepsis due to postprocedural infection.*

Note: The term urosepsis is a nonspecific term. If that is the only term documented then only code 599.0 should be assigned based on the default for the term in the ICD-9-CM index, in addition to the code for the causal organism if known.

4) **Bacterial Sepsis and Septicemia**

In most cases, it will be a code from category 038, Septicemia, that will be used in conjunction with a code from subcategory 995.9 such as the following:

(a) **Streptococcal sepsis**

If the documentation in the record states streptococcal sepsis, codes 038.0, Streptococcal septicemia, and code 995.91 should be used, in that sequence.

(b) **Streptococcal septicemia**

If the documentation states streptococcal septicemia, only code 038.0 should be assigned, however, the provider should be queried whether the patient has sepsis, an infection with SIRS.

5) **Acute organ dysfunction that is not clearly associated with the sepsis**

If a patient has sepsis and an acute organ dysfunction, but the medical record documentation indicates that the acute organ dysfunction is related to a medical condition other than the sepsis, do not assign code 995.92, Severe sepsis. An acute organ dysfunction must be associated with the sepsis in order to assign the severe sepsis code. If the documentation is not clear as to whether an acute organ dysfunction is related to the sepsis or another medical condition, query the provider.

6) **Septic shock**

   (a) **Sequencing of septic shock**
   Septic shock generally refers to circulatory failure associated with severe sepsis, and, therefore, it represents a type of acute organ dysfunction.

   For all cases of septic shock, the code for the systemic infection should be sequenced first, followed by codes 995.92 and 785.52. Any additional codes for other acute organ dysfunctions should also be assigned. As noted in the sequencing instructions in the Tabular List, the code for septic shock cannot be assigned as a principal diagnosis.

   (b) **Septic Shock without documentation of severe sepsis**
   Septic shock indicates the presence of severe sepsis.

   Code 995.92, Severe sepsis, must be assigned with code 785.52, Septic shock, even if the term severe sepsis is not documented in the record. The "use additional code" note and the "code first" note in the tabular support this guideline.

7) **Sepsis and septic shock complicating abortion and pregnancy**
   Sepsis and septic shock **complicating** abortion, ectopic pregnancy, and molar pregnancy are classified to category codes in Chapter 11 (630-639).
   See section I.C.11.

8) **Negative or inconlusive blood cultures**
   Negative or inconclusive blood cultures do not preclude a diagnosis of septicemia or sepsis in patients with clinical evidence of the condition, however, the provider should be queried.

9) **Newborn sepsis**
   See Section I.C.15.j for information on the coding of newborn sepsis.

10) **Sepsis due to a Postprocedural Infection**

    (a) **Documentation of causal relationship**
    As with all postprocedural complications, code assignment is based on the provider's

documentation of the relationship between the infection and the procedure.

(b) Sepsis due to postprocedural infection

In cases of postprocedural sepsis, the complication code, such as code 998.59, Other postoperative infection, or 674.3x, Other complications of obstetrical surgical wounds should be coded first followed by the appropriate sepsis codes (systemic infection code and either code 995.91or 995.92). An additional code(s) for any acute organ dysfunction should also be assigned for cases of severe sepsis.

11) External cause of injury codes with SIRS

Refer to Section I.C.19.a.7 for instruction on the use of external cause of injury codes with codes for SIRS resulting from trauma.

12) Sepsis and Severe Sepsis Associated with Non-infectious Process

In some cases, a non-infectious process, such as trauma, may lead to an infection which can result in sepsis or severe sepsis. If sepsis or severe sepsis is documented as associated with a non-infectious condition, such as a burn or serious injury, and this condition meets the definition for principal diagnosis, the code for the non-infectious condition should be sequenced first, followed by the code for the systemic infection and either code 995.91, Sepsis, or 995.92, Severe sepsis. Additional codes for any associated acute organ dysfunction(s) should also be assigned for cases of severe sepsis. If the sepsis or severe sepsis meets the definition of principal diagnosis, the systemic infection and sepsis codes should be sequenced before the non-infectious condition. When both the associated non-infectious condition and the sepsis or severe sepsis meet the definition of principal diagnosis, either may be assigned as principal diagnosis.

See Section I.C.1.b.2)(a) for guidelines pertaining to sepsis or severe sepsis as the principal diagnosis.

Only one code from subcategory 995.9 should be assigned. Therefore, when a non-infectious condition leads to an infection resulting in sepsis or severe sepsis, assign either code 995.91 or 995.92. Do not additionally assign code 995.93, Systemic inflammatory response syndrome due to non-infectious process without acute organ dysfunction, or 995.94, Systemic inflammatory response syndrome with acute organ dysfunction.

See Section I.C.17.g for information on the coding of SIRS due to trauma/burns or other non-infectious disease processes.

c. **Methicillin Resistant *Staphylococcus aureus* (MRSA) Conditions**

1) **Selection and sequencing of MRSA codes**

   (a) **Combination codes for MRSA infection**

   When a patient is diagnosed with an infection that is due to methicillin resistant *Staphylococcus aureus* (MRSA), and that infection has a combination code that includes the causal organism (e.g., septicemia, pneumonia) assign the appropriate code for the condition (e.g., code 038.12, Methicillin resistant Staphylococcus aureus septicemia or code 482.42, Methicillin resistant pneumonia due to Staphylococcus aureus). Do not assign code 041.12, Methicillin resistant Staphylococcus aureus, as an additional code because the code includes the type of infection and the MRSA organism. Do not assign a code from subcategory V09.0, Infection with microorganisms resistant to penicillins, as an additional diagnosis.

   See Section C.1.b.1 for instructions on coding and sequencing of septicemia.

   (b) **Other codes for MRSA infection**

   When there is documentation of a current infection (e.g., wound infection, stitch abscess, urinary tract infection) due to MRSA, and that infection does not have a combination code that includes the causal organism, select the appropriate code to identify the condition along with code 041.12, Methicillin resistant Staphylococcus aureus, for the MRSA infection. Do not assign a code from subcategory V09.0, Infection with microorganisms resistant to penicillins.

   (c) **Methicillin susceptible Staphylococcus aureus (MSSA) and MRSA colonization**

   The condition or state of being colonized or carrying MSSA or MRSA is called colonization or carriage, while an individual person is described as being colonized or being a carrier. Colonization means that MSSA or MSRA is present on or in the body without necessarily causing illness. A positive MRSA colonization test might be documented by the provider as "MRSA screen positive" or "MRSA nasal swab positive".

Assign code V02.54, Carrier or suspected carrier, Methicillin resistant Staphylococcus aureus, for patients documented as having MRSA colonization. Assign code V02.53, Carrier or suspected carrier, Methicillin susceptible Staphylococcus aureus, for patient documented as having MSSA colonization. Colonization is not necessarily indicative of a disease process or as the cause of a specific condition the patient may have unless documented as such by the provider.

Code V02.59, Other specified bacterial diseases, should be assigned for other types of staphylococcal colonization (e.g., S. *epidermidis*, S. *saprophyticus*). Code V02.59 should not be assigned for colonization with any type of *Staphylococcus aureus* (MRSA, MSSA).

(d) **MRSA colonization and infection**
If a patient is documented as having both MRSA colonization and infection during a hospital admission, code V02.54, Carrier or suspected carrier, Methicillin resistant *Staphylococcus aureus,* and a code for the MRSA infection may both be assigned.

2. **Chapter 2: Neoplasms (140-239)**

<u>General guidelines</u>

Chapter 2 of the ICD-9-CM contains the codes for most benign and all malignant neoplasms. Certain benign neoplasms, such as prostatic adenomas, may be found in the specific body system chapters. To properly code a neoplasm it is necessary to determine from the record if the neoplasm is benign, in-situ, malignant, or of uncertain histologic behavior. If malignant, any secondary (metastatic) sites should also be determined.

The neoplasm table in the Alphabetic Index should be referenced first. However, if the histological term is documented, that term should be referenced first, rather than going immediately to the Neoplasm Table, in order to determine which column in the Neoplasm Table is appropriate. For example, if the documentation indicates "adenoma," refer to the term in the Alphabetic Index to review the entries under this term and the instructional note to "see also neoplasm, by site, benign." The table provides the proper code based on the type of neoplasm and the site. It is important to select the proper column in the table that corresponds to the type of neoplasm. The tabular should then be referenced to verify that the correct code has been selected from the table and that a more specific site code does not exist.

See Section I. C. 18.d.4. for information regarding V codes for genetic susceptibility to cancer.

a. **Treatment directed at the malignancy**

If the treatment is directed at the malignancy, designate the malignancy as the principal diagnosis.

The only exception to this guideline is if a patient admission/encounter is solely for the administration of chemotherapy, immunotherapy or radiation therapy, assign the appropriate V58.x code as the first-listed or principal diagnosis, and the diagnosis or problem for which the service is being performed as a secondary diagnosis.

b. **Treatment of secondary site**

When a patient is admitted because of a primary neoplasm with metastasis and treatment is directed toward the secondary site only, the secondary neoplasm is designated as the principal diagnosis even though the primary malignancy is still present.

c. **Coding and sequencing of complications**

Coding and sequencing of complications associated with the malignancies or with the therapy thereof are subject to the following guidelines:

1) **Anemia associated with malignancy**

When admission/encounter is for management of an anemia associated with the malignancy, and the treatment is only for anemia, the appropriate anemia code (such as code 285.22, Anemia in neoplastic disease) is designated as the principal diagnosis and is followed by the appropriate code(s) for the malignancy.

Code 285.22 may also be used as a secondary code if the patient suffers from anemia and is being treated for the malignancy.

2) **Anemia associated with chemotherapy, immunotherapy and radiation therapy**

When the admission/encounter is for management of an anemia associated with chemotherapy, immunotherapy or radiotherapy and the only treatment is for the anemia, the anemia is sequenced first followed by code E933.1. The appropriate neoplasm code should be assigned as an additional code.

3) **Management of dehydration due to the malignancy**

When the admission/encounter is for management of dehydration due to the malignancy or the therapy, or a combination of both, and only the dehydration is being treated (intravenous rehydration), the dehydration is sequenced first, followed by the code(s) for the malignancy.

4) **Treatment of a complication resulting from a surgical procedure**

When the admission/encounter is for treatment of a complication resulting from a surgical procedure, designate the complication as the principal or first-listed diagnosis if treatment is directed at resolving the complication.

d. **Primary malignancy previously excised**

When a primary malignancy has been previously excised or eradicated from its site and there is no further treatment directed to that site and there is no evidence of any existing primary malignancy, a code from category V10, Personal history of malignant neoplasm, should be used to indicate the former site of the malignancy. Any mention of extension, invasion, or metastasis to another site is coded as a secondary malignant neoplasm to that site. The secondary site may be the principal or first-listed with the V10 code used as a secondary code.

e. **Admissions/Encounters involving chemotherapy, immunotherapy and radiation therapy**

1) **Episode of care involves surgical removal of neoplasm**

When an episode of care involves the surgical removal of a neoplasm, primary or secondary site, followed by adjunct chemotherapy or radiation treatment during the same episode of care, the neoplasm code should be assigned as principal or first-listed diagnosis, using codes in the 140-198 series or where appropriate in the 200-203 series.

2) **Patient admission/encounter solely for administration of chemotherapy, immunotherapy and radiation therapy**

If a patient admission/encounter is solely for the administration of chemotherapy, immunotherapy or radiation therapy assign code V58.0, Encounter for radiation therapy, or V58.11, Encounter for antineoplastic chemotherapy, or V58.12, Encounter for antineoplastic immunotherapy as the first-listed or principal diagnosis. If a patient receives more than one of these therapies during the same admission more than one of these codes may be assigned, in any sequence.

The malignancy for which the therapy is being administered should be assigned as a secondary diagnosis.

3) **Patient admitted for radiotherapy/ chemotherapy and immunotherapy and develops complications**

When a patient is admitted for the purpose of radiotherapy, immunotherapy or chemotherapy and develops complications such as uncontrolled nausea and vomiting or dehydration, the principal or first-listed diagnosis is V58.0, Encounter for radiotherapy, or V58.11, Encounter for antineoplastic chemotherapy, or V58.12, Encounter for antineoplastic immunotherapy followed by any codes for the complications.

f. **Admission/encounter to determine extent of malignancy**

When the reason for admission/encounter is to determine the extent of the malignancy, or for a procedure such as paracentesis or thoracentesis, the primary malignancy or appropriate metastatic site is designated as the principal or first-listed diagnosis, even though chemotherapy or radiotherapy is administered.

g. **Symptoms, signs, and ill-defined conditions listed in Chapter 16 <u>associated with neoplasms</u>**

Symptoms, signs, and ill-defined conditions listed in Chapter 16 characteristic of, or associated with, an existing primary or secondary site malignancy cannot be used to replace the malignancy as principal or first-listed diagnosis, regardless of the number of admissions or encounters for treatment and care of the neoplasm.

See section I.C.18.d.14, Encounter for prophylactic organ removal.

h. **Admission/encounter for pain control/management**

See Section I.C.6.a.5 for information on coding admission/encounter for pain control/management.

i. **Malignant neoplasm associated with transplanted organ**

A malignant neoplasm of a transplanted organ should be coded as a transplant complication. Assign first the appropriate code from subcategory 996.8, Complications of transplanted organ, followed by code 199.2, Malignant neoplasm associated with transplanted organ. Use an additional code for the specific malignancy.

3. **Chapter 3: Endocrine, Nutritional, and Metabolic Diseases and Immunity Disorders (240-279)**

a. **Diabetes mellitus**

Codes under category 250, Diabetes mellitus, identify complications/manifestations associated with diabetes mellitus. A fifth-digit is required for all category 250 codes to identify the type of diabetes mellitus and whether the diabetes is controlled or uncontrolled.

See I.C.3.a.7 for secondary diabetes.

1) **Fifth-digits for category 250:**

The following are the fifth-digits for the codes under category 250:

0   type II or unspecified type, not stated as uncontrolled

1   type I, [juvenile type], not stated as uncontrolled

2   type II or unspecified type, uncontrolled

3   type I, [juvenile type], uncontrolled

The age of a patient is not the sole determining factor, though most type I diabetics develop the condition before reaching puberty. For this reason type I diabetes mellitus is also referred to as juvenile diabetes.

2) **Type of diabetes mellitus not documented**

If the type of diabetes mellitus is not documented in the medical record the default is type II.

3) **Diabetes mellitus and the use of insulin**

All type I diabetics must use insulin to replace what their bodies do not produce. However, the use of insulin does not mean that a patient is a type I diabetic. Some patients with type II diabetes mellitus are unable to control their blood sugar through diet and oral medication alone and do require insulin. If the documentation in a medical record does not indicate the type of diabetes but does indicate that the patient uses insulin, the appropriate fifth-digit for type II must be used. For type II patients who routinely use insulin, code V58.67, Long-term (current) use of insulin, should also be assigned to indicate that the patient uses insulin. Code V58.67 should not be assigned if insulin is given temporarily to bring a type II patient's blood sugar under control during an encounter.

4) **Assigning and sequencing diabetes codes and associated conditions**

When assigning codes for diabetes and its associated conditions, the code(s) from category 250 must be sequenced before the codes for the associated conditions. The diabetes codes and the secondary codes that correspond to them are paired codes that follow the etiology/manifestation convention of the classification *(See Section I.A.6., Etiology/manifestation convention).* Assign as many codes from category 250 as needed to identify all of the associated conditions that the patient has. The corresponding secondary codes are listed under each of the diabetes codes.

(a) **Diabetic retinopathy/diabetic macular edema**

Diabetic macular edema, code 362.07, is only present with diabetic retinopathy. Another code from subcategory 362.0, Diabetic retinopathy, must be used with code 362.07. Codes under subcategory 362.0 are diabetes manifestation codes, so they must be used following the appropriate diabetes code.

5) **Diabetes mellitus in pregnancy and gestational diabetes**

   (a) For diabetes mellitus complicating pregnancy, see Section I.C.11.f., Diabetes mellitus in pregnancy.

   (b) For gestational diabetes, see Section I.C.11, g., Gestational diabetes.

6) **Insulin pump malfunction**

   (a) **Underdose of insulin due insulin pump failure**

   An underdose of insulin due to an insulin pump failure should be assigned 996.57, Mechanical complication due to insulin pump, as the principal or first listed code, followed by the appropriate diabetes mellitus code based on documentation.

   (b) **Overdose of insulin due to insulin pump failure**

   The principal or first listed code for an encounter due to an insulin pump malfunction resulting in an overdose of insulin, should also be 996.57, Mechanical complication due to insulin pump, followed by code 962.3, Poisoning by insulins and antidiabetic agents, and the appropriate diabetes mellitus code based on documentation.

7) **Secondary Diabetes Mellitus**
   Codes under category 249, Secondary diabetes mellitus, identify complications/manifestations associated with secondary diabetes mellitus. Secondary diabetes is always caused by another condition or event (e.g., cystic fibrosis, malignant neoplasm of pancreas, pancreatectomy, adverse effect of drug, or poisoning).

   (a) Fifth-digits for category 249:
   A fifth-digit is required for all category 249 codes to identify whether the diabetes is controlled or uncontrolled.

   (b) Secondary diabetes mellitus and the use of insulin
   For patients who routinely use insulin, code V58.67, Long-term (current) use of insulin, should also be assigned. Code V58.67 should not be assigned if insulin is given temporarily to bring a patient's blood sugar under control during an encounter.

   (c) Assigning and sequencing secondary diabetes codes and associated conditions
   When assigning codes for secondary diabetes and its associated conditions (e.g. renal manifestations), the code(s) from category 249 must be sequenced before the codes for the associated conditions. The secondary diabetes codes and the diabetic manifestation codes that correspond to them

are paired codes that follow the etiology/manifestation convention of the classification. Assign as many codes from category 249 as needed to identify all of the associated conditions that the patient has. The corresponding codes for the associated conditions are listed under each of the secondary diabetes codes. For example, secondary diabetes with diabetic nephrosis is assigned to code 249.40, followed by 581.81.

(d) Assigning and sequencing secondary diabetes codes and its causes

The sequencing of the secondary diabetes codes in relationship to codes for the cause of the diabetes is based on the reason for the encounter, applicable ICD-9-CM sequencing conventions, and chapter-specific guidelines.

If a patient is seen for treatment of the secondary diabetes or one of its associated conditions, a code from category 249 is sequenced as the principal or first-listed diagnosis, with the cause of the secondary diabetes (e.g. cystic fibrosis) sequenced as an additional diagnosis.

If, however, the patient is seen for the treatment of the condition causing the secondary diabetes (e.g., malignant neoplasm of pancreas), the code for the cause of the secondary diabetes should be sequenced as the principal or first-listed diagnosis followed by a code from category 249.

(i) Secondary diabetes mellitus due to pancreatectomy

For postpancreatectomy diabetes mellitus (lack of insulin due to the surgical removal of all or part of the pancreas), assign code 251.3, Postsurgical hypoinsulinemia. A code from subcategory 249 should not be assigned for secondary diabetes mellitus due to pancreatectomy. Code also any diabetic manifestations (e.g. diabetic nephrosis 581.81).

(ii) Secondary diabetes due to drugs

Secondary diabetes may be caused by an adverse effect of correctly administered medications, poisoning or late effect of poisoning.

See section I.C.17.e for coding of adverse effects and poisoning, and section I.C.19 for E code reporting

4. **Chapter 4: Diseases of Blood and Blood Forming Organs (280-289)**

a. **Anemia of chronic disease**

Subcategory 285.2, Anemia in chronic illness, has codes for anemia in chronic kidney disease, code

285.21; anemia in neoplastic disease, code 285.22; and anemia in other chronic illness, code 285.29. These codes can be used as the principal/first listed code if the reason for the encounter is to treat the anemia. They may also be used as secondary codes if treatment of the anemia is a component of an encounter, but not the primary reason for the encounter. When using a code from subcategory 285 it is also necessary to use the code for the chronic condition causing the anemia.

1) **Anemia in chronic kidney disease**

When assigning code 285.21, Anemia in chronic kidney disease, it is also necessary to assign a code from category 585, Chronic kidney disease, to indicate the stage of chronic kidney disease.
See I.C.10.a. Chronic kidney disease (CKD).

2) **Anemia in neoplastic disease**

When assigning code 285.22, Anemia in neoplastic disease, it is also necessary to assign the neoplasm code that is responsible for the anemia. Code 285.22 is for use for anemia that is due to the malignancy, not for anemia due to antineoplastic chemotherapy drugs, which is an adverse effect.
See I.C.2.c.1 Anemia associated with malignancy.
See I.C.2.c.2 Anemia associated with chemotherapy, immunotherapy and radiation therapy.
See I.C.17.e.1. Adverse effects.

5. **Chapter 5: Mental Disorders (290-319)**
Reserved for future guideline expansion

6. **Chapter 6: Diseases of Nervous System and Sense Organs (320-389)**

a. **Pain - Category 338**

1) **General coding information**
Codes in category 338 may be used in conjunction with codes from other categories and chapters to provide more detail about acute or chronic pain and neoplasm-related pain, **unless otherwise indicated below.**

If the pain is not specified as acute or chronic, do not assign codes from category 338, except for post-thoracotomy pain, postoperative pain or neoplasm related pain, **or central pain syndrome.**

A code from subcategories 338.1 and 338.2 should not be assigned if the underlying (definitive) diagnosis is known, unless the reason for the encounter is pain control/ management and not management of the underlying condition.

(a) **Category 338 Codes as Principal or First-Listed Diagnosis**
Category 338 codes are acceptable as principal diagnosis or the first-listed code:

• When pain control or pain management is the reason for the admission/encounter (e.g., a patient with displaced intervertebral disc, nerve impingement and severe back pain presents for injection of steriod into the spinal canal). The underlying cause of the pain should be reported as an additional diagnosis, if known.

- When an admission or encounter is for a procedure aimed at treating the underlying condition (e.g., spinal fusion, kyphoplasty), a code for the underlying condition (e.g., vertebral fracture, spinal stenosis) should be assigned as the principal diagnosis. No code from category 338 should be assigned.

- When a patient is admitted for the insertion of a neurostimulator for pain control, assign the appropriate pain code as the principal or first listed diagnosis. When an admission or encounter is for a procedure aimed at treating the underlying condition and a neurostimulator is inserted for pain control during the same admission/encounter, a code for the underlying condition should be assigned as the principal diagnosis and the appropriate pain code should be assigned as a secondary diagnosis.

(b) **Use of Category 338 Codes in Conjunction with Site Specific Pain Codes**

(i) **Assigning Category 338 Codes and Site-Specific Pain Codes**
Codes from category 338 may be used in conjunction with codes that identify the site of pain (including codes from chapter 16) if the category 338 code provides additional information. For example, if the code describes the site of the pain, but does not fully describe whether the pain is acute or chronic, then both codes should be assigned.

(ii) **Sequencing of Category 338 Codes with Site-Specific Pain Codes**
The sequencing of category 338 codes with site-specific pain codes (including chapter 16 codes), is dependent on the circumstances of the encounter/admission as follows:

- If the encounter is for pain control or pain management, assign the code from category 338 followed by the code identifying the specific site of pain (e.g., encounter for pain management for acute neck pain from trauma is assigned code 338.11, Acute pain due to trauma, followed by code 723.1, Cervicalgia, to identify the site of pain).

- If the encounter is for any other reason except pain control or pain management, and a related definitive diagnosis has not been established (confirmed) by the provider, assign the code for the specific site of pain first, followed by the appropriate code from category 338.

2) **Pain due to devices, <u>implants and grafts</u>**

Pain associated with devices, implants or grafts left in a surgical site (for example painful hip prosthesis) is assigned to the appropriate code(s) found in Chapter 17, Injury and Poisoning. Use additional code(s) from category 338 to identify acute or chronic pain due to presence of the device, implant or graft (338.18-338.19 or 338.28-338.29).

3) **Postoperative Pain**

Post-thoracotomy pain and other postoperative pain are classified to subcategories 338.1 and 338.2, depending on whether the pain is acute or chronic. The default for post-thoracotomy and other postoperative pain not specified as acute or chronic is the code for the acute form.

<u>**Routine or expected postoperative pain immediately after surgery should not be coded.**</u>

(a) **Postoperative pain not associated with specific postoperative complication**

Postoperative pain not associated with a specific postoperative complication is assigned to the appropriate postoperative pain code in category 338.

(b) **Postoperative pain associated with specific postoperative complication**

Postoperative pain associated with a specific postoperative complication (such as **painful suture wires**) is assigned to the appropriate code(s) found in Chapter 17, Injury and Poisoning. **If appropriate, use additional code(s) from category 338 to identify acute or chronic pain (338.18 or 338.28).** If pain control/management is the reason for the encounter, a code from category 338 should be assigned as the principal or first-listed diagnosis in accordance with *Section I.C.6.a.1.a above.*

(c) **Postoperative pain as principal or first-listed diagnosis**

Postoperative pain may be reported as the principal or first-listed diagnosis when the stated reason for the admission/encounter is documented as postoperative pain control/management.

(d) Postoperative pain as secondary diagnosis

Postoperative pain may be reported as a secondary diagnosis code when a patient presents for outpatient surgery and develops an unusual or inordinate amount of postoperative pain.

Routine or expected postoperative pain immediately after surgery should not be coded.

The provider's documentation should be used to guide the coding of postoperative pain, as well as *Section III. Reporting Additional Diagnoses and Section IV. Diagnostic Coding and Reporting in the Outpatient Setting.*

See Section II.I.2 for information on sequencing of diagnoses for patients admitted to hospital inpatient care following post-operative observation.

See Section II.J for information on sequencing of diagnoses for patients admitted to hospital inpatient care from outpatient surgery.

See Section IV.A.2 for information on sequencing of diagnoses for patients admitted for observation.

4) Chronic pain

Chronic pain is classified to subcategory 338.2. There is no time frame defining when pain becomes chronic pain. The provider's documentation should be used to guide use of these codes.

5) Neoplasm Related Pain

Code 338.3 is assigned to pain documented as being related, associated or due to cancer, primary or secondary malignancy, or tumor. This code is assigned regardless of whether the pain is acute or chronic.

This code may be assigned as the principal or first-listed code when the stated reason for the admission/encounter is documented as pain control/pain management. The underlying neoplasm should be reported as an additional diagnosis.

When the reason for the admission/ encounter is management of the neoplasm and the pain associated with the neoplasm is also documented, code 338.3 may be assigned as an additional diagnosis.

See Section I.C.2 for instructions on the sequencing of neoplasms for all other stated reasons for the admission/encounter (except for pain control/pain management).

6) Chronic pain syndrome

This condition is different than the term "chronic pain," and therefore this code should only be used when the provider has specifically documented this condition.

7. **Chapter 7: Diseases of Circulatory System (390-459)**

   a. **Hypertension**

   <u>Hypertension Table</u>

   The Hypertension Table, found under the main term, "Hypertension", in the Alphabetic Index, contains a complete listing of all conditions due to or associated with hypertension and classifies them according to malignant, benign, and unspecified.

   1) **Hypertension, Essential, or NOS**

      Assign hypertension (arterial) (essential) (primary) (systemic) (NOS) to category code 401 with the appropriate fourth digit to indicate malignant (.0), benign (.1), or unspecified (.9). Do not use either .0 malignant or .1 benign unless medical record documentation supports such a designation.

   2) **Hypertension with Heart Disease**

      Heart conditions (425.8, 429.0-429.3, 429.8, 429.9) are assigned to a code from category 402 when a causal relationship is stated (due to hypertension) or implied (hypertensive). Use an additional code from category 428 to identify the type of heart failure in those patients with heart failure. More than one code from category 428 may be assigned if the patient has systolic or diastolic failure and congestive heart failure.

      The same heart conditions (425.8, 429.0-429.3, 429.8, 429.9) with hypertension, but without a stated causal relationship, are coded separately. Sequence according to the circumstances of the admission/encounter.

   3) **Hypertensive Chronic Kidney Disease**

      Assign codes from category 403, Hypertensive chronic kidney disease, when conditions classified to **category** 585 are present. Unlike hypertension with heart disease, ICD-9-CM presumes a cause-and-effect relationship and classifies chronic kidney disease (CKD) with hypertension as hypertensive chronic kidney disease.

      Fifth digits for category 403 should be assigned as follows:

      • 0 with CKD stage I through stage IV, or unspecified.

      • 1 with CKD stage V or end stage renal disease.

      The appropriate code from category 585, Chronic kidney disease, should be used as a secondary code with a code from category 403 to identify the stage of chronic kidney disease. *See Section I.C.10.a for information on the coding of chronic kidney disease.*

   4) **Hypertensive Heart and Chronic Kidney Disease**

Assign codes from combination category 404, Hypertensive heart and chronic kidney disease, when both hypertensive kidney disease and hypertensive heart disease are stated in the diagnosis. Assume a relationship between the hypertension and the chronic kidney disease, whether or not the condition is so designated. Assign an additional code from category 428, to identify the type of heart failure. More than one code from category 428 may be assigned if the patient has systolic or diastolic failure and congestive heart failure.

Fifth digits for category 404 should be assigned as follows:

- 0 without heart failure and with chronic kidney disease (CKD) stage I through stage IV, or unspecified

- 1 with heart failure and with CKD stage I through stage IV, or unspecified

- 2 without heart failure and with CKD stage V or end stage renal disease

- 3 with heart failure and with CKD stage V or end stage renal disease

The appropriate code from category 585, Chronic kidney disease, should be used as a secondary code with a code from category 404 to identify the stage of kidney disease.
See Section I.C.10.a for information on the coding of chronic kidney disease.

5) **Hypertensive Cerebrovascular Disease**
First assign codes from 430-438, Cerebrovascular disease, then the appropriate hypertension code from categories 401-405.

6) **Hypertensive Retinopathy**
Two codes are necessary to identify the condition. First assign the code from subcategory 362.11, Hypertensive retinopathy, then the appropriate code from categories 401-405 to indicate the type of hypertension.

7) **Hypertension, Secondary**
Two codes are required: one to identify the underlying etiology and one from category 405 to identify the hypertension. Sequencing of codes is determined by the reason for admission/encounter.

8) **Hypertension, Transient**
Assign code 796.2, Elevated blood pressure reading without diagnosis of hypertension, unless patient has an established diagnosis of hypertension. Assign code 642.3x for transient hypertension of pregnancy.

9) **Hypertension, Controlled**
Assign appropriate code from categories 401-405. This diagnostic statement usually refers to

an existing state of hypertension under control by therapy.

10) Hypertension, Uncontrolled

Uncontrolled hypertension may refer to untreated hypertension or hypertension not responding to current therapeutic regimen. In either case, assign the appropriate code from categories 401-405 to designate the stage and type of hypertension. Code to the type of hypertension.

11) Elevated Blood Pressure

For a statement of elevated blood pressure without further specificity, assign code 796.2, Elevated blood pressure reading without diagnosis of hypertension, rather than a code from category 401.

b. Cerebral infarction/stroke/cerebrovascular accident (CVA)

The terms stroke and CVA are often used interchangeably to refer to a cerebral infarction. The terms stroke, CVA, and cerebral infarction NOS are all indexed to the default code 434.91, Cerebral artery occlusion, unspecified, with infarction. Code 436, Acute, but ill-defined, cerebrovascular disease, should not be used when the documentation states stroke or CVA.

See Section I.C.18.d.3 for information on coding status post administration of tPA in a different facility within the last 24 hours.

c. Postoperative cerebrovascular accident

A cerebrovascular hemorrhage or infarction that occurs as a result of medical intervention is coded to 997.02, Iatrogenic cerebrovascular infarction or hemorrhage. Medical record documentation should clearly specify the cause- and-effect relationship between the medical intervention and the cerebrovascular accident in order to assign this code. A secondary code from the code range 430-432 or from a code from subcategories 433 or 434 with a fifth digit of "1" should also be used to identify the type of hemorrhage or infarct.

This guideline conforms to the use additional code note instruction at category 997. Code 436, Acute, but ill-defined, cerebrovascular disease, should not be used as a secondary code with code 997.02.

d. Late Effects of Cerebrovascular Disease

1) Category 438, Late Effects of Cerebrovascular disease

Category 438 is used to indicate conditions classifiable to categories 430-437 as the causes of late effects (neurologic deficits), themselves classified elsewhere. These "late effects" include neurologic deficits that persist after initial onset of conditions classifiable to 430-437. The neurologic deficits caused by cerebrovascular disease may be present from the onset or may arise at any time after the onset of the condition classifiable to 430-437.

2) Codes from category 438 with codes from 430-437

Codes from category 438 may be assigned on a health care record with codes from 430-437, if the patient has a current cerebrovascular accident (CVA) and deficits from an old CVA.

3) Code V12.54

Assign code V12.**54, Transient ischemic attack (TIA), and cerebral infarction without residual deficits** (and not a code from category 438) as an additional code for history of cerebrovascular disease when no neurologic deficits are present.

e. **Acute myocardial infarction (AMI)**

1) ST elevation myocardial infarction (STEMI) and non ST elevation myocardial infarction (NSTEMI)

The ICD-9-CM codes for acute myocardial infarction (AMI) identify the site, such as anterolateral wall or true posterior wall. Subcategories 410.0-410.6 and 410.8 are used for ST elevation myocardial infarction (STEMI). Subcategory 410.7, Subendocardial infarction, is used for non ST elevation myocardial infarction (NSTEMI) and nontransmural MIs.

2) Acute myocardial infarction, unspecified

Subcategory 410.9 is the default for the unspecified term acute myocardial infarction. If only STEMI or transmural MI without the site is documented, query the provider as to the site, or assign a code from subcategory 410.9.

3) AMI documented as nontransmural or subendocardial but site provided

If an AMI is documented as nontransmural or subendocardial, but the site is provided, it is still coded as a subendocardial AMI. If NSTEMI evolves to STEMI, assign the STEMI code. If STEMI converts to NSTEMI due to thrombolytic therapy, it is still coded as STEMI.

See Section I.C.18.d.3 for information on coding status post administration of tPA in a different facility within the last 24 hours.

8. **Chapter 8: Diseases of Respiratory System (460-519)**

a. **Chronic Obstructive Pulmonary Disease [COPD] and Asthma**

See I.C.17.f for ventilator-associated pneumonia.

1) Conditions that comprise COPD and Asthma

The conditions that comprise COPD are obstructive chronic bronchitis, subcategory 491.2, and emphysema, category 492. All asthma codes are under category 493, Asthma. Code 496, Chronic airway obstruction, not elsewhere classified, is a nonspecific code that should only be used when the documentation in a medical record does not specify the type of COPD being treated.

2) **Acute exacerbation of chronic obstructive bronchitis and asthma**

The codes for chronic obstructive bronchitis and asthma distinguish between uncomplicated cases and those in acute exacerbation. An acute exacerbation is a worsening or a decompensation of a chronic condition. An acute exacerbation is not equivalent to an infection superimposed on a chronic condition, though an exacerbation may be triggered by an infection.

3) **Overlapping nature of the conditions that comprise COPD and asthma**

Due to the overlapping nature of the conditions that make up COPD and asthma, there are many variations in the way these conditions are documented. Code selection must be based on the terms as documented. When selecting the correct code for the documented type of COPD and asthma, it is essential to first review the index, and then verify the code in the tabular list. There are many instructional notes under the different COPD subcategories and codes. It is important that all such notes be reviewed to assure correct code assignment.

4) **Acute exacerbation of asthma and status asthmaticus**

An acute exacerbation of asthma is an increased severity of the asthma symptoms, such as wheezing and shortness of breath. Status asthmaticus refers to a patient's failure to respond to therapy administered during an asthmatic episode and is a life threatening complication that requires emergency care. If status asthmaticus is documented by the provider with any type of COPD or with acute bronchitis, the status asthmaticus should be sequenced first. It supersedes any type of COPD including that with acute exacerbation or acute bronchitis. It is inappropriate to assign an asthma code with 5th digit 2, with acute exacerbation, together with an asthma code with 5th digit 1, with status asthmatics. Only the 5th digit 1 should be assigned.

b. **Chronic Obstructive Pulmonary Disease [COPD] and Bronchitis**

1) **Acute bronchitis with COPD**

Acute bronchitis, code 466.0, is due to an infectious organism. When acute bronchitis is documented with COPD, code 491.22, Obstructive chronic bronchitis with acute bronchitis, should be assigned. It is not necessary to also assign code 466.0. If a medical record documents acute bronchitis with COPD with acute exacerbation, only code 491.22 should be assigned. The acute bronchitis included in code 491.22 supersedes the acute exacerbation. If a medical record documents COPD with acute exacerbation without mention of acute bronchitis, only code 491.21 should be assigned.

c. **Acute Respiratory Failure**

1) **Acute respiratory failure as principal diagnosis**
   Code 518.81, Acute respiratory failure, may be assigned as a principal diagnosis when it is the condition established after study to be chiefly responsible for occasioning the admission to the hospital, and the selection is supported by the Alphabetic Index and Tabular List. However, chapter-specific coding guidelines (such as obstetrics, poisoning, HIV, newborn) that provide sequencing direction take precedence.

2) **Acute respiratory failure as secondary diagnosis**
   Respiratory failure may be listed as a secondary diagnosis if it occurs after admission, or if it is present on admission, but does not meet the definition of principal diagnosis.

3) **Sequencing of acute respiratory failure and another acute condition**
   When a patient is admitted with respiratory failure and another acute condition, (e.g., myocardial infarction, cerebrovascular accident, **aspiration pneumonia**), the principal diagnosis will not be the same in every situation. **This applies whether the other acute condition is a respiratory or nonrespiratory condition.**
   Selection of the principal diagnosis will be dependent on the circumstances of admission. If both the respiratory failure and the other acute condition are equally responsible for occasioning the admission to the hospital, and there are no chapter-specific sequencing rules, the guideline regarding two or more diagnoses that equally meet the definition for principal diagnosis *(Section II, C.)* may be applied in these situations.
   If the documentation is not clear as to whether acute respiratory failure and another condition are equally responsible for occasioning the admission, query the provider for clarification.

d. **Influenza due to identified avian influenza virus (avian influenza)**

   Code only confirmed cases of avian influenza. This is an exception to the hospital inpatient guideline Section II, H. (Uncertain Diagnosis).
   In this context, "confirmation" does not require documentation of positive laboratory testing specific for avian influenza. However, coding should be based

on the provider's diagnostic statement that the patient has avian influenza.

If the provider records "suspected or possible or probable avian influenza," the appropriate influenza code from category 487 should be assigned. Code 488, Influenza due to identified avian influenza virus, should not be assigned.

9. **Chapter 9: Diseases of Digestive System (520-579)**
Reserved for future guideline expansion

10. **Chapter 10: Diseases of Genitourinary System (580-629)**

   a. **Chronic kidney disease**

   1) **Stages of chronic kidney disease (CKD)**
   The ICD-9-CM classifies CKD based on severity. The severity of CKD is designated by stages I-V. Stage II, code 585.2, equates to mild CKD; stage III, code 585.3, equates to moderate CKD; and stage IV, code 585.4, equates to severe CKD. Code 585.6, End stage renal disease (ESRD), is assigned when the provider has documented end-stage-renal disease (ESRD).

   If both a stage of CKD and ESRD are documented, assign code 585.6 only.

   2) **Chronic kidney disease and kidney transplant status**
   Patients who have undergone kidney transplant may still have some form of CKD, because the kidney transplant may not fully restore kidney function. Therefore, the presence of CKD alone does not constitute a transplant complication. Assign the appropriate 585 code for the patient's stage of CKD and code V42.0. If a transplant complication such as failure or rejection is documented, see section I.C.17.f.2.b for information on coding complications of a kidney transplant. If the documentation is unclear as to whether the patient has a complication of the transplant, query the provider.

   3) **Chronic kidney disease with other conditions**
   Patients with CKD may also suffer from other serious conditions, most commonly diabetes mellitus and hypertension. The sequencing of the CKD code in relationship to codes for other contributing conditions is based on the conventions in the tabular list.
   See I.C.3.a.4 for sequencing instructions for diabetes.
   See I.C.4.a.1 for anemia in CKD.
   See I.C.7.a.3 for hypertensive chronic kidney disease.
   See I.C.17.f.2.b, Kidney transplant complications, for instructions on coding of documented rejection or failure.

11. **Chapter 11: Complications of Pregnancy, Childbirth, and the Puerperium (630-679)**

   a. **General Rules for Obstetric Cases**

1) **Codes from chapter 11 and sequencing priority**
Obstetric cases require codes from chapter 11, codes in the range 630-679, Complications of Pregnancy, Childbirth, and the Puerperium. Chapter 11 codes have sequencing priority over codes from other chapters. Additional codes from other chapters may be used in conjunction with chapter 11 codes to further specify conditions. Should the provider document that the pregnancy is incidental to the encounter, then code V22.2 should be used in place of any chapter 11 codes. It is the provider's responsibility to state that the condition being treated is not affecting the pregnancy.

2) **Chapter 11 codes used only on the maternal record**
Chapter 11 codes are to be used only on the maternal record, never on the record of the newborn.

3) **Chapter 11 fifth-digits**
Categories 640-648, 651-676 have required fifth-digits, which indicate whether the encounter is antepartum, postpartum and whether a delivery has also occurred.

4) **Fifth-digits, appropriate for each code**
The fifth-digits, which are appropriate for each code number, are listed in brackets under each code. The fifth-digits on each code should all be consistent with each other. That is, should a delivery occur all of the fifth-digits should indicate the delivery.

b. **Selection of OB Principal or First-listed Diagnosis**

1) **Routine outpatient prenatal visits**
For routine outpatient prenatal visits when no complications are present codes V22.0, Supervision of normal first pregnancy, and V22.1, Supervision of other normal pregnancy, should be used as the first-listed diagnoses. These codes should not be used in conjunction with chapter 11 codes.

2) **Prenatal outpatient visits for high-risk patients**
For prenatal outpatient visits for patients with high-risk pregnancies, a code from category V23, Supervision of high-risk pregnancy, should be used as the principal or first-listed diagnosis. Secondary chapter 11 codes may be used in conjunction with these codes if appropriate.

3) **Episodes when no delivery occurs**
In episodes when no delivery occurs, the principal diagnosis should correspond to the principal complication of the pregnancy, which necessitated the encounter. Should more than one complication exist, all of which are treated or monitored, any of the complications codes may be sequenced first.

4) When a delivery occurs

When a delivery occurs, the principal diagnosis should correspond to the main circumstances or complication of the delivery. In cases of cesarean delivery, the selection of the principal diagnosis should correspond to the reason the cesarean delivery was performed unless the reason for admission/encounter was unrelated to the condition resulting in the cesarean delivery.

5) Outcome of delivery

An outcome of delivery code, V27.0-V27.9, should be included on every maternal record when a delivery has occurred. These codes are not to be used on subsequent records or on the newborn record.

c. Fetal Conditions Affecting the Management of the Mother

1) Codes from category 655

Known or suspected fetal abnormality affecting management of the mother, and category 656, Other fetal and placental problems affecting the management of the mother, are assigned only when the fetal condition is actually responsible for modifying the management of the mother, i.e., by requiring diagnostic studies, additional observation, special care, or termination of pregnancy. The fact that the fetal condition exists does not justify assigning a code from this series to the mother's record.

See I.C.18.d for suspected maternal and fetal conditions not found.

2) In utero surgery

In cases when surgery is performed on the fetus, a diagnosis code from category 655, Known or suspected fetal abnormalities affecting management of the mother, should be assigned identifying the fetal condition. Procedure code 75.36, Correction of fetal defect, should be assigned on the hospital inpatient record.

No code from Chapter 15, the perinatal codes, should be used on the mother's record to identify fetal conditions. Surgery performed in utero on a fetus is still to be coded as an obstetric encounter.

d. HIV Infection in Pregnancy, Childbirth and the Puerperium

During pregnancy, childbirth or the puerperium, a patient admitted because of an HIV-related illness should receive a principal diagnosis of 647.6X, Other specified infectious and parasitic diseases in the mother classifiable elsewhere, but complicating the pregnancy, childbirth or the puerperium, followed by 042 and the code(s) for the HIV-related illness(es).

Patients with asymptomatic HIV infection status admitted during pregnancy, childbirth, or the puerperium should receive codes of 647.6X and V08.

e. **Current Conditions Complicating Pregnancy**

Assign a code from subcategory 648.x for patients that have current conditions when the condition affects the management of the pregnancy, childbirth, or the puerperium. Use additional secondary codes from other chapters to identify the conditions, as appropriate.

f. **Diabetes mellitus in pregnancy**

Diabetes mellitus is a significant complicating factor in pregnancy. Pregnant women who are diabetic should be assigned code 648.0x, Diabetes mellitus complicating pregnancy, and a secondary code from category 250, Diabetes mellitus, **or category 249, Secondary diabetes** to identify the type of diabetes.

Code V58.67, Long-term (current) use of insulin, should also be assigned if the diabetes mellitus is being treated with insulin.

g. **Gestational diabetes**

Gestational diabetes can occur during the second and third trimester of pregnancy in women who were not diabetic prior to pregnancy. Gestational diabetes can cause complications in the pregnancy similar to those of pre-existing diabetes mellitus. It also puts the woman at greater risk of developing diabetes after the pregnancy. Gestational diabetes is coded to 648.8x, Abnormal glucose tolerance. Codes 648.0x and 648.8x should never be used together on the same record.

Code V58.67, Long-term (current) use of insulin, should also be assigned if the gestational diabetes is being treated with insulin.

h. **Normal Delivery, Code 650**

1) **Normal delivery**

Code 650 is for use in cases when a woman is admitted for a full-term normal delivery and delivers a single, healthy infant without any complications antepartum, during the delivery, or postpartum during the delivery episode. Code 650 is always a principal diagnosis. It is not to be used if any other code from chapter 11 is needed to describe a current complication of the antenatal, delivery, or perinatal period. Additional codes from other chapters may be used with code 650 if they are not related to or are in any way complicating the pregnancy.

2) **Normal delivery with resolved antepartum complication**

Code 650 may be used if the patient had a complication at some point during her pregnancy, but the complication is not present at the time of the admission for delivery.

3) **V27.0, Single liveborn, outcome of delivery**

V27.0, Single liveborn, is the only outcome of delivery code appropriate for use with 650.

i. **The Postpartum and Peripartum Periods**

1) **Postpartum and peripartum periods**

The postpartum period begins immediately after delivery and continues for six weeks following delivery. The peripartum period is defined as the last month of pregnancy to five months postpartum.

2) **Postpartum complication**

A postpartum complication is any complication occurring within the six-week period.

3) **Pregnancy-related complications after 6 week period**

Chapter 11 codes may also be used to describe pregnancy-related complications after the six-week period should the provider document that a condition is pregnancy related.

4) **Postpartum complications occurring during the same admission as delivery**

Postpartum complications that occur during the same admission as the delivery are identified with a fifth digit of "2." Subsequent admissions/encounters for postpartum complications should be identified with a fifth digit of "4."

5) **Admission for routine postpartum care following delivery outside hospital**

When the mother delivers outside the hospital prior to admission and is admitted for routine postpartum care and no complications are noted, code V24.0, Postpartum care and examination immediately after delivery, should be assigned as the principal diagnosis.

6) **Admission following delivery outside hospital with postpartum conditions**

A delivery diagnosis code should not be used for a woman who has delivered prior to admission to the hospital. Any postpartum conditions and/or postpartum procedures should be coded.

j. **Code 677, Late effect of complication of pregnancy**

1) **Code 677**

Code 677, Late effect of complication of pregnancy, childbirth, and the puerperium is for use in those cases when an initial complication of a pregnancy develops a sequelae requiring care or treatment at a future date.

2) **After the initial postpartum period**

This code may be used at any time after the initial postpartum period.

3) **Sequencing of Code 677**

This code, like all late effect codes, is to be sequenced following the code describing the sequelae of the complication.

k. Abortions

1) **Fifth-digits required for abortion categories**
   Fifth-digits are required for abortion categories 634-637. Fifth-digit 1, incomplete, indicates that all of the products of conception have not been expelled from the uterus. Fifth-digit 2, complete, indicates that all products of conception have been expelled from the uterus.

2) **Code from categories 640-648 and 651-659**
   A code from categories 640-648 and 651-659 may be used as additional codes with an abortion code to indicate the complication leading to the abortion.
   Fifth digit 3 is assigned with codes from these categories when used with an abortion code because the other fifth digits will not apply. Codes from the 660-669 series are not to be used for complications of abortion.

3) **Code 639 for complications**
   Code 639 is to be used for all complications following abortion. Code 639 cannot be assigned with codes from categories 634-638.

4) **Abortion with Liveborn Fetus**
   When an attempted termination of pregnancy results in a liveborn fetus assign code 644.21, Early onset of delivery, with an appropriate code from category V27, Outcome of Delivery. The procedure code for the attempted termination of pregnancy should also be assigned.

5) **Retained Products of Conception following an abortion**
   Subsequent admissions for retained products of conception following a spontaneous or legally induced abortion are assigned the appropriate code from category 634, Spontaneous abortion, or 635 Legally induced abortion, with a fifth digit of "1" (incomplete). This advice is appropriate even when the patient was discharged previously with a discharge diagnosis of complete abortion.

12. Chapter 12: Diseases Skin and Subcutaneous Tissue (680-709)

a. Pressure ulcer stage codes

1) **Pressure ulcer stages**
   Two codes are needed to completely describe a pressure ulcer: A code from subcategory 707.0, Pressure ulcer, to identify the site of the pressure ulcer and a code from subcategory 707.2, Pressure ulcer stages.
   The codes in subcategory 707.2, Pressure ulcer stages, are to be used as an additional

diagnosis with a code(s) from subcategory 707.0, Pressure Ulcer. Codes from 707.2, Pressure ulcer stages, may not be assigned as a principal or first-listed diagnosis. The pressure ulcer stage codes should only be used with pressure ulcers and not with other types of ulcers (e.g., stasis ulcer).

The ICD-9-CM classifies pressure ulcer stages based on severity, which is designated by stages I-IV and unstageable.

2) Unstageable pressure ulcers
Assignment of code 707.25, Pressure ulcer, unstageable, should be based on the clinical documentation. Code 707.25 is used for pressure ulcers whose stage cannot be clinically determined (e.g., the ulcer is covered by eschar or has been treated with a skin or muscle graft) and pressure ulcers that are documented as deep tissue injury but not documented as due to trauma. This code should not be confused with code 707.20, Pressure ulcer, stage unspecified. Code 707.20 should be assigned when there is no documentation regarding the stage of the pressure ulcer.

3) Documented pressure ulcer stage
Assignment of the pressure ulcer stage code should be guided by clinical documentation of the stage or documentation of the terms found in the index. For clinical terms describing the stage that are not found in the index, and there is no documentation of the stage, the provider should be queried.

4) Bilateral pressure ulcers with same stage
When a patient has bilateral pressure ulcers (e.g., both buttocks) and both pressure ulcers are documented as being the same stage, only the code for the site and one code for the stage should be reported.

5) Bilateral pressure ulcers with different stages
When a patient has bilateral pressure ulcers at the same site (e.g., both buttocks) and each pressure ulcer is documented as being at a different stage, assign one code for the site and the appropriate codes for the pressure ulcer stage.

6) Multiple pressure ulcers of different sites and stages
When a patient has multiple pressure ulcers at different sites (e.g., buttock, heel, shoulder) and each pressure ulcer is documented as being at different stages (e.g., stage 3 and stage 4), assign the appropriate codes for each different site and a code for each different pressure ulcer stage.

7) **Patients admitted with pressure ulcers documented as healed**
No code is assigned if the documentation states that the pressure ulcer is completely healed.

8) **Patients admitted with pressure ulcers documented as healing**
Pressure ulcers described as healing should be assigned the appropriate pressure ulcer stage code based on the documentation in the medical record. If the documentation does not provide information about the stage of the healing pressure ulcer, assign code 707.20, Pressure ulcer stage, unspecified.

   If the documentation is unclear as to whether the patient has a current (new) pressure ulcer or if the patient is being treated for a healing pressure ulcer, query the provider.

9) **Patient admitted with pressure ulcer evolving into another stage during the admission**
If a patient is admitted with a pressure ulcer at one stage and it progresses to a higher stage, assign the code for highest stage reported for that site.

13. **Chapter 13: Diseases of Musculoskeletal and Connective Tissue (710-739)**

   a. **Coding of Pathologic Fractures**

   1) **Acute Fractures vs. Aftercare**
   Pathologic fractures are reported using subcategory 733.1, when the fracture is newly diagnosed. Subcategory 733.1 may be used while the patient is receiving active treatment for the fracture. Examples of active treatment are: surgical treatment, emergency department encounter, evaluation and treatment by a new physician.

   Fractures are coded using the aftercare codes (subcategories V54.0, V54.2, V54.8 or V54.9) for encounters after the patient has completed active treatment of the fracture and is receiving routine care for the fracture during the healing or recovery phase. Examples of fracture aftercare are: cast change or removal, removal of external or internal fixation device, medication adjustment, and follow up visits following fracture treatment.

   Care for complications of surgical treatment for fracture repairs during the healing or recovery phase should be coded with the appropriate complication codes.

   Care of complications of fractures, such as malunion and nonunion, should be reported with the appropriate codes.

See Section I. C. 17.b for information on the coding of traumatic fractures.

14. **Chapter 14: Congenital Anomalies (740-759)**

   a. **Codes in categories 740-759, Congenital Anomalies**

   Assign an appropriate code(s) from categories 740-759, Congenital Anomalies, when an anomaly is documented. A congenital anomaly may be the principal/first listed diagnosis on a record or a secondary diagnosis.

   When a congenital anomaly does not have a unique code assignment, assign additional code(s) for any manifestations that may be present.

   When the code assignment specifically identifies the congenital anomaly, manifestations that are an inherent component of the anomaly should not be coded separately. Additional codes should be assigned for manifestations that are not an inherent component.

   Codes from Chapter 14 may be used throughout the life of the patient. If a congenital anomaly has been corrected, a personal history code should be used to identify the history of the anomaly. Although present at birth, a congenital anomaly may not be identified until later in life. Whenever the condition is diagnosed by the physician, it is appropriate to assign a code from codes 740-759.

   For the birth admission, the appropriate code from category V30, Liveborn infants, according to type of birth should be sequenced as the principal diagnosis, followed by any congenital anomaly codes, 740-759.

15. **Chapter 15: Newborn (Perinatal) Guidelines (760-779)**

   For coding and reporting purposes the perinatal period is defined as before birth through the 28th day following birth. The following guidelines are provided for reporting purposes. Hospitals may record other diagnoses as needed for internal data use.

   a. **General Perinatal Rules**

   1) **Chapter 15 Codes**

      They are <u>never</u> for use on the maternal record. Codes from Chapter 11, the obstetric chapter, are never permitted on the newborn record. Chapter 15 code may be used throughout the life of the patient if the condition is still present.

   2) **Sequencing of perinatal codes**

      Generally, codes from Chapter 15 should be sequenced as the principal/first-listed diagnosis on the newborn record, with the exception of the appropriate V30 code for the birth episode, followed by codes from any other chapter that provide additional detail. The "use additional code" note at the beginning of the chapter supports this guideline. If the index does not provide a specific code for a perinatal condition, assign code 779.89, Other specified conditions originating in the perinatal period, followed by the code from another chapter that specifies the condition. Codes for signs and symptoms may be assigned when a definitive diagnosis has not been established.

3) **Birth process or community acquired conditions**

If a newborn has a condition that may be either due to the birth process or community acquired and the documentation does not indicate which it is, the default is due to the birth process and the code from Chapter 15 should be used. If the condition is community-acquired, a code from Chapter 15 should not be assigned.

4) **Code all clinically significant conditions**

All clinically significant conditions noted on routine newborn examination should be coded. A condition is clinically significant if it requires:

- clinical evaluation; or
- therapeutic treatment; or
- diagnostic procedures; or
- extended length of hospital stay; or
- increased nursing care and/or monitoring; or
- has implications for future health care needs

Note: The perinatal guidelines listed above are the same as the general coding guidelines for "additional diagnoses", except for the final point regarding implications for future health care needs. Codes should be assigned for conditions that have been specified by the provider as having implications for future health care needs. Codes from the perinatal chapter should not be assigned unless the provider has established a definitive diagnosis.

b. **Use of codes V30-V39**

When coding the birth of an infant, assign a code from categories V30-V39, according to the type of birth. A code from this series is assigned as a principal diagnosis, and assigned only once to a newborn at the time of birth.

c. **Newborn transfers**

If the newborn is transferred to another institution, the V30 series is not used at the receiving hospital.

d. **Use of category V29**

1) **Assigning a code from category V29**

Assign a code from category V29, Observation and evaluation of newborns and infants for suspected conditions not found, to identify those instances when a healthy newborn is evaluated for a suspected condition that is determined after study not to be present. Do not use a code from category V29 when the patient has identified signs or symptoms of a suspected problem; in such cases, code the sign or symptom.

A code from category V29 may also be assigned as a principal code for readmissions or encounters when the V30 code no longer applies. Codes from category V29 are for use only for healthy newborns and infants for which no condition after study is found to be present.

2) **V29 code on a birth record**

A V29 code is to be used as a secondary code after the V30, Outcome of delivery, code.

e. **Use of other V codes on perinatal records**

V codes other than V30 and V29 may be assigned on a perinatal or newborn record code. The codes may be used as a principal or first-listed diagnosis for specific types of encounters or for readmissions or encounters when the V30 code no longer applies.

See Section I.C.18 for information regarding the assignment of V codes.

f. **Maternal Causes of Perinatal Morbidity**

Codes from categories 760-763, Maternal causes of perinatal morbidity and mortality, are assigned only when the maternal condition has actually affected the fetus or newborn. The fact that the mother has an associated medical condition or experiences some complication of pregnancy, labor or delivery does not justify the routine assignment of codes from these categories to the newborn record.

g. **Congenital Anomalies in Newborns**

For the birth admission, the appropriate code from category V30, Liveborn infants according to type of birth, should be used, followed by any congenital anomaly codes, categories 740-759. Use additional secondary codes from other chapters to specify conditions associated with the anomaly, if applicable.

Also, see Section I.C.14 for information on the coding of congenital anomalies.

h. **Coding Additional Perinatal Diagnoses**

1) **Assigning codes for conditions that require treatment**

Assign codes for conditions that require treatment or further investigation, prolong the length of stay, or require resource utilization.

2) **Codes for conditions specified as having implications for future health care needs**

Assign codes for conditions that have been specified by the provider as having implications for future health care needs.

Note: This guideline should not be used for adult patients.

3) Codes for newborn conditions originating in the perinatal period

Assign a code for newborn conditions originating in the perinatal period (categories 760-779), as well as complications arising during the current episode of care classified in other chapters, only if the diagnoses have been documented by the responsible provider at the time of transfer or discharge as having affected the fetus or newborn.

i. Prematurity and Fetal Growth Retardation

Providers utilize different criteria in determining prematurity. A code for prematurity should not be assigned unless it is documented. The 5th digit assignment for codes from category 764 and subcategories 765.0 and 765.1 should be based on the recorded birth weight and estimated gestational age.

A code from subcategory 765.2, Weeks of gestation, should be assigned as an additional code with category 764 and codes from 765.0 and 765.1 to specify weeks of gestation as documented by the provider in the record.

j. Newborn sepsis

Code 771.81, Septicemia [sepsis] of newborn, should be assigned with a secondary code from category 041, Bacterial infections in conditions classified elsewhere and of unspecified site, to identify the organism. A code from category 038, Septicemia, should not be used on a newborn record. **Do not assign code 995.91, Sepsis, as** code 771.81 describes the sepsis. **If applicable, use additional codes to identify severe sepsis (995.92) and any associated acute organ dysfunction.**

16. Chapter 16: Signs, Symptoms and Ill-Defined Conditions (780-799)

Reserved for future guideline expansion

17. Chapter 17: Injury and Poisoning (800-999)

a. Coding of Injuries

When coding injuries, assign separate codes for each injury unless a combination code is provided, in which case the combination code is assigned. Multiple injury codes are provided in ICD-9-CM, but should not be assigned unless information for a more specific code is not available. These codes are not to be used for normal, healing surgical wounds or to identify complications of surgical wounds.

The code for the most serious injury, as determined by the provider and the focus of treatment, is sequenced first.

1) Superficial injuries

Superficial injuries such as abrasions or contusions are not coded when associated with more severe injuries of the same site.

2) **Primary injury with damage to nerves/blood vessels**

When a primary injury results in minor damage to peripheral nerves or blood vessels, the primary injury is sequenced first with additional code(s) from categories 950-957, Injury to nerves and spinal cord, and/or 900-904, Injury to blood vessels. When the primary injury is to the blood vessels or nerves, that injury should be sequenced first.

b. **Coding of Traumatic Fractures**

The principles of multiple coding of injuries should be followed in coding fractures. Fractures of specified sites are coded individually by site in accordance with both the provisions within categories 800-829 and the level of detail furnished by medical record content. Combination categories for multiple fractures are provided for use when there is insufficient detail in the medical record (such as trauma cases transferred to another hospital), when the reporting form limits the number of codes that can be used in reporting pertinent clinical data, or when there is insufficient specificity at the fourth-digit or fifth-digit level. More specific guidelines are as follows:

1) **Acute Fractures vs. Aftercare**

Traumatic fractures are coded using the acute fracture codes (800-829) while the patient is receiving active treatment for the fracture. Examples of active treatment are: surgical treatment, emergency department encounter, and evaluation and treatment by a new physician.

Fractures are coded using the aftercare codes (subcategories V54.0, V54.1, V54.8, or V54.9) for encounters after the patient has completed active treatment of the fracture and is receiving routine care for the fracture during the healing or recovery phase. Examples of fracture aftercare are: cast change or removal, removal of external or internal fixation device, medication adjustment, and follow up visits following fracture treatment.

Care for complications of surgical treatment for fracture repairs during the healing or recovery phase should be coded with the appropriate complication codes.

Care of complications of fractures, such as malunion and nonunion, should be reported with the appropriate codes.

Pathologic fractures are not coded in the 800-829 range, but instead are assigned to subcategory 733.1. *See Section I.C.13.a for additional information.*

2) **Multiple fractures of same limb**

Multiple fractures of same limb classifiable to the same three-digit or four-digit category are coded to that category.

3) **Multiple unilateral or bilateral fractures of same bone**

Multiple unilateral or bilateral fractures of same bone(s) but classified to different fourth-digit subdivisions (bone part) within the same three-digit category are coded individually by site.

4) **Multiple fracture categories 819 and 828**

Multiple fracture categories 819 and 828 classify bilateral fractures of both upper limbs (819) and both lower limbs (828), but without any detail at the fourth-digit level other than open and closed type of fractures.

5) **Multiple fractures sequencing**

Multiple fractures are sequenced in accordance with the severity of the fracture. The provider should be asked to list the fracture diagnoses in the order of severity.

c. **Coding of Burns**

Current burns (940-948) are classified by depth, extent and by agent (E code). Burns are classified by depth as first degree (erythema), second degree (blistering), and third degree (full-thickness involvement).

1) **Sequencing of burn and related condition codes**

Sequence first the code that reflects the highest degree of burn when more than one burn is present.

a. When the reason for the admission or encounter is for treatment of external multiple burns, sequence first the code that reflects the burn of the highest degree.

b. When a patient has both internal and external burns, the circumstances of admission govern the selection of the principal diagnosis or first-listed diagnosis.

c. When a patient is admitted for burn injuries and other related conditions such as smoke inhalation and/or respiratory failure, the circumstances of admission govern the selection of the principal or first-listed diagnosis.

2) **Burns of the same local site**

Classify burns of the same local site (three-digit category level, 940-947) but of different degrees to the subcategory identifying the highest degree recorded in the diagnosis.

3) **Non-healing burns**

Non-healing burns are coded as acute burns. Necrosis of burned skin should be coded as a non-healed burn.

4) **Code 958.3, Posttraumatic wound infection**
Assign code 958.3, Posttraumatic wound infection, not elsewhere classified, as an additional code for any documented infected burn site.

5) **Assign separate codes for each burn site**
When coding burns, assign separate codes for each burn site. Category 946 Burns of Multiple specified sites, should only be used if the location of the burns are not documented. Category 949, Burn, unspecified, is extremely vague and should rarely be used.

6) **Assign codes from category 948, Burns**
Burns classified according to extent of body surface involved, when the site of the burn is not specified or when there is a need for additional data. It is advisable to use category 948 as additional coding when needed to provide data for evaluating burn mortality, such as that needed by burn units. It is also advisable to use category 948 as an additional code for reporting purposes when there is mention of a third-degree burn involving 20 percent or more of the body surface.

In assigning a code from category 948:

Fourth-digit codes are used to identify the percentage of total body surface involved in a burn (all degree).

Fifth-digits are assigned to identify the percentage of body surface involved in third-degree burn.

Fifth-digit zero (0) is assigned when less than 10 percent or when no body surface is involved in a third-degree burn.

Category 948 is based on the classic "rule of nines" in estimating body surface involved: head and neck are assigned nine percent, each arm nine percent, each leg 18 percent, the anterior trunk 18 percent, posterior trunk 18 percent, and genitalia one percent. Providers may change these percentage assignments where necessary to accommodate infants and children who have proportionately larger heads than adults and patients who have large buttocks, thighs, or abdomen that involve burns.

7) **Encounters for treatment of late effects of burns**
Encounters for the treatment of the late effects of burns (i.e., scars or joint contractures) should be coded to the residual condition (sequelae) followed by the appropriate late effect code (906.5-906.9). A late effect E code may also be used, if desired.

8) Sequelae with a late effect code and current burn

When appropriate, both a sequelae with a late effect code, and a current burn code may be assigned on the same record (when both a current burn and sequelae of an old burn exist).

d. Coding of Debridement of Wound, Infection, or Burn

Excisional debridement involves surgical removal or cutting away, as opposed to a mechanical (brushing, scrubbing, washing) debridement.

For coding purposes, excisional debridement is assigned to code 86.22.

Nonexcisional debridement is assigned to code 86.28.

e. Adverse Effects, Poisoning and Toxic Effects

The properties of certain drugs, medicinal and biological substances or combinations of such substances, may cause toxic reactions. The occurrence of drug toxicity is classified in ICD-9-CM as follows:

1) Adverse Effect

When the drug was correctly prescribed and properly administered, code the reaction plus the appropriate code from the E930-E949 series. Codes from the E930-E949 series must be used to identify the causative substance for an adverse effect of drug, medicinal and biological substances, correctly prescribed and properly administered. The effect, such as tachycardia, delirium, gastrointestinal hemorrhaging, vomiting, hypokalemia, hepatitis, renal failure, or respiratory failure, is coded and followed by the appropriate code from the E930-E949 series.

Adverse effects of therapeutic substances correctly prescribed and properly administered (toxicity, synergistic reaction, side effect, and idiosyncratic reaction) may be due to (1) differences among patients, such as age, sex, disease, and genetic factors, and (2) drug-related factors, such as type of drug, route of administration, duration of therapy, dosage, and bioavailability.

2) Poisoning

(a) Error was made in drug prescription

Errors made in drug prescription or in the administration of the drug by provider, nurse, patient, or other person, use the appropriate poisoning code from the 960-979 series.

(b) Overdose of a drug intentionally taken

If an overdose of a drug was intentionally taken or administered and resulted in drug toxicity, it would be coded as a poisoning (960-979 series).

(c) **Nonprescribed drug taken with correctly prescribed and properly administered drug**
If a nonprescribed drug or medicinal agent was taken in combination with a correctly prescribed and properly administered drug, any drug toxicity or other reaction resulting from the interaction of the two drugs would be classified as a poisoning.

(d) **Interaction of drug(s) and alcohol**
When a reaction results from the interaction of a drug(s) and alcohol, this would be classified as poisoning.

(e) **Sequencing of poisoning**
When coding a poisoning or reaction to the improper use of a medication (e.g., wrong dose, wrong substance, wrong route of administration) the poisoning code is sequenced first, followed by a code for the manifestation. If there is also a diagnosis of drug abuse or dependence to the substance, the abuse or dependence is coded as an additional code.
See Section I.C.3.a.6.b. if poisoning is the result of insulin pump malfunctions and Section I.C.19 for general use of E-codes.

3) **Toxic Effects**

(a) **Toxic effect codes**
When a harmful substance is ingested or comes in contact with a person, this is classified as a toxic effect. The toxic effect codes are in categories 980-989.

(b) **Sequencing toxic effect codes**
A toxic effect code should be sequenced first, followed by the code(s) that identify the result of the toxic effect.

(c) **External cause codes for toxic effects**
An external cause code from categories E860-E869 for accidental exposure, codes E950.6 or E950.7 for intentional self-harm, category E962 for assault, or categories E980-E982, for undetermined, should also be assigned to indicate intent.

f. **Complications of care**

1) **Complications of care**

(a) **Documentation of complications of care**
As with all procedural or postprocedural complications, code assignment is based on the provider's documentation of the relationship between the condition and the procedure.

2) **Transplant complications**

(a) **Transplant complications other than kidney**

Codes under subcategory 996.8, Complications of transplanted organ, are for use for both complications and rejection of transplanted organs. A transplant complication code is only assigned if the complication affects the function of the transplanted organ. Two codes are required to fully describe a transplant complication, the appropriate code from subcategory 996.8 and a secondary code that identifies the complication.

Pre-existing conditions or conditions that develop after the transplant are not coded as complications unless they affect the function of the transplanted organs.
See I.C.18.d.3) for transplant organ removal status
See I.C.2.i for malignant neoplasm associated with transplant organ.

(b) **Chronic kidney disease and kidney transplant complications**
Patients who have undergone kidney transplant may still have some form of chronic kidney disease (CKD) because the kidney transplant may not fully restore kidney function.

Code 996.81 should be assigned for documented complications of a kidney transplant, such as transplant failure or rejection **or other transplant complication.** Code 996.81 should not be assigned for post kidney transplant patients who have chronic kidney (CKD) unless a transplant complication such as transplant failure or rejection is documented. If the documentation is unclear as to whether the patient has a complication of the transplant, query the provider.

For patients with CKD following a kidney transplant, but who do not have a complication such as failure or rejection, *see section I.C.10.a.2, Chronic kidney disease and kidney transplant status.*

3) **Ventilator associated pneumonia**

(a) **Documentation of Ventilator associated Pneumonia**
As with all procedural or postprocedural complications, code assignment is based on the provider's documentation of the relationship between the condition and the procedure.

Code 997.31, Ventilator associated pneumonia, should be assigned only when the provider has documented ventilator associated pneumonia (VAP). An additional code to identify the organism (e.g., Pseudomonas aeruginosa, code 041.7) should also be assigned. Do not assign an additional code from categories 480-484 to identify the type of pneumonia.

Code 997.31 should not be assigned for cases where the patient has pneumonia and is on a mechanical ventilator but the provider has not specifically stated that the pneumonia is ventilator-associated pneumonia.

If the documentation is unclear as to whether the patient has a pneumonia that is a complication attributable to the mechanical ventilator, query the provider.

(b) Patient admitted with pneumonia and develops VAP

A patient may be admitted with one type of pneumonia (e.g., code 481, Pneumococcal pneumonia) and subsequently develop VAP. In this instance, the principal diagnosis would be the appropriate code from categories 480-484 for the pneumonia diagnosed at the time of admission. Code 997.31, Ventilator associated pneumonia, would be assigned as an additional diagnosis when the provider has also documented the presence of ventilator associated pneumonia.

g. **SIRS due to Non-infectious Process**

The systemic inflammatory response syndrome (SIRS) can develop as a result of certain non-infectious disease processes, such as trauma, malignant neoplasm, or pancreatitis. When SIRS is documented with a noninfectious condition, and no subsequent infection is documented, the code for the underlying condition, such as an injury, should be assigned, followed by code 995.93, Systemic inflammatory response syndrome due to noninfectious process without acute organ dysfunction, or 995.94, Systemic inflammatory response syndrome due to non-infectious process with acute organ dysfunction. If an acute organ dysfunction is documented, the appropriate code(s) for the associated acute organ dysfunction(s) should be assigned in addition to code 995.94. If acute organ dysfunction is documented, but it cannot be determined if the acute organ dysfunction is associated with SIRS or due to another condition (e.g., directly due to the trauma), the provider should be queried.

When the non-infectious condition has led to an infection that results in SIRS, *see Section I.C.1.b.12 for the guideline for sepsis and severe sepsis associated with a non-infectious process.*

18. **Classification of Factors Influencing Health Status and Contact with Health Service (Supplemental V01-V89)**

Note: The chapter specific guidelines provide additional information about the use of V codes for specified encounters.

a. **Introduction**

ICD-9-CM provides codes to deal with encounters for circumstances other than a disease or injury. The Supplementary Classification of Factors Influencing Health Status and Contact with Health Services (V01.0 - **V89.09**) is provided to deal with occasions when circumstances other than a disease or injury (codes 001-999) are recorded as a diagnosis or problem.

There are four primary circumstances for the use of V codes:

1) A person who is not currently sick encounters the health services for some specific reason, such as to act as an organ donor, to receive prophylactic care, such as inoculations or health screenings, or to receive counseling on health related issues.

2) A person with a resolving disease or injury, or a chronic, long-term condition requiring continuous care, encounters the health care system for specific aftercare of that disease or injury (e.g., dialysis for renal disease; chemotherapy for malignancy; cast change). A diagnosis/symptom code should be used whenever a current, acute, diagnosis is being treated or a sign or symptom is being studied.

3) Circumstances or problems influence a person's health status but are not in themselves a current illness or injury.

4) Newborns, to indicate birth status

b. **V codes use in any healthcare setting**

V codes are for use in any healthcare setting. V codes may be used as either a first listed (principal diagnosis code in the inpatient setting) or secondary code, depending on the circumstances of the encounter. Certain V codes may only be used as first listed, others only as secondary codes. *See Section I.C.18.e, V Code Table.*

c. **V Codes indicate a reason for an encounter**

They are not procedure codes. A corresponding procedure code must accompany a V code to describe the procedure performed.

d. **Categories of V Codes**

1) **Contact/Exposure**

Category V01 indicates contact with or exposure to communicable diseases. These codes are for patients who do not show any sign or symptom of a disease but have been exposed to it by close personal contact with an infected individual or are in an area where a disease is epidemic. These codes may be used as a first listed code to explain an encounter for testing, or, more commonly, as a secondary code to identify a potential risk.

2) **Inoculations and vaccinations**

Categories V03-V06 are for encounters for inoculations and vaccinations. They indicate that a patient is being seen to receive a prophylactic inoculation against a disease. The injection itself must be represented by the appropriate procedure code. A code from V03-V06 may be used as a secondary code if the inoculation is given as a routine part of preventive health care, such as a well-baby visit.

3) **Status**

Status codes indicate that a patient is either a carrier of a disease or has the sequelae or residual of a past disease or condition. This includes such things as the presence of prosthetic or mechanical devices resulting from past treatment. A status code is informative, because the status may affect the course of treatment and its outcome. A status code is distinct from a history code. The history code indicates that the patient no longer has the condition.

A status code should not be used with a diagnosis code from one of the body system chapters, if the diagnosis code includes the information provided by the status code. For example, code V42.1, Heart transplant status, should not be used with code 996.83, Complications of transplanted heart. The status code does not provide additional information. The complication code indicates that the patient is a heart transplant patient.

The status V codes/categories are:

V02   Carrier or suspected carrier of infectious diseases

Carrier status indicates that a person harbors the specific organisms of a disease without manifest symptoms and is capable of transmitting the infection.

V07.5X Prophylactic use of agents affecting estrogen receptors and estrogen level This code indicates when a patient is receiving a drug that affects estrogen receptors and estrogen levels for prevention of cancer.

V08   Asymptomatic HIV infection status

This code indicates that a patient has tested positive for HIV but has manifested no signs or symptoms of the disease.

V09   Infection with drug-resistant microorganisms

This category indicates that a patient has an infection that is resistant to drug treatment.

Sequence the infection code first.

V21   Constitutional states in development

V22.2   Pregnant state, incidental

This code is a secondary code only for use when the pregnancy is in no way complicating the reason for visit. Otherwise, a code from the obstetric chapter is required.

V26.5x   Sterilization status

V42   Organ or tissue replaced by transplant

V43   Organ or tissue replaced by other means

V44   Artificial opening status

V45   Other postsurgical states

Assign code V45.87, Transplant organ removal status, to indicate that a transplanted organ has been previously removed. This code should not be assigned for the encounter in which the transplanted organ is removed. The complication necessitating removal of the transplant organ should be assigned for that encounter.

See section I.C17.f.2. for information on the coding of organ transplant complications.

Assign code V45.88, Status post administration of tPA (rtPA) in a different facility within the last 24 hours prior to admission to the current facility, as a secondary diagnosis when a patient is received by transfer into a facility and documentation indicates they were administered tissue plasminogen activator (tPA) within the last 24 hours prior to admission to the current facility.

This guideline applies even if the patient is still receiving the tPA at the time they are received into the current facility.

The appropriate code for the condition for which the tPA was administered (such as cerebrovascular disease or myocardial infarction) should be assigned first.

Code V45.88 is only applicable to the receiving facility record and not to the transferring facility record.

V46   Other dependence on machines

V49.6   Upper limb amputation status

V49.7   Lower limb amputation status
Note: Categories V42-V46, and subcategories V49.6, V49.7 are for use only if there are no complications or malfunctions of the organ or tissue replaced, the amputation site or the equipment on which the patient is dependent.

V49.81 Postmenopausal status

V49.82 Dental sealant status

V49.83 Awaiting organ transplant status

V58.6x Long-term (current) drug use
Codes from this subcategory indicate a patient's continuous use of a prescribed drug (including such things as aspirin therapy) for the long-term treatment of a condition or for prophylactic use. It is not for use for patients who have addictions to drugs. **This subcategory is not for use of medications for detoxification or maintenance programs to prevent withdrawal symptoms in patients with drug dependence (e.g., methadone maintenance for opiate dependence). Assign the appropriate code for the drug dependence instead.**

Assign a code from subcategory V58.6, Long-term (current) drug use, if the patient is receiving a medication for an extended period as a prophylactic measure (such as for the prevention of deep vein thrombosis) or as treatment of a chronic condition (such as arthritis) or a disease requiring a lengthy course of treatment (such as cancer). Do not assign a code from subcategory V58.6 for medication being administered for a brief period of time to treat an acute illness or injury (such as a course of antibiotics to treat acute bronchitis)

V83   Genetic carrier status
Genetic carrier status indicates that a person carries a gene, associated with a particular disease, which may be passed to offspring who may develop that disease. The person does not have the disease and is not at risk of developing the disease.

V84   Genetic susceptibility status
Genetic susceptibility indicates that a person has a gene that increases the risk of that person developing the disease.

Codes from category V84, Genetic susceptibility to disease, should not be used as principal or first-listed codes. If the patient has the condition to which he/she is susceptible, and that condition is the reason for the encounter, the code for the current condition should be sequenced first. If the patient is being seen for follow-up after completed treatment for this condition, and the condition no longer exists, a follow-up code should be sequenced first, followed by the appropriate personal history and genetic susceptibility codes. If the purpose of the encounter is genetic counseling associated with procreative management, a code from subcategory V26.3, Genetic counseling and testing, should be assigned as the first-listed code, followed by a code from category V84. Additional codes should be assigned for any applicable family or personal history. *See Section I.C. 18.d.14 for information on prophylactic organ removal due to a genetic susceptibility.*

V86   Estrogen receptor status

V88   Acquired absence of other organs and tissue

4) **History (of)**
There are two types of history V codes, personal and family. Personal history codes explain a patient's past medical condition that no longer exists and is not receiving any treatment, but that has the potential for recurrence, and therefore may require continued monitoring. The exceptions to this general rule are category V14, Personal history of allergy to medicinal agents, and subcategory V15.0, Allergy, other than to medicinal agents. A person who has had an allergic episode to a substance or food in the past should always be considered allergic to the substance.

Family history codes are for use when a patient has a family member(s) who has had a particular disease that causes the patient to be at higher risk of also contracting the disease.

Personal history codes may be used in conjunction with follow-up codes and family history codes may be used in conjunction with screening codes to explain the need for a test or procedure. History codes are also acceptable on any medical record regardless of the reason for visit. A history of an illness, even if no longer present, is important information that may alter the type of treatment ordered.

The history V code categories are:

V10	Personal history of malignant neoplasm
V12	Personal history of certain other diseases
V13	Personal history of other diseases

Except: V13.4, Personal history of arthritis, and V13.6, Personal history of congenital malformations. These conditions are life-long so are not true history codes.

V14	Personal history of allergy to medicinal agents
V15	Other personal history presenting hazards to health

Except: V15.7, Personal history of contraception.

V16	Family history of malignant neoplasm
V17	Family history of certain chronic disabling diseases
V18	Family history of certain other specific diseases
V19	Family history of other conditions
V87	**Other specified personal exposures and history presenting hazards to health**

5) **Screening**

Screening is the testing for disease or disease precursors in seemingly well individuals so that early detection and treatment can be provided for those who test positive for the disease. Screenings that are recommended for many subgroups in a population include: routine mammograms for women over 40, a fecal occult blood test for everyone over 50, an amniocentesis to rule out a fetal anomaly for pregnant women over 35, because the incidence of breast cancer and colon cancer in these subgroups is higher than in the general population, as is the incidence of Down's syndrome in older mothers.

The testing of a person to rule out or confirm a suspected diagnosis because the patient has some sign or symptom is a diagnostic examination, not a screening. In these cases, the sign or symptom is used to explain the reason for the test.

A screening code may be a first listed code if the reason for the visit is specifically the screening exam. It may also be used as an additional code if the screening is done during an office visit for other health problems. A screening code is not necessary if the screening is inherent to a routine examination, such as a pap smear done during a routine pelvic examination.

Should a condition be discovered during the screening then the code for the condition may be assigned as an additional diagnosis.

The V code indicates that a screening exam is planned. A procedure code is required to confirm that the screening was performed.

The screening V code categories:

V28   Antenatal screening

V73-V82   Special screening examinations

6) **Observation**

There are three observation V code categories. They are for use in very limited circumstances when a person is being observed for a suspected condition that is ruled out. The observation codes are not for use if an injury or illness or any signs or symptoms related to the suspected condition are present. In such cases the diagnosis/symptom code is used with the corresponding E code to identify any external cause.

The observation codes are to be used as principal diagnosis only. The only exception to this is when the principal diagnosis is required to be a code from the V30, Live born infant, category. Then the V29 observation code is sequenced after the V30 code. Additional codes may be used in addition to the observation code but only if they are unrelated to the suspected condition being observed.

Codes from subcategory V89.0, Suspected maternal and fetal conditions not found, may either be used as a first listed or as an additional code assignment depending on the case. They are for use in very limited circumstances on a maternal record when an encounter is for a suspected maternal or fetal condition that is ruled out during that encounter (for example, a maternal or fetal condition may be suspected due to an abnormal test result). These codes should not be used when the condition is confirmed. In those cases, the confirmed condition should be coded. In addition, these codes are not for use if an illness or any signs or symptoms related to the suspected condition or problem are present. In such cases the diagnosis/symptom code is used.

Additional codes may be used in addition to the code from subcategory V89.0, but only if they are unrelated to the suspected condition being evaluated.

Codes from subcategory V89.0 may not be used for encounters for antenatal screening of mother. *See Section I.C.18.d., Screening).*

For encounters for suspected fetal condition that are inconclusive following testing and

evaluation, assign the appropriate code from category 655, 656, 657 or 658.

The observation V code categories:

V29   Observation and evaluation of newborns for suspected condition not found

For the birth encounter, a code from category V30 should be sequenced before the V29 code.

V71   Observation and evaluation for suspected condition not found

V89   Suspected maternal and fetal conditions not found

7) **Aftercare**

Aftercare visit codes cover situations when the initial treatment of a disease or injury has been performed and the patient requires continued care during the healing or recovery phase, or for the long-term consequences of the disease. The aftercare V code should not be used if treatment is directed at a current, acute disease or injury. The diagnosis code is to be used in these cases. Exceptions to this rule are codes V58.0, Radiotherapy, and codes from subcategory V58.1, Encounter for chemotherapy and immunotherapy for neoplastic conditions. These codes are to be first listed, followed by the diagnosis code when a patient's encounter is solely to receive radiation therapy or chemotherapy for the treatment of a neoplasm. Should a patient receive both chemotherapy and radiation therapy during the same encounter code V58.0 and V58.1 may be used together on a record with either one being sequenced first.

The aftercare codes are generally first listed to explain the specific reason for the encounter. An aftercare code may be used as an additional code when some type of aftercare is provided in addition to the reason for admission and no diagnosis code is applicable. An example of this would be the closure of a colostomy during an encounter for treatment of another condition.

Aftercare codes should be used in conjunction with any other aftercare codes or other diagnosis codes to provide better detail on the specifics of an aftercare encounter visit, unless otherwise directed by the classification. The sequencing of multiple aftercare codes is discretionary.

Certain aftercare V code categories need a secondary diagnosis code to describe the resolving condition or sequelae, for others, the condition is inherent in the code title.

Additional V code aftercare category terms include, fitting and adjustment, and attention to artificial openings.

Status V codes may be used with aftercare V codes to indicate the nature of the aftercare. For example code V45.81, Aortocoronary bypass status, may be used with code V58.73, Aftercare following surgery of the circulatory system, NEC, to indicate the surgery for which the aftercare is being performed. Also, a transplant status code may be used following code V58.44, Aftercare following organ transplant, to identify the organ transplanted. A status code should not be used when the aftercare code indicates the type of status, such as using V55.0, Attention to tracheostomy with V44.0, Tracheostomy status. *See Section I. B.16 Admissions/Encounter for Rehabilitation*

The aftercare V category/codes:

V51   **Encounter for breast reconstruction following mastectomy**

V52   Fitting and adjustment of prosthetic device and implant

V53   Fitting and adjustment of other device

V54   Other orthopedic aftercare

V55   Attention to artificial openings

V56   Encounter for dialysis and dialysis catheter care

V57   Care involving the use of rehabilitation procedures

V58.0   Radiotherapy

V58.11   Encounter for antineoplastic chemotherapy

V58.12   Encounter for antineoplastic immunotherapy

V58.3x   Attention to dressings and sutures

V58.41   Encounter for planned post-operative wound closure

V58.42   Aftercare, surgery, neoplasm

V58.43   Aftercare, surgery, trauma

V58.44   Aftercare involving organ transplant

V58.49   Other specified aftercare following surgery

V58.7x   Aftercare following surgery

V58.81   Fitting and adjustment of vascular catheter

V58.82   Fitting and adjustment of non-vascular catheter

V58.83   Monitoring therapeutic drug

V58.89   Other specified aftercare

8) Follow-up

The follow-up codes are used to explain continuing surveillance following completed treatment of a disease, condition, or injury.

They imply that the condition has been fully treated and no longer exists. They should not be confused with aftercare codes that explain current treatment for a healing condition or its sequelae. Follow-up codes may be used in conjunction with history codes to provide the full picture of the healed condition and its treatment. The follow-up code is sequenced first, followed by the history code.

A follow-up code may be used to explain repeated visits. Should a condition be found to have recurred on the follow-up visit, then the diagnosis code should be used in place of the follow-up code.

The follow-up V code categories:

V24   Postpartum care and evaluation

V67   Follow-up examination

9) Donor

Category V59 is the donor codes. They are used for living individuals who are donating blood or other body tissue. These codes are only for individuals donating for others, not for self donations. They are not for use to identify cadaveric donations.

10) Counseling

Counseling V codes are used when a patient or family member receives assistance in the aftermath of an illness or injury, or when support is required in coping with family or social problems. They are not necessary for use in conjunction with a diagnosis code when the counseling component of care is considered integral to standard treatment.

The counseling V categories/codes:

V25.0   General counseling and advice for contraceptive management

V26.3   Genetic counseling

V26.4   General counseling and advice for procreative management

V61.X   Other family circumstances

V65.1   Person consulted on behalf of another person

V65.3   Dietary surveillance and counseling

V65.4   Other counseling, not elsewhere classified

11) Obstetrics and related conditions

See Section I.C.11., the Obstetrics guidelines for further instruction on the use of these codes.

V codes for pregnancy are for use in those circumstances when none of the problems or complications included in the codes from the Obstetrics chapter exist (a routine prenatal visit or postpartum care). Codes V22.0, Supervision of normal first pregnancy, and V22.1,

Supervision of other normal pregnancy, are always first listed and are not to be used with any other code from the OB chapter.

The outcome of delivery, category V27, should be included on all maternal delivery records. It is always a secondary code.

V codes for family planning (contraceptive) or procreative management and counseling should be included on an obstetric record either during the pregnancy or the postpartum stage, if applicable.

Obstetrics and related conditions V code categories:

V22	Normal pregnancy
V23	Supervision of high-risk pregnancy Except: V23.2, Pregnancy with history of abortion. Code 646.3, Habitual aborter, from the OB chapter is required to indicate a history of abortion during a pregnancy.
V24	Postpartum care and evaluation
V25	Encounter for contraceptive management Except V25.0x *(See Section I.C.18.d.11, Counseling)*
V26	Procreative management Except V26.5x, Sterilization status, V26.3 and V26.4 *(See Section I.C.18.d.11., Counseling)*
V27	Outcome of delivery
V28	Antenatal screening *(See Section I.C.18.d.6., Screening)*

12) Newborn, infant and child

See Section I.C.15, the Newborn guidelines for further instruction on the use of these codes.

Newborn V code categories:

V20	Health supervision of infant or child
V29	Observation and evaluation of newborns for suspected condition not found *(See Section I.C.18.d.7, Observation)*
V30-V39	Liveborn infant according to type of birth

13) Routine and administrative examinations

The V codes allow for the description of encounters for routine examinations, such as, a general check-up, or, examinations for administrative purposes, such as, a pre-employment physical. The codes are not to be used if the examination is for diagnosis of a suspected condition or for treatment purposes. In such cases the diagnosis code is used. During a routine exam, should a diagnosis or condition be discovered, it should be coded as an additional code. Pre-existing and chronic conditions and history codes may also be included as additional codes as long as the examination is for administrative purposes and not focused on any particular condition.

Pre-operative examination V codes are for use only in those situations when a patient is being cleared for surgery and no treatment is given.

The V codes categories/code for routine and administrative examinations:

V20.2   Routine infant or child health check
        Any injections given should have a corresponding procedure code.

V70   General medical examination

V72   Special investigations and examinations
        Codes V72.5 and V72.6 may be used if the reason for the patient encounter is for routine laboratory/radiology testing in the absence of any signs, symptoms, or associated diagnosis. If routine testing is performed during the same encounter as a test to evaluate a sign, symptom, or diagnosis, it is appropriate to assign both the V code and the code describing the reason for the non-routine test.

14) Miscellaneous V codes

The miscellaneous V codes capture a number of other health care encounters that do not fall into one of the other categories. Certain of these codes identify the reason for the encounter, others are for use as additional codes that provide useful information on circumstances that may affect a patient's care and treatment.

Prophylactic Organ Removal

For encounters specifically for prophylactic removal of breasts, ovaries, or another organ due to a genetic susceptibility to cancer or a family history of cancer, the principal or first listed code should be a code from subcategory V50.4, Prophylactic organ removal, followed by the appropriate genetic susceptibility code and the appropriate family history code.

If the patient has a malignancy of one site and is having prophylactic removal at another site to prevent either a new primary malignancy or metastatic disease, a code for the malignancy should also be assigned in addition to a code from subcategory V50.4. A V50.4 code should not be assigned if the patient is having organ removal for treatment of a malignancy, such as the removal of the testes for the treatment of prostate cancer.

Miscellaneous V code categories/codes:

V07   Need for isolation and other prophylactic measures

Except V07.5 Prophylactic use of agents affecting estrogen receptors and estrogen levels

V50   Elective surgery for purposes other than remedying health states

V58.5   Orthodontics

V60   Housing, household, and economic circumstances

V62   Other psychosocial circumstances

V63   Unavailability of other medical facilities for care

V64   Persons encountering health services for specific procedures, not carried out

V66   Convalescence and Palliative Care

V68   Encounters for administrative purposes

V69   Problems related to lifestyle

V85   Body Mass Index

15) Nonspecific V codes

Certain V codes are so non-specific, or potentially redundant with other codes in the classification, that there can be little justification for their use in the inpatient setting. Their use in the outpatient setting should be limited to those instances when there is no further documentation to permit more precise coding. Otherwise, any sign or symptom or any other reason for visit that is captured in another code should be used.

Nonspecific V code categories/codes:

V11   Personal history of mental disorder A code from the mental disorders chapter, with an in remission fifth-digit, should be used.

V13.4   Personal history of arthritis

V13.6   Personal history of congenital malformations

V15.7   Personal history of contraception

V23.2   Pregnancy with history of abortion

V40   Mental and behavioral problems

V41   Problems with special senses and other special functions

V47   Other problems with internal organs

V48   Problems with head, neck, and trunk

V49   Problems with limbs and other problems
Exceptions:

    V49.6   Upper limb amputation status

    V49.7   Lower limb amputation status

    V49.81   Postmenopausal status

    V49.82   Dental sealant status

V49.83 Awaiting organ transplant status

V51.8 **Other a**ftercare involving the use of plastic surgery

V58.2 Blood transfusion, without reported diagnosis

V58.9 Unspecified aftercare

See Section IV.K. and Section IV.L. of the Outpatient guidelines.

TABLE 1

V CODE TABLE

October 1, 2008 (FY2009)
Items in bold indicate a new entry or change from the October 2007 table
Items underlined have been moved within the table since November 2006

The V code table below contains columns for 1st listed, 1st or additional, additional only, and non-specific. Each code or category is listed in the left hand column and the allowable sequencing of the code or codes within the category is noted under the appropriate column.

As indicated by the footnote in the "1st Dx Only" column, the V codes designated as first-listed only are generally intended to be limited for use as a first-listed only diagnosis, but may be reported as an additional diagnosis in those situations when the patient has more than one encounter on a single day and the codes for the multiple encounters are combined, or when there is more than one V code that meets the definition of principal diagnosis (e.g., a patient is admitted to home healthcare for both aftercare and rehabilitation and they equally meet the definition of principal diagnosis). The V codes designated as first-listed only should not be reported if they do not meet the definition of principal or first-listed diagnosis.

See Section II and Section IV.A for information on selection of principal and first-listed diagnosis.

See Section II.C for information on two or more diagnoses that equally meet the definition for principal diagnosis.

Code(s)	Description	1st Dx Only[1]	1st or Add'l Dx[2]	Add'l Dx Only[3]	Non-Specific Diagnosis[4]
V01.X	Contact with or exposure to communicable diseases		X		
V02.X	Carrier or suspected carrier of infectious diseases		X		
V03.X	Need for prophylactic vaccination and inoculation against bacterial diseases		X		
V04.X	Need for prophylactic vaccination and inoculation against certain diseases		X		
V05.X	Need for prophylactic vaccination and inoculation against single diseases		X		
V06.X	Need for prophylactic vaccination and inoculation against combinations of diseases		X		
V07.0	Isolation		X		
V07.1	Desensitization to allergens		X		
V07.2	Prophylactic immunotherapy		X		
V07.3X	Other prophylactic chemotherapy		X		
V07.4	Hormone replacement therapy (postmenopausal)			X	
V07.5X	Prophylactic use of agents affecting estrogen receptors and estrogen levels			X	
V07.8	Other specified prophylactic measure		X		
V07.9	Unspecified prophylactic measure				X
V08	Asymptomatic HIV infection status		X		

[1]Generally for use as first listed only but may be used as additional if patient has more than one encounter on one day or there is more than one reason for the encounter
[2]These codes may be used as first listed or additional codes
[3]These codes are only for use as additional codes
[4]These codes are primarily for use in the nonacute setting and should be limited to encounters for which no sign or symptom or reason for visit is documented in the record. Their use may be as either a first listed or additional code.

TABLE 1

V CODE TABLE (Continued)

Code(s)	Description	1st Dx Only[1]	1st or Add'l Dx[2]	Add'l Dx Only[3]	Non-Specific Diagnosis[4]
V09.X	Infection with drug resistant organisms			X	
V10.X	Personal history of malignant neoplasm		X		
V11.X	Personal history of mental disorder				X
V12.X	Personal history of certain other diseases		X		
V13.0X	Personal history of other disorders of urinary system		X		
V13.1	Personal history of trophoblastic disease		X		
V13.2X	Personal history of other genital system and obstetric disorders		X		
V13.3	Personal history of diseases of skin and subcutaneous tissue		X		
V13.4	Personal history of arthritis				X
V13.5X	Personal history of other musculoskeletal disorders		X		
V13.61	Personal history of hypospadias			X	
V13.69	Personal history of congenital malformations				X
V13.7	Personal history of perinatal problems		X		
V13.8	Personal history of other specified diseases		X		
V13.9	Personal history of unspecified disease				X
V14.X	Personal history of allergy to medicinal agents			X	
V15.0X	Personal history of allergy, other than to medicinal agents			X	
V15.1	Personal history of surgery to heart and great vessels			X	
V15.2X	**Personal history of surgery to other organs**			X	
V15.3	Personal history of irradiation			X	
V15.4X	Personal history of psychological trauma			X	
V15.5X	Personal history of injury			X	
V15.6	Personal history of poisoning			X	
V15.7	Personal history of contraception				X
V15.81	Personal history of noncompliance with medical treatment			X	
V15.82	Personal history of tobacco use			X	
V15.84	Personal history of exposure to asbestos			X	
V15.85	Personal history of exposure to potentially hazardous body fluids			X	
V15.86	Personal history of exposure to lead			X	
V15.87	Personal history of extracorporeal membrane oxygenation [ECMO]			X	
V15.88	History of fall		X		
V15.89	Other specified personal history presenting hazards to health			X	
V16.X	Family history of malignant neoplasm		X		
V17.X	Family history of certain chronic disabling diseases		X		
V18.X	Family history of certain other specific conditions		X		
V19.X	Family history of other conditions		X		
V20.X	Health supervision of infant or child	X			
V21.X	Constitutional states in development			X	
V22.0	Supervision of normal first pregnancy	X			
V22.1	Supervision of other normal pregnancy	X			
V22.2	Pregnancy state, incidental			X	

Table continued on following page

TABLE 1

V CODE TABLE (Continued)

Code(s)	Description	1st Dx Only[1]	1st or Add'l Dx[2]	Add'l Dx Only[3]	Non-Specific Diagnosis[4]
V23.X	Supervision of high-risk pregnancy		X		
V24.X	Postpartum care and examination	X			
V25.X	Encounter for contraceptive management		X		
V26.0	Tuboplasty or vasoplasty after previous sterilization		X		
V26.1	Artificial insemination		X		
V26.2X	Procreative management investigation and testing		X		
V26.3X	Procreative management, genetic counseling and testing		X		
V26.4X	Procreative management, genetic counseling and advice		X		
V26.5X	Procreative management, sterilization status			X	
V26.81	Encounter for assisted reproductive fertility procedure cycle	X			
V26.89	Other specified procreative management		X		
V26.9	Unspecified procreative management		X		
V27.X	Outcome of delivery			X	
V28.X	Encounter for antenatal screening of mother		X		
V29.X	Observation and evaluation of newborns for suspected condition not found		X		
V30.X	Single liveborn	X			
V31.X	Twin, mate liveborn	X			
V32.X	Twin, mate stillborn	X			
V33.X	Twin, unspecified	X			
V34.X	Other multiple, mates all liveborn	X			
V35.X	Other multiple, mates all stillborn	X			
V36.X	Other multiple, mates live- and stillborn	X			
V37.X	Other multiple, unspecified	X			
V39.X	Unspecified	X			
V40.X	Mental and behavioral problems				X
V41.X	Problems with special senses and other special functions				X
V42.X	Organ or tissue replaced by transplant			X	
V43.0	Organ or tissue replaced by other means, eye globe			X	
V43.1	Organ or tissue replaced by other means, lens			X	
V43.21	Organ or tissue replaced by other means, heart assist device			X	
V43.22	Fully implantable artificial heart status		X		
V43.3	Organ or tissue replaced by other means, heart valve			X	
V43.4	Organ or tissue replaced by other means, blood vessel			X	
V43.5	Organ or tissue replaced by other means, bladder			X	
V43.6X	Organ or tissue replaced by other means, joint			X	
V43.7	Organ or tissue replaced by other means, limb			X	
V43.8X	Other organ or tissue replaced by other means			X	
V44.X	Artificial opening status			X	

[1]Generally for use as first listed only but may be used as additional if patient has more than one encounter on one day or there is more than one reason for the encounter
[2]These codes may be used as first listed or additional codes
[3]These codes are only for use as additional codes
[4]These codes are primarily for use in the nonacute setting and should be limited to encounters for which no sign or symptom or reason for visit is documented in the record. Their use may be as either a first listed or additional code.

TABLE 1

V CODE TABLE (Continued)

Code(s)	Description	1st Dx Only[1]	1st or Add'l Dx[2]	Add'l Dx Only[3]	Non-Specific Diagnosis[4]
V45.0X	Cardiac device in situ			X	
V45.1X	Renal dialysis status			X	
V45.2	Presence of cerebrospinal fluid drainage device			X	
V45.3	Intestinal bypass or anastomosis status			X	
V45.4	Arthrodesis status			X	
V45.5X	Presence of contraceptive device			X	
V45.6X	States following surgery of eye and adnexa			X	
V45.7X	Acquired absence of organ		X		
V45.8X	Other postprocedural status			X	
V46.0	Other dependence on machines, aspirator			X	
V46.11	Dependence on respiratory, status			X	
V46.12	Encounter for respirator dependence during power failure	X			
V46.13	Encounter for weaning from respirator [ventilator]	X			
V46.14	Mechanical complication of respirator [ventilator]		X		
V46.2	Other dependence on machines, supplemental oxygen			X	
V46.3	**Wheelchair dependence**			X	
V46.8	Other dependence on other enabling machines			X	
V46.9	Unspecified machine dependence				X
V47.X	Other problems with internal organs				X
V48.X	Problems with head, neck and trunk				X
V49.0	Deficiencies of limbs				X
V49.1	Mechanical problems with limbs				X
V49.2	Motor problems with limbs				X
V49.3	Sensory problems with limbs				X
V49.4	Disfigurements of limbs				X
V49.5	Other problems with limbs				X
V49.6X	Upper limb amputation status		X		
V49.7X	Lower limb amputation status		X		
V49.81	Asymptomatic postmenopausal status (age-related) (natural)		X		
V49.82	Dental sealant status			X	
V49.83	Awaiting organ transplant status			X	
V49.84	Bed confinement status		X		
V49.85	**Dual sensory impairment**			X	
V49.89	Other specified conditions influencing health status		X		
V49.9	Unspecified condition influencing health status				X
V50.X	Elective surgery for purposes other than remedying health states		X		
V51.0	**Encounter for breast reconstruction following mastectomy**	X			
V51.8	**Other aftercare involving the use of plastic surgery**				X
V52.X	Fitting and adjustment of prosthetic device and implant		X		
V53.X	Fitting and adjustment of other device		X		
V54.X	Other orthopedic aftercare		X		

Table continued on following page

TABLE 1

V CODE TABLE (Continued)

Code(s)	Description	1st Dx Only[1]	1st or Add'l Dx[2]	Add'l Dx Only[3]	Non-Specific Diagnosis[4]
V55.X	Attention to artificial openings		X		
V56.0	Extracorporeal dialysis	X			
V56.1	Encounter for fitting and adjustment of extracorporeal dialysis catheter		X		
V56.2	Encounter for fitting and adjustment of peritoneal dialysis catheter		X		
V56.3X	Encounter for adequacy testing for dialysis		X		
V56.8	Encounter for other dialysis and dialysis catheter care		X		
V57.X	Care involving use of rehabilitation procedures	X			
V58.0	Radiotherapy	X			
V58.11	Encounter for antineoplastic chemotherapy	X			
V58.12	Encounter for antineoplastic immunotherapy	X			
V58.2	Blood transfusion without reported diagnosis				X
V58.3X	Attention to dressings and sutures		X		
V58.4X	Other aftercare following surgery		X		
V58.5	Encounter for orthodontics				X
V58.6X	Long term (current) drug use			X	
V58.7X	Aftercare following surgery to specified body systems, not elsewhere classified		X		
V58.8X	Other specified procedures and aftercare		X		
V58.9	Unspecified aftercare				X
V59.X	Donors	X			
V60.X	Housing, household, and economic circumstances			X	
V61.X	Other family circumstances		X		
V62.X	Other psychosocial circumstances			X	
V63.X	Unavailability of other medical facilities for care		X		
V64.X	Persons encountering health services for specified procedure, not carried out			X	
V65.X	Other persons seeking consultation without complaint or sickness		X		
V66.0	Convalescence and palliative care following surgery	X			
V66.1	Convalescence and palliative care following radiotherapy	X			
V66.2	Convalescence and palliative care following chemotherapy	X			
V66.3	Convalescence and palliative care following psychotherapy and other treatment for mental disorder	X			
V66.4	Convalescence and palliative care following treatment of fracture	X			
V66.5	Convalescence and palliative care following other treatment	X			
V66.6	Convalescence and palliative care following combined treatment	X			
V66.7	Encounter for palliative care			X	

[1]Generally for use as first listed only but may be used as additional if patient has more than one encounter on one day or there is more than one reason for the encounter

[2]These codes may be used as first listed or additional codes

[3]These codes are only for use as additional codes

[4]These codes are primarily for use in the nonacute setting and should be limited to encounters for which no sign or symptom or reason for visit is documented in the record. Their use may be as either a first listed or additional code.

TABLE 1

V CODE TABLE (Continued)

Code(s)	Description	1st Dx Only[1]	1st or Add'l Dx[2]	Add'l Dx Only[3]	Non-Specific Diagnosis[4]
V66.9	Unspecified convalescence	X			
V67.X	Follow-up examination		X		
V68.X	Encounters for administrative purposes	X			
V69.X	Problems related to lifestyle		X		
V70.0	Routine general medical examination at a health care facility	X			
V70.1	General psychiatric examination, requested by the authority	X			
V70.2	General psychiatric examination, other and unspecified	X			
V70.3	Other medical examination for administrative purposes	X			
V70.4	Examination for medicolegal reasons	X			
V70.5	Health examination of defined subpopulations	X			
V70.6	Health examination in population surveys	X			
V70.7	Examination of participant in clinical trial		X		
V70.8	Other specified general medical examinations	X			
V70.9	Unspecified general medical examination	X			
V71.X	Observation and evaluation for suspected conditions not found	X			
V72.0	Examination of eyes and vision		X		
V72.1X	Examination of ears and hearing		X		
V72.2	Dental examination		X		
V72.3X	Gynecological examination		X		
V72.4X	Pregnancy examination or test		X		
V72.5	Radiological examination, NEC		X		
V72.6	Laboratory examination		X		
V72.7	Diagnostic skin and sensitization tests		X		
V72.81	Preoperative cardiovascular examination		X		
V72.82	Preoperative respiratory examination		X		
V72.83	Other specified preoperative examination		X		
V72.84	Preoperative examination, unspecified		X		
V72.85	Other specified examination		X		
V72.86	Encounter for blood typing		X		
V72.9	Unspecified examination				X
V73.X	Special screening examination for viral and chlamydial diseases		X		
V74.X	Special screening examination for bacterial and spirochetal diseases		X		
V75.X	Special screening examination for other infectious diseases		X		
V76.X	Special screening examination for malignant neoplasms		X		
V77.X	Special screening examination for endocrine, nutritional, metabolic and immunity disorders		X		
V78.X	Special screening examination for disorders of blood and blood-forming organs		X		
V79.X	Special screening examination for mental disorders and developmental handicaps		X		

Table continued on following page

TABLE 1

V CODE TABLE (Continued)					
Code(s)	Description	1st Dx Only[1]	1st or Add'l Dx[2]	Add'l Dx Only[3]	Non-Specific Diagnosis[4]
V80.X	Special screening examination for neurological, eye, and ear diseases		X		
V81.X	Special screening examination for cardiovascular, respiratory, and genitourinary diseases		X		
V82.X	Special screening examination for other conditions		X		
V83.X	Genetic carrier status		X		
V84.X	Genetic susceptibility to disease			X	
V85	Body mass index			X	
V86	Estrogen receptor status			X	
V87.0X	**Contact with and (suspected) exposure to hazardous metals**		X		
V87.1X	**Contact with and (suspected) exposure to hazardous aromatic compounds**		X		
V87.2	**Contact with and (suspected) exposure to other potentially hazardous chemicals**		X		
V87.3X	**Contact with and (suspected) exposure to other potentially hazardous substances**		X		
V87.4X	**Personal history of drug therapy**			X	
V88.0X	**Acquired absence of cervix and uterus**			X	
V89.0X	**Suspected maternal and fetal anomalies not found**		X		

[1]Generally for use as first listed only but may be used as additional if patient has more than one encounter on one day or there is more than one reason for the encounter

[2]These codes may be used as first listed or additional codes

[3]These codes are only for use as additional codes

[4]These codes are primarily for use in the nonacute setting and should be limited to encounters for which no sign or symptom or reason for visit is documented in the record. Their use may be as either a first listed or additional code.

19. **Supplemental Classification of External Causes of Injury and Poisoning (E-codes, E800-E999)**

Introduction: These guidelines are provided for those who are currently collecting E codes in order that there will be standardization in the process. If your institution plans to begin collecting E codes, these guidelines are to be applied. The use of E codes is supplemental to the application of ICD-9-CM diagnosis codes. E codes are never to be recorded as principal diagnoses (first-listed in non-inpatient setting) and are not required for reporting to CMS.

External causes of injury and poisoning codes (E codes) are intended to provide data for injury research and evaluation of injury prevention strategies. E codes capture how the injury or poisoning happened (cause), the intent (unintentional or accidental; or intentional, such as suicide or assault), and the place where the event occurred.

Some major categories of E codes include:

transport accidents

poisoning and adverse effects of drugs, medicinal substances and biologicals accidental falls

accidents caused by fire and flames

accidents due to natural and environmental factors

late effects of accidents, assaults or self injury

assaults or purposely inflicted injury

suicide or self inflicted injury

These guidelines apply for the coding and collection of E codes from records in hospitals, outpatient clinics, emergency departments, other ambulatory care settings and provider offices, and nonacute care settings, except when other specific guidelines apply.

a. **General E Code Coding Guidelines**

1) **Used with any code in the range of 001-V89**
   An E code may be used with any code in the range of 001-**V89**, which indicates an injury, poisoning, or adverse effect due to an external cause.

2) **Assign the appropriate E code for all initial treatments**
   Assign the appropriate E code for the initial encounter of an injury, poisoning, or adverse effect of drugs, not for subsequent treatment. External cause of injury codes (E-codes) may be assigned while the acute fracture codes are still applicable.
   See Section I.C.17.b.1 for coding of acute fractures.

3) **Use the full range of E codes**
   Use the full range of E codes to completely describe the cause, the intent and the place of occurrence, if applicable, for all injuries, poisonings, and adverse effects of drugs.

4) **Assign as many E codes as necessary**
   Assign as many E codes as necessary to fully explain each cause. If only one E code can be recorded, assign the E code most related to the principal diagnosis.

5) **The selection of the appropriate E code**
   The selection of the appropriate E code is guided by the Index to External Causes, which is located after the alphabetical index to diseases and by Inclusion and Exclusion notes in the Tabular List.

6) **E code can never be a principal diagnosis**
   An E code can never be a principal (first listed) diagnosis.

7) **External cause code(s) with systemic inflammatory response syndrome (SIRS)**
   An external cause code is not appropriate with a code from subcategory 995.9, unless the patient also has an injury, poisoning, or adverse effect of drugs.

b. **Place of Occurrence Guideline**

Use an additional code from category E849 to indicate the Place of Occurrence for injuries and poisonings. The Place of Occurrence describes the place where the event occurred and not the patient's activity at the time of the event.

Do not use E849.9 if the place of occurrence is not stated.

c. **Adverse Effects of Drugs, Medicinal and Biological Substances Guidelines**

1) **Do not code directly from the Table of Drugs**

Do not code directly from the Table of Drugs and Chemicals. Always refer back to the Tabular List.

2) **Use as many codes as necessary to describe**

Use as many codes as necessary to describe completely all drugs, medicinal or biological substances.

3) **If the same E code would describe the causative agent**

If the same E code would describe the causative agent for more than one adverse reaction, assign the code only once.

4) **If two or more drugs, medicinal or biological substances**

If two or more drugs, medicinal or biological substances are reported, code each individually unless the combination code is listed in the Table of Drugs and Chemicals. In that case, assign the E code for the combination.

5) **When a reaction results from the interaction of a drug(s)**

When a reaction results from the interaction of a drug(s) and alcohol, use poisoning codes and E codes for both.

6) **If the reporting format limits the number of E codes**

If the reporting format limits the number of E codes that can be used in reporting clinical data, code the one most related to the principal diagnosis. Include at least one from each category (cause, intent, place) if possible.

If there are different fourth digit codes in the same three digit category, use the code for "Other specified" of that category. If there is no "Other specified" code in that category, use the appropriate "Unspecified" code in that category.

If the codes are in different three digit categories, assign the appropriate E code for other multiple drugs and medicinal substances.

7) **Codes from the E930-E949 series**

Codes from the E930-E949 series must be used to identify the causative substance for an adverse effect of drug, medicinal and biological substances, correctly prescribed and properly administered. The effect, such as tachycardia, delirium, gastrointestinal hemorrhaging, vomiting, hypokalemia, hepatitis, renal failure, or respiratory failure, is coded and followed by the appropriate code from the E930-E949 series.

d. **Multiple Cause E Code Coding Guidelines**

If two or more events cause separate injuries, an E code should be assigned for each cause. The first listed E code will be selected in the following order:

E codes for child and adult abuse take priority over all other E codes.

See Section I.C.19.e., Child and Adult abuse guidelines.

E codes for terrorism events take priority over all other E codes except child and adult abuse

E codes for cataclysmic events take priority over all other E codes except child and adult abuse and terrorism.

E codes for transport accidents take priority over all other E codes except cataclysmic events and child and adult abuse and terrorism.

The first-listed E code should correspond to the cause of the most serious diagnosis due to an assault, accident, or self-harm, following the order of hierarchy listed above.

e. **Child and Adult Abuse Guideline**

1) **Intentional injury**

When the cause of an injury or neglect is intentional child or adult abuse, the first listed E code should be assigned from categories E960-E968, Homicide and injury purposely inflicted by other persons, (except category E967). An E code from category E967, Child and adult battering and other maltreatment, should be added as an additional code to identify the perpetrator, if known.

2) **Accidental intent**

In cases of neglect when the intent is determined to be accidental E code E904.0, Abandonment or neglect of infant and helpless person, should be the first listed E code.

f. **Unknown or Suspected Intent Guideline**

1) **If the intent (accident, self-harm, assault) of the cause of an injury or poisoning is unknown**

If the intent (accident, self-harm, assault) of the cause of an injury or poisoning is unknown or unspecified, code the intent as undetermined E980-E989.

2) **If the intent (accident, self-harm, assault) of the cause of an injury or poisoning is questionable**

If the intent (accident, self-harm, assault) of the cause of an injury or poisoning is questionable, probable or suspected, code the intent as undetermined E980-E989.

g. Undetermined Cause

When the intent of an injury or poisoning is known, but the cause is unknown, use codes: E928.9, Unspecified accident, E958.9, Suicide and self-inflicted injury by unspecified means, and E968.9, Assault by unspecified means.

These E codes should rarely be used, as the documentation in the medical record, in both the inpatient outpatient and other settings, should normally provide sufficient detail to determine the cause of the injury.

h. Late Effects of External Cause Guidelines

1) **Late effect E codes**

Late effect E codes exist for injuries and poisonings but not for adverse effects of drugs, misadventures and surgical complications.

2) **Late effect E codes (E929, E959, E969, E977, E989, or E999.1)**

A late effect E code (E929, E959, E969, E977, E989, or E999.1) should be used with any report of a late effect or sequela resulting from a previous injury or poisoning (905-909).

3) **Late effect E code with a related current injury**

A late effect E code should never be used with a related current nature of injury code.

4) **Use of late effect E codes for subsequent visits**

Use a late effect E code for subsequent visits when a late effect of the initial injury or poisoning is being treated. There is no late effect E code for adverse effects of drugs. Do not use a late effect E code for subsequent visits for follow-up care (e.g., to assess healing, to receive rehabilitative therapy) of the injury or poisoning when no late effect of the injury has been documented.

i. Misadventures and Complications of Care Guidelines

1) **Code range E870-E876**

Assign a code in the range of E870-E876 if misadventures are stated by the provider.

2) **Code range E878-E879**

Assign a code in the range of E878-E879 if the provider attributes an abnormal reaction or later complication to a surgical or medical procedure, but does not mention misadventure at the time of the procedure as the cause of the reaction.

j. Terrorism Guidelines

1) **Cause of injury identified by the Federal Government (FBI) as terrorism**

When the cause of an injury is identified by the Federal Government (FBI) as terrorism, the first-listed E-code should be a code from category E979, Terrorism. The definition of terrorism employed by the FBI is found at the inclusion note at E979. The terrorism E-code is the only E-code that should be assigned. Additional E codes from the assault categories should not be assigned.

2) **Cause of an injury is suspected to be the result of terrorism**

When the cause of an injury is suspected to be the result of terrorism a code from category E979 should not be assigned. Assign a code in the range of E codes based circumstances on the documentation of intent and mechanism.

3) **Code E979.9, Terrorism, secondary effects**

Assign code E979.9, Terrorism, secondary effects, for conditions occurring subsequent to the terrorist event. This code should not be assigned for conditions that are due to the initial terrorist act.

4) **Statistical tabulation of terrorism codes**

For statistical purposes these codes will be tabulated within the category for assault, expanding the current category from E960-E969 to include E979 and E999.1.

SECTION II. ■ *Selection of Principal Diagnosis*

The circumstances of inpatient admission always govern the selection of principal diagnosis. The principal diagnosis is defined in the Uniform Hospital Discharge Data Set (UHDDS) as "that condition established after study to be chiefly responsible for occasioning the admission of the patient to the hospital for care."

The UHDDS definitions are used by hospitals to report inpatient data elements in a standardized manner. These data elements and their definitions can be found in the July 31, 1985, Federal Register (Vol. 50, No, 147), pp. 31038-40.

Since that time the application of the UHDDS definitions has been expanded to include all non-outpatient settings (acute care, short term, long term care and psychiatric hospitals; home health agencies; rehab facilities; nursing homes, etc).

In determining principal diagnosis the coding conventions in the ICD-9-CM, Volumes I and II take precedence over these official coding guidelines. *(See Section I.A., Conventions for the ICD-9-CM)*

The importance of consistent, complete documentation in the medical record cannot be overemphasized. Without such documentation the application of all coding guidelines is a difficult, if not impossible, task.

A. **Codes for symptoms, signs, and ill-defined conditions**

Codes for symptoms, signs, and ill-defined conditions from Chapter 16 are not to be used as principal diagnosis when a related definitive diagnosis has been established.

B. **Two or more interrelated conditions, each potentially meeting the definition for principal diagnosis.**

When there are two or more interrelated conditions (such as diseases in the same ICD-9-CM chapter or manifestations characteristically associated with a certain disease) potentially meeting the definition of principal diagnosis, either condition may be sequenced first, unless the circumstances of the admission, the therapy provided, the Tabular List, or the Alphabetic Index indicate otherwise.

C. **Two or more diagnoses that equally meet the definition for principal diagnosis**
In the unusual instance when two or more diagnoses equally meet the criteria for principal diagnosis as determined by the circumstances of admission, diagnostic workup and/or therapy provided, and the Alphabetic Index, Tabular List, or another coding guidelines does not provide sequencing direction, any one of the diagnoses may be sequenced first.

D. **Two or more comparative or contrasting conditions.**
In those rare instances when two or more contrasting or comparative diagnoses are documented as "either/or" (or similar terminology), they are coded as if the diagnoses were confirmed and the diagnoses are sequenced according to the circumstances of the admission. If no further determination can be made as to which diagnosis should be principal, either diagnosis may be sequenced first.

E. **A symptom(s) followed by contrasting/comparative diagnoses**
When a symptom(s) is followed by contrasting/comparative diagnoses, the symptom code is sequenced first. All the contrasting/comparative diagnoses should be coded as additional diagnoses.

F. **Original treatment plan not carried out**
Sequence as the principal diagnosis the condition, which after study occasioned the admission to the hospital, even though treatment may not have been carried out due to unforeseen circumstances.

G. **Complications of surgery and other medical care**
When the admission is for treatment of a complication resulting from surgery or other medical care, the complication code is sequenced as the principal diagnosis. If the complication is classified to the 996-999 series and the code lacks the necessary specificity in describing the complication, an additional code for the specific complication should be assigned.

H. **Uncertain Diagnosis**
If the diagnosis documented at the time of discharge is qualified as "probable", "suspected", "likely", "questionable", "possible", or "still to be ruled out", or other similar terms indicating uncertainty, code the condition as if it existed or was established. The bases for these guidelines are the diagnostic workup, arrangements for further workup or observation, and initial therapeutic approach that correspond most closely with the established diagnosis.

Note: This guideline is applicable only to <u>inpatient admissions to</u> short-term, acute, long-term care and psychiatric hospitals.

I. **Admission from Observation Unit**

1. **Admission Following Medical Observation**

   When a patient is admitted to an observation unit for a medical condition, which either worsens or does not improve, and is subsequently admitted as an inpatient of the same hospital for this same medical condition, the principal diagnosis would be the medical condition which led to the hospital admission.

2. **Admission Following Post-Operative Observation**

   When a patient is admitted to an observation unit to monitor a condition (or complication) that develops following outpatient surgery, and then is subsequently admitted as an inpatient of the same hospital, hospitals should apply the Uniform Hospital Discharge Data Set (UHDDS) definition of principal diagnosis as "that condition established after study to be chiefly responsible for occasioning the admission of the patient to the hospital for care."

J. **Admission from Outpatient Surgery**

When a patient receives surgery in the hospital's outpatient surgery department and is subsequently admitted for continuing inpatient care at the same hospital, the following guidelines should be followed in selecting the principal diagnosis for the inpatient admission:

- If the reason for the inpatient admission is a complication, assign the complication as the principal diagnosis.

- If no complication, or other condition, is documented as the reason for the inpatient admission, assign the reason for the outpatient surgery as the principal diagnosis.

- If the reason for the inpatient admission is another condition unrelated to the surgery, assign the unrelated condition as the principal diagnosis.

SECTION III. ■ *Reporting Additional Diagnoses*

GENERAL RULES FOR OTHER (ADDITIONAL) DIAGNOSES

For reporting purposes the definition for "other diagnoses" is interpreted as additional conditions that affect patient care in terms of requiring:

clinical evaluation; or

therapeutic treatment; or

diagnostic procedures; or

extended length of hospital stay; or

increased nursing care and/or monitoring.

The UHDDS item #11-b defines Other Diagnoses as "all conditions that coexist at the time of admission, that develop subsequently, or that affect the treatment received and/or the length of stay. Diagnoses that relate to an earlier episode which have no bearing on the current hospital stay are to be excluded." UHDDS definitions apply to inpatients in acute care, short-term, long term care and psychiatric hospital setting. The UHDDS definitions are used by acute care short-term hospitals to report inpatient data elements in a standardized manner. These data elements and their definitions can be found in the July 31, 1985, Federal Register (Vol. 50, No, 147), pp. 31038-40.

Since that time the application of the UHDDS definitions has been expanded to include all non-outpatient settings (acute care, short term, long term care and psychiatric hospitals; home health agencies; rehab facilities; nursing homes, etc).

The following guidelines are to be applied in designating "other diagnoses" when neither the Alphabetic Index nor the Tabular List in ICD-9-CM provide direction. The listing of the diagnoses in the patient record is the responsibility of the attending provider.

A.   Previous conditions

If the provider has included a diagnosis in the final diagnostic statement, such as the discharge summary or the face sheet, it should ordinarily be coded. Some providers include in the diagnostic statement resolved conditions or diagnoses and status-post procedures from previous admission that have no bearing on the current stay. Such conditions are not to be reported and are coded only if required by hospital policy.

However, history codes (V10-V19) may be used as secondary codes if the historical condition or family history has an impact on current care or influences treatment.

B.   Abnormal findings

Abnormal findings (laboratory, x-ray, pathologic, and other diagnostic results) are not coded and reported unless the provider indicates their clinical significance. If the findings are outside the normal range and the attending provider has ordered other tests to evaluate the condition or prescribed treatment, it is appropriate to ask the provider whether the abnormal finding should be added.

Please note: This differs from the coding practices in the outpatient setting for coding encounters for diagnostic tests that have been interpreted by a provider.

C.   Uncertain Diagnosis

If the diagnosis documented at the time of discharge is qualified as "probable", "suspected", "likely", "questionable", "possible", or "still to be ruled out" or other similar terms indicating uncertainty, code the condition as if it existed or was established. The bases for these guidelines are the diagnostic workup, arrangements for further workup or observation, and initial therapeutic approach that correspond most closely with the established diagnosis.

Note: This guideline is applicable only to <u>inpatient admissions to</u> short-term, acute, long-term care and psychiatric hospitals.

SECTION IV. ▪ *Diagnostic Coding and Reporting Guidelines for Outpatient Services*

These coding guidelines for outpatient diagnoses have been approved for use by hospitals/providers in coding and reporting hospital-based outpatient services and provider-based office visits.

Information about the use of certain abbreviations, punctuation, symbols, and other conventions used in the ICD-9-CM Tabular List (code numbers and titles), can be found in Section IA of these guidelines, under "Conventions Used in the Tabular List." Information about the correct sequence to use in finding a code is also described in Section I.

The terms encounter and visit are often used interchangeably in describing outpatient service contacts and, therefore, appear together in these guidelines without distinguishing one from the other.

Though the conventions and general guidelines apply to all settings, coding guidelines for outpatient and provider reporting of diagnoses will vary in a number of instances from those for inpatient diagnoses, recognizing that:

The Uniform Hospital Discharge Data Set (UHDDS) definition of principal diagnosis applies only to inpatients in acute, short-term, long-term care and psychiatric hospitals.

Coding guidelines for inconclusive diagnoses (probable, suspected, rule out, etc.) were developed for inpatient reporting and do not apply to outpatients.

A. **Selection of first-listed condition**

In the outpatient setting, the term first-listed diagnosis is used in lieu of principal diagnosis.

In determining the first-listed diagnosis the coding conventions of ICD-9-CM, as well as the general and disease specific guidelines take precedence over the outpatient guidelines.

Diagnoses often are not established at the time of the initial encounter/visit. It may take two or more visits before the diagnosis is confirmed.

The most critical rule involves beginning the search for the correct code assignment through the Alphabetic Index. Never begin searching initially in the Tabular List as this will lead to coding errors.

1. **Outpatient Surgery**

When a patient presents for outpatient surgery, code the reason for the surgery as the first-listed diagnosis (reason for the encounter), even if the surgery is not performed due to a contraindication.

2. **Observation Stay**

When a patient is admitted for observation for a medical condition, assign a code for the medical condition as the first-listed diagnosis.

When a patient presents for outpatient surgery and develops complications requiring admission to observation, code the reason for the surgery as the first reported diagnosis (reason for the encounter), followed by codes for the complications as secondary diagnoses.

B. **Codes from 001.0 through V89**

The appropriate code or codes from 001.0 through **V89** must be used to identify diagnoses, symptoms, conditions, problems, complaints, or other reason(s) for the encounter/visit.

C. **Accurate reporting of ICD-9-CM diagnosis codes**

For accurate reporting of ICD-9-CM diagnosis codes, the documentation should describe the patient's condition, using terminology which includes specific diagnoses as well as symptoms, problems, or reasons for the encounter. There are ICD-9-CM codes to describe all of these.

D. **Selection of codes 001.0 through 999.9**

The selection of codes 001.0 through 999.9 will frequently be used to describe the reason for the encounter. These codes are from the section of ICD-9-CM for the classification of diseases and injuries (e.g. infectious and parasitic diseases; neoplasms; symptoms, signs, and ill-defined conditions, etc.).

E. **Codes that describe symptoms and signs**

Codes that describe symptoms and signs, as opposed to diagnoses, are acceptable for reporting purposes when a diagnosis has not been established (confirmed) by the provider. Chapter 16 of ICD-9-CM, Symptoms, Signs, and Ill-defined conditions (codes 780.0 - 799.9) contain many, but not all codes for symptoms.

F. **Encounters for circumstances other than a disease or injury**

ICD-9-CM provides codes to deal with encounters for circumstances other than a disease or injury. The Supplementary Classification of factors Influencing Health Status and Contact with Health Services (V01.0- **V89**) is provided to deal with occasions when circumstances other than a disease or injury are recorded as diagnosis or problems. *See Section I.C. 18 for information on V-codes*

G. **Level of Detail in Coding**

1. **ICD-9-CM codes with 3, 4, or 5 digits**

ICD-9-CM is composed of codes with either 3, 4, or 5 digits. Codes with three digits are included in ICD-9-CM as the heading of a category of codes that may be further subdivided by the use of fourth and/or fifth digits, which provide greater specificity.

2. **Use of full number of digits required for a code**

A three-digit code is to be used only if it is not further subdivided. Where fourth-digit subcategories and/or fifth-digit subclassifications are provided, they must be assigned. A code is invalid if it has not been coded to the full number of digits required for that code.

See also discussion under Section I.b.3., General Coding Guidelines, Level of Detail in Coding.

H. **ICD-9-CM code for the diagnosis, condition, problem, or other reason for encounter/visit**

List first the ICD-9-CM code for the diagnosis, condition, problem, or other reason for encounter/visit shown in the medical record to be chiefly responsible for the services provided. List additional codes that describe any coexisting conditions. In some cases the first-listed diagnosis may be a symptom when a diagnosis has not been established (confirmed) by the physician.

I. **Uncertain diagnosis**

Do not code diagnoses documented as "probable", "suspected," "questionable," "rule out," or "working diagnosis" or other similar terms indicating uncertainty. Rather, code the condition(s) to the highest degree of certainty for that encounter/visit, such as symptoms, signs, abnormal test results, or other reason for the visit.

Please note: This differs from the coding practices used by short-term, acute care, long-term care and psychiatric hospitals.

J. Chronic diseases

Chronic diseases treated on an ongoing basis may be coded and reported as many times as the patient receives treatment and care for the condition(s)

K. Code all documented conditions that coexist

Code all documented conditions that coexist at the time of the encounter/visit, and require or affect patient care treatment or management. Do not code conditions that were previously treated and no longer exist. However, history codes (V10-V19) may be used as secondary codes if the historical condition or family history has an impact on current care or influences treatment.

L. Patients receiving diagnostic services only

For patients receiving diagnostic services only during an encounter/visit, sequence first the diagnosis, condition, problem, or other reason for encounter/visit shown in the medical record to be chiefly responsible for the outpatient services provided during the encounter/visit. Codes for other diagnoses (e.g., chronic conditions) may be sequenced as additional diagnoses.

For encounters for routine laboratory/radiology testing in the absence of any signs, symptoms, or associated diagnosis, assign V72.5 and V72.6. If routine testing is performed during the same encounter as a test to evaluate a sign, symptom, or diagnosis, it is appropriate to assign both the V code and the code describing the reason for the non-routine test.

For outpatient encounters for diagnostic tests that have been interpreted by a physician, and the final report is available at the time of coding, code any confirmed or definitive diagnosis(es) documented in the interpretation. Do not code related signs and symptoms as additional diagnoses.

Please note: This differs from the coding practice in the hospital inpatient setting regarding abnormal findings on test results.

M. Patients receiving therapeutic services only

For patients receiving therapeutic services only during an encounter/visit, sequence first the diagnosis, condition, problem, or other reason for encounter/visit shown in the medical record to be chiefly responsible for the outpatient services provided during the encounter/visit. Codes for other diagnoses (e.g., chronic conditions) may be sequenced as additional diagnoses.

The only exception to this rule is that when the primary reason for the admission/encounter is chemotherapy, radiation therapy, or rehabilitation, the appropriate V code for the service is listed first, and the diagnosis or problem for which the service is being performed listed second.

N. Patients receiving preoperative evaluations only

For patients receiving preoperative evaluations only, sequence first a code from category V72.8, Other specified examinations, to describe the pre-op consultations. Assign a code for the condition to describe the reason for the surgery as an additional diagnosis. Code also any findings related to the pre-op evaluation.

O. Ambulatory surgery

For ambulatory surgery, code the diagnosis for which the surgery was performed. If the postoperative diagnosis is known to be different from the preoperative diagnosis at the time the diagnosis is confirmed, select the postoperative diagnosis for coding, since it is the most definitive.

P. Routine outpatient prenatal visits

For routine outpatient prenatal visits when no complications are present, codes V22.0, Supervision of normal first pregnancy, or V22.1, Supervision of other normal pregnancy, should be used as the principal diagnosis. These codes should not be used in conjunction with chapter 11 codes.

APPENDIX I ▪ *Present on Admission Reporting Guidelines*

INTRODUCTION

These guidelines are to be used as a supplement to the *ICD-9-CM Official Guidelines for Coding and Reporting* to facilitate the assignment of the Present on Admission (POA) indicator for each diagnosis and external cause of injury code reported on claim forms (UB-04 and 837 Institutional).

These guidelines are not intended to replace any guidelines in the main body of the *ICD-9-CM Official Guidelines for Coding and Reporting*. The POA guidelines are not intended to provide guidance on when a condition should be coded, but rather, how to apply the POA indicator to the final set of diagnosis codes that have been assigned in accordance with Sections I, II, and III of the official coding guidelines. Subsequent to the assignment of the ICD-9-CM codes, the POA indicator should then be assigned to those conditions that have been coded.

As stated in the Introduction to the ICD-9-CM Official Guidelines for Coding and Reporting, a joint effort between the healthcare provider and the coder is essential to achieve complete and accurate documentation, code assignment, and reporting of diagnoses and procedures. The importance of consistent, complete documentation in the medical record cannot be overemphasized. Medical record documentation from any provider involved in the care and treatment of the patient may be used to support the determination of whether a condition was present on admission or not. In the context of the official coding guidelines, the term "provider" means a physician or any qualified healthcare practitioner who is legally accountable for establishing the patient's diagnosis.

These guidelines are not a substitute for the provider's clinical judgment as to the determination of whether a condition was/was not present on admission. The provider should be queried regarding issues related to the linking of signs/symptoms, timing of test results, and the timing of findings.

GENERAL REPORTING REQUIREMENTS

All claims involving inpatient admissions to general acute care hospitals or other facilities that are subject to a law or regulation mandating collection of present on admission information.

Present on admission is defined as present at the time the order for inpatient admission occurs—conditions that develop during an outpatient encounter, including emergency department, observation, or outpatient surgery, are considered as present on admission.

POA indicator is assigned to principal and secondary diagnoses (as defined in Section II of the Official Guidelines for Coding and Reporting) and the external cause of injury codes.

Issues related to inconsistent, missing, conflicting or unclear documentation must still be resolved by the provider.

If a condition would not be coded and reported based on UHDDS definitions and current official coding guidelines, then the POA indicator would not be reported.

Reporting Options	Y - Yes
	N - No
	U - Unknown
	W – Clinically undetermined
	Unreported/Not used **(or "1" for Medicare usage)** – (Exempt from POA reporting)

For more specific instructions on Medicare POA indicator reporting options, refer to <u>http://www.cms.hhs.gov/HospitalAcqCond/02_Statute_Regulations_Program_Instructions.asp#TopOfPage</u>

Reporting Definitions

Y = present at the time of inpatient admission
N = not present at the time of inpatient admission

U = documentation is insufficient to determine if condition is present on admission

W = provider is unable to clinically determine whether condition was present on admission or not

Timeframe for POA Identification and Documentation

There is no required timeframe as to when a provider (per the definition of "provider" used in these guidelines) must identify or document a condition to be present on admission. In some clinical situations, it may not be possible for a provider to make a definitive diagnosis (or a condition may not be recognized or reported by the patient) for a period of time after admission. In some cases it may be several days before the provider arrives at a definitive diagnosis. This does not mean that the condition was not present on admission. Determination of whether the condition was present on admission or not will be based on the applicable POA guideline as identified in this document, or on the provider's best clinical judgment.

If at the time of code assignment the documentation is unclear as to whether a condition was present on admission or not, it is appropriate to query the provider for clarification.

Assigning the POA Indicator

Condition is on the "Exempt from Reporting" list

Leave the "present on admission" field blank if the condition is on the list of ICD-9-CM codes for which this field is not applicable. This is the only circumstance in which the field may be left blank.

POA Explicitly Documented

Assign Y for any condition the provider explicitly documents as being present on admission.

Assign N for any condition the provider explicitly documents as not present at the time of admission.

Conditions diagnosed prior to inpatient admission

Assign "Y" for conditions that were diagnosed prior to admission (example: hypertension, diabetes mellitus, asthma)

Conditions diagnosed during the admission but clearly present before admission

Assign "Y" for conditions diagnosed during the admission that were clearly present but not diagnosed until after admission occurred.

Diagnoses subsequently confirmed after admission are considered present on admission if at the time of admission they are documented as suspected, possible, rule out, differential diagnosis, or constitute an underlying cause of a symptom that is present at the time of admission.

Condition develops during outpatient encounter prior to inpatient admission

Assign Y for any condition that develops during an outpatient encounter prior to a written order for inpatient admission.

Documentation does not indicate whether condition was present on admission

Assign "U" when the medical record documentation is unclear as to whether the condition was present on admission. "U" should not be routinely assigned and used only in very limited circumstances. Coders are encouraged to query the providers when the documentation is unclear.

Documentation states that it cannot be determined whether the condition was or was not present on admission

Assign "W" when the medical record documentation indicates that it cannot be clinically determined whether or not the condition was present on admission.

Chronic condition with acute exacerbation during the admission

If the code is a combination code that identifies both the chronic condition and the acute exacerbation, see POA guidelines pertaining to combination codes.

If the combination code only identifies the chronic condition and not the acute exacerbation (e.g., acute exacerbation of CHF), assign "Y."

Conditions documented as possible, probable, suspected, or rule out at the time of discharge

If the final diagnosis contains a possible, probable, suspected, or rule out diagnosis, and this diagnosis was suspected at the time of inpatient admission, assign "Y."

If the final diagnosis contains a possible, probable, suspected, or rule out diagnosis, and this diagnosis was based on symptoms or clinical findings that were not present on admission, assign "N".

Conditions documented as impending or threatened at the time of discharge

If the final diagnosis contains an impending or threatened diagnosis, and this diagnosis is based on symptoms or clinical findings that were present on admission, assign "Y".

If the final diagnosis contains an impending or threatened diagnosis, and this diagnosis is based on symptoms or clinical findings that were not present on admission, assign "N".

Acute and Chronic Conditions

Assign "Y" for acute conditions that are present at time of admission and N for acute conditions that are not present at time of admission.

Assign "Y" for chronic conditions, even though the condition may not be diagnosed until after admission.

If a single code identifies both an acute and chronic condition, see the POA guidelines for combination codes.

Combination Codes

Assign "N" if any part of the combination code was not present on admission (e.g., obstructive chronic bronchitis with acute exacerbation and the exacerbation was not present on admission; gastric ulcer that does not start bleeding until after admission; asthma patient develops status asthmaticus after admission)

Assign "Y" if all parts of the combination code were present on admission (e.g., patient with diabetic nephropathy is admitted with uncontrolled diabetes)

If the final diagnosis includes comparative or contrasting diagnoses, and both were present, or suspected, at the time of admission, assign "Y".

For infection codes that include the causal organism, assign "Y" if the infection (or signs of the infection) was present on admission, even though the culture results may not be known until after admission (e.g., patient is admitted with pneumonia and the provider documents pseudomonas as the causal organism a few days later).

Same Diagnosis Code for Two or More Conditions

When the same ICD-9-CM diagnosis code applies to two or more conditions during the same encounter (e.g. bilateral condition, or two separate conditions classified to the same ICD-9-CM diagnosis code):

Assign "Y" if all conditions represented by the single ICD-9-CM code were present on admission (e.g. bilateral fracture of the same bone, same site, and both fractures were present on admission)

Assign "N" if any of the conditions represented by the single ICD-9-CM code was not present on admission (e.g. dehydration with hyponatremia is assigned to code 276.1, but only one of these conditions was present on admission).

Obstetrical conditions

Whether or not the patient delivers during the current hospitalization does not affect assignment of the POA indicator. The determining factor for POA assignment is whether the pregnancy complication or obstetrical condition described by the code was present at the time of admission or not.

If the pregnancy complication or obstetrical condition was present on admission (e.g., patient admitted in preterm labor), assign "Y".

If the pregnancy complication or obstetrical condition was not present on admission (e.g., 2nd degree laceration during delivery, postpartum hemorrhage that occurred during current hospitalization, fetal distress develops after admission), assign "N".

If the obstetrical code includes more than one diagnosis and any of the diagnoses identified by the code were not present on admission assign "N".

> (e.g., Code 642.7, Pre-eclampsia or eclampsia superimposed on pre-existing hypertension).

If the obstetrical code includes information that is not a diagnosis, do not consider that information in the POA determination.

(e.g. Code 652.1x, Breech or other malpresentation successfully converted to cephalic presentation should be reported as present on admission if the fetus was breech on admission but was converted to cephalic presentation after admission (since the conversion to cephalic presentation does not represent a diagnosis, the fact that the conversion occurred after admission has no bearing on the POA determination).

Perinatal conditions

Newborns are not considered to be admitted until after birth. Therefore, any condition present at birth or that developed in utero is considered present at admission and should be assigned "Y". This includes conditions that occur during delivery (e.g., injury during delivery, meconium aspiration, exposure to streptococcus B in the vaginal canal).

Congenital conditions and anomalies

Assign "Y" for congenital conditions and anomalies. Congenital conditions are always considered present on admission.

External cause of injury codes

Assign "Y" for any E code representing an external cause of injury or poisoning that occurred prior to inpatient admission (e.g., patient fell out of bed at home, patient fell out of bed in emergency room prior to admission)

Assign "N" for any E code representing an external cause of injury or poisoning that occurred during inpatient hospitalization (e.g., patient fell out of hospital bed during hospital stay, patient experienced an adverse reaction to a medication administered after inpatient admission)

CATEGORIES AND CODES EXEMPT FROM DIAGNOSIS PRESENT ON ADMISSION REQUIREMENT

Effective Date: October 1, 2008

Note: "Diagnosis present on admission" for these code categories are exempt because they represent circumstances regarding the healthcare encounter or factors influencing health status that do not represent a current disease or injury or are always present on admission

137-139, Late effects of infectious and parasitic diseases

268.1, Rickets, late effect

326, Late effects of intracranial abscess or pyogenic infection

412, Old myocardial infarction

438, Late effects of cerebrovascular disease

650, Normal delivery

660.7, Failed forceps or vacuum extractor, unspecified

677, Late effect of complication of pregnancy, childbirth, and the puerperium

905-909, Late effects of injuries, poisonings, toxic effects, and other external causes

V02, Carrier or suspected carrier of infectious diseases

V03, Need for prophylactic vaccination and inoculation against bacterial diseases

V04, Need for prophylactic vaccination and inoculation against certain viral diseases

V05, Need for other prophylactic vaccination and inoculation against single diseases

V06, Need for prophylactic vaccination and inoculation against combinations of diseases

V07, Need for isolation and other prophylactic measures

V10, Personal history of malignant neoplasm

V11, Personal history of mental disorder

V12, Personal history of certain other diseases

V13, Personal history of other diseases

V14, Personal history of allergy to medicinal agents

V15.01-V15.09, Other personal history, Allergy, other than to medicinal agents

V15.1, Other personal history, Surgery to heart and great vessels

V15.2, Other personal history, Surgery to other major organs

V15.3, Other personal history, Irradiation

V15.4, Other personal history, Psychological trauma

V15.5, Other personal history, Injury

V15.6, Other personal history, Poisoning

V15.7, Other personal history, Contraception

V15.81, Other personal history, Noncompliance with medical treatment

V15.82, Other personal history, History of tobacco use

V15.88, Other personal history, History of fall

V15.89, Other personal history, Other

V15.9 Unspecified personal history presenting hazards to health

V16, Family history of malignant neoplasm

V17, Family history of certain chronic disabling diseases

V18, Family history of certain other specific conditions

V19, Family history of other conditions

V20, Health supervision of infant or child

V21, Constitutional states in development

V22, Normal pregnancy

V23, Supervision of high-risk pregnancy

V24, Postpartum care and examination

V25, Encounter for contraceptive management

V26, Procreative management

V27, Outcome of delivery

V28, Antenatal screening

V29, Observation and evaluation of newborns for suspected condition not found

V30-V39, Liveborn infants according to type of birth

V42, Organ or tissue replaced by transplant

V43, Organ or tissue replaced by other means

V44, Artificial opening status

V45, Other postprocedural states

V46, Other dependence on machines

V49.60-V49.77, Upper and lower limb amputation status

V49.81-V49.84, Other specified conditions influencing health status

V50, Elective surgery for purposes other than remedying health states

V51, Aftercare involving the use of plastic surgery

V52, Fitting and adjustment of prosthetic device and implant

V53, Fitting and adjustment of other device

V54, Other orthopedic aftercare

V55, Attention to artificial openings

V56, Encounter for dialysis and dialysis catheter care

V57, Care involving use of rehabilitation procedures

V58, Encounter for other and unspecified procedures and aftercare

V59, Donors

V60, Housing, household, and economic circumstances

V61, Other family circumstances

V62, Other psychosocial circumstances

V64, Persons encountering health services for specific procedures, not carried out

V65, Other persons seeking consultation

V66, Convalescence and palliative care

V67, Follow-up examination

V68, Encounters for administrative purposes

V69, Problems related to lifestyle

V70, General medical examination

V71, Observation and evaluation for suspected condition not found

V72, Special investigations and examinations

V73, Special screening examination for viral and chlamydial diseases

V74, Special screening examination for bacterial and spirochetal diseases

V75, Special screening examination for other infectious diseases

V76, Special screening for malignant neoplasms

V77, Special screening for endocrine, nutritional, metabolic, and immunity disorders

V78, Special screening for disorders of blood and blood-forming organs

V79, Special screening for mental disorders and developmental handicaps

V80, Special screening for neurological, eye, and ear diseases

V81, Special screening for cardiovascular, respiratory, and genitourinary diseases

V82, Special screening for other conditions

V83, Genetic carrier status

V84, Genetic susceptibility to disease

V85, Body Mass Index

V86 Estrogen receptor status

V87.4, Personal history of drug therapy

V88, Acquired absence of cervix and uterus

V89, Suspected maternal and fetal conditions not found

E800-E807, Railway accidents

E810-E819, Motor vehicle traffic accidents

E820-E825, Motor vehicle nontraffic accidents

E826-E829, Other road vehicle accidents

E830-E838, Water transport accidents

E840-E845, Air and space transport accidents

E846-E848, Vehicle accidents not elsewhere classifiable

E849.0-E849.6, Place of occurrence

E849.8-E849.9, Place of occurrence

E883.1, Accidental fall into well

E883.2, Accidental fall into storm drain or manhole

E884.0, Fall from playground equipment

E884.1, Fall from cliff

E885.0, Fall from (nonmotorized) scooter

E885.1, Fall from roller skates

E885.2, Fall from skateboard

E885.3, Fall from skis

E885.4, Fall from snowboard

E886.0, Fall on same level from collision, pushing, or shoving, by or with other person, In sports

E890.0-E89.9, Conflagration in private dwelling

E893.0, Accident caused by ignition of clothing, from controlled fire in private dwelling

E893.2, Accident caused by ignition of clothing, from controlled fire not in building or structure

E894, Ignition of highly inflammable material

E895, Accident caused by controlled fire in private dwelling

E897, Accident caused by controlled fire not in building or structure

E898.0-E898.1, Accident caused by other specified fire and flames

E917.0, Striking against or struck accidentally by objects or persons, in sports without subsequent fall

E917.1, Striking against or struck accidentally by objects or persons, caused by a crowd, by collective fear or panic without subsequent fall

E917.2, Striking against or struck accidentally by objects or persons, in running water without subsequent fall

E917.5, Striking against or struck accidentally by objects or persons, object in sports with subsequent fall

E917.6, Striking against or struck accidentally by objects or persons, caused by a crowd, by collective fear or panic with subsequent fall

E919.0-E919.1, Accidents caused by machinery

E919.3-E919.9, Accidents caused by machinery

E921.0-E921.9, Accident caused by explosion of pressure vessel

E922.0-E922.9, Accident caused by firearm and air gun missile

E924.1, Caustic and corrosive substances

E926.2, Visible and ultraviolet light sources

E927, Overexertion and strenuous movements

E928.0-E928.8, Other and unspecified environmental and accidental causes

E929.0-E929.9, Late effects of accidental injury

E959, Late effects of self-inflicted injury

E970-E978, Legal intervention

E979, Terrorism

E981.0-E981.8, Poisoning by gases in domestic use, undetermined whether accidentally or purposely inflicted

E982.0-E982.9, Poisoning by other gases, undetermined whether accidentally or purposely inflicted

E985.0-E985.7, Injury by firearms, air guns and explosives, undetermined whether accidentally or purposely inflicted

E987.0, Falling from high place, undetermined whether accidentally or purposely inflicted, residential premises

E987.2, Falling from high place, undetermined whether accidentally or purposely inflicted, natural sites

E989, Late effects of injury, undetermined whether accidentally or purposely inflicted

E990-E999, Injury resulting from operations of war

POA Examples

General Medical Surgical

1. Patient is admitted for diagnostic work-up for cachexia. The final diagnosis is malignant neoplasm of lung with metastasis.
    Assign "Y" on the POA field for the malignant neoplasm. The malignant neoplasm was clearly present on admission, although it was not diagnosed until after the admission occurred.

2. A patient undergoes outpatient surgery. During the recovery period, the patient develops atrial fibrillation and the patient is subsequently admitted to the hospital as an inpatient.
    Assign "Y" on the POA field for the atrial fibrillation since it developed prior to a written order for inpatient admission.

3. A patient is treated in observation and while in Observation, the patient falls out of bed and breaks a hip. The patient is subsequently admitted as an inpatient to treat the hip fracture.
    Assign "Y" on the POA field for the hip fracture since it developed prior to a written order for inpatient admission.

4. A patient with known congestive heart failure is admitted to the hospital after he develops decompensated congestive heart failure.
    Assign "Y" on the POA field for the congestive heart failure. The ICD-9-CM code identifies the chronic condition and does not specify the acute exacerbation.

5. A patient undergoes inpatient surgery. After surgery, the patient develops fever and is treated aggressively. The physician's final diagnosis documents "possible postoperative infection following surgery."
    Assign "N" on the POA field for the postoperative infection since final diagnoses that contain the terms "possible", "probable", "suspected" or "rule out" and that are based on symptoms or clinical findings that were not present on admission should be reported as "N".

6. A patient with severe cough and difficulty breathing was diagnosed during his hospitalization to have lung cancer.
    Assign "Y" on the POA field for the lung cancer. Even though the cancer was not diagnosed until after admission, it is a chronic condition that was clearly present before the patient's admission.

7. A patient is admitted to the hospital for a coronary artery bypass surgery. Postoperatively he developed a pulmonary embolism.
    Assign "N" on the POA field for the pulmonary embolism. This is an acute condition that was not present on admission.

8. A patient is admitted with a known history of coronary atherosclerosis, status post myocardial infarction five years ago is now admitted for treatment of impending myocardial infarction. The final diagnosis is documented as "impending myocardial infarction."
    Assign "Y" to the impending myocardial infarction because the condition is present on admission.

9. A patient with diabetes mellitus developed uncontrolled diabetes on day 3 of the hospitalization.
    Assign "N" to the diabetes code because the "uncontrolled" component of the code was not present on admission.

10. A patient is admitted with high fever and pneumonia. The patient rapidly deteriorates and becomes septic. The discharge diagnosis lists sepsis and pneumonia. The documentation is unclear as to whether the sepsis was present on admission or developed shortly after admission.
    Query the physician as to whether the sepsis was present on admission, developed shortly after admission, or it cannot be clinically determined as to whether it was present on admission or not.

11. A patient is admitted for repair of an abdominal aneurysm. However, the aneurysm ruptures after hospital admission.
    Assign "N" for the ruptured abdominal aneurysm. Although the aneurysm was present on admission, the "ruptured" component of the code description did not occur until after admission.

12. A patient with viral hepatitis B progresses to hepatic coma after admission.
    Assign "N" for the viral hepatitis B with hepatic coma because part of the code description did not develop until after admission.

13. A patient with a history of varicose veins and ulceration of the left lower extremity strikes the area against the side of his hospital bed during an inpatient hospitalization. It bleeds profusely. The final diagnosis lists varicose veins with ulcer and hemorrhage.
    Assign "Y" for the varicose veins with ulcer. Although the hemorrhage occurred after admission, the code description for varicose veins with ulcer does not mention hemorrhage.

14. The nursing initial assessment upon admission documents the presence of a decubitus ulcer. There is no mention of the decubitus ulcer in the physician documentation until several days after admission.
    Query the physician as to whether the decubitus ulcer was present on admission, or developed after admission. Both diagnosis code assignment and determination of whether a condition was present on admission must be based on provider documentation in the medical record (per the definition of "provider" found at the beginning of these POA guidelines and in the introductory section of the ICD-9-CM Official Guidelines for Coding and Reporting). If it cannot be determined from the provider documentation whether or not a condition was present on admission, the provider should be queried.

15. **A urine culture is obtained on admission. The provider documents urinary tract infection when the culture results become available a few days later.**
    Assign "Y" to the urinary tract infection since the diagnosis is based on test results from a specimen obtained on admission. It may not be possible for a provider to make a definitive diagnosis for a period of

time after admission. There is no required timeframe as to when a provider must identify or document a condition to be present on admission.

16. A patient tested positive for Methicillin resistant Staphylococcus (MRSA) on routine nasal culture on admission to the hospital. During the hospitalization, he underwent insertion of a central venous catheter and later developed an infection and was diagnosed with MRSA sepsis due to central venous catheter infection.
    Assign "Y" to the positive MRSA colonization. Assign "N" for the MRSA sepsis due to central venous catheter infection since the patient did not have a MRSA infection at the time of admission.

Obstetrics

1. A female patient was admitted to the hospital and underwent a normal delivery.
   Leave the "present on admission" (POA) field blank. Code 650, Normal delivery, is on the "exempt from reporting" list.

2. Patient admitted in late pregnancy due to excessive vomiting and dehydration. During admission patient goes into premature labor
   Assign "Y" for the excessive vomiting and the dehydration.
   Assign "N" for the premature labor

3. Patient admitted in active labor. During the stay, a breast abscess is noted when mother attempted to breast feed. Provider is unable to determine whether the abscess was present on admission
   Assign "W" for the breast abscess.

4. Patient admitted in active labor. After 12 hours of labor it is noted that the infant is in fetal distress and a Cesarean section is performed
   Assign "N" for the fetal distress.

5. **Pregnant female was admitted in labor and fetal nuchal cord entanglement was diagnosed. Physician is queried, but is unable to determine whether the cord entanglement was present on admission or not.**
   Assign "W" for the fetal nuchal cord entanglement.

Newborn

1. A single liveborn infant was delivered in the hospital via Cesarean section. The physician documented fetal bradycardia during labor in the final diagnosis in the newborn record.
   Assign "Y" because the bradycardia developed prior to the newborn admission (birth).

2. A newborn developed diarrhea which was believed to be due to the hospital baby formula.
   Assign "N" because the diarrhea developed after admission.

3. **A newborn born in the hospital, birth complicated by nuchal cord entanglement.**
   Assign "Y" for the nuchal cord entanglement on the baby's record. Any condition that is present at birth or that developed in utero is considered present at admission, including conditions that occur during delivery.

Exercise Answers

CHAPTER 1

Exercise 1-1
1. American Medical Association
2. Current Procedural Terminology
3. services
4. 1966
5. 1983

Exercise 1-2
1. c
2. a
3. g
4. b
5. d
6. e
7. f
8. Appendix B
9. Appendix E
10. Appendix D

Exercise 1-3
1. Surgery
2. Respiratory System
3. Nose
4. Excision

Exercise 1-4
1. A concise statement describing the symptom, problem, condition, diagnosis, or other factor that is the reason for the encounter, usually stated in the patient's words
2. different
3. interpreting physician

4. a physician
5. **99070**

Exercise 1-5

1. those codes that have full description (or similar wording)
2. those codes that include their own description as well as that portion of the stand-alone code description found before the semicolon in a preceding code (or similar wording)
3. alternative anatomic site, alternative procedure, or description of the extent of service (in any order and similar wording)

Exercise 1-6

1. -62
2. **43820-62**
3. -50
4. -78
5. -57
6. -51
7. -66
8. -80

Exercise 1-7

1. **69799, 29999, 43499**
2. **88299, 81099, 84999**
3. **99199**
4. **77799, 78999**

Exercise 1-8

1. **49900**
2. **27303**
3. **27786-27814, 27792**

Exercise 1-9

1. a. Emergency
   b. **99288** (Emergency Department Services, Physician Direction of Advanced Life Support)
2. a. Fracture
   b. **27238** (Fracture, Femur, Intertrochanteric, Closed Treatment)
3. a. Removal
   b. **47480** (Removal, Calculi, Gallbladder)
4. a. Lung
   b. **32141** (Excision, Bullae, Lung)

Exercise 1-10

1. *See* Dialysis
2. *See* Antinuclear Antibodies (ANA)
3. *See* Radius; Ulna; Wrist

CHAPTER 2

Exercise 2-1

1. office
2. office visit or other outpatient service
3. new

4. **99201**
5. five
6. five

Exercise 2-2
1. problem focused
2. expanded problem focused
3. detailed
4. comprehensive
5. comprehensive

Exercise 2-3
1. problem focused
2. expanded problem focused
3. detailed
4. comprehensive
5. comprehensive

Exercise 2-4
1. OS
2. BA
3. OS
4. OS
5. OS
6. OS
7. OS
8. BA
9. BA
10. BA
11. OS
12. OS
13. BA
14. OS
15. OS
16. BA
17. OS
18. OS
19. OS
20. OS

Note: Some terms—thorax, lungs, heart, vagina, blood vessels, neurologic—are specifically presented in the text as being a body area or an organ system. For other terms, you have to make the connection; for example, the thorax is examined as a body area but the lungs are examined as an organ system.

21. a. problem focused
    b. problem focused
22. CC: Cold
    HPI: Quality (dry, hacking)
          Location (nasal)

Duration (9 days)

Associated Signs and Symptoms (sleeplessness)

4 HPI ELEMENTS = COMPREHENSIVE

PFSH: Personal

           Family

2 PFSH ELEMENTS = COMPREHENSIVE

ROS: Constitutional (fever, aching)

          Respiratory (coughing)

2 ROS ELEMENTS = DETAILED

a. This is a detailed (Level 3) history

Examination

General survey: Minor distress

Vital signs: Temperature, BP, pulse

1 CONSTITUTIONAL (no matter how many elements checked off it only counts as 1)

Body Areas: Head

1 BODY AREA

Organ Systems: Respiratory (mucous membranes, lungs clear to percussion and auscultation), Otolaryngologic (ears, nose)

2 ORGAN SYSTEMS

b. 5 Elements = Expanded Problem Focused examination

Detailed history

EPF Exam

Exercise 2-5

1. limited (Some chart audit forms classify a new problem to a physician with no further follow-up planned as moderate.)
2. limited (The data could be moderate if the patient has brought records that the physician would have to review.)
3. moderate
4. low
5. **99203**
6. straightforward or low
7. low (risks are increased for the elderly)

Exercise 2-6

1. b or c
2. d or e
3. e
4. c
5. a
6. b

Exercise 2-7

1. detailed, detailed, low
2. comprehensive, comprehensive, moderate
3. comprehensive, comprehensive, high
4. **99203** (Office and/or Other Outpatient Services, Office Visit, New Patient)
5. **99201** (Office and/or Other Outpatient Services, Office Visit, New Patient)

6. **99205** (Office and/or Other Outpatient Services, Office Visit, New Patient) (Note that some coders may use 90801, Psychiatric Diagnostic or Evaluation Interview Procedures, subject to the credentials of the provider.) (Based on time—"more than an hour is spent discussing . . ." The History element is not comprehensive and would not meet this level on that basis.)

7. **99203** (Office and/or Other Outpatient Services, Office Visit, New Patient)

8. **99202** (Office and/or Other Outpatient Services, Office Visit, New Patient)

Exercise 2-8

1. yes

2. **99212** (Office and/or Other Outpatient Services, Office Visit, Established Patient) (Note some chart audit forms would indicate 99213 because of the antibiotic prescription.)

3. **99211** (Office and/or Other Outpatient Services, Office Visit, Established Patient)

4. **99215** (Office and/or Other Outpatient Services, Office Visit, Established Patient)

5. **99213** (Office and/or Other Outpatient Services, Office Visit, Established Patient) (Note: Although the MDM complexity is at the level of code 99214, the history and examination were at the level of code 99213; because two of the three key components must be documented in order to use 99214, you must assign the lower level, 99213.)

6. **99212** (Office and/or Other Outpatient Services, Office Visit, Established Patient)

7. **99213** (Office and/or Other Outpatient Services, Office Visit, Established Patient)

Exercise 2-9

1. **99219** (Hospital Services, Observation, Initial Care)

Exercise 2-10

1. **99221** (Hospital Service, Initial Hospital Care)

2. **99223** (Hospital Service, Initial Hospital Care)

3. comprehensive, moderate

4. **99221** (Hospital Service, Inpatient Services, Initial Hospital Care)

Exercise 2-11

1. 30 minutes or less, more than 30 minutes

2. no

Exercise 2-12

1. **99244** (Consultation, Office and/or Other Outpatient)

2. **99241** (Consultation, Office and/or Other Outpatient)

3. **99242** (Consultation, Office and/or Other Outpatient)

4. **99241** (Consultation, Office and/or Other Outpatient)

5. **99244** (Consultation, Office and/or Other Outpatient)

6. **99252** (Consultation, Inpatient)

7. **99255** (Consultation, Inpatient) (Modifier -57 would also be used to indicate the decision to perform surgery, depending on the third-party payer.)

8. **99252** (Consultation, Inpatient)

9. **99255** (Consultation, Inpatient)

10. **99233** (Hospital Inpatient Services, Subsequent Hospital Care)

11. **99233** (Hospital Inpatient Services, Subsequent Hospital Care)

12. **99244** (Consultation, Office)

13. **99242-32** (Consultation, Office) (Modifier -32, insurance company requested)

14. **99244-32** (Consultation, Office) (Modifier -32 indicates a mandatory consultation.)

Exercise 2-13

1. self-limited or minor
2. high
3. moderate
4. low to moderate
5. **99285** (Emergency Department Services)
6. **99285** (Emergency Department Services)
7. **99283** (Emergency Department Services)
8. **99288** (Emergency Department, Physician Direction of Advanced Life Support)

Exercise 2-14

1. **99291** (Critical Care Services)
2. no
3. **99291** and **99292 × 4** (180 minutes of care) (Critical Care Services)

Exercise 2-15

1. moderate
2. **99306** (Nursing Facility Services, Initial Care)
3. c
4. b
5. a
6. **99308** (Nursing Facility Services, Subsequent Care)

Exercise 2-16

1. **99347** (Home Services, Established Patient)

Exercise 2-17

1. no
2. no
3. no
4. whether the patient is an inpatient or an outpatient
5. no
6. no

Exercise 2-18

1. 30 minutes or more
2. 99366, 99367, 99368

Exercise 2-19

1. Age
2. -25

Exercise 2-20

1. Basic Life and/or Disability Evaluation Services
2. Work-Related or Medical Disability Evaluation Services
3. whether the treating physician or a physician other than the treating physician conducted the evaluation
4. **99455** (Insurance Exam)

Exercise 2-21	1. Very low birth weight
	2. **99466** (Critical Care Servics, Pediatric, Interfacility Transport)
	3. **99463** (Newborn Care, Normal)
	4. **99476** (Critical Care Services, Pediatric, Subsequent)
	5. **99478** (Critical Care Services, Neonatal, Low Birth Weight Infant)
Exercise 2-22	1. **99201** (Office and/or Other Outpatient Services, Office Visits, New Patient)
	2. **99212** (Office and Other Outpatient Visits, Office Visits, Established Patient)
	3. **99211** (Office and/or Other Outpatient Services, Office Visits, Established Patient)
	4. **99306** (Nursing Facility Services, Initial Care)
	5. **99202** (Office and/or Other Outpatient Services, Office Visits, New Patient)
	6. **99211** (Office and/or Other Outpatient Services, Office Visits, Established Patient)
	7. **99285** (Emergency Department Services)
	8. **99291** (Critical Care Services)
	9. **99291** (Critical Care Services) and **99292** (Critical Care Services)
	10. **99214** (Office and/or Other Outpatient Services, Established Patient)
	11. **99254** (Consultation, Inpatient)

CHAPTER 3

Exercise 3-1	1. Head; Neck; Thorax (Chest Wall and Shoulder Girdle); Intrathoracic; Spine and Spinal Cord; Upper Abdomen; Lower Abdomen; Perineum; Pelvis (Except Hip); Upper Leg (Except Knee); Knee and Popliteal Area; Lower Leg (Below Knee, Includes Ankle and Foot); Shoulder and Axilla; Upper Arm and Elbow; Forearm, Wrist, and Hand; Radiological Procedures; Burn Excisions or Debridement; Obstetric; Other Procedures.
	2. Radiologic Procedures, Burn Excisions or Debridement, Obstetrics, and Other Procedures
	3. absence of pain
	4. induction or administration of a drug to obtain partial or complete loss of sensation (or similar wording)
	5. general, regional, local, sacral, caudal, lumbar, endotracheal, epidural, and patient controlled.
	6. moderate or conscious sedation
	7. Medicine
Exercise 3-2	1. P2
	2. P3
	3. **99116**
Exercise 3-3	1. -22
	2. -23
	3. -22
	4. -23

Exercise 3-4

1. **01999** (Anesthesia, Unlisted Services and Procedures)
2. Anesthesia, Thyroid, **00322**
3. Anesthesia, Cesarean Delivery, **01961**
4. Anesthesia, Prostate, **00914**
5. Anesthesia, Cleft Palate Repair, **00172**
6. Anesthesia, Achilles Tendon Repair, **01472**
7. **$94.30** (B = 3, T = 1, M = 1; total = 5; 5 × $18.86)
8. a. **$180.27** (B = 5, T = 4, M = 0; total = 9; 9 × $20.03)
   b. ~~**$169.74**~~ (B = 5, T = 4, M = 0; total = 9; 9 × $18.86) $173.07
9. a. **$190.90** (B = 7, T = 2, M = 1; total = 10; 10 × $19.09)
   b. **$209.99** (B = 7, T = 3, M = 1; total = 11; 11 × $19.09)

Exercise 3-5

1. **57270-22**
2. **54535-22**
3. -23
4. -24
5. -25
6. -26

Exercise 3-6

1. -32
2. -47
3. -50
4. **17274** and **17264-51** (Since 17274 is more resource-intensive it is therefore listed first and without the modifier.)
5. **61250** and **61250-50** or **61250-50**
6. **28450** and **28450-51** or **28450** × **2**
7. **27447** and **27447-50** (Arthroplasty, Knee) or **27447-RT** and **27447-LT** or **27447-50**
8. **24006** and **24006-50** or **24006-50** or **24006-RT** and **24006-LT**
9. **19305-50** or **19305** and **19305-50** or **19305-RT** and **19305-LT**
10. -52

Exercise 3-7

1. -58
2. **43124-54**
3. **19306-55**
4. **19306-56**

Exercise 3-8

1. -62
2. -66
3. -80
4. -81
5. -78
6. -79
7. -77

Exercise 3-9	1. -99
	2. -90
	3. -91

CHAPTER 4

Exercise 4-1	1. General
	2. Integumentary System
	3. Musculoskeletal System
	4. Respiratory System
	5. Cardiovascular System
	6. Hemic and Lymphatic Systems
	7. Mediastinum and Diaphragm
	8. Digestive System
	9. Urinary System
	10. Male Genital System
	11. Reproductive System Procedures
	12. Intersex Surgery
	13. Female Genital System
	14. Maternity Care and Delivery
	15. Endocrine System
	16. Nervous System
	17. Eye and Ocular Adnexa
	18. Auditory System
	19. Operating Microscope

Exercise 4-2	1. **20999**
	2. **69949**
	3. **17999**
	4. **27899**
	5. **64999**
	6. **67999**

Exercise 4-3	1. pre-, intra-, and postoperative services, or similar wording
	2. no
	3. no

Exercise 4-4	1. **11056** (Lesion, Skin, Paring/Curettement)
	2. **11200** (Lesion, Skin Tags, Removal)
	3. **11311** (Lesion, Skin, Shaving)

Exercise 4-5	1. **13121** (Repair, Wound, Complex)
	2. **13101** for complex repair of abdomen (Repair, Wound, Complex); **12004-51** for 12-cm simple repair of back, forearm, and neck added together (Repair, Wound, Simple). (Note that the same types of repair are combined—back (trunk), forearm (extremities), and neck are all included in the code description for 12004.)

3. **12034** for the 10.7-cm intermediate forearm repair (Wound, Repair, Intermediate); **12002-51** for the 3.1-cm scalp repair (Repair, Wound, Simple).

4. **Cheek graft: 15120** (Skin Grafts and Flaps, Split Grafts)
   Upper chest graft: 15100-51 (Skin Grafts and Flaps, Split Grafts)
   Site preparation, cheek, 100 cm²: **15004-51, 15101** (Skin Grafts and Flaps, Recipient Site Preparation) [no modifier on add-on code 15101], chest, 200 cm²: **15002-51, 15003** (Skin Grafts and Flaps, Recipient Site Preparation) [no modifier on add-on code 15103]
   Note that if this claim were submitted to Medicare, modifier -51 would not be applied to the preparation codes.

5. **14041** (Skin, Adjacent Tissue Transfer)

6. **14040** (Skin, Adjacent Tissue Transfer) (Note that a Z-plasty is a form of adjacent tissue transfer. The excision is included in the adjacent tissue transfer code.)

7. **15732** (Skin, Myocutaneous) (Note that modifier -58 may also be used if the procedure was a staged procedure.)

8. **16025 × 5** debridement of medium area, 10% for each day of the first week, and **16025 × 6** for debridement of medium area, 10% for every other day of the next 2 weeks (Burn, Dressings) or **16025 × 11**

Exercise 4-6
1. **17110** (Destruction, Skin, Lesion, Benign) (If a specific anatomic area was indicated, you could report the destruction with a more specific code. For example, 56501 for destruction of a lesion of the vulva.)

2. **17000** (Destruction, Skin, Benign), **17003 × 13** (Destruction, Skin, Benign)

3. **17311** (Mohs', First Stage)

Exercise 4-7
1. **19000** (Breast, Cyst, Puncture Aspiration)

2. **19303** and **19303-50** or **19303-50** (Breast; Removal; Simple, Complete)

3. **19307** or **19307-RT** (Breast, Removal, Modified Radical)

4. **19290-LT** (Breast, Needle Wire Placement)

5. **19350-RT** (Breast, Reconstruction, Nipple, Areola)

CHAPTER 5

Exercise 5-1
1. **21310** (Nasal Bone, Fracture, Closed Treatment)

2. **21800** (Rib, Fracture, Closed Treatment)

3. **28675** (Dislocation, Interphalangeal Joint, Toe, Open Treatment)

4. **27792** (Fracture, Fibula, Open Treatment)

5. **27500** (Fracture, Femur, Closed Treatment)

6. **27235** (Fracture, Femur, Percutaneous Fixation)

7. **23670** (Fracture, Humerus, with Dislocation, Open Treatment)

8. **21453** (Fracture, Mandible, Closed Treatment, Interdental Fixation)

9. **25606** (Fracture, Radius, Percutaneous Fixation)

10. **27840** (Ankle, Dislocation, Closed Treatment)

Exercise 5-2
1. **20103** (Wound, Exploration, Extremity)
2. **20838** (Replantation, Foot)
3. **21015** (Tumor, Resection, Face)
4. **20974** (Electrical Stimulation, Bone Healing, Noninvasive)
5. **20206** (Biopsy, Muscle)
6. **20600** (Aspiration, Joint)

Exercise 5-3
1. **29065** (Cast, Long Arm); **99070** or **A4580-A4590** or **Q4005-Q4008** (Supply, Materials)
2. **29425** (Cast, Walking)
3. **29705** (Cast, Removal)
4. **29530** (Strapping, Knee)
5. **29345** (Cast, Long Leg); **99070** or **A4580-A4590** or **Q4005-Q4008** (Supply, Materials)

Exercise 5-4
1. **29898** (Arthroscopy, Surgical, Ankle)
2. **29870** (Arthroscopy, Diagnostic, Knee)
3. **29805** (Arthroscopy, Shoulder)
4. **29850** (Fracture, Knee, Arthroscopic Treatment)
5. **29891** (Arthroscopy, Surgical, Ankle)

CHAPTER 6

Exercise 6-1
1. **31256** (Antrostomy, Sinus, Maxillary)
2. **31530** (Laryngoscopy, Direct)
3. **31628** (Bronchoscopy, Biopsy)
4. **32605** (Thoracoscopy, Diagnostic, without Biopsy)
5. **32663** (Thoracoscopy, Surgical, with Lobectomy)

Exercise 6-2
1. **30100** (Biopsy, Nose, Intranasal)
2. **30420** (Rhinoplasty, Primary)
3. **30901** (Epistaxis)
4. **30520** (Septoplasty)
5. **30300** (Removal, Foreign Bodies, Nose)

Exercise 6-3
1. **31000** and **31000-50** (Sinuses, Maxillary, Irrigation)
2. **31070** (Sinusotomy, Frontal Sinus, Exploratory)
3. **31090** (Sinusotomy, Combined)
4. **31030** (Sinusotomy, Maxillary)
5. **31040** (Ptergomaxillary Fossa, Incision)

Exercise 6-4
1. **31320** (Laryngotomy, Diagnostic)
2. **31580** (Laryngoplasty, Laryngeal Web)
3. **31500** (Endotracheal Tube, Intubation)
4. **31368** (Laryngectomy, Partial)
5. **31390** (Pharyngolaryngectomy)

Exercise 6-5
1. **31605** (Tracheostomy, Emergency)
2. **31785** (Trachea; Tumor; Excision, Cervical)
3. **31715** (Bronchography; Injection, Transtracheal)
4. **31600** (Tracheostomy, Planned)
5. **31717** (Bronchial Brush Biopsy, with Catheterization)

Exercise 6-6
1. **32095** (Biopsy, Lung, Thoracotomy)
2. **32405** (Biopsy, Lung, Needle)
3. **32480** (Lobectomy, Lung) and **32501** (Bronchoplasty). (Note that code 32501 is an add-on code and does not need modifier -51.)
4. **32503** (Resection, Lung)
5. **32200** (Pneumonostomy)

CHAPTER 7

Exercise 7-1
1. invasive
2. internal
3. Medicine, Surgery, Radiology
4. invasive
5. electrophysiology
6. angiography or angiogram

Exercise 7-2
1. **33207** (Pacemaker, Heart, Insertion)
2. **33216-78** (Pacemaker, Heart, Insertion, Electrode) Note that -78 is appended because the patient is in a postoperative period. The patient had a single chamber pacemaker implanted. The replacement of the lead wire is reported as insertion of a new electrode, the removal of the defective electrode is not separately reported.
3. **33214** (Pacemaker, Conversion)
4. **33010** (Pericardiocentesis)
5. **33120** (Tumor, Heart, Excision)

Exercise 7-3
1. **33430** (Mitral Valve, Replacement)
2. **33405** (Aorta, Valve, Replacement) (Note that a prosthetic valve, and not a homograft valve, is used.)
3. **33251** (Heart, Arrhythmogenic Focus, Destruction)
4. **33282** (Implantation, Cardiac Event Recorder)

Exercise 7-4
1. **33511** (Bypass Graft, Coronary Artery, Venous Graft)
2A. **33534** (Coronary Artery Bypass Graft, Arterial)
2B. **33519** (Coronary Artery Bypass Graft, Arterial-Venous)
3. **33533** (Bypass Graft, Coronary Artery, Arterial) and **33519** (Coronary Artery, Bypass Graft, Arterial-Venous)

Exercise 7-5
1. **34201** (Thrombectomy, Aortoiliac Artery)
2. **34001** (Embolectomy, Carotid Artery)
3. **35875** (Thrombectomy, Bypass Graft, Other Than Hemodialysis Graft or Fistula)

Exercise 7-6
1. **35506** (Bypass Graft, Carotid Artery)
2. **35556** (Bypass Graft, Femoral Artery)
3. **35650** (Bypass Graft, Axillary Artery)
4. **35141** (Aneurysm Repair, Femoral Artery)
5. **36246** or **36246-LT** (Catheterization); **75716-26** (Angiography)

Exercise 7-7
1. **92950** (CPR)
2. **93015** (Stress Tests, Cardiovascular)
3. **92982** and **92984** × **2** (Angioplasty, Percutaneous Transluminal Angioplasty)
4. **93278-26** (Electrocardiography, Signal-Averaged)

Exercise 7-8
1. Catheterization procedure **93501** (Catheterization, Cardiac, Right Heart); Injection procedure **93542-51** (Catheterization, Cardiac, Injection); Supervision, interpretation, and report for injection procedure **93555** (Catheterization, Cardiac, Imaging)
2. **93511** (Catheterization, Cardiac, Left Heart); **93543-51** (Catheterization, Cardiac, Injection); **93555** (Catheterization, Cardiac, Imaging)
3. False; they are already bundled into the codes.
4. True
5. False; some codes are modifier -51-exempt.

Exercise 7-9
1. **93600** (Electrophysiology Procedure)
2. **93620, 93622** (Electrophysiology Procedure)
3. **93720** (Plethysmography, Total Body)

Exercise 7-10
1. Injection procedure for angiography **36215** (Catheterization, Brachio-cephalic Artery); angiography **75658** (Angiography, Brachial Artery); contrast material **99070** (Supply, Materials)
2. **36215-LT** (Artery, Carotid, Catheterization); **75660** (Angiography, Carotid, Artery)
3. **36216** (Artery, Carotid, Catheterization); **75660** (Aortography, Carotid)
4. **75563** (MRI, Heart)

CHAPTER 8

Exercise 8-1
1. **57061** (Destruction, Lesion, Vagina, Simple)
2. **56605, 56606** × **2** (Vulva, Perineum, Biopsy) (Note that the code 56605 is for the first lesion, and 56606 is for *each* additional lesion.)
3. **57305** (Vagina, Repair, Fistula, Rectovaginal)
4. **57520** (Cervix, Conization) (Note that dilation and curettage is not coded separately because it is included in the description of the conization.)
5. **58662** (Cystectomy, Ovarian, Laparoscopic)
6. c
7. b
8. d
9. a

Exercise 8-2

1. **59151** (Laparoscopy, Ectopic Pregnancy with Salpingectomy and/or Oophorectomy)
2. **59409** (Vaginal Delivery, Delivery only); **59412** (External Cephalic Version) (Note that the version is stated "list in addition"; therefore, modifier -51 is not necessary.)
3. **59320** (Cerclage, Cervix, Vaginal)

CHAPTER 9

Exercise 9-1

1. **54520** (Orchiectomy, Simple) (Note that the terms "simple" and "radical" are based on the interpretation of the physician.)
2. **54865** (Epididymis, Exploration, Biopsy) (Note that even though the question states without biopsy, the CPT code states with or without biopsy, so this would be the correct code to assign.)
3. **55000** (Tunica Vaginalis, Hydrocele, Aspiration)
4. **54065** (Penis, Lesion, Destruction, Extensive)
5. **55400-50** (Vas Deferens, Repair, Suture) (Note: This procedure could also be done with an operating microscope, in which case you would code 55400 and 69990 [Operating Microscope].)
6. **55845** (Prostatectomy, Retropubic, Radical)
7. **54505-50** or **54505, 54505-50** (Biopsy, Testes)
8. **53852** (Transurethral Procedure, Prostate, Radiofrequency)
9. **54415** (Removal, Prosthesis, Penis)

Exercise 9-2

1. **51100** (Aspiration, Bladder)
2. **52332** (Cystourethroscopy, Insertion, Indwelling Ureteral Stent)
3. **50065** (Nephrolithotomy) (Note that the term "secondary" means that the procedure is being repeated. Some may code this 50060-76, but this would not be correct because there is a more accurate code to assign.)
4. **53520** (Urethra, Repair, Fistula)
5. **53405** (Urethra, Repair, Fistula)
6. **50398-LT** (Nephrostomy, Change Tube)
7. **50590-RT** (Lithotripsy, Kidney), **52310** (Cystourethroscopy, Removal, Urethral Stent)
8. **51840** (Urethropexy)
9. **52320-LT** (Ureter, Endoscopy, Removal Calculus), **74420-50-26** or **74420-26-LT, 74420-26-RT** (Urography, Retrograde)
10. **52332-LT** (Ureter, Endoscopy, Insertion, Stent), **74420-26** (Urography, Retrograde)

Exercise 9-3

1. surgical communication from the colon to the rectum
2. surgical communication from the ileum to the body surface
3. surgical communication from the large intestine to the body surface
4. surgical communication between segments of intestine
5. **44141** (Colon, Excision, Partial)
6. **44120** (Enterectomy)

7. **46257** (Hemorrhoidectomy, Simple, with Fissurectomy) Note that **46220-51** (Papillectomy) and **46080-51** (Sphincterotomy, Anal) are not reported as they are both bundled into the 46257 because they are designated "separate procedure" in the CPT.

8. **45331** (Endoscopy, Colon-Sigmoid, Biopsy)

Exercise 9-4

1. **43255** (Hemorrhage; Gastrointestinal, Upper; Endoscopic Control)

2. **45331** (Sigmoidoscopy, Biopsy); the description states biopsy, single or multiple, so only one code is used for multiple (three) biopsies.

3. **45385** (Colonoscopy, Removal, Polyp)

Exercise 9-5

1. **47562** (Cholecystectomy) (Note that the exploratory laparotomy is not coded, as it turns into the surgical approach once the cholecystectomy is performed.)

2. **47480** (Cholecystotomy)

3. **49565** (Hernia, Repair, Abdominal Recurrent); **49568** (Implantation, Mesh, Hernia Repair) (Note that the mesh code can be used only with incisional hernias, and it is stated to "list separately," so a -51 modifier is not necessary.)

4. **49507** (Hernia, Repair, Inguinal, Incarcerated)

5. **40490** (Biopsy, Lip)

Exercise 9-6

1. **39502** (Diaphragm, Repair, Hernia)

2. **39000** (Mediastinum, Exploration)

3. **39220** (Mediastinum, Tumor, Excision)

4. **39520** (Diaphragm, Repair, Hernia)

CHAPTER 10

Exercise 10-1

1. **38550** (Lymph Nodes, Hygroma Cystic Axillary/Cervical, Excision)

2. **38100** (Splenectomy, Total)

3. **38200** (Splenoportography, Injection Procedure)

4. **38241** (Transplantation, Bone Marrow)

Exercise 10-2

1. **60200** (Thyroid Gland, Cyst, Excision)

2. **60280** (Thyroglossal Duct, Cyst, Excision)

3. **60522** (Thymectomy, Sternal Split/Transthoracic Approach)

4. **60600** (Carotid Body, Lesion, Excision)

5. **60210** (Thyroid Gland, Excision, Partial)

Exercise 10-3

1. **61154** (Burr Hole, Skull, Drainage, Hematoma)

2. **61312** (Craniectomy, Surgical)

3. **61607** (Skull Base Surgery, Middle Cranial Fossa, Extradural); **61605** Definitive procedure (Skull Base Surgery, Middle Cranial Fossa, Extradural); **61590-51** Approach procedure (Skull Base Surgery, Middle Cranial Fossa, Infratemporal Approach)

4. **62258** (Shunt, Brain, Replacement)

Exercise 10-4

1. **65930-LT** (Eye, Removal, Blood Clot)
2. **67318-RT** (Strabismus, Repair, Superior Oblique Muscle)
3. **67145-LT** (Retina, Repair, Prophylaxis, Detachment)
4. **65772-RT** (Cornea, Repair, Astigmatism)
5. **65105-LT** (Eye, with Muscle or Myocutaneous Flap, Muscles Attached)

Exercise 10-5

1. **69801-LT** (Labyrinthotomy, with/without Cryosurgery)
2. **69436** and **69436-50** (Tympanostomy)
3. **69950-LT** (Vestibular Nerve, Section, Transcranial Approach)
4. **69310-RT** (Reconstruction, Auditory Canal, External)
5. **69820-RT** (Ear, Inner, Incision)

CHAPTER 11

Exercise 11-1

1. aorta
2. joint
3. biliary system or pancreas
4. bile ducts
5. urinary bladder
6. lacrimal sac or tear duct sac
7. duodenum or first part of the small intestine
8. heart or heart walls or neighboring tissues
9. subarachnoid space and ventricles of the brain
10. epididymis with contrast material
11. liver
12. uterine cavity and fallopian tubes
13. larynx
14. lymphatic vessels and node
15. spinal cord
16. ureter and renal pelvis
17. salivary duct and branches
18. sinus or sinus tract
19. spleen
20. any part of the urinary system
21. vein and tributaries
22. seminal vesicles

Exercise 11-2

1. position
2. projection
3. anteroposterior
4. posteroanterior
5. right anterior oblique
6. left posterior oblique
7. dorsal
8. ventral

9. right lateral recumbent

10. dorsal decubitus, left lateral

Exercise 11-3

1. separate

2. MUE, Medically Unlikely Edits, or Medically Unbelievable Edits

3. Diagnostic Radiology, Diagnostic Ultrasound, Radiologic Guidance, Breast Mammography, Bone/Joint Studies, Radiation Oncology, and Nuclear Medicine (in any order)

Exercise 11-4

1. **77056** (Mammography)

2. **76499** (Radiology, Diagnostic; Unlisted Services and Procedures); also see Unlisted Service or Procedure in the index listing.

3. **75605** (Aortography)

Exercise 11-5

1. Head and Neck

2. Chest

3. Abdomen and Retroperitoneum

4. Spinal Canal

5. Pelvis

6. Genitalia

7. Extremities

8. Ultrasonic Guidance Procedures

9. Other Procedures

Exercise 11-6

1. **76800** (Ultrasound, Spine)

2. **76604** (Ultrasound, Chest)

3. **76700** (Ultrasound, Abdomen)

4. **76816** (Ultrasound, Pregnant Uterus)

5. **76818** (Ultrasound, Fetus)

Exercise 11-7

1. **77290** (Radiation Therapy, Field Set-Up)

2. **77261** (Radiation Therapy, Planning)

Exercise 11-8

1. **77333** (Radiation Therapy, Treatment Device)

2. **77326** (Radiation Therapy, Dose Plan, Brachytherapy)

3. **77305** (Radiation Therapy, Dose Plan, Teletherapy)

Exercise 11-9

1. **77402** (Radiation Therapy, Treatment Delivery, Single Area)

2. **77401** (Radiation Therapy, Treatment Delivery, Superficial)

3. **77412** (Radiation Therapy, Treatment Delivery, Three or More Areas)

4. **77407** (Radiation Therapy, Treatment Delivery, Two Areas)

5. **77412** (Radiation Therapy, Treatment Delivery, Three or More Areas)

Exercise 11-10

1. **77427** (Radiation Therapy, Treatment Delivery, Weekly)

2. **77499** (Radiation Therapy, Treatment Management, Unlisted Services and Procedures)

Exercise 11-11	1. **77761** (Brachytherapy)
	2. **77776** (Brachytherapy)
	3. **77789** (Brachytherapy)
Exercise 11-12	1. Gastrointestinal System
	2. Endocrine System
	3. Hematopoietic, Reticuloendothelial, and Lymphatic System
	4. Musculoskeletal System
	5. Nervous System

CHAPTER 12

Exercise 12-1	1. **80076** (Organ or Disease Oriented Panel, Hepatic Function Panel)
	2. seven
	3. yes
	4. yes
Exercise 12-2	1. **80102** (Drug, Confirmation)
	2. **80162** (Drug Assay, Digoxin)
	3. **80150** (Drug Assay, Amikacin)
	4. **80178** (Drug Assay, Lithium)
Exercise 12-3	1. **81003** (Urinalysis, Automated)
	2. **81015** (Urinalysis, Microscopic)
	3. **82040** (Albumin, Serum)
	4. **82247** (Bilirubin, Total, Direct)
	5. **82800** (Blood Gases, pH)
	6. **84300** (Sodium, Urine)
	7. **84550** (Uric Acid, Blood)
Exercise 12-4	1. **85027** (Hemogram, Automated)
	2. **85025** (Hemogram, Automated)
	3. **85041** (Red Blood Cell, Count)
	4. **85097** (Bone Marrow, Smear)
Exercise 12-5	1. **86039** (Antibody, Antinuclear)
	2. **86063** (Antibody, Antistreptolysin O)
	3. **86156** (Cold Agglutinin)
Exercise 12-6	1. **86900** (Blood Typing, ABO only); **86901** (Blood Typing, Rh)
	2. **86945 × 3** (Blood Products, Irradiation)
Exercise 12-7	1. **87536** (Microbiology)
	2. **87651** (Microbiology)
	3. **87512** (Microbiology); **87530** (Microbiology); **87482** (Microbiology)
	4. **87555** (Microbiology); **87528** (Microbiology); **87490** (Microbiology)

5. **87086** (Microbiology)

6. to identify each organism present in a microbacterial culture

Exercise 12-8

1. **88309** (Pathology, Surgical, Gross and Micro Exam Level VI)

2. **88309** (Pathology, Surgical, Gross and Micro Exam Level VI)

3. **88305** (Pathology, Surgical, Gross and Micro Exam Level IV)

4. **88302** (Pathology, Surgical, Gross and Micro Exam Level II)

CHAPTER 13

Exercise 13-1

1. **90712** (Vaccines, Poliovirus, Live, Oral); **90473** (Immunization Administration, One Vaccine/Toxoid), **99211-25** (Evaluation and Management) Note that Medicare does not allow an E/M service to be submitted when the only service is the administration of a vaccine.

2. a. **90701** (Vaccines, Diphtheria, Tetanus, Whole Cell Pertussis); **90712** (Vaccines, Polio Virus, Live, Oral); **90471** for first injection; and **90474** for the administration service (Immunization Administration), **99211-25** (Evaluation and Management)

    b. **99392-25** (Preventive Medicine); **90713** (Vaccines, Poliovirus, Inactivated, Intramuscular or Subcutaneous); **90702** (Vaccines, Diphtheria, Tetanus); **90465** for the first injection; and **90466** for the second injection (Immunization Administration, with Counseling) (Note that E/M code 99392 is used here because the well-baby checkup service provided is significant and separate from the injection service.)

    c. **90658** (Vaccines, Influenza); **90471** (Immunization Administration, One Vaccine/Toxoid), **99211-25** (Evaluation and Management) Note that Medicare does not allow an E/M service to be submitted when the only service is the administration of a vaccine.

    d. **99202-25** (Office and/or Other Outpatient Services, New Patient); **90720,** combination code for DTP and Hib (Vaccines, Diphtheria); and **90471** (Immunization Administration) (Note: E/M code 99202 is used here because the E/M service provided was significant and separate from the injection service.)

3. **99392-25** (Preventive Medicine, Established Patient); **90702** (Vaccines, Diphtheria, Tetanus); **90465** (Immunization Administration, One Vaccine/Toxoid) (Note that an E/M code, 99392, is used here because the E/M service provided was significant and was separate from the injection service.)

Exercise 13-2

1. **96372** (Injection, Intramuscular, Therapeutic) (Note that the injection code does not include the drug provided, so 99070 would also be used to identify the drug supplied) or J3420 (Note that an E/M code is not used here because the service provided is not a significant and separate service from the injection service.)

2. **90658** (Vaccines, Influenza) **90471** (Administration, One Vaccine/Toxoid)

Exercise 13-3

1. **90804** (Psychiatric Treatment, Individual Insight-Oriented, Office or Outpatient)

2. **96101 × 2** (Psychiatric Diagnosis, Psychological Testing)

3. **90885** (Psychiatric Diagnosis, Evaluation of Records or Reports)

4. **90801** (Psychiatric Diagnosis, Interview and Evaluation)

Exercise 13-4
1. **90875** (Biofeedback, Psychiatric Treatment)
2. **90901** (Training, Biofeedback)

Exercise 13-5
1. **90955** (Dialysis, End-Stage Renal Disease)
2. **90935** (Dialysis, Hemodialysis)
3. **90947** (Dialysis, Peritoneal)
4. within the lining of the abdominal cavity
5. filtration of blood and waste products through a filter outside the body
6. end-stage renal disease

Exercise 13-6
1. **91038** (Esophagus, Acid Reflux Tests)
2. **91105** (Intubation, Gastric)
3. **91055** (Intubation, Specimen Collection, Stomach)
4. spontaneous movement study
5. pressure measurements

Exercise 13-7
1. **92014** (Ophthalmology, Diagnostic; Eye Exam; Established Patient)
2. **92070** (Contact Lens Services, Fitting and Prescription)
3. **92120** (Ophthalmology, Diagnostic; Tonography)
4. **92004** (Ophthalmology, Diagnostic; Eye Exam, New Patient)

Exercise 13-8
1. **92592** (Hearing Aid, Check)
2. **92551** (Audiologic Function Tests, Screening)
3. **92511** (Nasopharyngoscopy)
4. **92512** (Nasal Function Study)

Exercise 13-9
1. **93965** (Plethysmography, Extremities, Veins)
2. **93980** (Vascular Studies, Penile Vessels)

Exercise 13-10
1. **94620** (Pulmonology, Diagnostic; Stress Test, Pulmonary)
2. **94150** (Vital Capacity Measurement)
3. **94060** (Pulmonology, Diagnostic; Spirometry)

Exercise 13-11
1. **95065** (Allergy Tests, Nose Allergy)
2. **95004 × 10** (Allergy Tests, Skin Tests, Allergen Extract) (Note that one unit is used for each test.)
3. **95115** (Allergen Immunotherapy, Allergen, Injection)

Exercise 13-12
1. nasal continuous positive airway pressure
2. electroencephalogram
3. electromyogram
4. electro-oculogram
5. **95816** (Electroencephalography)
6. **95863** (Electromyography, Needle; Extremities)
7. **95851 × 2** (both legs) (Range of Motion Test, Extremities or Trunk)

Exercise 13-13
1. **96110** (Developmental Testing)
2. **96101** (MMPI)
3. **96116** (Cognitive Function Tests)

Exercise 13-14
1. **96440** (Chemotherapy, Pleural Cavity)
2. **96521** (Chemotherapy, Pump Services, Portable)
3. **96401** (Chemotherapy, Subcutaneous)
4. **96413** (Chemotherapy, Intravenous)
5. **96450** (Chemotherapy, CNS)

Exercise 13-15
1. **99241-25** (Consultation, Office and/or Other Outpatient); **96900** (Ultraviolet Light Therapy, for Dermatology)
2. **99244-25** (Consultation, Office and/or Other Outpatient); **96913** (Photo-chemotherapy)

Exercise 13-16
1. **97010** (Physical Medicine/Therapy/Occupational Therapy, Modalities, Hot or Cold Pack)
2. **97761 × 2** (Physical Medicine/Therapy/Occupational Therapy, Prosthetic Training)
3. **97116 × 2** (Physical Medicine/Therapy/Occupational Therapy, Procedures, Gait Training) (Note that the stand-alone code 97110 specifies "each 15 minutes.")

Exercise 13-17
1. **98940** (Chiropractic Treatment, Spinal, Extraspinal)
2. **98925** (Osteopathic Manipulation)

Exercise 13-18
1. **99050** (Special Services, After Hours Medical Services)
2. **99000** (Special Services, Specimen Handling)
3. **99070** (Special Services, Supply of Materials)

Exercise 13-19
1. into the subarachnoid space
2. into a vein
3. into a muscle
4. under the skin
5. through the respiratory system

Exercise 13-20
1. a. Current Procedural Terminology, Level I
   b. National Codes, Level II
2. K, G, Q, S
3. No
4. J codes
5. oral
6. E codes
7. a. NU
   b. E2
   c. AM

8. IM
9. up to 5 mg
10. J1730
11. E0950

CHAPTER 14

Exercise 14-1

1. morbidity or sickness; mortality or death rate
2. ICD-9
3. Clinical Modification
4. Any four of the following six:
   a. facilitate payment of health services
   b. evaluate patients' use of health care facilities (utilization patterns)
   c. study health care costs
   d. research the quality of health care
   e. predict health care trends
   f. plan for future health care needs
5. diagnosis, procedure

Exercise 14-2

1. f
2. g
3. a
4. i
5. h
6. l
7. j
8. e
9. d
10. k
11. b
12. c
13. false
14. true

Exercise 14-3

1. f
2. b
3. c
4. d
5. a
6. e
7. g
8. *See also*

Exercise 14-4

1. 175.0
2. 217

Exercise 14-5	1. 980.0, E980.9
	2. 989.89, E980.9
	3. 969.4, E853.2
	4. Due to drugs and medicines
Exercise 14-6	1. Endocrine, Nutritional and Metabolic Disease, and Immunity Disorders
	2. Disorders of Thyroid Gland
	3. Simple and unspecified goiter
	4. Goiter, specified as simple
Exercise 14-7	1. **711.06**
	2. no
	3. by adding fourth and fifth digits to the codes
Exercise 14-8	1. Contact, smallpox; **V01.3**
	2. Vaccination, prophylactic, smallpox; **V04.1**
	3. History, personal, malignant neoplasm, tongue; **V10.01**
Exercise 14-9	1. Derailment, railway; **E802.0**
	2. Accident, motor vehicle, not involving collision; **E816.0**
	3. Collision, off-road vehicle and other object, fixed; **E821.1**
	4. Collision, animal being ridden; **E828.2**
	5. Collision, watercraft, causing, injury; **E831.1**
Exercise 14-10	1. a. Appendix B
	b. Appendix D
	c. Appendix A
	d. Appendix E
	e. Appendix C
	2. Appendix D: Industrial Accidents
Exercise 14-11	1. Obstetrical Procedures
	2. Miscellaneous Diagnostic and Therapeutic Procedures
	3. Procedures and Interventions, Not Elsewhere Classified
Exercise 14-12	1. referring to a vein
	2. pertaining to the lungs or pulmonary artery
	3. the joining together of two openings
	4. pertaining to the heart and lungs
	5. circulation that occurs outside of the body
	6. a surgical procedure that joins the superior vena cava and pulmonary artery
	7. takes over the heart and lung functions of the patient during the surgical procedure
Exercise 14-13	1. **45.24** (Sigmoidoscopy, flexible)
	2. **63.73** (Vasectomy)
	3. **76.73** (Reduction, fracture, maxilla)

4. **99.04** (Transfusion, packed cells)

5. **21.03** (Cauterization, nose)

CHAPTER 15

Exercise 15-1

1. category code, subcategory code, subclassification code
2. category code, subcategory code, subclassification code

Exercise 15-2

1. **482.2** (Pneumonia, due to, *Haemophilus influenzae*)
2. **112.0** (Thrush)
3. **008.45** (Enteritis, *Clostridium difficile*)
4. **437.2** (Hypertension, cerebrovascular disease)
5. **823.82** (Fracture, tibia (closed), with fibula)

Exercise 15-3

1. **601.1** (Prostatitis, chronic); **041.00** (Infection, streptococcal) [in this order]
2. **466.0** (Bronchitis, with acute or subacute); **041.7** (Infection, *Pseudomonas* NEC) [in this order]
3. **250.71** (Diabetes, with gangrene); **785.4** (Gangrene) [in this order]
4. **599.0** (Infection, urinary [tract] NEC); **041.4** (Infection, *Escherichia coli* NEC) [in this order]
5. **277.39** (Cardiomyopathy, amyloid); **425.7** (Cardiomyopathy, metabolic NEC, amyloid)

Exercise 15-4

1. **434.91** (Stroke, in evolution)
2. **291.0** (Impending, delirium tremens)
3. **640.03** (Threatened, miscarriage)
4. **644.13** (Labor, threatened)
5. **411.1** (Impending, coronary, syndrome)

Exercise 15-5

1. No answer required
2. a. Pyelonephritis, acute
   b. Acute, **590.10**
   c. **590,** Infections of kidney
   d. no
   e. **590.10**
   f. because flank pain and hematuria are symptoms of pyelonephritis

Exercise 15-6

1. No answer required
2. a. disseminated lupus erythematosus 710.0 [*424.91*]
   b. **710.0** and **[*424.91*]**
   c. Diffuse disease of connective tissue
   d. all collagen diseases whose effects are not mainly confined to a single system
   e. endocarditis **[*424.91*]**
   f. **710.0**
   g. **710.0, 424.91**

Exercise 15-7
1. No answer required
2. a. open fracture of the right humerus and distal femur
   b. Fracture
   c. humerus
   d. (closed); **812.30** (Note that "open 812.30" is a subterm under "humerus open")
   e. Yes, because the patient record did not specify the exact location of the fracture of the humerus, so the "unspecified part of the humerus, open" is as specific as you can get with the information that you have available.
   f. femur
   g. (closed)
   h. distal or distal end
   i. see Fracture, femur, lower end
   j. open
   k. 821.30
   l. yes

Exercise 15-8
1. No answer necessary
2. a. menometrorrhagia
   b. **626.2**
   c. anemia
   d. **285.1**

Exercise 15-9
1. No answer necessary
2. a. Fracture
   b. *see also* Fracture, by site
   c. **198.5**

Exercise 15-10
1. a. **719.46**
   b. **717.0**
   c. **717.6**

Exercise 15-11
1. a. **V71.4**
   b. **913.0**
2. a. **V71.5** (Rape)

Exercise 15-12
1. a. **574.10** (Cholelithiasis with cholecystitis, chronic, with, calculus, gallbladder)
   b. **486** (Pneumonia)
   c. Contraindicated
   d. **V64.1** (Procedure not done because of, contraindicated)
2. a. 2; sterilization and surgery not done
   b. **V25.2** (Admission for sterilization)
   c. Procedure not done because of, patient's decision *V64.2*

Exercise 15-13
1. **V53.31** (Cardiac, device, pacemaker, cardiac, fitting or adjustment)
2. **V25.5** (Insertion, subdermal implantable contraceptive)

    3. **V10.46** (History, personal, malignant neoplasm, prostate)

    4. **V06.4** (Vaccination, mumps, with measles and rubella [MMR])

    5. **V76.12** (Screening, mammogram)

    6. **V70.5** (Examination, medical, pre-employment)

Exercise 15-14

1. scars, face; third-degree burns
2. constrictive pericarditis; tuberculosis infection
3. foreign body, femur; gunshot injury, femur
4. mental retardation; poliomyelitis
5. leg pain; fracture, femur

Exercise 15-15

1. arthritis, ankle, traumatic, **716.17** (Arthritis, traumatic); fracture, ankle, **905.4** (Late, effect(s) (of), fracture, extremity, lower)
2. aphasia (Note that there is no code for residual because there is one code for residual and cause); cerebrovascular accident, **438.11** (Late effect(s) (of), cerebrovascular disease with aphasia)
3. deafness, sensorineural, **389.10** (Deafness, sensorineural); meningitis, **326** (Late effect(s) (of), Meningitis, unspecified cause)

Exercise 15-16

1. **008.8** (Gastroenteritis, viral NEC)
2. **038.43** (Septicemia, *Pseudomonas*); **995.92** (Sepsis); **785.52** (Septic, shock)
3. **045.90** (Poliomyelitis, unspecified type)
4. **112.1** (Candidiasis, vagina)

Exercise 15-17

1. i
2. c
3. h
4. g
5. a
6. b
7. e
8. f
9. d

Exercise 15-18

1. **V58.11** (Chemotherapy, encounter for); **183.0** (Neoplasm, ovary, primary) (Although you were not directed to code the procedure, the code for the injection of the chemotherapy agent would be 99.25.)
2. **V58.0** (Admission, radiation management); **198.5** (Neoplasm, bone, secondary); **V10.3** (History (of), malignant neoplasm (of), breast) (Although you were not directed to code the procedure, the code for the radiation would be 99.29.)
3. a. metastatic carcinoma of bronchus

    b. primary, unknown

    c. secondary

    d. **197.0** (Neoplasm, lung, main bronchus, secondary); **199.1** (Neoplasm, unknown site or unspecified, primary)

4. a. Two, plus an E code

   b. Uncontrolled nausea and vomiting

   c. Lung cancer

   d. **787.01** (Nausea, with vomiting)

   e. **162.9** (Neoplasm, lung, primary); **E933.1** (Table of Drugs and Chemicals, Antineoplastic agents, Therapeutic Use)

Exercise 15-19

1. **203.00** (Myeloma, multiple); **M9730/3** (Myeloma)

2. **233.1** (Neoplasm, cervix); **M8010/2** (Carcinoma, in situ)

3. **153.3** (Neoplasm, intestinal, colon, sigmoid, primary); **M8000/3** (Cancer); **197.6** (Neoplasm, peritoneum, secondary); **M8000/6** (Metastasis, cancer, to specified site)

4. **185** (Neoplasm, prostate, primary); **M8140/3** (Adenocarcinoma, primary); **198.5** (Neoplasm, bone, secondary); **M8140/6** (Adenocarcinoma)

5. **198.3** (Neoplasm, brain, secondary); **M8000/6** (Metastasis, cancer, to specified site); **199.1** (Neoplasm, unknown, primary); **M8000/3** (Cancer primary)

6. **197.0** (Neoplasm, lung, secondary); **V10.3** (History (of), malignant neoplasm (of), breast (Note: This is personal history, not family history [V16.3])); **M8010/6** (Carcinoma, secondary)

Exercise 15-20

1. **255.41** (Disease, Addison's)

2. **276.51** (Dehydration)

3. **250.30** (Diabetes, coma, hypoglycemic)

4. **242.01** (Goiter, toxic, with mention of thyrotoxic crisis or storm)

Exercise 15-21

1. **281.0** (Anemia, pernicious)

2. **286.6** (Coagulation, intravascular)

3. **286.0** (Hemophilia)

4. **285.1** (Anemia, blood loss, acute)

5. **289.6** (Polycythemia, familial)

Exercise 15-22

1. **331.0** (Alzheimer's, disease or sclerosis); **294.11** (Alzheimer's, dementia, with behavior disturbance) [in this order]

2. **300.4** (Depression, anxiety)

3. **318.2** (Retardation, mental, profound, IQ under 20)

4. **307.1** (Anorexia, nervosa)

5. **291.0** (Delirium, withdrawal, alcoholic, acute); **303.91** (Dependence, alcohol, alcoholic)

Exercise 15-23

1. **320.82** (Meningitis, *Proteus morganii*)

2. **340** (Sclerosis, multiple)

3. **382.9** (Otitis, media, acute)

4. **365.11** (Glaucoma, chronic, open angle)

5. **351.0** (Palsy, Bell's)

Exercise 15-24
1. **428.0** (Failure, heart, congestive)
2. **410.71** (Infarction, subendocardial)
3. **446.0** (Periarteritis); **405.99** (Hypertension, due to, periarteritis nodosa)
4. **434.01** (Infarction, brain, thrombotic)
5. **430** (Hemorrhage, subarachnoid)

Exercise 15-25
1. **464.4** (Croup)
2. **428.0** (Failure, heart, congestive); **518.81** (Respiratory, failure)
3. **491.20** (Disease, lung, obstructive with, bronchitis)
4. **487.1** (Influenza, with, bronchitis)
5. **482.2** (Pneumonia, due to, *Hemophilus influenzae*)

Exercise 15-26
1. **540.0** (Appendicitis, with perforation, peritonitis or rupture)
2. **532.00** (Ulcer, duodenum, acute, with hemorrhage)
3. **574.00** (Cholelithiasis, with cholecystitis, acute); **574.10** (Cholelithiasis, with cholecystitis, chronic) Note acute before chronic.
4. **558.9** (Gastroenteritis)
5. **530.81** (Reflux, gastroesophageal)

Exercise 15-27
1. **614.9** (Disease, pelvis, inflammatory)
2. **599.70** (Hematuria)
3. **590.10** (Pyelonephritis, acute); **590.00** (Pyelonephritis, chronic) Note acute before chronic.
4. **600.00** (Hypertrophy, prostatic, benign)
5. **610.1** (Disease, breast, fibrocystic)

Exercise 15-28
1. **631** (Blighted ovum)
2. **634.91** (Abortion, spontaneous); hospital would also report **69.02** (Dilation and curettage, uterus, after, abortion)
3. **644.13** (Labor, false)
4. **664.31** (Laceration, perineum, complicating delivery, fourth degree); **V27.0** (Outcome of delivery, single, liveborn); hospital would also report **75.69** (Repair, perineum, laceration, obstetric, current)
5. **660.11** (Delivery, complicated by, deformity, fetus, causing obstructed labor); **653.41** (Delivery, complicated, cephalopelvic disproportion); **V27.0** (Outcome of delivery, single, liveborn); hospital would also report **74.1** (Cesarean section, lower uterine segment)

Exercise 15-29
1. **698.9** (Pruritus)
2. **705.1** (Rash, heat)
3. **696.1** (Psoriasis)
4. **707.05** (Ulcer, skin, decubitus buttock)
5. **692.6** (Dermatitis, due to, poison ivy)

Exercise 15-30
1. **714.0** (Arthritis, rheumatoid)
2. **723.1** (Pain, neck)

3. **718.31** (Dislocation, shoulder, recurrent)

4. **733.11** (Fracture, pathologic, humerus); **198.5** (Neoplasm, bone, secondary); **V10.3** (History (of), malignant neoplasm, breast)

Exercise 15-31

1. **744.21** (Absence, ear, lobe)

2. **V30.00** (Newborn, single, born in hospital, without mention of cesarean delivery or section); **752.51** (Undescended, testis)

3. **759.83** (Syndrome, fragile X)

4. **754.30** (Dislocation, hip, congenital)

Exercise 15-32

1. **780.91** (Fussy infant)

2. **786.52** (Pain, chest, wall)

3. **793.80** (Abnormal, mammogram)

4. **780.39** (Seizure)

5. **796.2** (Blood, pressure, high, incidental reading, without diagnosis of hypertension)

Exercise 15-33

1. **942.33** (Burn, abdomen, third degree); **945.26** (Burn, thigh, second degree); **E924.0** (Burning, hot, liquid); **948.11**—15% with 10% 3rd degree

2. **945.36** (Burn, thigh, third degree); **958.3** (Burn, infected); **948.00**—4½% (No E code is required for subsequent treatment.)

3. **945.22** (Burn, foot, second degree) (Note that only the highest level burn is coded when burns are in the same area); **E897** (Fire, controlled, bonfire); **948.00**—2¼%

4. **944.30** (Burn, hand, third degree); **948.00**—2¼% (No E code is required for subsequent treatment.)

5. **942.32** (Burn, chest wall, third degree); **943.21** (Burn, forearm, second degree); **944.11** (Burn, finger, first degree); **948.00**—5% [in this order] (No E code is required for subsequent treatment.)

Exercise 15-34

1. **996.69** (Complications, breast implants, infection or inflammation)

2. **996.85** (Rejection, transplant, bone marrow)

3. **998.59** (Abscess, stitch)

4. **996.01** (Complications, mechanical, implant, electrode NEC, cardiac)

Exercise 15-35

1. history of hysterectomy

2. history of peptic ulcer disease

Exercise 15-36

1. chest pain, shortness of breath

2. hip pain, contusion of hip

3. No; the patient did not require any of the five items that would substantiate use of additional resources (unless hospital policy dictates otherwise).

4. Yes; additional laboratory studies were done, and treatment (transfusion) was provided.

5. No; diagnoses are not made from laboratory values

Exercise 15-37	1. 9
	2. 1
	3. 5
	4. 0
	5. 7
	6. 0

Exercise 15-38	1. 7
	2. L
	3. M
	4. G
	5. N
	6. 1
	7. R
	8. 4
	9. T
	10. 8

Exercise 15-39	1. transfer
	2. resection
	3. inspection
	4. transplantation
	5. insertion
	6. removal
	7. fragmentation
	8. occlusion
	9. revision
	10. release

Exercise 15-40	1. complete
	2. expandable
	3. multiaxial
	4. standardized in terminology
	5. 7
	6. alphanumeric
	7. 34
	8. O and I
	9. procedure

CHAPTER 16

Exercise 16-1	1. the government
	2. 1965
	3. A
	4. B

Exercise 16-2
1. October
2. November or December
3. Department of Health and Human Services
4. ~~January 29, 2008~~ *Mar 24, 2008*
5. Long-term care hospitals
6. Tzui Hefter

Exercise 16-3
1. No (because 850.11 has 851.32 listed as a C/C)
2. No (because 839.03 has 847.0 listed as a C/C)
3. Yes (because 839.16 does not have 900.02 listed as a C/C)
4. Yale
5. New Jersey

Exercise 16-4
1. TEFRA
2. Medicare beneficiaries
3. Medically, setting, coded
4. MACs

Exercise 16-5
1. Resource-Based Relative Value Scale
2. the *Federal Register*
3. OBRA

Exercise 16-6
1. Ambulatory Payment Classification
2. 2000
3. 20%
4. Discontinued

1995 Guidelines for E/M Services

I. INTRODUCTION

What Is Documentation and Why Is It Important?

Medical record documentation is required to record pertinent facts, findings, and observations about an individual's health history including past and present illnesses, examinations, tests, treatments, and outcomes. The medical record chronologically documents the care of the patient and is an important element contributing to high quality care. The medical record facilitates:

- the ability of the physician and other health care professionals to evaluate and plan the patient's immediate treatment, and to monitor his/her health care over time.
- communication and continuity of care among physicians and other health care professionals involved in the patient's care;
- accurate and timely claims review and payment;
- appropriate utilization review and quality of care evaluations; and
- collection of data that may be useful for research and education.

An appropriately documented medical record can reduce many of the "hassles" associated with claims processing and may serve as a legal document to verify the care provided, if necessary.

What Do Payers Want and Why?

Because payers have a contractual obligation to enrollees, they may require reasonable documentation that services are consistent with the insurance coverage provided. They may request information to validate:

- the site of service;
- the medical necessity and appropriateness of the diagnostic and/or therapeutic services provided; and/or
- that services provided have been accurately reported.

II. GENERAL PRINCIPLES OF MEDICAL RECORD DOCUMENTATION

The principles of documentation listed below are applicable to all types of medical and surgical services in all settings. For Evaluation and Management (E/M) services, the nature and amount of physician work and documentation varies by type of service, place of service and the patient's status. The general principles listed below may be modified to account for these variable circumstances in providing E/M services.

1. The medical record should be complete and legible.

2. The documentation of each patient encounter should include:

   ▪ reason for the encounter and relevant history, physical examination findings and prior diagnostic test results;

   ▪ assessment, clinical impression or diagnosis;

   ▪ plan for care; and

   ▪ date and legible identity of the observer.

3. If not documented, the rationale for ordering diagnostic and other ancillary services should be easily inferred.

4. Past and present diagnoses should be accessible to the treating and/or consulting physician.

5. Appropriate health risk factors should be identified.

6. The patient's progress, response to and changes in treatment, and revision of diagnosis should be documented.

7. The CPT and ICD-9-CM codes reported on the health insurance claim form or billing statement should be supported by the documentation in the medical record.

III. DOCUMENTATION OF E/M SERVICES

This publication provides definitions and documentation guidelines for the three **key** components of E/M services and for visits which consist predominately of counseling or coordination of care. The three key components—history, examination, and medical decision making—appear in the descriptors for office and other outpatient services, hospital observation services, hospital inpatient services, consultations, emergency department services, nursing facility services, domiciliary care services, and home services. While some of the text of CPT has been repeated in this publication, the reader should refer to CPT for the complete descriptors for E/M services and instructions for selecting a level of service.

Documentation guidelines are identified by the symbol •DG.

The descriptors for the levels of E/M services recognize seven components which are used in defining the levels of E/M services. These components are:

▪ history;

▪ examination;

▪ medical decision making;

▪ counseling;

▪ coordination of care;

▪ nature of presenting problem; and

▪ time.

The first three of these components (i.e., history, examination and medical decision making) are the **key** components in selecting the level of E/M services. An exception to this rule is the case of visits which consist predominantly of counseling or coordination of care; for these services time is the key or controlling factor to qualify for a particular level of E/M service.

For certain groups of patients, the recorded information may vary slightly from that described here. Specifically, the medical records of infants, children, adolescents and pregnant women may have additional or modified information recorded in each history and examination area.

As an example, newborn records may include under history of the present illness (HPI) the details of mother's pregnancy and the infant's status at birth; social history will focus on family structure; family history will focus on congenital anomalies and hereditary disorders in the family. In addition, information on growth and development and/or nutrition will be recorded. Although not specifically defined in these documentation guidelines, these patient group variations on history and examination are appropriate.

A. Documentation of History

The levels of E/M services are based on four types of history (Problem Focused, Expanded Problem Focused, Detailed, and Comprehensive.) Each type of history includes some or all of the following elements:

- Chief complaint (CC);
- History of present illness (HPI);
- Review of systems (ROS); and
- Past, family and/or social history (PFSH).

The extent of history of present illness, review of systems and past, family and/or social history that is obtained and documented is dependent upon clinical judgement and the nature of the presenting problem(s).

The chart below shows the progression of the elements required for each type of history. To qualify for a given type of history, **all three elements in the table must be met.** (A chief complaint is indicated at all levels.)

MEDICAL AND SURGICAL ROOT OPERATIONS

History of Present Illness (HPI)	Review of Systems (ROS)	Past, Family, and/ or Social History (PFSH)	Type of History
Brief	N/A	N/A	*Problem Focused*
Brief	Problem Pertinent	N/A	*Expanded Problem Focused*
Extended	Extended	Pertinent	*Detailed*
Extended	Complete	Complete	*Comprehensive*

•*DG: The CC, ROS and PFSH may be listed as separate elements of history, or they may be included in the description of the history of the present illness.*

•*DG: A ROS and/or a PFSH obtained during an earlier encounter does not need to be re-recorded if there is evidence that the physician reviewed and updated the previous information. This may occur when a physician updates his or her own record or in an institutional setting or group practice where many physicians use a common record. The review and update may be documented by:*

- *describing any new ROS and/or PFSH information or noting there has been no change in the information; and*
- *noting the date and location of the earlier ROS and/or PFSH.*

•*DG: The ROS and/or PFSH may be recorded by ancillary staff or on a form completed by the patient. To document that the physician reviewed the information, there must be a notation supplementing or confirming the information recorded by others.*

•*DG: If the physician is unable to obtain a history from the patient or other source, the record should describe the patient's condition or other circumstance which precludes obtaining a history.*

Definitions and specific documentation guidelines for each of the elements of history are listed below.

Chief Complaint (CC). The CC is a concise statement describing the symptom, problem, condition, diagnosis, physician recommended return, or other factor that is the reason for the encounter.

•*DG: The medical record should clearly reflect the chief complaint.*

History of Present Illness (HPI). The HPI is a chronological description of the development of the patient's present illness from the first sign and/or symptom or from the previous encounter to the present. It includes the following elements:

- location,
- quality,
- severity,
- duration,
- timing,
- context,
- modifying factors, and
- associated signs and symptoms.

Brief and ***extended*** HPIs are distinguished by the amount of detail needed to accurately characterize the clinical problem(s).

A ***brief*** HPI consists of one to three elements of the HPI.

•*DG:* The medical record should describe one to three elements of the present illness (HPI).

An ***extended*** HPI consists of four or more elements of the HPI.

•*DG: The medical record should describe four or more elements of the present illness (HPI) or associated comorbidities.*

Review of Systems (ROS). A ROS is an inventory of body systems obtained through a series of questions seeking to identify signs and/or symptoms which the patient may be experiencing or has experienced. For purposes of ROS, the following systems are recognized:

- Constitutional symptoms (e.g., fever, weight loss)
- Eyes
- Ears, Nose, Mouth, Throat
- Cardiovascular
- Respiratory
- Gastrointestinal
- Genitourinary
- Musculoskeletal
- Integumentary (skin and/or breast)
- Neurological
- Psychiatric
- Endocrine
- Hematologic/Lymphatic
- Allergic/Immunologic

A ***problem pertinent*** ROS inquires about the system directly related to the problem(s) identified in the HPI.

•*DG: The patient's positive responses and pertinent negatives for the system related to the problem should be documented.*

An ***extended*** ROS inquires about the system directly related to the problem(s) identified in the HPI and a limited number of additional systems.

•*DG: The patient's positive responses and pertinent negatives for two to nine systems should be documented.*

A ***complete*** ROS inquires about the system(s) directly related to the problem(s) identified in the HPI <u>plus</u> all additional body systems.

•*DG: At least ten organ systems must be reviewed. Those systems with positive or pertinent negative responses must be individually documented. For the remaining systems, a notation indicating all other systems are negative is permissible. In the absence of such a notation, at least ten systems must be individually documented.*

Past, Family and/or Social History (PFSH). The PFSH consists of a review of three areas:

- past history (the patient's past experiences with illnesses, operations, injuries and treatments);
- family history (a review of medical events in the patient's family, including diseases which may be hereditary or place the patient at risk); and
- social history (an age appropriate review of past and current activities).

For the categories of subsequent hospital care, follow-up inpatient consultations and subsequent nursing facility care, CPT requires only an "interval" history. It is not necessary to record information about the PFSH.

A ***pertinent*** PFSH is a review of the history area(s) directly related to the problem(s) identified in the HPI.

•*DG: At least one specific item from <u>any</u> of the three history areas must be documented for a pertinent PFSH .*

A ***complete*** PFSH is of a review of two or all three of the PFSH history areas, depending on the category of the E/M service. A review of all three history areas is required for services that by their nature include a comprehensive assessment or reassessment of the patient. A review of two of the three history areas is sufficient for other services.

•*DG At least one specific item from <u>two</u> of the three history areas must be documented for a complete PFSH for the following categories of E/M services: office or other outpatient services, established patient; emergency department; subsequent nursing facility care; domiciliary care, established patient; and home care, established patient.*

•*DG: At least one specific item from <u>each</u> of the three history areas must be documented for a complete PFSH for the following categories of E/M services: office or other outpatient services, new patient; hospital observation services; hospital inpatient services, initial care; consultations; comprehensive nursing facility assessments; domiciliary care, new patient; and home care, new patient.*

B. Documentation of Examination

The levels of E/M services are based on four types of examination that are defined as follows:

- ***Problem Focused***—a limited examination of the affected body area or organ system.
- ***Expanded Problem Focused***—a limited examination of the affected body area or organ system and other symptomatic or related organ system(s).

- **Detailed**—an extended examination of the affected body area(s) and other symptomatic or related organ system(s).
- **Comprehensive**—a general multi-system examination or complete examination of a single organ system.

For purposes of examination, the following **body areas** are recognized:

- Head, including the face
- Neck
- Chest, including breasts and axillae
- Abdomen
- Genitalia, groin, buttocks
- Back, including spine
- Each extremity

For purposes of examination, the following **organ systems** are recognized:

- Constitutional (e.g., vital signs, general appearance)
- Eyes
- Ears, nose, mouth and throat
- Cardiovascular
- Respiratory
- Gastrointestinal
- Genitourinary
- Musculoskeletal
- Skin
- Neurologic
- Psychiatric
- Hematologic/lymphatic/immunologic

The extent of examinations performed and documented is dependent upon clinical judgement and the nature of the presenting problem(s). They range from limited examinations of single body areas to general multi-system or complete single organ system examinations.

•*DG: Specific abnormal and relevant negative findings of the examination of the affected or symptomatic body area(s) or organ system(s) should be documented. A notation of "abnormal" without elaboration is insufficient.*

•*DG: Abnormal or unexpected findings of the examination of the unaffected or asymptomatic body area(s) or organ system(s) should be described.*

•*DG: A brief statement or notation indicating "negative" or "normal" is sufficient to document normal findings related to unaffected area(s) or asymptomatic organ system(s).*

•*DG: The medical record for a general multi-system examination should include findings about 8 or more of the 12 organ systems.*

C. Documentation of the Complexity of Medical Decision Making

The levels of E/M services recognize four types of medical decision making (straight-forward, low complexity, moderate complexity and high complexity). Medical decision making refers to the complexity of establishing a diagnosis and/or selecting a management option as measured by:

- the number of possible diagnoses and/or the number of management options that must be considered;
- the amount and/or complexity of medical records, diagnostic tests, and /or other information that must be obtained, reviewed and analyzed; and

- the risk of significant complications, morbidity and/or mortality, as well as comorbidities, associated with the patient's presenting problem(s), the diagnostic procedure(s) and/or the possible management options.

The chart below shows the progression of the elements required for each level of medical decision making. To qualify for a given type of decision making, **two of the three elements in the table must be either met or exceeded**. Each of the elements of medical decision making is described below.

MEDICAL AND SURGICAL ROOT OPERATIONS

Number of diagnoses or management options	Amount and/or complexity of data to be reviewed	Risk of complications and/or morbidity or mortality	Type of decision making
Minimal	Minimal or None	Minimal	*Straightforward*
Limited	Limited	Low	*Low Complexity*
Multiple	Moderate	Moderate	*Moderate Complexity*
Extensive	Extensive	High	*High Complexity*

Number of Diagnoses or Management Options. The number of possible diagnoses and/or the number of management options that must be considered is based on the number and types of problems addressed during the encounter, the complexity of establishing a diagnosis and the management decisions that are made by the physician.

Generally, decision making with respect to a diagnosed problem is easier than that for an identified but undiagnosed problem. The number and type of diagnostic tests employed may be an indicator of the number of possible diagnoses. Problems which are improving or resolving are less complex than those which are worsening or failing to change as expected. The need to seek advice from others is another indicator of complexity of diagnostic or management problems.

> •DG: For each encounter, an assessment, clinical impression, or diagnosis should be documented. It may be explicitly stated or implied in documented decisions regarding management plans and/or further evaluation.
>
> - For a presenting problem with an established diagnosis the record should reflect whether the problem is: a) improved, well controlled, resolving or resolved; or, b) inadequately controlled, worsening, or failing to change as expected.
> - For a presenting problem without an established diagnosis, the assessment or clinical impression may be stated in the form of a differential diagnoses or as "possible", "probable", or "rule out" (R/O) diagnoses.
>
> •DG: The initiation of, or changes in, treatment should be documented. Treatment includes a wide range of management options including patient instructions, nursing instructions, therapies, and medications.
>
> •DG: If referrals are made, consultations requested or advice sought, the record should indicate to whom or where the referral or consultation is made or from whom the advice is requested.

Amount and/or Complexity of Data to be Reviewed. The amount and complexity of data to be reviewed is based on the types of diagnostic testing ordered or reviewed. A decision to obtain and review old medical records and/or obtain history from sources other than the patient increases the amount and complexity of data to be reviewed.

Discussion of contradictory or unexpected test results with the physician who performed or interpreted the test is an indication of the complexity of data being reviewed. On occasion the physician who ordered a test may personally review the image, tracing or specimen to supplement information from the physician who prepared the test report or interpretation; this is another indication of the complexity of data being reviewed.

•*DG: If a diagnostic service (test or procedure) is ordered, planned, scheduled, or performed at the time of the E/M encounter, the type of service, eg, lab or x-ray, should be documented.*

•*DG: The review of lab, radiology and/or other diagnostic tests should be documented. An entry in a progress note such as "WBC elevated" or "chest x-ray unremarkable" is acceptable. Alternatively, the review may be documented by initialing and dating the report containing the test results.*

•*DG: A decision to obtain old records or decision to obtain additional history from the family, caretaker or other source to supplement that obtained from the patient should be documented.*

•*DG: Relevant finding from the review of old records, and/or the receipt of additional history from the family, caretaker or other source should be documented. If there is no relevant information beyond that already obtained, that fact should be documented. A notation of "Old records reviewed" or "additional history obtained from family" without elaboration is insufficient.*

•*DG: The results of discussion of laboratory, radiology or other diagnostic tests with the physician who performed or interpreted the study should be documented.*

•*DG: The direct visualization and independent interpretation of an image, tracing or specimen previously or subsequently interpreted by another physician should be documented.*

Risk of Significant Complications, Morbidity, and/or Mortality. The risk of significant complications, morbidity, and/or mortality is based on the risks associated with the presenting problem(s), the diagnostic procedure(s), and the possible management options.

•*DG: Comorbidities/underlying diseases or other factors that increase the complexity of medical decision making by increasing the risk of complications, morbidity, and/or mortality should be documented.*

•*DG: If a surgical or invasive diagnostic procedure is ordered, planned or scheduled at the time of the E/M encounter, the type of procedure, eg, laparoscopy, should be documented.*

•*DG: If a surgical or invasive diagnostic procedure is performed at the time of the E/M encounter, the specific procedure should be documented.*

•*DG: The referral for or decision to perform a surgical or invasive diagnostic procedure on an urgent basis should be documented or implied.*

The following table may be used to help determine whether the risk of significant complications, morbidity, and/or mortality is *minimal, low, moderate,* or *high*. Because the determination of risk is complex and not readily quantifiable, the table includes common clinical examples rather than absolute measures of risk. The assessment of risk of the presenting problem(s) is based on the risk related to the disease process anticipated between the present encounter and the next one. The assessment of risk of selecting diagnostic procedures and management options is based on the risk during and immediately following any procedures or treatment. The highest level of risk in any one category (presenting problem(s), diagnostic procedure(s), or management options) determines the overall risk.

TABLE OF RISK

Level of Risk	Presenting Problem(s)	Diagnostic Procedure(s) Ordered	Management Options Selected
Minimal	• One self-limited or minor problem, eg, cold, insect bite, tinea corporis	• Laboratory tests requiring venipuncture • Chest x-rays • EKG/EEG • Urinalysis • Ultrasound, eg, echocardiography • KOH prep	• Rest • Gargles • Elastic bandages • Superficial dressings
Low	• Two or more self-limited or minor problems • One stable chronic illness, eg, well controlled hypertension, non-insulin dependent diabetes, cataract, BPH • Acute uncomplicated illness or injury, eg, cystitis, allergic rhinitis, simple sprain	• Physiologic tests not under stress, eg, pulmonary function tests • Non-cardiovascular imaging studies with contrast, eg, barium enema • Superficial needle biopsies • Clinical laboratory tests requiring arterial puncture • Skin biopsies	• Over-the-counter drugs • Minor surgery with no identified risk factors • Physical therapy • Occupational therapy • IV fluids without additives
Moderate	• One or more chronic illnesses with mild exacerbation, progression, or side effects of treatment • Two or more stable chronic illnesses • Undiagnosed new problem with uncertain prognosis, eg, lump in breast • Acute illness with systemic symptoms, eg, pyelonephritis, pneumonitis, colitis • Acute complicated injury, eg, head injury with brief loss of consciousness	• Physiologic tests under stress, eg, cardiac stress test, fetal contraction stress test • Diagnostic endoscopies with no identified risk factors • Deep needle or incisional biopsy • Cardiovascular imaging studies with contrast and no identified risk factors, eg, arteriogram, cardiac catheterization • Obtain fluid from body cavity, eg, lumbar puncture, thoracentesis, culdocentesis	• Minor surgery with identified risk factors • Elective major surgery (open, percutaneous or endoscopic) with no identified risk factors • Prescription drug management • Therapeutic nuclear medicine • IV fluids with additives • Closed treatment of fracture or dislocation without manipulation
High	• One or more chronic illnesses with severe exacerbation, progression, or side effects of treatment • Acute or chronic illnesses or injuries that pose a threat to life or bodily function, eg, multiple trauma, acute MI, pulmonary embolus, severe respiratory distress, progressive severe rheumatoid arthritis, psychiatric illness with potential threat to self or others, peritonitis, acute renal failure • An abrupt change in neurologic status, eg, seizure, TIA, weakness, sensory loss	• Cardiovascular imaging studies with contrast with identified risk factors • Cardiac electrophysiological tests • Diagnostic endoscopies with identified risk factors • Discography	• Elective major surgery (open, percutaneous or endoscopic) with identified risk factors • Emergency major surgery (open, percutaneous or endoscopic) • Parenteral controlled substances • Drug therapy requiring intensive monitoring for toxicity • Decision not to resuscitate or to de-escalate care because of poor prognosis

D. Documentation of an Encounter Dominated by Counseling or Coordination of Care

In the case where counseling and/or coordination of care dominates (more than 50%) of the physician/patient and/or family encounter (face-to-face time in the office or other outpatient setting or floor/unit time in the hospital or nursing facility), time is considered the key or controlling factor to qualify for a particular level of E/M services.

•*DG: If the physician elects to report the level of service based on counseling and/or coordination of care, the total length of time of the encounter (face-to-face or floor time, as appropriate) should be documented and the record should describe the counseling and/or activities to coordinate care.*

1997 Documentation Guidelines for Evaluation and Management Services*

Table of Contents

*Developed jointly by the American Medical Association (AMA) and the Health Care Financing Administration (HCFA) (now Centers for Medicare and Medicaid Services).

I. INTRODUCTION

What Is Documentation and Why Is It Important?

Medical record documentation is required to record pertinent facts, findings, and observations about an individual's health history including past and present illnesses, examinations, tests, treatments, and outcomes. The medical record chronologically documents the care of the patient and is an important element contributing to high quality care. The medical record facilitates:

- the ability of the physician and other health care professionals to evaluate and plan the patient's immediate treatment, and to monitor his/her health care over time.
- communication and continuity of care among physicians and other health care professionals involved in the patient's care;
- accurate and timely claims review and payment;
- appropriate utilization review and quality of care evaluations; and
- collection of data that may be useful for research and education.

An appropriately documented medical record can reduce many of the "hassles" associated with claims processing and may serve as a legal document to verify the care provided, if necessary.

What Do Payers Want and Why?

Because payers have a contractual obligation to enrollees, they may require reasonable documentation that services are consistent with the insurance coverage provided. They may request information to validate:

- the site of service;
- the medical necessity and appropriateness of the diagnostic and/or therapeutic services provided; and/or
- that services provided have been accurately reported.

II. GENERAL PRINCIPLES OF MEDICAL RECORD DOCUMENTATION

The principles of documentation listed below are applicable to all types of medical and surgical services in all settings. For Evaluation and Management (E/M) services, the nature and amount of physician work and documentation varies by type of service, place of service and the patient's status. The following list of general principles may be modified to account for these variable circumstances in providing E/M services.

1. The medical record should be complete and legible.
2. The documentation of each patient encounter should include:
   - reason for the encounter and relevant history, physical examination findings and prior diagnostic test results;
   - assessment, clinical impression or diagnosis;

> ▪ plan for care; and
>
> ▪ date and legible identity of the observer.

3. If not documented, the rationale for ordering diagnostic and other ancillary services should be easily inferred.

4. Past and present diagnoses should be accessible to the treating and/or consulting physician.

5. Appropriate health risk factors should be identified.

6. The patient's progress, response to and changes in treatment, and revision of diagnosis should be documented.

7. The CPT and ICD-9-CM codes reported on the health insurance claim form or billing statement should be supported by the documentation in the medical record.

III. DOCUMENTATION OF E/M SERVICES

This publication provides definitions and documentation guidelines for the three key components of E/M services and for visits which consist predominantly of counseling or coordination of care. The three *key* components—history, examination, and medical decision making—appear in the descriptors for office and other outpatient services, hospital observation services, hospital inpatient services, consultations, emergency department services, nursing facility services, domiciliary care services, and home services. While some of the text of CPT has been repeated in this publication, the reader should refer to CPT for the complete descriptors for E/M services and instructions for selecting a level of service. Documentation guidelines are identified by the symbol ▪ *DG*.

The descriptors for the levels of E/M services recognize seven components which are used in defining the levels of E/M services. These components are:

- history;
- examination;
- medical decision making;
- counseling;
- coordination of care;
- nature of presenting problem; and
- time.

The first three of these components (i.e., history, examination and medical decision making) are the key components in selecting the level of E/M services. In the case of visits which consist *predominantly* of counseling or coordination of care, time is the key or controlling factor to qualify for a particular level of E/M service.

Because the level of E/M service is dependent on two or three key components, performance and documentation of one component (e.g., examination) at the highest level does not necessarily mean that the encounter in its entirety qualifies for the highest level of E/M service.

These Documentation Guidelines for E/M services reflect the needs of the typical adult population. For certain groups of patients, the recorded information may vary slightly from that described here. Specifically, the medical records of infants, children, adolescents and pregnant women may have additional or modified information recorded in each history and examination area.

As an example, newborn records may include under history of the present illness (HPI) the details of mother's pregnancy and the infant's status at birth; social history will focus on family structure; family history will focus on congenital anomalies and hereditary disorders in the family. In addition, the content of a pediatric examination will vary with the age and development of the child. Although not specifically defined in these documentation guidelines, these patient group variations on history and examination are appropriate.

A. Documentation of History

The levels of E/M services are based on four types of history (Problem Focused, Expanded Problem Focused, Detailed, and Comprehensive). Each type of history includes some or all of the following elements:

- Chief complaint (CC);
- History of present illness (HPI);
- Review of systems (ROS); and
- Past, family and/or social history (PFSH).

The extent of history of present illness, review of systems and past, family and/or social history that is obtained and documented is dependent upon clinical judgment and the nature of the presenting problem(s).

The chart below shows the progression of the elements required for each type of history. To qualify for a given type of history all three elements in the table must be met. (A chief complaint is indicated at all levels.)

History of Present Illness	Review of Systems (ROS)	Past, Family, and/or Social History	Type of History
Brief	N/A	N/A	Problem Focused
Brief	Problem pertinent	N/A	Expanded Problem Focused
Extended	Extended	Pertinent	Detailed
Extended	Complete	Complete	Comprehensive

- DG: The CC, ROS, and PFSH may be listed as separate elements of history, or they may be included in the description of the history of the present illness.

- DG: A ROS and/or a PFSH obtained during an earlier encounter does not need to be re-recorded if there is evidence that the physician reviewed and updated the previous information. This may occur when a physician updates his or her own record or in an institutional setting or group practice where many physicians use a common record. The review and update may be documented by:

  - describing any new ROS and/or PFSH information or noting there has been no change in the information; and

  - noting the date and location of the earlier ROS and/or PFSH.

- DG: The ROS and/or PFSH may be recorded by ancillary staff or on a form completed by the patient. To document that the physician reviewed the information, there must be a notation supplementing or confirming the information recorded by others.

- DG: If the physician is unable to obtain a history from the patient or other source, the record should describe the patient's condition or other circumstance which precludes obtaining a history.

Definitions and specific documentation guidelines for each of the elements of history are in the following list.

Chief Complaint (CC). The CC is a concise statement describing the symptom, problem, condition, diagnosis, physician recommended return, or other factor that is the reason for the encounter, usually stated in the patient's words.

- DG: The medical record should clearly reflect the chief complaint.

History of Present Illness (HPI). The HPI is a chronological description of the development of the patient's present illness from the first sign and/or symptom or from the previous encounter to the present. It includes the following elements:

- location,
- quality,
- severity,
- duration,
- timing,
- context,
- modifying factors, and
- associated signs and symptoms.

Brief and *extended* HPIs are distinguished by the amount of detail needed to accurately characterize the clinical problem(s).

A *brief* HPI consists of one to three elements of the HPI.

- DG: The medical record should describe one to three elements of the present illness (HPI).

An *extended* HPI consists of at least four elements of the HPI or the status of at least three chronic or inactive conditions.

- DG: The medical record should describe at least four elements of the present illness (HPI), or the status of at least three chronic or inactive conditions.

Review of Systems (ROS). A ROS is an inventory of body systems obtained through a series of questions seeking to identify signs and/or symptoms which the patient may be experiencing or has experienced.

For purposes of ROS, the following systems are recognized:

- Constitutional symptoms (e.g., fever, weight loss)
- Eyes
- Ears, Nose, Mouth, Throat
- Cardiovascular
- Respiratory
- Gastrointestinal
- Genitourinary
- Musculoskeletal
- Integumentary (skin and/or breast)
- Neurological
- Psychiatric
- Endocrine
- Hematologic/Lymphatic
- Allergic/Immunologic

A *problem pertinent* ROS inquires about the system directly related to the problem(s) identified in the HPI.

    ▪ DG: The patient's positive responses and pertinent negatives for the system related to the problem should be documented.

An *extended* ROS inquires about the system directly related to the problem(s) identified in the HPI and a limited number of additional systems.

    ▪ DG: The patient's positive responses and pertinent negatives for two to nine systems should be documented.

A *complete* ROS inquires about the system(s) directly related to the problem(s) identified in the HPI *plus* all additional body systems.

    ▪ DG: At least ten organ systems must be reviewed. Those systems with positive or pertinent negative responses must be individually documented. For the remaining systems, a notation indicating all other systems are negative is permissible. In the absence of such a notation, at least ten systems must be individually documented.

Past, Family and/or Social History (PFSH). The PFSH consists of a review of three areas:

    ▪ past history (the patient's past experiences with illnesses, operations, injuries and treatments);

    ▪ family history (a review of medical events in the patient's family, including diseases which may be hereditary or place the patient at risk); and

    ▪ social history (an age appropriate review of past and current activities).

For certain categories of E/M services that include only an interval history, it is not necessary to record information about the PFSH. Those categories are subsequent hospital care, follow-up inpatient consultations and subsequent nursing facility care.

A *pertinent* PFSH is a review of the history area(s) directly related to the problem(s) identified in the HPI.

    ▪ DG: At least one specific item from any of the three history areas must be documented for a pertinent PFSH.

A *complete* PFSH is a review of two or all three of the PFSH history areas, depending on the category of the E/M service. A review of all three history areas is required for services that by their nature include a comprehensive assessment or reassessment of the patient. A review of two of the three history areas is sufficient for other services.

    ▪ DG: At least one specific item from two of the three history areas must be documented for a complete PFSH for the following categories of E/M services: office or other outpatient services, established patient; emergency department; domiciliary care, established patient; and home care, established patient.

    ▪ DG: At least one specific item from each of the three history areas must be documented for a complete PFSH for the following categories of E/M services: office or other outpatient services, new patient; hospital observation services; hospital inpatient services, initial care; consultations; comprehensive nursing facility assessments; domiciliary care, new patient; and home care, new patient.

B. Documentation of Examination

The levels of E/M services are based on four types of examination:

    ▪ *Problem Focused*—a limited examination of the affected body area or organ system.

    ▪ *Expanded Problem Focused*—a limited examination of the affected body area or organ system and any other symptomatic or related body area(s) or organ system(s).

- *Detailed*—an extended examination of the affected body area(s) or organ system(s) and any other symptomatic or related body area(s) or organ system(s).
- *Comprehensive*—a general multi-system examination, or complete examination of a single organ system and other symptomatic or related body area(s) or organ system(s).

These types of examinations have been defined for general multi-system and the following single organ systems:

- Cardiovascular
- Ears, Nose, Mouth and Throat
- Eyes
- Genitourinary (Female)
- Genitourinary (Male)
- Hematologic/Lymphatic/Immunologic
- Musculoskeletal
- Neurological
- Psychiatric
- Respiratory
- Skin

A general multi-system examination or a single organ system examination may be performed by any physician regardless of specialty. The type (general multi-system or single organ system) and content of examination are selected by the examining physician and are based upon clinical judgment, the patient's history, and the nature of the presenting problem(s).

The content and documentation requirements for each type and level of examination are summarized following and described in detail in tables beginning on page 571. In the tables, organ systems and body areas recognized by CPT for purposes of describing examinations are shown in the left column. The content, or individual elements, of the examination pertaining to that body area or organ system are identified by bullets (•) in the right column.

Parenthetical examples, "(e.g., . . .)," have been used for clarification and to provide guidance regarding documentation. Documentation for each element must satisfy any numeric requirements (such as "Measurement of *any three of the following seven . . .*") included in the description of the element. Elements with multiple components but with no specific numeric requirement (such as "Examination of *liver* and *spleen*") require documentation of at least one component. It is possible for a given examination to be expanded beyond what is defined here. When that occurs, findings related to the additional systems and/or areas should be documented.

- DG: Specific abnormal and relevant negative findings of the examination of the affected or symptomatic body area(s) or organ system(s) should be documented. A notation of "abnormal" without elaboration is insufficient.
- DG: Abnormal or unexpected findings of the examination of any asymptomatic body area(s) or organ system(s) should be described.
- DG: A brief statement or notation indicating "negative" or "normal" is sufficient to document normal findings related to unaffected area(s) or asymptomatic organ system(s).

General Multi-System Examinations. General multi-system examinations are described in detail beginning on page 571. To qualify for a given level of multi-system examination, the following content and documentation requirements should be met:

- *Problem Focused Examination*—should include performance and documentation of one to five elements identified by a bullet (•) in one or more organ system(s) or body area(s).

- *Expanded Problem Focused Examination*—should include performance and documentation of at least six elements identified by a bullet (•) in one or more organ system(s) or body area(s).

- *Detailed Examination*—should include at least six organ systems or body areas. For each system/area selected, performance and documentation of at least two elements identified by a bullet (•) is expected. Alternatively, a detailed examination may include performance and documentation of at least twelve elements identified by a bullet (•) in two or more organ systems or body areas.

- *Comprehensive Examination*—should include at least nine organ systems or body areas. For each system/area selected, all elements of the examination identified by a bullet (•) should be performed, unless specific directions limit the content of the examination. For each area/system, documentation of at least two elements identified by a bullet is expected.

Single Organ System Examinations. The single organ system examinations recognized by CPT are described in detail beginning on page 574. Variations among these examinations in the organ systems and body areas identified in the left columns and in the elements of the examinations described in the right columns reflect differing emphases among specialties. To qualify for a given level of single organ system examination, the following content and documentation requirements should be met:

- *Problem Focused Examination*—should include performance and documentation of one to five elements identified by a bullet (•), whether in a box with a shaded or unshaded border.

- *Expanded Problem Focused Examination*—should include performance and documentation of at least six elements identified by a bullet (•), whether in a box with a shaded or unshaded border.

- *Detailed Examination*—examinations other than the eye and psychiatric examinations should include performance and documentation of at least twelve elements identified by a bullet (•), whether in box with a shaded or unshaded border.

- Eye and psychiatric examinations should include the performance and documentation of at least nine elements identified by a bullet (•), whether in a box with a shaded or unshaded border.

- *Comprehensive Examination*—should include performance of all elements identified by a bullet (•), whether in a shaded or unshaded box. Documentation of every element in each box with a shaded border and at least one element in each box with an unshaded border is expected.

Content and Documentation Requirements

GENERAL MULTI-SYSTEM EXAMINATION	
System/Body Area	**Elements of Examination**
Constitutional	• Measurement of **any three of the following seven** vital signs: 1) sitting or standing blood pressure, 2) supine blood pressure, 3) pulse rate and regularity, 4) respiration, 5) temperature, 6) height, 7) weight (may be measured and recorded by ancillary staff)
	• General appearance of patient (e.g., development, nutrition, body habitus, deformities, attention to grooming)
Eyes	• Inspection of conjunctivae and lids
	• Examination of pupils and irises (e.g., reaction to light and accommodation, size and symmetry)
	• Ophthalmoscopic examination of optic discs (e.g., size, C/D ratio, appearance) and posterior segments (e.g., vessel changes, exudates, hemorrhages)
Ears, Nose, Mouth and Throat	• External inspection of ears and nose (e.g., overall appearance, scars, lesions, masses
	• Otoscopic examination of external auditory canals and tympanic membranes
	• Assessment of hearing (e.g., whispered voice, finger rub, tuning fork)
	• Inspection of nasal mucosa, septum and turbinates
	• Inspection of lips, teeth and gums
	• Examination of oropharynx: oral mucosa, salivary glands, hard and soft palates, tongue, tonsils and posterior pharynx
Neck	• Examination of neck (e.g., masses, overall appearance, symmetry, tracheal position, crepitus)
	• Examination of thyroid (e.g., enlargement, tenderness, mass)
Respiratory	• Assessment of respiratory effort (e.g., intercostal retractions, use of accessory muscles, diaphragmatic movement)
	• Percussion of chest (e.g., dullness, flatness, hyperresonance)
	• Palpation of chest (e.g., tactile fremitus)
	• Auscultation of lungs (e.g., breath sounds, adventitious sounds, rubs)
Cardiovascular	• Palpation of heart (e.g., location, size, thrills)
	• Auscultation of heart with notation of abnormal sounds and murmurs
	Examination of:
	• carotid arteries (e.g., pulse amplitude, bruits)
	• abdominal aorta (e.g., size, bruits)
	• femoral arteries (e.g., pulse amplitude, bruits)
	• pedal pulses (e.g., pulse amplitude)
	• extremities for edema and/or varicosities
Chest (Breasts)	• Inspection of breasts (e.g., symmetry, nipple discharge)
	• Palpation of breasts and axillae (e.g., masses or lumps, tenderness)
Gastrointestinal (Abdomen)	• Examination of abdomen with notation of presence of masses or tenderness
	• Examination of liver and spleen
	• Examination for presence or absence of hernia
	• Examination (when indicated) of anus, perineum and rectum, including sphincter tone, presence of hemorrhoids, rectal masses
	• Obtain stool sample for occult blood test when indicated
Genitourinary	**Male:**
	• Examination of the scrotal contents (e.g., hydrocele, spermatocele, tenderness of cord, testicular mass)
	• Examination of the penis

Table continued on following page

GENERAL MULTI-SYSTEM EXAMINATION (Continued)

System/Body Area	Elements of Examination
Genitourinary	**Male:** (Cont'd) • Digital rectal examination of prostate gland (e.g., size, symmetry, nodularity, tenderness) **Female:** Pelvic examination (with or without specimen collection for smears and cultures), including • Examination of external genitalia (e.g., general appearance, hair distribution, lesions) and vagina (e.g., general appearance, estrogen effect, discharge, lesions, pelvic support, cystocele, rectocele) • Examination of urethra (e.g., masses, tenderness, scarring) • Examination of bladder (e.g., fullness, masses, tenderness) • Cervix (e.g., general appearance, lesions, discharge) • Uterus (e.g., size, contour, position, mobility, tenderness, consistency, descent or support) • Adnexa/parametria (e.g., masses, tenderness, organomegaly, nodularity)
Lymphatic	Palpation of lymph nodes in **two or more** areas: • Neck • Axillae • Groin • Other
Musculoskeletal	• Examination of gait and station • Inspection and/or palpation of digits and nails (e.g., clubbing, cyanosis, inflammatory conditions, petechiae, ischemia, infections, nodes) Examination of joints, bones and muscles of **one or more of the following six** areas: 1) head and neck; 2) spine, ribs and pelvis; 3) right upper extremity; 4) left upper extremity; 5) right lower extremity; and 6) left lower extremity. The examination of a given area includes: • Inspection and/or palpation with notation of presence of any misalignment, asymmetry, crepitation, defects, tenderness, masses, effusions • Assessment of range of motion with notation of any pain, crepitation orcontracture • Assessment of stability with notation of any dislocation (luxation), subluxation or laxity • Assessment of muscle strength and tone (e.g., flaccid, cog wheel, spastic) with notation of any atrophy or abnormal movements
Skin	• Inspection of skin and subcutaneous tissue (e.g., rashes, lesions, ulcers) • Palpation of skin and subcutaneous tissue (e.g., induration, subcutaneous nodules, tightening)
Neurologic	• Test cranial nerves with notation of any deficits • Examination of deep tendon reflexes with notation of pathological reflexes (e.g., Babinski) • Examination of sensation (e.g., by touch, pin, vibration, proprioception)
Psychiatric	• Description of patient's judgment and insight Brief assessment of mental status including: • orientation to time, place and person • recent and remote memory • mood and affect (e.g., depression, anxiety, agitation)

Content and Documentation Requirements

LEVEL OF EXAM	PERFORM AND DOCUMENT
Problem Focused	**One to five** elements identified by a bullet.
Expanded Problem Focused	**At least six** elements identified by a bullet.
Detailed	**At least two** elements identified by a bullet **from each of six areas/systems** OR **at least twelve** elements identified by a bullet **in two or more areas/systems.**
Comprehensive	Perform **all elements** identified by a bullet in **at least nine** organ systems or body areas and document **at least two** elements identified by a bullet **from each of nine areas/systems.**

CARDIOVASCULAR EXAMINATION

System/Body Area	Elements of Examination
Constitutional	• Measurement of **any three of the following seven** vital signs: 1) sitting or standing blood pressure, 2) supine blood pressure, 3) pulse rate and regularity, 4) respiration, 5) temperature, 6) height, 7) weight (may be measured and recorded by ancillary staff) • General appearance of patient (e.g., development, nutrition, body habitus, deformities, attention to grooming)
Head and Face	
Eyes	• Inspection of conjunctivae and lids (e.g., xanthelasma)
Ears, Nose, Mouth and Throat	• Inspection of teeth, gums and palate • Inspection of oral mucosa with notation of presence of pallor or cyanosis
Neck	Examination of jugular veins (e.g., distension; a, v or cannon a waves) • Examination of thyroid (e.g., enlargement, tenderness, mass)
Respiratory	• Assessment of respiratory effort (e.g., intercostal retractions, use of accessory muscles, diaphragmatic movement) • Auscultation of lungs (e.g., breath sounds, adventitious sounds, rubs)
Cardiovascular	• Palpation of heart (e.g., location, size and forcefulness of the point of maximal impact; thrills; lifts; palpable S3 or S4) • Auscultation of heart including sounds, abnormal sounds and murmurs • Measurement of blood pressure in two or more extremities when indicated (e.g., aortic dissection, coarctation) Examination of: • Carotid arteries (e.g., waveform, pulse amplitude, bruits, apical-carotid delay) • Abdominal aorta (e.g., size, bruits) • Femoral arteries (e.g., pulse amplitude, bruits) • Pedal pulses (e.g., pulse amplitude) • Extremities for peripheral edema and/or varicosities
Chest (Breasts)	
Gastrointestinal (Abdomen)	• Examination of abdomen with notation of presence of masses or tenderness • Examination of liver and spleen • Obtain stool sample for occult blood from patients who are being considered for thrombolytic or anticoagulant therapy

Table continued on following page

CARDIOVASCULAR EXAMINATION (Continued)

System/Body Area	Elements of Examination
Lymphatic	
Musculoskeletal	• Examination of the back with notation of kyphosis or scoliosis
	• Examination of gait with notation of ability to undergo exercise testing and/or participation in exercise programs
	• Assessment of muscle strength and tone (e.g., flaccid, cog wheel, spastic) with notation of any atrophy and abnormal movements
Extremities	• Inspection and palpation of digits and nails (e.g., clubbing, cyanosis, inflammation, petechiae, ischemia, infections, Osler's nodes)
Skin	• Inspection and/or palpation of skin and subcutaneous tissue (e.g., stasis dermatitis, ulcers, scars, xanthomas)
Neurologic/ Psychiatric	Brief assessment of mental status including
	• Orientation to time, place and person
	• Mood and affect (e.g., depression, anxiety, agitation)

Content and Documentation Requirements

LEVEL OF EXAM	PERFORM AND DOCUMENT
Problem Focused	**One to five** elements identified by a bullet.
Expanded Problem Focused	**At least six** elements identified by a bullet.
Detailed	**At least twelve** elements identified by a bullet.
Comprehensive	Perform **all** elements identified by a bullet; document every element in each box with ashaded border and at least one element in each box with an unshaded border.

EARS, NOSE AND THROAT EXAMINATION

System/Body Area	Elements of Examination
Constitutional	• Measurement of **any three of the following seven** vital signs: 1) sitting or standing blood pressure, 2) supine blood pressure, 3) pulse rate and regularity, 4) respiration, 5) temperature, 6) height, 7) weight (may be measured and recorded by ancillary staff)
	• General appearance of patient (e.g., development, nutrition, body habitus, deformities, attention to grooming)
	• Assessment of ability to communicate (e.g., use of sign language or other communication aids) and quality of voice
Head and Face	• Inspection of head and face (e.g., overall appearance, scars, lesions and masses)
	• Palpation and/or percussion of face with notation of presence or absence of sinus tenderness
	• Examination of salivary glands
	• Assessment of facial strength
Eyes	• Test ocular motility including primary gaze alignment
Ears, Nose, Mouth and Throat	• Otoscopic examination of external auditory canals and tympanic membranes including pneumo-otoscopy with notation of mobility of membranes
	• Assessment of hearing with tuning forks and clinical speech reception thresholds (e.g., whispered voice, finger rub)
	• External inspection of ears and nose (e.g., overall appearance, scars, lesions and masses)

EARS, NOSE AND THROAT EXAMINATION (Continued)

System/Body Area	Elements of Examination
Ears, Nose, Mouth and Throat (Cont'd)	• Inspection of nasal mucosa, septum and turbinates • Inspection of lips, teeth and gums • Examination of oropharynx: oral mucosa, hard and soft palates, tongue, tonsils and posterior pharynx (e.g., asymmetry, lesions, hydration of mucosal surfaces) • Inspection of pharyngeal walls and pyriform sinuses (e.g., pooling of saliva, asymmetry, lesions) • Examination by mirror of larynx including the condition of the epiglottis, false vocal cords, true vocal cords and mobility of larynx (use of mirror not required in children) • Examination by mirror of nasopharynx including appearance of the mucosa, adenoids, posterior choanae and eustachian tubes (use of mirror not required in children)
Neck	• Examination of neck (e.g., masses, overall appearance, symmetry, tracheal position, crepitus) • Examination of thyroid (e.g., enlargement, tenderness, mass)
Respiratory	• Inspection of chest including symmetry, expansion and/or assessment of respiratory effort (e.g., intercostal retractions, use of accessory muscles, diaphragmatic movement) • Auscultation of lungs (e.g., breath sounds, adventitious sounds, rubs)
Cardiovascular	• Auscultation of heart with notation of abnormal sounds and murmurs • Examination of peripheral vascular system by observation (e.g., swelling, varicosities) and palpation (e.g., pulses, temperature, edema, tenderness)
Chest (Breasts)	
Gastrointestinal (Abdomen)	
Genitourinary	
Lymphatic	• Palpation of lymph nodes in neck, axillae, groin and/or other location
Musculoskeletal	
Extremities	
Skin	
Neurological/ Psychiatric	• Test cranial nerves with notation of any deficits Brief assessment of mental status including • Orientation to time, place and person • Mood and affect (e.g., depression, anxiety, agitation)

Content and Documentation Requirements

LEVEL OF EXAM	PERFORM AND DOCUMENT
Problem Focused	**One to five** elements identified by a bullet.
Expanded Problem Focused	**At least six** elements identified by a bullet.
Detailed	**At least twelve** elements identified by a bullet.
Comprehensive	Perform **all** elements identified by a bullet; document every element in each box with a shaded border and at least one element in each box with an unshaded border.

EYE EXAMINATION

System/Body Area	Elements of Examination
Constitutional	
Head and Face	
Eyes	• Test visual acuity (does not include determination of refractive error)
	• Gross visual field testing by confrontation
	• Test ocular motility including primary gaze alignment
	• Inspection of bulbar and palpebral conjunctivae
	• Examination of ocular adnexae including lids (e.g., ptosis or lagophthalmos), lacrimal glands, lacrimal drainage, orbits and preauricular lymph nodes
	• Examination of pupils and irises including shape, direct and consensual reaction (afferent pupil), size (e.g., anisocoria) and morphology
	• Slit lamp examination of the corneas including epithelium, stroma, endothelium, and tear film
	• Slit lamp examination of the anterior chambers including depth, cells, and flare
	• Slit lamp examination of the lenses including clarity, anterior and posterior capsule, cortex, and nucleus
	• Measurement of intraocular pressures (except in children and patients with trauma or infectious disease)
	Ophthalmoscopic examination through dilated pupils (unless contraindicated) of
	• Optic discs including size, C/D ratio, appearance (e.g., atrophy, cupping, tumor elevation) and nerve fiber layer
	• Posterior segments including retina and vessels (e.g., exudates and hemorrhages)
Ears, Nose, Mouth and Throat	
Neck	
Respiratory	
Cardiovascular	
Chest (Breasts)	
Gastrointestinal (Abdomen)	
Genitourinary	
Lymphatic	
Musculoskeletal	
Extremities	
Skin	
Neurological/ Psychiatric	Brief assessment of mental status including
	• Orientation to time, place and person
	• Mood and affect (e.g., depression, anxiety, agitation)

Content and Documentation Requirements

LEVEL OF EXAM	PERFORM AND DOCUMENT
Problem Focused	**One to five** elements identified by a bullet.
Expanded Problem Focused	**At least six** elements identified by a bullet.
Detailed	**At least nine** elements identified by a bullet.
Comprehensive	Perform **all** elements identified by a bullet; document every element in each box with a shaded border and at least one element in each box with an unshaded border.

GENITOURINARY EXAMINATION

System/Body Area	Elements of Examination
Constitutional	• Measurement of **any three of the following seven** vital signs: 1) sitting or standing blood pressure, 2) supine blood pressure, 3) pulse rate and regularity, 4) respiration, 5) temperature, 6) height, 7) weight (may be measured and recorded by ancillary staff)
	• General appearance of patient (e.g., development, nutrition, body habitus, deformities, attention to grooming)
Head and Face	
Eyes	
Ears, Nose, Mouth and Throat	
Neck	• Examination of neck (e.g., masses, overall appearance, symmetry, tracheal position, crepitus)
	• Examination of thyroid (e.g., enlargement, tenderness, mass)
Respiratory	• Assessment of respiratory effort (e.g., intercostal retractions, use of accessory muscles, diaphragmatic movement)
	• Auscultation of lungs (e.g., breath sounds, adventitious sounds, rubs)
Cardiovascular	• Auscultation of heart with notation of abnormal sounds and murmurs
	• Examination of peripheral vascular system by observation (e.g., swelling, varicosities) and palpation (e.g., pulses, temperature, edema, tenderness)
Chest (Breasts)	[See genitourinary (female).]
Gastrointestinal (Abdomen)	• Examination of abdomen with notation of presence of masses or tenderness
	• Examination for presence or absence of hernia
	• Examination of liver and spleen
	• Obtain stool sample for occult blood test when indicated
Genitourinary	**Male:**
	• Inspection of anus and perineum
	Examination (with or without specimen collection for smears and cultures) of genitalia including:
	• Scrotum (e.g., lesions, cysts, rashes)
	• Epididymides (e.g., size, symmetry, masses)
	• Testes (e.g., size, symmetry, masses)
	• Urethral meatus (e.g., size, location, lesions, discharge)
	• Penis (e.g., lesions, presence or absence of foreskin, foreskin retractability, plaque, masses, scarring, deformities)

Table continued on following page

GENITOURINARY EXAMINATION (Continued)

System/Body Area	Elements of Examination
Genitourinary	**Male:** (Cont'd) Digital rectal examination including: • Prostate gland (e.g., size, symmetry, nodularity, tenderness) • Seminal vesicles (e.g., symmetry, tenderness, masses, enlargement) • Sphincter tone, presence of hemorrhoids, rectal masses **Female:** Includes **at least seven of the following** eleven elements identified by bullets: • Inspection and palpation of breasts (e.g., masses or lumps, tenderness, symmetry, nipple discharge) • Digital rectal examination including sphincter tone, presence of hemorrhoids, rectal masses Pelvic examination (with or without specimen collection for smears and cultures) including: • External genitalia (e.g., general appearance, hair distribution, lesions) • Urethral meatus (e.g., size, location, lesions, prolapse) • Urethra (e.g., masses, tenderness, scarring) • Bladder (e.g., fullness, masses, tenderness) • Vagina (e.g., general appearance, estrogen effect, discharge, lesions, pelvic support, cystocele, rectocele) • Cervix (e.g., general appearance, lesions, discharge) • Uterus (e.g., size, contour, position, mobility, tenderness, consistency, descent or support) • Adnexa/parametria (e.g., masses, tenderness, organomegaly, nodularity) • Anus and perineum
Lymphatic	• Palpation of lymph nodes in neck, axillae, groin and/or other location
Musculoskeletal	
Extremities	
Skin	• Inspection and/or palpation of skin and subcutaneous tissue (e.g., rashes, lesions, ulcers)
Neurological/ Psychiatric	Brief assessment of mental status including • Orientation (e.g., time, place and person) and • Mood and affect (e.g., depression, anxiety, agitation)

Content and Documentation Requirements

LEVEL OF EXAM	PERFORM AND DOCUMENT
Problem Focused	**One to five** elements identified by a bullet.
Expanded Problem Focused	**At least six** elements identified by a bullet.
Detailed	**At least twelve** elements identified by a bullet.
Comprehensive	Perform **all** elements identified by a bullet; document every element in each box with a shaded border and at least one element in each box with an unshaded border.

HEMATOLOGIC/LYMPHATIC/IMMUNOLOGIC EXAMINATION

System/Body Area	Elements of Examination
Constitutional	• Measurement of **any three of the following seven** vital signs: 1) sitting or standing blood pressure, 2) supine blood pressure, 3) pulse rate and regularity, 4) respiration, 5) temperature, 6) height, 7) weight (may be measured and recorded by ancillary staff)
	• General appearance of patient (e.g., development, nutrition, body habitus, deformities, attention to grooming)
Head and Face	• Palpation and/or percussion of face with notation of presence or absence of sinus tenderness
Eyes	• Inspection of conjunctivae and lids
Ears, Nose, Mouth and Throat	• Otoscopic examination of external auditory canals and tympanic membranes
	• Inspection of nasal mucosa, septum and turbinates
	• Inspection of teeth and gums
	• Examination of oropharynx (e.g., oral mucosa, hard and soft palates, tongue, tonsils, posterior pharynx)
Neck	• Examination of neck (e.g., masses, overall appearance, symmetry, tracheal position, crepitus)
	• Examination of thyroid (e.g., enlargement, tenderness, mass)
Respiratory	• Assessment of respiratory effort (e.g., intercostal retractions, use of accessory muscles, diaphragmatic movement)
	• Auscultation of lungs (e.g., breath sounds, adventitious sounds, rubs)
Cardiovascular	• Auscultation of heart with notation of abnormal sounds and murmurs
	• Examination of peripheral vascular system by observation (e.g., swelling, varicosities) and palpation (e.g., pulses, temperature, edema, tenderness)
Chest (Breasts)	
Gastrointestinal (Abdomen)	• Examination of abdomen with notation of presence of masses or tenderness
	• Examination of liver and spleen
Genitourinary	
Lymphatic	• Palpation of lymph nodes in neck, axillae, groin, and/or other location
Musculoskeletal	
Extremities	• Inspection and palpation of digits and nails (e.g., clubbing, cyanosis, inflammation, petechiae, ischemia, infections, nodes)
Skin	• Inspection and/or palpation of skin and subcutaneous tissue (e.g., rashes, lesions, ulcers, ecchymoses, bruises)
Neurological/ Psychiatric	Brief assessment of mental status including
	• Orientation to time, place and person
	• Mood and affect (e.g., depression, anxiety, agitation)

Content and Documentation Requirements

LEVEL OF EXAM	PERFORM AND DOCUMENT
Problem Focused	**One to five** elements identified by a bullet.
Expanded Problem Focused	**At least six** elements identified by a bullet.
Detailed	**At least twelve** elements identified by a bullet.
Comprehensive	Perform **all** elements identified by a bullet; document every element in each box with a shaded border and at least one element in each box with an unshaded border.

MUSCULOSKELETAL EXAMINATION

System/Body Area	Elements of Examination
Constitutional	• Measurement of **any three of the following seven** vital signs: 1) sitting or standing blood pressure, 2) supine blood pressure, 3) pulse rate and regularity, 4) respiration, 5) temperature, 6) height, 7) weight (may be measured and recorded by ancillary staff) • General appearance of patient (e.g., development, nutrition, body habitus, deformities, attention to grooming)
Head and Face	
Eyes	
Ears, Nose, Mouth and Throat	
Neck	
Respiratory	
Cardiovascular	• Examination of peripheral vascular system by observation (e.g., swelling, varicosities) and palpation (e.g., pulses, temperature, edema, tenderness)
Chest (Breasts)	
Gastrointestinal (Abdomen)	
Genitourinary	
Lymphatic	• Palpation of lymph nodes in neck, axillae, groin and/or other location
Musculoskeletal	• Examination of gait and station Examination of joint(s), bone(s) and muscle(s)/tendon(s) **of four of the following six** areas: 1) head and neck; 2) spine, ribs and pelvis; 3) right upper extremity; 4) left upper extremity; 5) right lower extremity; and 6) left lower extremity. The examination of a given area includes: • Inspection, percussion and/or palpation with notation of any misalignment, asymmetry, crepitation, defects, tenderness, masses or effusions • Assessment of range of motion with notation of any pain (e.g., straight leg raising), crepitation or contracture • Assessment of stability with notation of any dislocation (luxation), subluxation or laxity • Assessment of muscle strength and tone (e.g., flaccid, cog wheel, spastic) with notation of any atrophy or abnormal movements *Note:* For the comprehensive level of examination, all four of the elements identified by a bullet must be performed and documented for each of four anatomic areas. For the three lower levels of examination, each element is counted separately for each body area. For example, assessing range of motion in two extremities constitutes two elements.
Extremities	[See musculoskeletal and skin.]
Skin	• Inspection and/or palpation of skin and subcutaneous tissue (e.g., scars, rashes, lesions, cafe-au-lait spots, ulcers) **in four of the following six** areas: 1) head and neck; 2) trunk; 3) right upper extremity; 4) left upper extremity; 5) right lower extremity; and 6) left lower extremity. *Note:* For the comprehensive level, the examination of all four anatomic areas must be performed and documented. For the three lower levels of examination, each body area is counted separately. For example, inspection and/or palpation of the skin and subcutaneous tissue of two extremities constitutes two elements.
Neurological/ Psychiatric	• Test coordination (e.g., finger/nose, heel/knee/shin, rapid alternating movements in the upper and lower extremities, evaluation of fine motor coordination in young children) • Examination of deep tendon reflexes and/or nerve stretch test with notation of pathological reflexes (e.g., Babinski) • Examination of sensation (e.g., by touch, pin, vibration, proprioception)

MUSCULOSKELETAL EXAMINATION (Continued)	
System/Body Area	**Elements of Examination**
	Brief assessment of mental status including
	• Orientation to time, place and person
	• Mood and affect (e.g., depression, anxiety, agitation)

Content and Documentation Requirements

LEVEL OF EXAM	PERFORM AND DOCUMENT
Problem Focused	**One to five** elements identified by a bullet.
Expanded Problem Focused	**At least six** elements identified by a bullet.
Detailed	**At least twelve** elements identified by a bullet.
Comprehensive	Perform **all** elements identified by a bullet; document every element in each box with a shaded border and at least one element in each box with an unshaded border.

NEUROLOGICAL EXAMINATION	
System/Body Area	**Elements of Examination**
Constitutional	• Measurement of **any three of the following seven** vital signs: 1) sitting or standing blood pressure, 2) supine blood pressure, 3) pulse rate and regularity, 4) respiration, 5) temperature, 6) height, 7) weight (may be measured and recorded by ancillary staff)
	• General appearance of patient (e.g., development, nutrition, body habitus, deformities, attention to grooming)
Head and Face	
Eyes	• Ophthalmoscopic examination of optic discs (e.g., size, C/D ratio, appearance) and posterior segments (e.g., vessel changes, exudates, hemorrhages)
Ears, Nose, Mouth and Throat	
Neck	
Respiratory	
Cardiovascular	• Examination of carotid arteries (e.g., pulse amplitude, bruits)
	• Auscultation of heart with notation of abnormal sounds and murmurs
	• Examination of peripheral vascular system by observation (e.g., swelling, varicosities) and palpation (e.g., pulses, temperature, edema, tenderness)
Chest (Breasts)	
Gastrointestinal (Abdomen)	
Genitourinary	
Lymphatic	
Musculoskeletal	• Examination of gait and station
	Assessment of motor function including:
	• Muscle strength in upper and lower extremities
	• Muscle tone in upper and lower extremities (e.g., flaccid, cog wheel, spastic) with notation of any atrophy or abnormal movements (e.g., fasciculation, tardive dyskinesia)
Extremities	[See musculoskeletal.]

Table continued on following page

NEUROLOGICAL EXAMINATION (Continued)

System/Body Area	Elements of Examination
Skin	
Neurological	Evaluation of higher integrative functions including:
	• Orientation to time, place and person
	• Recent and remote memory
	• Attention span and concentration
	• Language (e.g., naming objects, repeating phrases, spontaneous speech)
	• Fund of knowledge (e.g., awareness of current events, past history, vocabulary)
	Test the following cranial nerves:
	• 2nd cranial nerve (e.g., visual acuity, visual fields, fundi)
	• 3rd, 4th and 6th cranial nerves (e.g., pupils, eye movements)
	• 5th cranial nerve (e.g., facial sensation, corneal reflexes)
	• 7th cranial nerve (e.g., facial symmetry, strength)
	• 8th cranial nerve (e.g., hearing with tuning fork, whispered voice and/or finger rub)
	• 9th cranial nerve (e.g., spontaneous or reflex palate movement)
	• 11th cranial nerve (e.g., shoulder shrug strength)
	• 12th cranial nerve (e.g., tongue protrusion)
	• Examination of sensation (e.g., by touch, pin, vibration, proprioception)
	• Examination of deep tendon reflexes in upper and lower extremities with notation of pathological reflexes (e.g., Babinski)
	• Test coordination (e.g., finger/nose, heel/knee/shin, rapid alternating movements in the upper and lower extremities, evaluation of fine motor coordination in young children)
Psychiatric	

Content and Documentation Requirements

LEVEL OF EXAM	PERFORM AND DOCUMENT
Problem Focused	**One to five** elements identified by a bullet.
Expanded Problem Focused	**At least six** elements identified by a bullet.
Detailed	**At least twelve** elements identified by a bullet.
Comprehensive	Perform **all** elements identified by a bullet; document every element in each box with a shaded border and at least one element in each box with an unshaded border.

PSYCHIATRIC EXAMINATION

System/Body Area	Elements of Examination
Constitutional	• Measurement of **any three of the following seven** vital signs: 1) sitting or standing blood pressure, 2) supine blood pressure, 3) pulse rate and regularity, 4) respiration, 5) temperature, 6) height, 7) weight (may be measured and recorded by ancillary staff) • General appearance of patient (e.g., development, nutrition, body habitus, deformities, attention to grooming)
Head and Face	
Eyes	
Ears, Nose, Mouth and Throat	
Neck	
Respiratory	
Cardiovascular	
Chest (Breasts)	
Gastrointestinal (Abdomen)	
Genitourinary	
Lymphatic	
Musculoskeletal	• Assessment of muscle strength and tone (e.g., flaccid, cog wheel, spastic) with notation of any atrophy and abnormal movements • Examination of gait and station
Extremities	
Skin	
Neurological	
Psychiatric	• Description of speech including: rate; volume; articulation; coherence; and spontaneity with notation of abnormalities (e.g., perseveration, paucity of language) • Description of thought processes including: rate of thoughts; content of thoughts (e.g., logical vs. illogical, tangential); abstract reasoning; and computation • Description of associations (e.g., loose, tangential, circumstantial, intact) • Description of abnormal or psychotic thoughts including: hallucinations; delusions; preoccupation with violence; homicidal or suicidal ideation; and obsessions • Description of the patient's judgment (e.g., concerning everyday activities and social situations) and insight (e.g., concerning psychiatric condition) Complete mental status examination including • Orientation to time, place and person • Recent and remote memory • Attention span and concentration • Language (e.g., naming objects, repeating phrases) • Fund of knowledge (e.g., awareness of current events, past history, vocabulary) • Mood and affect (e.g., depression, anxiety, agitation, hypomania, lability)

Content and Documentation Requirements

LEVEL OF EXAM	PERFORM AND DOCUMENT
Problem Focused	**One to five** elements identified by a bullet.
Expanded Problem Focused	**At least six** elements identified by a bullet.
Detailed	**At least nine** elements identified by a bullet.
Comprehensive	Perform **all** elements identified by a bullet; document every element in each box with a shaded border and at least one element in each box with an unshaded border.

RESPIRATORY EXAMINATION

System/Body Area	Elements of Examination
Constitutional	• Measurement of **any three of the following seven** vital signs: 1) sitting or standing blood pressure, 2) supine blood pressure, 3) pulse rate and regularity, 4) respiration, 5) temperature, 6) height, 7) weight (may be measured and recorded by ancillary staff)
	• General appearance of patient (e.g., development, nutrition, body habitus, deformities, attention to grooming)
Head and Face	
Eyes	
Ears, Nose, Mouth and Throat	• Inspection of nasal mucosa, septum and turbinates
	• Inspection of teeth and gums
	• Examination of oropharynx (e.g., oral mucosa, hard and soft palates, tongue, tonsils and posterior pharynx)
Neck	• Examination of neck (e.g., masses, overall appearance, symmetry, tracheal position, crepitus)
	• Examination of thyroid (e.g., enlargement, tenderness, mass)
	• Examination of jugular veins (e.g., distension; a, v or cannon a waves)
Respiratory	• Inspection of chest with notation of symmetry and expansion
	• Assessment of respiratory effort (e.g., intercostal retractions, use of accessory muscles, diaphragmatic movement)
	• Percussion of chest (e.g., dullness, flatness, hyperresonance)
	• Palpation of chest (e.g., tactile fremitus)
	• Auscultation of lungs (e.g., breath sounds, adventitious sounds, rubs)
Cardiovascular	• Auscultation of heart including sounds, abnormal sounds and murmurs
	• Examination of peripheral vascular system by observation (e.g., swelling, varicosities) and palpation (e.g., pulses, temperature, edema, tenderness)
Chest (Breasts)	
Gastrointestinal (Abdomen)	• Examination of abdomen with notation of presence of masses or tenderness
	• Examination of liver and spleen
Genitourinary	
Lymphatic	• Palpation of lymph nodes in neck, axillae, groin and/or other location
Musculoskeletal	• Assessment of muscle strength and tone (e.g., flaccid, cog wheel, spastic) with notation of any atrophy and abnormal movements
	• Examination of gait and station
Extremities	• Inspection and palpation of digits and nails (e.g., clubbing, cyanosis, inflammation, petechiae, ischemia, infections, nodes)
Skin	• Inspection and/or palpation of skin and subcutaneous tissue (e.g., rashes, lesions, ulcers)
Neurological/ Psychiatric	Brief assessment of mental status including
	• Orientation to time, place and person
	• Mood and affect (e.g., depression, anxiety, agitation)

Content and Documentation Requirements

LEVEL OF EXAM	PERFORM AND DOCUMENT
Problem Focused	**One to five** elements identified by a bullet.
Expanded Problem Focused	**At least six** elements identified by a bullet.
Detailed	**At least twelve** elements identified by a bullet.
Comprehensive	Perform **all** elements identified by a bullet; document every element in each box with a shaded border and at least one element in each box with an unshaded border.

SKIN EXAMINATION

System/Body Area	Elements of Examination
Constitutional	• Measurement of any **three of the following seven** vital signs: 1) sitting or standing blood pressure, 2) supine blood pressure, 3) pulse rate and regularity, 4) respiration, 5) temperature, 6) height, 7) weight (may be measured and recorded by ancillary staff)
	• General appearance of patient (e.g., development, nutrition, body habitus, deformities, attention to grooming)
Head and Face	
Eyes	• Inspection of conjunctivae and lids
Ears, Nose, Mouth and Throat	• Inspection of lips, teeth and gums
	• Examination of oropharynx (e.g., oral mucosa, hard and soft palates, tongue, tonsils, posterior pharynx)
Neck	• Examination of thyroid (e.g., enlargement, tenderness, mass)
Respiratory	
Cardiovascular	• Examination of peripheral vascular system by observation (e.g., swelling, varicosities) and palpation (e.g., pulses, temperature, edema, tenderness)
Chest (Breasts)	
Gastrointestinal (Abdomen)	• Examination of liver and spleen
	• Examination of anus for condyloma and other lesions
Genitourinary	
Lymphatic	• Palpation of lymph nodes in neck, axillae, groin and/or other location
Musculoskeletal	
Extremities	• Inspection and palpation of digits and nails (e.g., clubbing, cyanosis, inflammation, petechiae, ischemia, infections, nodes)
Skin	• Palpation of scalp and inspection of hair of scalp, eyebrows, face, chest, pubic area (when indicated) and extremities
	• Inspection and/or palpation of skin and subcutaneous tissue (e.g., rashes, lesions, ulcers, susceptibility to and presence of photo damage) in **eight of the following ten** areas
	• Head, including the face and neck
	• Chest, including breasts and axillae
	• Abdomen
	• Genitalia, groin, buttocks
	• Back
	• Right upper extremity
	• Left upper extremity
	• Right lower extremity
	• Left lower extremity

Note: For the comprehensive level, the examination of at least eight anatomic areas must be performed and documented. For the three lower levels of examination, each body area is counted separately. For example, inspection and/or palpation of the skin and subcutaneous tissue of the right upper extremity and the left upper extremity constitutes two elements.

Table continued on following page

SKIN EXAMINATION (Continued)	
System/Body Area	**Elements of Examination**
	• Inspection of eccrine and apocrine glands of skin and subcutaneous tissue with identification and location of any hyperhidrosis, chromhidroses or bromhidrosis
Neurological/ Psychiatric	Brief assessment of mental status including
	• Orientation to time, place and person
	• Mood and affect (e.g., depression, anxiety, agitation)

Content and Documentation Requirements

LEVEL OF EXAM	PERFORM AND DOCUMENT
Problem Focused	**One to five** elements identified by a bullet.
Expanded Problem Focused	**At least six** elements identified by a bullet.
Detailed	**At least twelve** elements identified by a bullet.
Comprehensive	Perform **all** elements identified by a bullet; document every element in each box with a shaded border and at least one element in each box with an unshaded border.

C. Documentation of the Complexity of Medical Decision-Making

The levels of E/M services recognize four types of medical decision-making (straightforward, low complexity, moderate complexity and high complexity). Medical decision-making refers to the complexity of establishing a diagnosis and/or selecting a management option as measured by:

- the number of possible diagnoses and/or the number of management options that must be considered;
- the amount and/or complexity of medical records, diagnostic tests, and/or other information that must be obtained, reviewed and analyzed; and
- the risk of significant complications, morbidity and/or mortality, as well as comorbidities, associated with the patient's presenting problem(s), the diagnostic procedure(s) and/or the possible management options.

The following chart shows the progression of the elements required for each level of medical decision-making. To qualify for a given type of decision-making, **two of the three elements in the table must be either met or exceeded.**

Each of the elements of medical decision-making is described following.

Number of diagnoses or management options	Amount and/or complexity of data to be reviewed	Risk of complications and/or morbidity or mortality	Type of decision making
Minimal	Minimal or None	Minimal	*Straightforward*
Limited	Limited	Low	*Low Complexity*
Multiple	Moderate	Moderate	*Moderate Complexity*
Extensive	Extensive	High	*High Complexity*

Number of Diagnoses or Management Options. The number of possible diagnoses and/or the number of management options that must be considered is based on the number and types of problems addressed during the encounter, the complexity of establishing a diagnosis and the management decisions that are made by the physician.

Generally, decision-making with respect to a diagnosed problem is easier than that for an identified but undiagnosed problem. The number and type of diagnostic tests employed may be an indicator of the number of possible diagnoses. Problems which are improving or resolving are less complex than those which are worsening or failing to change as expected. The need to seek advice from others is another indicator of complexity of diagnostic or management problems.

- DG: For each encounter, an assessment, clinical impression, or diagnosis should be documented. It may be explicitly stated or implied in documented decisions regarding management plans and/or further evaluation.

  - For a presenting problem with an established diagnosis the record should reflect whether the problem is: a) improved, well controlled, resolving or resolved; or, b) inadequately controlled, worsening, or failing to change as expected.

  - For a presenting problem without an established diagnosis, the assessment or clinical impression may be stated in the form of differential diagnoses or as a "possible," "probable," or "rule out" (R/O) diagnosis.

- DG: The initiation of, or changes in, treatment should be documented. Treatment includes a wide range of management options including patient instructions, nursing instructions, therapies, and medications.

- DG: If referrals are made, consultations requested or advice sought, the record should indicate to whom or where the referral or consultation is made or from whom the advice is requested.

Amount and/or Complexity of Data to Be Reviewed. The amount and complexity of data to be reviewed is based on the types of diagnostic testing ordered or reviewed. A decision to obtain and review old medical records and/or obtain history from sources other than the patient increases the amount and complexity of data to be reviewed.

Discussion of contradictory or unexpected test results with the physician who performed or interpreted the test is an indication of the complexity of data being reviewed. On occasion the physician who ordered a test may personally review the image, tracing or specimen to supplement information from the physician who prepared the test report or interpretation; this is another indication of the complexity of data being reviewed.

- DG: If a diagnostic service (test or procedure) is ordered, planned, scheduled, or performed at the time of the E/M encounter, the type of service, eg, lab or x-ray, should be documented.

- DG: The review of lab, radiology and/or other diagnostic tests should be documented. A simple notation such as "WBC elevated" or "chest x-ray unremarkable" is acceptable. Alternatively, the review may be documented by initialing and dating the report containing the test results.

- DG: A decision to obtain old records or decision to obtain additional history from the family, caretaker or other source to supplement that obtained from the patient should be documented.

- DG: Relevant findings from the review of old records, and/or the receipt of additional history from the family, caretaker or other source to supplement that obtained from the patient should be documented. If there is no relevant information beyond that already obtained, that fact should be documented. A notation of "Old records reviewed" or "additional history obtained from family" without elaboration is insufficient.

- DG: The results of discussion of laboratory, radiology or other diagnostic tests with the physician who performed or interpreted the study should be documented.

- DG: The direct visualization and independent interpretation of an image, tracing or specimen previously or subsequently interpreted by another physician should be documented.

Risk of Significant Complications, Morbidity, and/or Mortality. The risk of significant complications, morbidity, and/or mortality is based on the risks associated with the presenting problem(s), the diagnostic procedure(s), and the possible management options.

- DG: Comorbidities/underlying diseases or other factors that increase the complexity of medical decision making by increasing the risk of complications, morbidity, and/or mortality should be documented.

- DG: If a surgical or invasive diagnostic procedure is ordered, planned or scheduled at the time of the E/M encounter, the type of procedure, eg, laparoscopy, should be documented.

- DG: If a surgical or invasive diagnostic procedure is performed at the time of the E/M encounter, the specific procedure should be documented.

- DG: The referral for or decision to perform a surgical or invasive diagnostic procedure on an urgent basis should be documented or implied.

The following table may be used to help determine whether the risk of significant complications, morbidity, and/or mortality is *minimal, low, moderate,* or *high.* Because the determination of risk is complex and not readily quantifiable, the table includes common clinical examples rather than absolute measures of risk. The assessment of risk of the presenting problem(s) is based on the risk related to the disease process anticipated between the present encounter and the next one. The assessment of risk of selecting diagnostic procedures and management options is based on the risk during and immediately following any procedures or treatment. **The highest level of risk in any one category (presenting problem(s), diagnostic procedure(s), or management options) determines the overall risk.**

TABLE OF RISK

Level of Risk	Presenting Problem(s)	Diagnostic Procedure(s) Ordered	Management Options Selected
Minimal	• One self-limited or minor problem, eg, cold, insect bite, tinea corporis	• Laboratory tests requiring venipuncture • Chest x-rays • EKG/EEG • Urinalysis • Ultrasound, eg, echocardiography • KOH prep	• Rest • Gargles • Elastic bandages • Superficial dressings
Low	• Two or more self-limited or minor problems • One stable chronic illness, eg, well controlled hypertension, non-insulin dependent diabetes, cataract, BPH • Acute uncomplicated illness or injury, eg, cystitis, allergic rhinitis, simple sprain	• Physiologic tests not under stress, eg, pulmonary function tests • Non-cardiovascular imaging studies with contrast, eg, barium enema • Superficial needle biopsies • Clinical laboratory tests requiring arterial puncture • Skin biopsies	• Over-the-counter drugs • Minor surgery with no identified risk factors • Physical therapy • Occupational therapy • IV fluids without additives
Moderate	• One or more chronic illnesses with mild exacerbation, progression, or side effects of treatment • Two or more stable chronic illnesses • Undiagnosed new problem with uncertain prognosis, eg, lump in breast • Acute illness with systemic symptoms, eg, pyelonephritis, pneumonitis, colitis, • Acute complicated injury, eg, head injury with brief loss of consciousness	• Physiologic tests under stress, eg, cardiac stress test, fetal contraction stress test • Diagnostic endoscopies with no identified risk factors • Deep needle or incisional biopsy • Cardiovascular imaging studies with contrast and no identified risk factors, eg, arteriogram, cardiac catheterization • Obtain fluid from body cavity, eg, lumbar puncture, thoracentesis, uldocentesis	• Minor surgery with identified risk factors • Elective major surgery (open, percutaneous or endoscopic) with no identified risk factors • Prescription drug management • Therapeutic nuclear medicine • IV fluids with additives • Closed treatment of fracture or dislocation without manipulation
High	• One or more chronic illnesses with severe exacerbation, progression, or side effects of treatment • Acute or chronic illnesses or injuries that pose a threat to life or bodily function, eg, multiple trauma, acute MI, pulmonary embolus, severe respiratory distress, progressive severe rheumatoid arthritis, psychiatric illness with potential threat to self or others, peritonitis, acute renal failure • An abrupt change in neurologic status, eg, seizure, TIA, weakness, sensory loss	• Cardiovascular imaging studies with contrast with identified risk factors • Cardiac electrophysiological tests • Diagnostic endoscopies with identified risk factors • Discography	• Elective major surgery (open, percutaneous or endoscopic) with identified risk factors • Emergency major surgery (open, percutaneous or endoscopic) • Parenteral controlled substances • Drug therapy requiring intensive monitoring for toxicity • Decision not to resuscitate or to de-escalate care because of poor prognosis

D. Documentation of an Encounter Dominated by Counseling or Coordination of Care

In the case where counseling and/or coordination of care dominates (more than 50%) of the physician/patient and/or family encounter (face-to-face time in the office or other or outpatient setting, floor/unit time in the hospital or nursing facility), time is considered the key or controlling factor to qualify for a particular level of E/M services.

- ▪ DG: If the physician elects to report the level of service based on counseling and/or coordination of care, the total length of time of the encounter (face-to-face or floor time, as appropriate) should be documented and the record should describe the counseling and/or activities to coordinate care.

Alpha II *i*Coder Exercises

Note: It is recommended that you wait to access this feature until you've finished working through the main text.

As an additional bonus feature, we have included 30-day access to Alpha II *i*Coder online code editor from UnicorMed.

CASES 1 THROUGH 15

Your supervisor has asked you to use the *i*Coder to check the accuracy of several cases that were coded by another coder.

CASES 16 THROUGH 20

For Cases 16 through 20, you are to assign the correct CPT and ICD-9-CM codes. Be sure to check the codes you assign with the *i*Coder. Once you have finished, your instructor will provide you with answers for Cases 16-20 so you can check your work.

USING ALPHA II ICODER ONLINE CODE EDITOR
Note: The User Name and Password will only be valid during the current coding year.

Also, if you are logged in to *i*Coder and leave without clicking on Sign Out, you will not be able to re-enter for 15 minutes. If you are logged in to *i*Coder and the system doesn't detect any input from you for 15 minutes, you will be automatically logged out, and you will not be able to re-enter for 15 minutes.

Here are some easy steps to start using your free trial of the Alpha II *i*Coder.
1. Start at the Evolve Learning Resources at
   http://evolve.elsevier.com/ Buck/step
2. Click on the *iCoder* section, and click on the link to be taken to the *iCoder login page.*
3. Enter your **User Name** and **Password** from the card you received with your textbook. (You may want to check the **Remember My User Name** box for faster access in subsequent logins.)
4. The first page that opens in *i*Coder is the main page. Click on **My Settings.** This will take you to a settings page.

5. Scroll down to **Change My Geographical Location.** Using the drop down box, choose the location that is correct for you (e.g., 31140: California—San Mateo). Some states do not have county-specific locations (e.g., 00510: Alabama—All Counties).

6. Click on *iCoder* **Main,** and enter your CPT codes, modifiers, and ICD codes in the spaces indicated.

7. Click on **Check Codes.** You will get all green lights if your coding is correct. You will get a yellow or red light if the coding is questionable.

8. Click on the **Help** button for explanations of any **Flags** you may get on Code Check.

9. Click on **Descriptions** for a full description of your CPT and ICD-9 codes.

10. Click on **Proc Notes for RVU schedule, global fee period, surgical team allowance,** and other information regarding a procedure. Click on the drop down box next to **Get Notes** and click on **ALL** if you have more than one CPT code.

11. Click on **Diagnosis** to find ICD-9 codes. There are five basic look-up criteria in *iCoder*:

   1. **Definitive Medical Term:** (e.g., arthritis, encephalitis, pericarditis, hemorrhage) After typing in the definitive medical diagnosis, a listing will appear in alphabetical order that will give all the different code numbers according to type, etiology, site, or situation. More criteria will make the search faster and will also search by partial words; the more complete the description, the more exact the search (e.g., arthritis tra vs. arthritis traumatic, hemorrhage brain, fracture tibia).

   2. **Proper Named Diseases, Conditions, or Syndromes:** (e.g., Downs for Down's Syndrome, Guillain for Guillain-Barre disease, Apert for Apert's Disease)

   3. **Medical Acronym:** (e.g., GERD, COPD, ASHD, CHF, CAD)

   4. **Anatomical Site:** (e.g., gallbladder disorder, heart block, ankle injury, rib separation, knee deformity)

   5. **Obvious Key Words or Exactly as Written in the Record:** (e.g., divorce, halo, pacemaker, knock knee, fructose intolerance, idiopathic hypertrophic subaortic stenosis, temporomandibular joint disorder)

      NOTE: When looking-up cancer codes if you enter the word "CANCER" you will be taken to the cancer screening codes. To find the proper "CANCER" diagnosis you should enter CA and the organ or anatomical site (e.g., CA BRAIN, CA LUNG, CA SPINE).

      Click on **E-Codes** for a list of E-Codes. You will be automatically directed to the E-Code menu from **Check Codes** if you enter a diagnosis code that may need an E-Code with it. Click on **Modifiers** for a list of modifiers that will fit with a particular CPT code. Any screen can be printed by clicking on the printer icon at the top of the screen.

      Caution: If you are logged-in to *iCoder* and leave without clicking on **Sign Out** you will not be able to re-enter for 15 minutes. If you are logged-in to *iCoder* and the system doesn't detect any input from you for 15 minutes, you will be automatically logged out, and you will not be able to re-enter for 15 minutes.

CASE 1

Cases 1 and 2 are ongoing services provided to the same patient by the same physician.

PREOPERATIVE DIAGNOSIS: Pyogenic granuloma, sinus tract, buttock.

POSTOPERATIVE DIAGNOSIS: Multiple sinus tracts, one extending inferiorly about 7 × 3 cm in diameter, one extending to the right approximately 4 × 3 cm, and one extending to the left for about 3 cm.

SURGICAL FINDINGS: As above, plus granulation tissue present in a capsule of multiple sinus tracts. Sinus tracts measured a total of about 15 × 8 cm in their total dimensions.

SURGICAL PROCEDURE: Partial unroofing of sinus tracts.

SURGEON: Tony Wellbed, MD

ANESTHESIA: General endotracheal.

DESCRIPTION OF PROCEDURE: The patient was intubated and turned in the prone position. A probe was inserted in the sinus cavity, and dissection was carried down to this. I encountered a piece of chronically infected granulation tissue coming out of a hole, in which I stuck the probe, but this continued for a distance longer than the probe and accordingly, I put my finger in this and this extended down the length of my index finger (about 7-8 cm by about 3 cm in width). I left this intact, because this would necessitate extensive dissection and we have no blood on this patient at this time. We then unroofed two other sinus cavities, and packed this opened with 2-inch vaginal packing and applied a dressing and Kerlix plus an Elastoplast. Estimated blood loss: 25 cc. The patient seemed to tolerate the procedure well and left the operating room in good condition.

CPT	Modifiers			ICD-9-CMs				
11041				686.1				

CASE 2

PREOPERATIVE DIAGNOSIS: Postop bleeding from sacral wound.

POSTOPERATIVE DIAGNOSIS: Same.

SURGICAL FINDINGS: One very active bleeder and one less active bleeder along the wound margin.

SURGICAL PROCEDURE: Wound exploration and cauterization of two bleeders of the wound edge.

SURGEON: Tony Wellbed, MD

ANESTHESIA: Local with plain 1% Xylocaine, approximately 10 cc along each suture line.

Following her unroofing of the sinus tracts yesterday, I was called by the Recovery Room nurse for a large spot of blood on the dressing. She also incidentally had this on the bed. I took the dressing down and called for some silver nitrate because the patient had a very active bleeder coming from the edge of the wound. I asked for some sterile Kerlix fluffs and light. Because we could not adequately visualize everything that was going on at the time, I took the patient back to the Operating Room where the bleeder was easily identified and cautery was used to stop the bleeding. There was also one other small bleeder cauterized. No other bleeders were noted. I sprayed the bed with topical thrombin and packed some Surgicel in the more proximal aspect of the wound and then packed thrombin-soaked 2-inch vaginal packing in the wound followed by Kerlix fluffs and a snug dressing covered by Elastoplast. The bleeding appeared to be controlled.

DESCRIPTION OF PROCEDURE: The patient was turned in the prone position and we injected more local anesthesia (1% Xylocaine and 1:100,000 epinephrine, having injected some in the Recovery Room). I cauterized the very active bleeder that was noted, and saw one more less-active bleeder along the suture line. Surgicel was in place at the depths of the wound in a pool of topical thrombin that we had placed in the proximal aspect of the wound from where the bleeding came. I then saturated a 2-inch vaginal gauze packing with topical thrombin and packed this in the wound followed by one box of Kerlix fluffs. The wound was then dressed with Elastoplast.

Coincidentally noted at the time of her surgery with the wound exploration was conversion of her electrocardiogram to a Mobitz Type I heart block. I did consult the cardiologist at the same time.

CPT	Modifiers			ICD-9-CMs				
17999				998.11				

CASE 3

Cases 3 and 4 are a continuation of care provided to the same patient by the same physician. The previous decompression fasciotomy was performed 1 day prior to Case 3.

PREOPERATIVE DIAGNOSIS: Status post-fasciotomy, lateral aspect of the right lower extremity.

POSTOPERATIVE DIAGNOSIS: Same.

SURGICAL PROCEDURE: Extension of fasciotomy, lateral aspect, right thigh and dressing change.

SURGEON: George M. Pathfinder, MD

ANESTHESIA: General endotracheal.

SURGICAL FINDINGS: Open wound, right thigh, with compression of the vastus lateralis laterally.

DESCRIPTION: The dressings were removed. The wound was inspected, and the muscle was quite clean. However, there was some constriction of the vastus lateralis by the tensor fascia lata laterally. The fasciotomy was further incised to extended beyond the original fasciotomy. Dressing of Xeroform, Kerlix fluffs, and a splint was then reapplied.

ESTIMATED BLOOD LOSS: 25 cc.

The patient tolerated the procedure well and left the operating room in good condition.

ADDENDUM: This patient was scheduled originally for skin graft, but we elected at this point to attempt wound vacuum suction on the thigh to see if it could be closed without a skin graft.

CPT	Modifiers			ICD-9-CMs				
27496	RT			958.8				
15852				958.8				

CASE 4

The same physician completes the decompression fasciotomy 3 days later.

PREOPERATIVE DIAGNOSIS: Status post-fasciotomy, right thigh, for compartment syndrome.

POSTOPERATIVE DIAGNOSIS: Same.

PROCEDURE PERFORMED: Irrigation and debridement with 12.5 cm closure, right thigh wound.

SURGEON: George M. Pathfinder, MD

ANESTHESIA: General.

FINDINGS: The wound vac seems to have reduced the volume of the thigh fairly nicely and we were able to close the skin without any undue tension. The wound itself looked clean and there was no evidence of any purulent material at all.

PROCEDURE: While under a general anesthetic, the patient was placed in the supine position on the operating room table. The wound vac was removed from the patient's thigh and the wound appeared to be very clean without any purulent material at all. We then prepped the patient's right leg with Betadine and draped it in a sterile fashion.

We then initially used a Surgilav device with saline and a sponge to scrub the incision and irrigated very thoroughly. After this, we attempted to see if the quadriceps would contract by pinching it with a forceps. We were able to pinch the quadriceps in several areas and it seemed to respond quite nicely.

We then began to close the subcutaneous tissue from each end using 2-0 Vicryl suture. We were actually able to pull the wound together quite nicely without any undue tension. We were then able to close the skin using skin staples. With the wound closed, we could flex the knee approximately 90 degrees.

We then dressed the wound with Xeroform gauze dressings under 4 × 4s, ABD pads, and an ACE wrap. The dorsalis pedis pulse was strong at the end of the procedure. He was taken from the operating room in good condition and breathing spontaneously. He was given IV Kefzol preoperatively and will be continued on IV Kefzol postoperatively as well. He tolerated the procedure very well.

CPT	Modifiers			ICD-9-CMs				
27496	RT			958.92				
12004	RT			958.92				

CASE 5

PREOPERATIVE DIAGNOSIS: Gun shot wound to left thigh.

POSTOPERATIVE DIAGNOSIS: Gun shot wound to left thigh with transection of superficial femoral artery and veins.

PROCEDURE PERFORMED: Exploratory laparotomy with control of left external iliac artery. Debridement of left thigh wound. Repair of left superficial femoral artery using a right greater saphenous vein interposition vein graft. Repair of left superficial femoral vein. Ligation of branch of left profunda femoris artery. Fasciotomy left lower leg.

SURGEON: Marsha Petros, MD

ANESTHESIA: General anesthesia.

INDICATIONS FOR SURGERY: This patient is a 27-year-old Caucasian male who was shot in the left thigh. The exact cause or how the accident occurred is unknown. The patient was initially seen in Anytown and was transferred to Central Hospital for treatment.

DESCRIPTION OF PROCEDURE: The patient was bleeding from the left thigh. The prep was just Betadine solution splashed on the skin. An abdominal incision was then made and the iliac artery on the left side was isolated with a vessel loop and clamp. This controlled the bleeding. The left thigh incision was then opened from the gunshot wound to the groin area. There was a large clot in this area and this whole area was opened. Upon examination there was oozing and bleeding from the torn muscle. The proximal and distal end of the superficial femoral artery was found. There was a large segment missing. The superficial femoral vein was also found and this was repaired. The holes that were in the vein were found and repaired. The nerves of the left thigh were not seen. A repair of the left superficial femoral artery was then done. The right groin area was dissected and the right greater saphenous vein on the upper thigh was excised. The branches of the vein were ligated with 3-0 silk sutures and divided. At the junction of the right femoral vein a vascular clamp was then placed across the saphenous vein. The saphenous vein was then transected. The saphenous vein was then oversewn with a running 4-0 Prolene suture. Clamp was then removed. The dissection was then carried out distally for at least 8 inches. The saphenous vein was then harvested. The distal end was tied with a 2-0 silk suture, and the vein was then removed. The vein was irrigated and was brought into the left wound area. The proximal end of the left superficial femoral artery was then trimmed back to normal tissue. The saphenous vein was then spatulated and sewn end-to-end to the artery using running 5-0 Prolene sutures. After this was completed the distal anastomosis was then done and again the vein in the artery was debrided back to normal tissue. The vein was cut to length and sutured end-to-end to the artery using 5-0 Prolene sutures. Just prior to completion of the closure the clamp on the artery was removed to allow the vein to be flushed, this was done and the closure was then completed. After examination it was noted that the vein was in spasm and even though it was reversed, the flow through the vein was marginal. Because of this the superficial femoral artery was clamped. An arteriotomy was then made in the proximal artery. The catheter was passed down through the graft. A LeMaitre valvulotome was also passed down through the graft and then opened and then all the valves were lysed. After this was completed the opening in the artery was closed with a running 5-0 Prolene suture. This allowed for excellent flow through the graft in the distal artery. Also, before the initial anastomosis of the superficial femoral artery there was some clotting present and so therefore a Fogarty catheter was passed down distally and all that clot was removed. Then the artery was flushed with heparinized saline. The patient did not receive any systemic heparin because his INR was elevated because of the transfusions and because of his extensive blood loss, which required multiple units of transfusion. After the anastomosis was completed and repairs were completed the operative area was irrigated. A small branch of the left profunda femoris artery was found and this was doubly ligated with 2-0 silk sutures. A JP drain was then left in the operative area and the fascia was closed over the drain and also covering the graft. The right groin incision and tissue thigh incision were also closed with a running 3-0 Vicryl suture and skin clips for the skin. The vessel loop on the external iliac artery in the abdomen was then removed and the abdominal incision was closed with a running looped #1 PDS suture. Subcutaneous tissue was irrigated and skin was closed with skin clips. The left thigh incision was then closed with initially figure-of-eight #1 Prolene sutures. After this was completed the left lower leg fasciotomy was then done. The left lower leg was then prepped and draped in the usual manner and fasciotomy was then done opening all compartments. There was marked venous hypertension noted and the muscle did protrude through the fascia indicating swelling. After this was completed the dressings were applied. By this time it was noted that the groin incision was leaking and oozing blood; because of this the incision was prepped and draped again and reopened. Upon reopening it was noted that the patient had pooled blood in the cavity which was created by the gunshot wound. This area was then irrigated and no obvious bleeding site could be found. There was some generalized oozing from the muscle. This space was then obliterated with figure-of-eight 0 Vicryl sutures. The JP drain was then left in the operative area again and the muscle was again closed around the drain using figure-of-eight 0 Vicryl sutures. Again, the fascia on the anterior layer was closed with interrupted 0 Vicryl sutures. A dressing was then applied. The oozing was now minimal and the patient was transferred to the intensive care unit in critical condition.

This patient is a 27-year-old Caucasian male who was shot in the left thigh. How the accident occurred I am not sure. He was sent from his hometown hospital to this hospital. Upon arriving, the patient was hypotensive with a systolic pressure of 60. He had bleeding from his left thigh wound. His lungs were clear. Heart was tachycardic.

IMPRESSION: Gunshot wound to left thigh.

PLAN: The patient was taken immediately to the operating room for control of his bleeding and exploration of his left thigh. The patient was in critical condition.

CPT	Modifiers			ICD-9-CMs				
35256				890.1	958.8	E922.9		
37618				890.1	958.8	E922.9		
35226				890.1	958.8	E922.9		
27496				958.8	E922.9			

CASE 6

Cases 6 and 7 are ongoing care provided by the same physician.

PREOPERATIVE DIAGNOSIS: Desmoplastic malignant melanoma, submucosal, left side of upper lip.

POSTOPERATIVE DIAGNOSIS: Same.

SURGICAL PROCEDURES:

1. Sentinel node biopsy, left submandibular region.
2. Wide V-excision (1 centimeter) of desmoplastic malignant melanoma, left side of upper lip with through-and-through excision and 1 centimeter margins on all sides.

SURGEON: Brian Wilson, MD

ANESTHESIA: General endotracheal with supplementary 2 cc of 1% Xylocaine and 1:800,000 epinephrine.

SURGICAL FINDINGS: The patient had a scar of the upper lip and a 5 millimeter linear, pigmented lesion near the mucosal junction. There was one submandibular lymph node identified that appeared to be benign. No occipital or posterior submandibular lymph nodes were identified despite assiduous search.

DESCRIPTION OF PROCEDURE: Following injection of radioactive dye in the Radiology Department, the patient was sent to the operating room where the face and neck were prepped with Betadine scrub and solution and draped in a routine sterile fashion.

Sentinal node biopsy: The sites that had been identified in Radiology were noted, and on the mastoid area, I detected 100 on the probe externally. I explored this, but when I got inside, I was unable to reproduce the external reading despite a vigorous exploration of the mastoid area and splitting of the sternocleidomastoid muscle over the site where most of the probe activity was evident. We made about a 3-centimeter incision in this area and explored it thoroughly in all areas indicated. I thought on occasion I palpated a lymph node, but upon deep dissection, it was noted that this was simply another fiber of the sternocleidomastoid muscle, and we abandoned this after a search of about 15 minutes. In the submandibular area, an incision was made, and activity was evident. The skin in the posterior mandibular area had a reading of 13 with an in vivo reading of 63. However, the ex vivo was only approximately 7 on the specimen itself. It may have been too small to have caused any reactivity. The background was 26 following removal of a small lymph node which was less than 1 centimeter diameter. No anterior mandibular lymph node was ever identified. Also, it should be noted that at no time did I, other than the small lymph node we removed, palpate lymphadenopathy in the mesenteric muscle region nor in the region of the external maxillary artery which crossed the marginal mandibular nerve.

Wide V-excision, left upper lip: I then marked out a margin of 1 centimeter around the previous scar, and in so doing, I noted that included within this resection was a 5-millimeter linear pigmented lesion. This was a wedge resection of the lip, and bleeding of the coronal arteries were clamped and ligated with 4-0 Vicryl. I then began closure of the mucosa, lining up the mucocutaneous junction and lining up the vermilion where it meets the white roll. After completion of the mucosal closure, the musculature was brought together. The orbicularis oculi musculature was brought together with 4-0 Vicryl suture, and interrupted 5-0 Prolene was used to reapproximate the skin. There was no evidence of residual tumor within the specimen submitted. A silk suture tagged the lip side of the specimen. Antibiotic ointment was applied, and 4 × 4 was used to cover the incision. The patient tolerated the procedure well and left the area in good condition.

Pathology report later indicated: Melanocarcinoma

CPT	Modifiers			ICD-9-CMs					
38500				172.0					
40520				172.0					

CASE 7

PREOPERATIVE DIAGNOSIS: Residual desmoplastic malignant melanoma, left side of upper lip.

POSTOPERATIVE DIAGNOSIS: Same.

SURGICAL FINDINGS: 1.5 cm healed incision, left side of upper lip through-and-through. No residual tumor seen in resected specimen.

PROCEDURE PERFORMED: Excision of residual malignant melanoma, left side upper lip, with 1 cm margins with reconstruction by flaps created by perialar crescentic incisions producing flaps of 4 × 4 cm and 2.5 × 2 cm.

SURGEON: Brian Wilson, MD

ANESTHESIA: General endotracheal anesthesia plus 7 cc of 1% Xylocaine with 1:800,000 epinephrine.

ESTIMATED BLOOD LOSS: 25 cc.

COMPLICATIONS: None.

SPONGE AND NEEDLE COUNTS: Correct

FINDINGS: It's been 3 weeks since I performed a wide excision of the malignant melanoma of the upper lip. This patient is back today for residual excision and flap creation.

DESCRIPTION: The patient's face was prepped with Betadine scrub and solution and draped in routine sterile fashion. I infiltrated the potential areas of resection with a total of 7 cc of 1% Xylocaine with 1:800,000 epinephrine, and made a left perialar crescentic incision that I excised in continuity with the specimen, which I excised by taking a cm margin on either side of it and up to the nostril sill, taking a block of tissue out through-and-through by using a number eleven knife blade from the skin through the mucosa. The top of the crescent was tagged with a silk suture and submitted for frozen section. Dr. Cooley examined the specimen and found no residual tumor at the site that it would be most likely to be located. After assurance there was no tumor in this area I returned to the operating room, and resected a little bit of apparent scar tissue more inferiorly in the wound than the specimen that had been tagged for microscopic examination. After resection of that tissue, I did a right perialar crescentic excision, creating a flap of about 4 × 4 cm, and on the left the resultant perialar crescentic excision resulting in a flap of about 2.5 × 2 cm. Mucosal incisions were made with about 5 mm away from the gingival margin, and the mucosa was advanced. I sutured the mucosa with interrupted 4-0 Vicryl, sutured the orbicularis oculi with 4-0 Vicryl and one 4-0 Monocryl, following which I closed the skin with interrupted 4-0 Prolene. Steri-Strips were applied to the lip. The patient tolerated the procedure well and left the operating room in good condition.

CPT	Modifiers			ICD-9-CMs				
40525				172.0				

CASE 8

PREOPERATIVE DIAGNOSIS: Anal fissure.

POSTOPERATIVE DIAGNOSIS: Same.

PROCEDURE PERFORMED:
1. Sphincterotomy.
2. One quadrant hemorrhoidectomy.

SURGEON: Meridian Casha, MD

ANESTHESIA: Spinal.

INDICATION: The patient is a pleasant 46-year-old female who is post three quadrant hemorrhoidectomy for severe external hemorrhoids. She has an anal fissure as well as the external hemorrhoid and that is quite tender. She presents today for elective sphincterotomy, excision of the external hemorrhoid, understands surgery and the risks of bleeding and infection, possible damage to the sphincter muscles and wishes to proceed.

DESCRIPTION OF PROCEDURE: The patient was brought to the operating room, given spinal anesthesia and placed in a jackknife position. We could see the enlarged hemorrhoid/sentinel tag at the 10 o'clock position and the fissure right at the base of this. Anoscope was placed and we placed a Kelly clamp behind the hypertrophied scarred band of muscle and divided the muscle. We then excised the external hemorrhoid and then closed the defect with interrupted 3-0 chromic sutures and running locked 3-0 chromic. There were no other hemorrhoids and there were no other fissures. We infiltrated the area with a total of 30 cc of 0.5% Sensorcaine with epinephrine solution, placed four gauze dressings in the area that we will remove in 30 minutes and she was taken to recovery in stable condition.

CPT	Modifiers			ICD-9-CMs				
46250				565.0				

CASE 9

PREOPERATIVE DIAGNOSES:
1. Respiratory failure.
2. Morbid obesity.
3. Excess cervical skin and adipose tissue.

POSTOPERATIVE DIAGNOSES:
1. Respiratory failure.
2. Morbid obesity.
3. Excess cervical skin and adipose tissue.

PROCEDURE PERFORMED:
1. Flap tracheostomy.
2. Bilateral cervical lipectomy.
3. Bilateral cervical skin resection, with intermediate closure, 10 cm.

SURGEON: Eda Seekong, MD

ANESTHESIA: General endotracheal anesthesia.

INDICATION: 68-year-old female, with respiratory failure, requiring ventilator support. She also has pancreatitis that will require long-term treatment, as well as ventilator therapy. She has morbid obesity. The patient is now prepared for tracheostomy placement for long-term ventilatory support. Due to her morbid obesity and excessive cervical adipose tissue and skin, lipectomy and skin resection are also necessary.

DESCRIPTION OF PROCEDURE: After written consent was obtained, the patient was taken to the operating room and placed on the operating room table in the supine position. The patient's neck was then prepped with Betadine prep and then draped in a sterile manner. An omega-shaped inferior flap was marked. The area was then infiltrated with 1% Xylocaine with 1:100,000 units epinephrine. After several minutes, sharp dissect was carried down through the skin and subcutaneous tissue. The platysma was identified. Excessive fat from the dermis down to the sternocleidomastoid muscle was removed bilaterally. Additional fat was removed off of the strap muscles. This was done from a level of the thyroid notch to the clavicle. Subsequently, the strap muscles were divided in the midline and retracted laterally. The thyroid was divided in the midline and then retracted laterally. Suture ligatures of 4-0 silk were used for the thyroid. The thyroid was then entered between the second and third tracheal rings. Superior and inferior tracheal cartilage flaps were then made. A #8 Shiley cuff tracheostomy tube was then placed. The superior and inferior skin flaps were secured to the cartilage flaps with 4-0 Vicryl suture in a half vertical mattress closure. Subsequently, the skin and adipose tissue excision was then marked in the submental and upper cervical region bilaterally. This area was then infiltrated with local solution. Sharp dissection was then carried down through the skin and subcutaneous tissue. This skin and excess adipose tissue were then removed. Hemostasis was achieved with the Bovie cautery. The wound was closed by reapproximating the subcutaneous tissue and dermis with interrupted 4-0 Vicryl suture. The skin was then approximated with skin staples. The tracheostomy tube was secured both with sutures and ties. Bacitracin ointment was applied to the upper incision. A dressing of 4 × 4s and Elastoplast was then placed over the submental area. The patient tolerated the procedure well, there was no break in technique, and the patient was taken back to the medical critical care unit in stable condition.

FLUIDS ADMINISTERED: 1800 cc of RL.

ESTIMATED BLOOD LOSS: 100 cc.

URINE OUTPUT: 175 cc.

CPT	Modifiers			ICD-9-CMs				
31610				278.01				
15838				278.01				

CASE 10

PREOPERATIVE DIAGNOSIS: Torn left lateral meniscus.

POSTOPERATIVE DIAGNOSES:
1. Torn left lateral meniscus.
2. Chondromalacia, left knee.

PROCEDURE PERFORMED:
1. Examination of left knee under anesthesia.
2. Arthroscopy of left knee with partial lateral meniscectomy and debridement of chondromalacia.

SURGEON: Pita Hortaga, MD

ANESTHESIA: General.

FINDINGS: The patient was found to have significant chondromalacia in all three compartments of her left knee. She has bare bone exposed on the weight-bearing surface of the medial and lateral femoral condyles and she has significant chondromalacia on the articular surface of the patella almost down to subchondral bone. She had a degenerative tear involving the lateral meniscus. The medial meniscus appeared to be intact. The anterior cruciate ligament was intact.

PROCEDURE: While under a general anesthetic, the patient's left knee was examined. The collateral ligaments were intact and Lachman's test was negative as was pivot shift. McMurray's test was negative.

We then prepped the patient's left leg with Betadine and draped it in a sterile fashion. An Esmarch bandage was used to exsanguinate the leg and a tourniquet on the thigh was inflated to 300 mmHg. We ended up deflating this tourniquet after about 5-10 minutes as the bleeding was not controlled. The total tourniquet time including the first and second tourniquet times was about 43 minutes.

We created three portals. The first was placed along the superior anterolateral aspect. The second was placed along the inferior anteromedial aspect and the third along the inferior anterolateral aspect of the knee. We distended the knee with lactated Ringer's solution. We examined the suprapatellar pouch and the medial and lateral gutters. She appeared to have somewhat hypertrophic synovium and was somewhat reddish and angry in appearance. We then examined the articular surface of the patella and found that she had significant chondromalacia characterized by fraying almost down to subchondral bone. We used a shaver to trim this area. The adjacent surface of the trochlea, however, appeared to be in relatively good condition.

We then examined the medial compartment and the medial meniscus appeared to be in relatively good condition with only minor fraying. We then examined the articular surface of the medial femoral condyle and noticed that she had raised a blister of articular cartilage. There was fissure over this and we could pass a probe underneath the articular cartilage. We gave some consideration to leaving this alone; however, we eventually elected to unroof this blister. This left an area of bare bone on the weightbearing surface of the medial femoral condyle. This blister was therefore made up of cartilage which had no attachment to the subchondral bone and was fairly easily debrided with a shaver. We tried to smooth this area as best as possible with the shaver and soften the edges around this area.

We then turned our attention to the notch area and probed the anterior cruciate ligament. It was intact. There was an obvious tear of the lateral meniscus as there was a fragment of the meniscus laying against the anterior cruciate ligament, which we removed. She had a degenerative tear involving the entire length of the lateral meniscus. We used a combination of basket forceps and the shaver to trim the lateral meniscus back to a stable rim. The lateral compartment has significant chondromalacia in both the femur and the tibia. The articular surface on the lateral femoral condyle has worn almost down to subchondral bone and subchondral bone actually could be seen through the thin layer of articular cartilage. We used the shaver to trim the chondromalacia as best as possible.

At this point, then, we would look for any remaining loose fragments and drain the knee. We then injected 80 mg of Depo-Medrol with 2 mL of 1% Xylocaine. The skin incisions were closed using 4-0 nylon suture and sterile dressings were applied under ABD pads and an ACE wrap. She was taken from the operating room in good condition breathing spontaneously. The final sponge and needle counts were correct. The prognosis for her left knee is only fair since she does have significant chondromalacia in all three compartments.

CPT	Modifiers			ICD-9-CMs				
29877	LT			733.92				

CASE 11

PREOPERATIVE DIAGNOSIS: Right knee medial meniscus old bucket handle tear.

POSTOPERATIVE DIAGNOSIS: Same.

PROCEDURES PERFORMED:
1. Diagnostic arthroscopy.
2. Right knee arthroscopy with partial medial meniscectomy.

SURGEON: Dennis M. Schaffer, MD

ANESTHESIA: General anesthesia

DRAINS: None

FINDINGS: 40-year-old male suffering with persistent pain in his knee following medial meniscus repair and ACL reconstruction of 1 year. He is taken back to surgery. After appropriate level of anesthesia was achieved the right knee was prepped and draped in an orthopaedic manner. We went through the previous portals sites. Sharp dissection was carried through the skin, blunt dissection was carried into the joint space. The patient had some scar tissue in the notch area and we went ahead and debrided this. The hamstring was probed and felt to be intact and functioning nicely. Immediately the patient's old meniscus repair was not functioning. The patient's meniscus was a little bit more complexly torn. I went ahead and debrided it. This was an essential bucket handle that would have been previously repaired. We debrided back to stable tissue. We explored the lateral compartment and it was felt to be intact. No loose bodies were noted. We explored the medial and lateral gutters, suprapatellar pouch, and no loose bodies were noted.

The articular surface was noted to be in good shape. There was some minimal grade two chondromalacia involving the medial femoral condyle area. The knee was irrigated copiously. 20 cc of 0.25% Marcaine was injected into the joint space and portal sites. We repaired the wounds with interrupted nylon sutures. We dressed the wound sterilely and the patient was placed in a knee immobilizer. The patient tolerated the procedure well and left the operating room in good condition.

CPT	Modifiers			ICD-9-CMs				
29881	59	RT		717.0				

CASE 12

PREOPERATIVE DIAGNOSES: Persistent hemoptysis and pneumonia and changes on x-ray.

POSTOPERATIVE DIAGNOSES: Same.

PROCEDURE: Transbronchial biopsy, bronchial biopsy, bronchoalveolar lavage, bronchial washings, and bronchial brushings.

PHYSICIAN: Hurada Maltose, MD

FINDINGS: The patient was sedated and preop'd while he was on the ventilator (status, ventilator dependent is reported with a V code) which did not really require much additional drug at all. Please see the drug sheet for further information.

PROCEDURE: The patient was monitored throughout the procedure with usual monitoring. There were no significant changes in blood pressure, oxygen saturation, or pulse rate, nor did any arrhythmias develop. No pneumothorax was discovered postprocedure by chest x-ray or by auscultation.

Once the patient was sedated, more than usual since he was maintained on a ventilator in the first place, the bronchoscope was introduced with a #9 endotracheal tube so it fit quite easily, and we were able to see the distal 2 centimeters of trachea, which was red and swollen, the carina, which was red and swollen, and all the airways were red and swollen and with white plaquing consistent with candidiasis on the left mainstem and going down toward the lower lobe. The area in question was biopsied, brushed and washed and subjected to bronchioalveolar lavage as well as bronchial brushings with sheath and non-sheath brushes as well as bronchial biopsies and transbronchial biopsies performed in that area. There were no complications. There was some blood seen in the left lower lobe, which was where most of the secretions were and they were bloody. There were excess secretions everywhere but most were in the left lower lobe. The specimens were sent for appropriate pathological, cytological, and bacteriological studies, including a tissue sample, which was sent for bacteriological studies. Followup will be done in the Intensive Care Unit when we get the information back from the Lab.

CPT	Modifiers			ICD-9-CMs				
31624				786	486	V46.11		
31623				786	486	V46.11		
31628				786	486	V46.11		

CASE 13

SAME DAY SURGERY

PREOPERATIVE DIAGNOSIS: Basal cell carcinoma, right side of nose.

POSTOPERATIVE DIAGNOSIS: Same.

SURGICAL FINDINGS: Healing 5-mm ulcer, right side of nose, with surrounding inflammatory response.

SURGICAL PROCEDURE: Excision of a 0.5 cm basal cell carcinoma, right side of nose, with reconstruction by 3 × 2.5 centimeter bilobed flap.

SURGEON: Bella Donald, MD

ANESTHESIA: Standby sedation with 5 cc of 1% Xylocaine with 1:100,000 epinephrine.

DESCRIPTION OF PROCEDURE: The patient's face was prepped with Betadine scrub and solution, and draped in a routine sterile fashion. The lesion and the surrounding tissue for the flap were both anesthetized with a total of 5 cc of 1% Xylocaine with 1:100,000 epinephrine. The lesion was excised circumferentially with a 5-mm margin. It was submitted for frozen section with a tag on the inferior aspect. The lesion was clear on all margins. Bleeding was electrocoagulated. We developed a 3 × 2.5 cm bilobed flap based on the left side, rotating it in place, and insetting it with 5-0 Prolene. Antibiotic ointment and Surgicel were applied followed by a 4 × 4. The patient tolerated the procedure well and left the area in good condition.

Pathology report later indicated: Carcinoma, basal cell.

CPT	Modifiers			ICD-9-CMs				
14060	52			173.3				

CASE 14

The procedures in Cases 14 and 15 are provided on the same day, to the same patient, by the same physician.

PREOPERATIVE DIAGNOSIS: Hematochezia.

POSTOPERATIVE DIAGNOSIS: Numerous diverticula in the descending sigmoid colon, burgundy and slight fresh blood present, but no active bleeding.

PROCEDURE PERFORMED: Flexible sigmoidoscopy.

SURGEON: Mohammad Kang, MD

INDICATION: 62-year-old white male, who was admitted with five episodes of dark red blood per rectum and then some melanotic stool. His hemoglobin was 14 on admission, dropped to 10.5 by yesterday evening and now is 10.0. He had a colonoscopy at the hospital. The report was reviewed, and there were numerous diverticula. He had previous radiation for prostate carcinoma. There was no mention of radiation proctitis.

PREOPERATIVE MEDICATIONS: Fentanyl 100 mcg IV with Versed 3 mg IV.

FINDINGS: The Pentax video colonoscope was inserted without difficulty to the mid descending colon. Inspection in the descending sigmoid revealed numerous diverticula and many that had wide openings. There was blood clot and burgundy throughout, but no active bleeding. The rectum was normal. Only a small amount of the rectal surface was visualized, and it was questionable whether there was any radiation proctitis. The patient tolerated the procedure well.

IMPRESSION: Burgundy and some fresh blood throughout the colon, numerous diverticula in the descending sigmoid colon, questionable radiation proctitis.

PLAN: The patient's bleeding is likely from diverticular disease, and it is certainly not due to radiation proctitis. Because of the melena, we are going to do an upper endoscopy. We would recommend a technetium RBC scan if he continues bleeding requiring further transfusion.

CPT	Modifiers			ICD-9-CMs				
45330				562.10				

CASE 15

PREOPERATIVE DIAGNOSIS: Question of melena.

POSTOPERATIVE DIAGNOSIS: Gastritis with erosions, duodenitis—mild, biopsy for *H. pylori*.

PROCEDURE PERFORMED: Esophagogastroduodenoscopy.

SURGEON: Mohammad Kang, MD

INDICATION: 62-year-old white male, who was admitted with five episodes of dark red blood per rectum and then some melanotic stool. His hemoglobin was 14 on admission, dropped to 10.5 by yesterday evening and now is 10.0. He had a colonoscopy at the hospital. The report was reviewed, and there were numerous diverticula. He has had previous radiation for prostate carcinoma. There was no mention of radiation proctitis.

PREOPERATIVE MEDICATION: Fentanyl 100 mcg IV, Versed 3 mg IV

FINDINGS: The Pentax video pediatric endoscope was passed without difficulty into the oropharynx. The gastroesophageal junction was seen at 42 cm. Inspection of the esophagus revealed no erythema, ulceration, exudate, friability, stricture, varices, or other mucosal abnormalities. The stomach proper was entered. The endoscope was advanced to the second duodenum. Inspection of the second duodenum and first duodenum revealed no abnormalities. The duodenal bulb revealed some mild erythema. The antrum revealed several small erosions, not bleeding. Biopsies were obtained for *H. pylori*. There was no active ulceration. No bleeding. Retroflexion revealed no lesions along the cardia or fundus. Inspection of the body revealed no abnormalities. The patient tolerated the procedure well.

IMPRESSION: Gastritis with erosions, duodenitis—mild, biopsy for *H. pylori*.

PLAN: The patient will be on Protonix and will be observed carefully and given a technetium RBC scan if he has continued lower GI bleeding.

CPT		Modifiers			ICD-9-CMs				
43239		58			535.40	535.60			

CASE 16

PREOPERATIVE DIAGNOSES:
1. Fat atrophy of the latissimus dorsi flap of right breast.
2. Asymmetry of the breasts.
3. Scar tissue, right side of back incision.

POSTOPERATIVE DIAGNOSIS: Same.

SURGICAL FINDINGS:
1. There was a clean and relatively avascular pectoralis submuscular pocket on the right side.
2. There was what appeared to be scar tissue mass with fat necrosis, also a cutaneous scar, of the more lateral aspect of the donor site from the previous latissimus dorsi flap.

SURGICAL PROCEDURES:
1. Insertion of submuscular breast implant, right breast. 150 cc implant was used.
2. Excision of scar tissue, donor area on latissimus dorsi flap, right side of back.

SURGEON: Mary Hallowell, MD

ANESTHESIA: Approximately 5 cc of 1% Xylocaine, 1:100,000 epinephrine.

DESCRIPTION OF PROCEDURE: The patient's chest and right side of the back were prepped with Betadine scrub and solution and draped in a routine sterile fashion. I injected a total of about 5 cc of 1% Xylocaine, 1:100,000 epinephrine in both the incision site of the medial aspect of the right breast and the back incision. The scar was excised from the lower aspect of the right breast, and a right pectoralis submuscular pocket was created using the balloon dissector to aid in dissection. Hemostasis was satisfactory, and following insertion of the balloon dissector, which we inflated to about 300 cc, I inserted a 230 cc Pfizer. This obviously was too large compared to the left side. In accordance with the patient's wishes, we put a 150 cc implant in, which made the right breast appear to be somewhat larger than the left, although they appeared the same with the patient in the recumbent position. The patient had expressly told us that she wished to have the right breast to be somewhat larger than the left breast and we tried to comply with the patient's wishes by insertion of the 150 cc implant. I felt that 100 cc would perhaps be too small, but the 150 cc did make the right breast larger than the left, although this may equilibrate more with the patient in the standing position. After insertion of the implant, I closed the wound with fascial sutures of 3-0 Monocryl and used interrupted twists of 5-0 Prolene. I excised the scar on the back in continuity with some scar tissue underneath and then excised a separate nodule of apparent scar tissue and fat necrosis, closing 6.8-cm wound with subcuticular 3-0 Monocryl in interrupted twists using some horizontal mattress twists of 4-0 Prolene. Xeroform and a 4 × 4 were applied to the back, and Kerlix fluffs and a support bra were used to dress the right breast reconstruction. Estimated blood loss was negligible. No drains were inserted. The patient tolerated the procedure well and left the operating room in good condition.

CPT   **Modifiers**   **ICD-9-CMs**

CASE 17

Code only Dr. Foxtrot's services.

PREOPERATIVE DIAGNOSES:
1. Bunion with hallux abductovalgus, right foot.
2. Severe diaphysitis with fat pad atrophy, right foot.

POSTOPERATIVE DIAGNOSES: Same.

PROCEDURES:
1. Bunionectomy with distal first metatarsal osteotomy with internal fixation, right foot.
2. Metatarsal head resection, 2 through 5, right foot.

SURGEON: Douglas Foxtrot, MD

ANESTHESIA: General.

HEMOSTASIS: Ankle tourniquet at 250 millimeters of mercury.

ESTIMATED BLOOD LOSS: Less than 20 cc.

MATERIALS: 4-0 Vicryl, 5-0 Prolene, 2.0 millimeter cortical stainless screws times two.

INJECTABLES: 18 cc of a 1:1 mix of 1% lidocaine plain, 0.5% Marcaine plain in postoperative anesthesia.

INDICATION FOR PROCEDURE: Patient had presented to my office upon consult from Dr. Bowler for complaint of right foot pain. In discussing and evaluating the patient, we discussed the possibility of conservative treatment versus surgical intervention. She would like to forego all conservative treatment at this point and proceed with surgical intervention to her right foot. I explained to her all the risks, benefits, and complications of the procedure with all questions answered to her satisfaction. No guarantees were given. She understands. She was consented for bunionectomy with distal first metatarsal osteotomy, internal fixation of the right foot with metatarsal head resections, 2 through 5, of the right foot secondary to severe long-term diaphysitis. This is going to be done in conjunction with Dr. Mathews' procedure where he is defatting a flap to her right heel. Her NPO status was confirmed. The surgical consent was signed and in the chart.

SURGERY IN DETAIL: Under mild IV sedation, the patient was brought back to the operating room and placed under general anesthesia and intubated. She was placed in the prone position. Dr. Mathews proceeded with defatting of a flap to the right heel. Following his procedure, which he did not use a tourniquet, she was replaced on the operating table in the supine position. A well-padded tourniquet was placed about her right ankle. Local anesthesia was infiltrated in the forefoot region, obtaining postoperative anesthesia with a total of 18 cc of a 1:1 mix of 1% lidocaine plain and 0.5 % Marcaine plain. The right foot was then rescrubbed, prepped and draped in the usual aseptic manner. The right foot was exsanguinated. The ankle tourniquet was elevated to 250 millimeters of mercury. Attention was directed to the dorsum of the right foot where a 2-centimeter linear longitudinal incision was made over the second metatarsophalangeal joint. Dissection was carried down through the subcutaneous tissues. All bleeders were cauterized and ligated. All vital neurovascular structures were identified and retracted. Capsulotomy of the second metatarsophalangeal joint was performed. A periosteal elevator was used to free the capsule and periosteum from the head and neck of the second metatarsal. An oscillating saw was used to resect the head of the second metatarsal just proximal to the articular cartilage, angled in a dorsal distal to planter proximal attitude. The metatarsal head was removed from the operative field through sharp dissection. The wound was irrigated with copious amounts of normal sterile saline. The periosteal and capsular structures were reapproximated with 4-0 Vicryl. The skin was reapproximated with 5-0 Prolene. The identical procedure was performed to the 3rd, 4th, and 5th metatarsophalangeal joints with the same type linear 2 centimeter incision with resection of the metatarsal heads, 3, 4, and 5. All wounds were irrigated in a similar fashion and closed in a similar fashion as that of the 2nd metatarsophalangeal joint. The tourniquet was then released after sterile 4 × 4s and a mildly compressive ACE bandage was placed over all the wounds to aid in re-nourishment of that flap per the request of Dr Matthews. The tourniquet was deflated and left deflated for 10 minutes. The foot was re-exsanguinated with elevation for 3 minutes, and the ankle tourniquet was then re-elevated to 250 millimeters of mercury. Attention was then directed to the bunion deformity of the right foot where a 6-centimeter linear longitudinal incision was made just medial to the extensor hallucis longus tendon. Dissection was carried down through the subcutaneous tissues. All bleeders were cauterized and ligated. All vital neurovascular structures were identified and retracted. Dissection was carried into the first interspace where the deep transverse intermetatarsal ligament was identified and transected. A lateral capsulotomy of the first metatarsophalangeal joint was performed. The fibular sesamoid was freed of all the soft tissue ligamentous structures proximally, distally and laterally. The conjoined tendon of the adductor hallucis muscle inserts at the base of the proximal phalanx was transected, and flexibility was then noted. Inverted L-capsulotomy of the first metatarsophalangeal joint was made dorsally and medially. The head of the first metatarsal was freed of all of its soft tissue and periosteal structures. Hypertrophic dorsal medial eminence of the first metatarsal head was resected and removed from the operative field. Chevron-style osteotomy was made from medial to lateral in the first metatarsal with the apex at the central most portion of the metatarsal head. Osteotomy exited dorsal-proximal and plantar-proximal, and a dorsal proximal osteotomy was made more proximal to aid in fixation. Capsular fragment was then moved laterally to the correct anatomical position. Utilizing proper AO technique in lag fashion, 2.0 millimeter cortical stainless steel screws × 2 were driven across the osteotomy utilizing proper AO technique in a lag fashion with excellent compression noted. The medial cortical bone shelf was resected and removed from the operative field. All rough edges were smoothed, utilizing back-brushing technique with the oscillating saw. Intraoperative fluoroscopy revealed that anatomical alignment of the first ray had been restored with good position of the screw fixation noted on multiple views. The wound was irrigated with copious amounts of normal sterile saline. Medial capsulorraphy was performed, resecting all redundant medial capsular tissue. The periosteal and capsular structures were reapproximated with 4-0 Vicryl. The skin was reapproximated with 5-0 Prolene. All surgical sites were dressed with Adaptic, sterile 4 × 4s, Kerlix roll, and an ACE bandage. The ankle tourniquet was deflated and prompt hyperemic response was noted to all digits of the right foot. The anatomical alignment of all digits were splinted in place with the soft dressing. The patient tolerated the procedure and anesthesia well with vital signs stable throughout. She was sent to the recovery room with vascular status intact to the right foot. Following a period of postoperative monitoring, she will be admitted under Dr's care for postoperative follow-up for the defatting of the flap to the aspect of her right heel.

I will see her postoperatively in the hospital and will follow-up with her when she is discharged in my office.

CPT	Modifiers			ICD-9-CMs				

CASE 18

PREOPERATIVE DIAGNOSIS: Urinary retention.

POSTOPERATIVE DIAGNOSIS: Recurrent prostatic hyperplasia.

PROCEDURE PERFORMED: Cystoscopy and transurethral resection of the prostate.

SURGEON: Edith Hopkins, MD

ANESTHESIA: Spinal.

CLINICAL NOTE: This is a 75-year-old gentleman who underwent right hip arthroplasty. Prior to need for hip procedure this gentleman had undergone a right transurethral resection of the prostate for urinary retention and has again developed urinary retention. He has had several trials of voiding with both alpha blockade and bethanechol. Cystoscopy revealed recurrent prostatic hyperplasia. There is a large piece of tissue acting as a ball valve.

PROCEDURE: The patient was given a spinal anesthetic, prepped and draped in the lithotomy position. 28-French resectoscope was passed under direct vision. Again, the prostate shows irregular ingrowth and obstruction. The bladder shows mild to moderate trabeculation. The prostate was thoroughly resected on the left and chips evacuated from the bladder and hemostasis achieved. A 22-French three-way catheter was inserted into the bladder and placed at continuous bladder irrigation. The patient tolerated the procedure well and was transferred to the recovery room in good condition.

CPT	Modifiers			ICD-9-CMs				

CASE 19

PREOPERATIVE DIAGNOSIS: Dysfunctional uterine bleeding.

POSTOPERATIVE DIAGNOSIS: Same.

PROCEDURE PERFORMED: Hysteroscopy with fractional dilation and curettage and lysis of intrauterine adhesions.

SURGEON: Timothy Canterwell, MD

ANESTHESIA: Laryngeal general mask anesthesia.

ESTIMATED BLOOD LOSS: Less than 10 cc.

COMPLICATIONS: None.

PROCEDURE: The patient was prepped and draped in the lithotomy position under general laryngeal mask anesthesia. The bladder was straight cathed. A weighted speculum was placed in the vagina. The anterior lip of the cervix was grasped with a single tooth tenaculum. Kevorkian curet was then used to obtain endocervical curettages. The uterus was then sounded to a depth of 6 cm. The cervical os was then serially dilated to allow passage of the hysteroscope. The hysteroscope was then passed and uterine contents were examined, documented, and photographed. No evidence of polyps or fibroids. There were some adhesions seen. These were broken down easily. The sharp curet was then used to thoroughly sample the endometrial cavity with return of a moderate amount of tissue. The tenaculum was removed from the cervix and the tenaculum site was over-sewn with 3-0 chromic figure-of-eight sutures. The instruments were removed from the vagina. All sponges and needles were accounted for upon completion of the procedure. The patient left the Operating Room in apparent good condition having tolerated the procedure well.

CPT	Modifiers			ICD-9-CMs				

CASE 20

PREOPERATIVE DIAGNOSIS: Phimosis.

POSTOPERATIVE DIAGNOSIS: Same.

PROCEDURE PERFORMED: Lysis of prepuce adhesions, meatotomy, and cystoscopy.

CLINICAL NOTE: This 4-year-old has voiding dysfunction and his urine sprays and goes up rather than down. He had had prior circumcision. There is a minimal amount of redundant foreskin.

SURGEON: Lucama Hitachi

ANESTHESIA: General mask.

PROCEDURE: The patient was given a general mask anesthetic, prepped and draped in the supine position. There were some adhesions between the glans and the prepuce. These were broken down easily. Meatus was quite stenotic and I believe this is a result of a congenital atresia of the ureter. Meatotomy was performed at the 6 o'clock position. A clamp was placed, skin divided and then reapproximating sutures using 5-0 chromic were then placed. The patient was then cystoscoped using a 9.2 rigid instrument. There was no evidence of urethral stricture posterior to the urethral valves. Bladder mucosa and ureteric orifices were all normal. Cystoscope was withdrawn. Bacitracin ointment was applied. The patient tolerated the procedure well and was transferred to the recovery room in good condition.

CPT	Modifiers			ICD-9-CMs					

A-mode: one-dimensional ultrasonic display reflecting the time it takes a sound wave to reach a structure and reflect back; maps the structure's outline

ablation: removal by cutting

abortion: termination of pregnancy

abscess: localized collection of pus that will result in the disintegration of tissue over time

abuse: misuse of substance

acquired: not genetic

actinotherapy: treatment of acne using ultraviolet rays

acute: of sudden onset and short duration

addiction: dependence on a drug

admission: attention to an acute illness or injury resulting in admission to a hospital

adrenal: glands, located at the top of the kidneys, that produce steroid hormones

AHA: American Hospital Association

AHIMA: American Health Information Management Association

allogenic: a graft that is from the same species, but genetically different

allograft: tissue graft between individuals who are not of the same genotype

allotransplantation: transplantation between individuals who are not of the same genotype

amniocentesis: percutaneous aspiration of amniotic fluid

anastomosis: surgical connection of two tubular structures, such as two pieces of the intestine

aneurysm: is an abnormal weakening of a vessel wall with outpouching beyond the normal confines of the vessel

angiography: taking of x-ray films of vessels after injection of contrast material

angioplasty: surgical or percutaneous procedure in a vessel to dilate the vessel opening; used in the treatment of atherosclerotic disease

angioscopy: studying the capillaries of the eyes

anomaloscope: instrument used to test color vision

anomaly: abnormality

anoscopy: procedure that uses a scope to examine the anus

antepartum: before childbirth

anterior (ventral): in front of

anterior segment: those parts of the eye in the front of and including the lens, orbit, extraocular muscles, and eyelid

anteroposterior: from front to back

antrum: sinus

aortography: radiographic recording of the aorta

apexcardiography: noninvasive graphic recording of the movement of the chest wall from the cardiac pulsations from the region of the apex of the heart, usually of the left ventricle

APC (Ambulatory Payment Classification): a patient classification that provides a payment system for outpatients

aphakia: absence of the lens of the eye

apicectomy: excision of a portion of the temporal bone

Appendix A: located near the back of the CPT manual; lists all modifiers with complete explanations for use

Appendix B: located near the back of the CPT manual; contains a complete list of additions to, deletions from, and revisions of the previous edition

Appendix C: located near the back of the CPT manual; presents clinical examples of Evaluation and Management (E/M)

Appendix D: located near the back of the CPT manual; contains a list of the CPT add-on codes

Appendix E: located near the back of the CPT manual; contains a list of modifier -51 exempt codes

Appendix F: located near the back of the CPT manual; contains information about modifier -63, Procedures Performed on Infants less than 4 kg

Appendix G: located near the back of the CPT manual; contains information about moderate (conscious) sedation

Appendix H: located near the back of the CPT manual; contains information about performance measures of Category II codes

Appendix I: located near the back of the CPT manual; contains information about Category II modifiers

Appendix J: located near the back of the CPT manual; contains information on sensory, motor, and mixed nerves and the corresponding conduction study code

Appendix K: located near the back of the CPT manual; contains the codes that are pending FDA (Food and Drug Administration) approval

Appendix L: located near the back of the CPT manual; contains the vascular families

Appendix M: located near the back of the CPT manual; contains a crosswalk of deleted CPT codes

arteriovenous fistula: direct communication (passage) between an artery and vein

artery: vessel that generally carries oxygenated blood from the heart to body tissues (pulmonary artery carries un-oxygenated blood)

arthrodesis: surgical immobilization of a joint

arthrography: radiographic recording of a joint

arthroplasty: reshaping or reconstruction of a joint

aspiration: use of a needle and a syringe to withdraw fluid

assignment: Medicare's payment for the service, which participating physicians agree to accept as payment in full

astigmatism: condition in which the refractive surfaces of the eye are unequal

asymptomatic: not showing any of the typical symptoms of a disease or condition

atrium: chamber in the upper part of the heart

attending physician: the physician with the primary responsibility for care of the patient

audi-: prefix meaning hearing

audiometry: hearing testing

aur-: prefix meaning ear

aural atresia: congenital absence of the external auditory canal

autogenous, autologous: from oneself

axillary nodes: lymph nodes located in the armpit

B-scan: two-dimensional display of tissues and organs

barium enema: radiographic contrast medium–enhanced examination of the colon

benign: not progressive

benign hypertension: hypertensive condition with a continuous, mild blood pressure elevation

bifocal: two focuses in eyeglasses, one usually for close work and the other for improvement of distance vision

bilateral: occurring on two sides

bilobectomy: surgical removal of two lobes of a lung

biofeedback: process of giving a person self-information

biometry: application of a statistical measure to a biologic fact

biopsy: removal of a small piece of living tissue for diagnostic purposes

blephar(o)-: prefix meaning eyelid

block: frozen piece of a sample

blood patch: a procedure in which a cerebrospinal fluid leak is closed by means of an injection of the patient's blood into the area used during spinal anesthesia

brachytherapy: therapy using radioactive sources that are placed inside the body

bronchography: radiographic recording of the lungs

bronchoplasty: surgical repair of the bronchi

bronchoscopy: inspection of the bronchial tree using a bronchoscope

bulbocavernosus: muscle that constricts the vagina in a female and the urethra in a male

bulbourethral gland: rounded mass of the urethra

bypass: to go around

calculus: concretion of mineral salts, also called a stone

calycoplasty: surgical reconstruction of a recess of the renal pelvis

calyx: recess of the renal pelvis

cannulation: insertion of a tube into a duct or cavity

carcinoma in situ: a cancerous tumor in its original place that has not invaded neighboring tissues

cardiopulmonary: refers to the heart and lungs

cardiopulmonary bypass: blood bypasses the heart through a heart-lung machine during open-heart surgery

cardioversion: electric shock to the heart to restore normal rhythm

cardioverter-defibrillator: surgically placed device that directs an electric current shock to the heart to restore rhythm

cataract: opaque covering on or in the lens

Category I: CPT codes approved by the FDA and representing widely used services and procedures

Category II: Supplemental codes that can be used for performance measurements

Category III: Temporary CPT codes

catheter: tube placed into the body to put fluid in or take fluid out

caudal: away from the head, or the lower part of the body; same as inferior

cauterization: destruction of tissue by the use of cautery

cavernosa–corpus spongiosum shunt: creation of a connection between a cavity of the penis and the urethra

cavernosa–glans penis fistulization: creation of a connection between a cavity of the penis and the glans penis, which overlaps the penis cavity

cavernos–saphenous vein shunt: creation of a connection between the cavity of the penis and a vein

cavernosography: radiographic recording of a cavity, e.g., the pulmonary cavity or the main part of the penis

cavernosometry: measurement of the pressure in a cavity, e.g., the penis

-centesis: suffix meaning puncture of a cavity

central nervous system (CNS): brain and spinal cord

cervical: pertaining to the neck or to the cervix of the uterus

cervix uteri: rounded, cone-shaped neck of the uterus

cesarean: surgical opening through abdominal wall for delivery

CF (conversion factor): national dollar amount that is applied to all services paid on the Medicare Fee Schedule basis

cholangiography: radiographic recording of the bile ducts

cholangiopancreatography (ERCP): radiographic recording of the biliary system and pancreas

chole-: prefix meaning bile

cholecystectomy: surgical removal of the gallbladder

cholecystoenterostomy: creation of a connection between the gallbladder and intestine

cholecystography: radiographic recording of the gallbladder

chordee: condition resulting in the penis' being bent downward

chorionic villus sampling (CVS): biopsy of the outermost part of the placenta

chronic: of long duration

Cloquet's node: also called a gland; it is the highest of the deep groin lymph nodes

closed treatment: fracture site that is not surgically opened and visualized

CMS: Centers for Medicare and Medicaid Services, formerly HCFA, Health Care Financing Administration

colonoscopy: fiberscopic examination of the entire colon that may include part of the terminal ileum

colostomy: artificial opening between the colon and the abdominal wall

combination code: single ICD-9-CM code used to identify etiology and manifestation of a disease

communicable disease: disease that can be transmitted from one person to another or one species to another

comparative conditions: patient conditions that are documented as "either/or" in the medical record

component: part

computed axial tomography (CAT or CT): procedure by which selected planes of tissue are pinpointed through computer enhancement, and images may be reconstructed by analysis of variance in absorption of the tissue

concurrent care: the provision of similar services (e.g., hospital visits) to the same patient by more than one physician on the same day. Each physician provides services for a separate condition, not reasonably expected to be managed by the attending physician. When concurrent care is provided, the diagnosis must reflect the medical necessity of different specialties

congenital: existing from birth

conjunctiva: the lining of the eyelids and the covering of the sclerae

conscious sedation: a decreased level of consciousness in which the patient is not completely asleep

consultation: includes those services rendered by a physician whose opinion or advice is requested by another physician or agency concerning the evaluation and/or treatment of a patient; a consultant is not an attending physician

contralateral: the opposite side

contributory factors: counseling, coordination of care, nature of the presenting problem, and time of an E/M service

cordectomy: surgical removal of the vocal cord(s)

cordocentesis: procedure to obtain a fetal blood sample; also called a percutaneous umbilical blood sampling

corneosclera: cornea and sclera of the eye

corpora cavernosa: the two cavities of the penis

corpus uteri: uterus

counseling: a discussion with a patient and/or family concerning one or more of the following areas: diagnostic results, impressions, and/or recommended diagnostic studies; prognosis; risks and benefits of treatment; instructions for treatment; importance of compliance with treatment; risk factor reduction; and patient and family education

CPT (Current Procedural Terminology): a coding system developed by the American Medical Association (AMA) to convert widely accepted, uniform descriptions of medical, surgical, and diagnostic services rendered by health care providers into five-digit codes

cranium: that part of the skeleton that encloses the brain

critical care: the care of critically ill patients in medical emergencies that requires the constant attendance of the physician (e.g., cardiac arrest, shock, bleeding, respiratory failure); critical care is usually, but not always, given in a critical care area, such as the coronary care unit (CCU) or the intensive care unit (ICU)

CRNA: certified registered nurse anesthetist

Crohn's disease: regional enteritis

cryosurgery: destruction of lesions using extreme cold

curettage: scraping of a cavity using a spoon-shaped instrument

cycl/o-: prefix meaning ciliary body or eye muscle

cyst: closed sac containing matter or fluid

cystic hygroma: congenital deformity or benign tumor of the lymphatic system

cystocele: herniation of the bladder into the vagina

cystography: radiographic recording of the urinary bladder

cystolithectomy: removal of a calculus (stone) from the urinary bladder

cystolithotomy: cystolithectomy

cystometrogram (CMG): measurement of the pressures and capacity of the urinary bladder

cystoplasty: surgical reconstruction of the bladder

cystorrhaphy: suture of the bladder

cystoscopy: use of a scope to view the bladder

cystostomy: surgical creation of an opening into the bladder

cystotomy: incision into the bladder

cystourethroplasty: surgical reconstruction of the bladder and urethra

cystourethroscopy: use of a scope to view the bladder and urethra

cytopathology: study of the diseases of cells

dacry/o-: prefix meaning tear or tear duct

dacryocyst/o-: prefix meaning pertaining to the lacrimal sac

dacryocystography: radiographic recording of the lacrimal sac or tear duct sac

debridement: cleansing of or removal of dead tissue from a wound

delivery: childbirth

Demerol: a narcotic analgesic

dermatoplasty: surgical repair of the skin

dermis: second layer of skin, holding blood vessels, nerve endings, sweat glands, and hair follicles

destruction: killing of tissue by means of electrocautery, laser, chemicals, or other means

DHHS: Department of Health and Human Services

diagnostic: that done to identify the cause, origin, or extent of a condition

diaphragm: muscular wall that separates the thoracic and abdominal cavities

diaphragmatic hernia: hernia of the diaphragm

dilation: expansion (of the cervix)

diskography: radiographic recording of an intervertebral joint

dislocation: placement in a location other than the original location

distal: farther from the point of attachment or origin

distinct procedure: one service or procedure that has no relationship to another service or procedure

Doppler: ultrasonic measure of blood movement

dosimetry: scientific calculation of radiation emitted from various radioactive sources

drainage: free flow or withdrawal of fluids from a wound or cavity

DRGs (Diagnosis Related Groups): a disease classification system that relates the type of inpatients a hospital treats (case mix) to the costs incurred by the hospital (now MS-DRGs)

dual-chamber pacemaker: electrodes of the pacemaker are placed in both the atria and the ventricle of the heart

duodenography: radiographic recording of the duodenum, or first part of the small intestine

E Codes: alphanumeric designations preceded by the letter "E," used to classify external causes

ear, parts of the external: auricle, pinna, external acoustic, meatus, and tympanic membrane

ear, parts of the inner: vestibule, semicircular canals, and cochlea

ear, parts of the middle: malleus, incus, and stapes

ECG: *see* electrocardiogram

echocardiography: radiographic recording of the heart or heart walls or surrounding tissues

echoencephalography: ultrasound of the brain

echography: ultrasound procedure in which sound waves are bounced off an internal organ and the resulting image is recorded

-ectomy: suffix meaning removal of part or all of an organ of the body

ectopic: pregnancy outside the uterus (i.e., in the fallopian tube)

EEG: *see* electroencephalogram

electrocardiogram (ECG): written record of the electrical activity of the heart

electrocochleography: stimulation of the cochlea to measure electrical activity

electrode: lead attached to a generator that carries the electric current from the generator to the atria or ventricles

electrodesiccation: destruction of a lesion by the use of electric current radiated through a needle

electroencephalogram (EEG): written record of the electrical activity of the brain

electromyogram (EMG): written record of the electrical activity of the skeletal muscles

electromyography (EMG): recording of the electrical impulses of muscles

electro-oculogram (EOG): written record of the electrical activity of the eye

electrophysiology: the study of the electrical system of the heart, including the study of arrhythmias

embolectomy: removal of blockage (embolism) from vessels

embolism: blockage of a blood vessel by a blood clot or other matter that has moved from another area of the body through the circulatory system

emergency care services: services that are provided by the physician in the emergency department for unplanned patient encounters; no distinction is made between new and established patients who are seen in the emergency department

encephalography: radiographic recording of the subarachnoid space and ventricles of the brain

endarterectomy: incision into an artery to remove the inner lining so as to eliminate disease or blockage

endomyocardial: pertaining to the inner and middle layers of the heart

endopyelotomy: procedure involving the bladder and ureters, including the insertion of a stent

endoscopy: inspection of body organs or cavities using a lighted scope that may be inserted through an existing opening or through a small incision

endotracheal tube: can be inserted through the nose or mouth and passed into the trachea for ventilation

enterocystoplasty: surgical reconstruction of the small intestine after the removal of a cyst and usually including a bowel anastomosis

enucleation: removal of an organ or organs from a body cavity

epicardial: over the heart

epidermis: outer layer of skin

epididymectomy: surgical removal of the epididymis

epididymis: tube located at the top of the testes that stores sperm

epididymography: radiographic recording of the epididymis

epididymovasostomy: creation of a new connection between the vas deferens and epididymis

epidural anesthesia: injection of an anesthesia agent into the spaces between the vertebrae. Also known as peridural anesthesia, epidural, epidural block, and intraspinal anesthesia

epiglottidectomy: excision of the covering of the larynx

ESRD: end-stage renal disease

established patient: a patient who has received face-to-face professional services from the physician or another physician of the same specialty in the same group within the past 3 years

etiology: study of causes of diseases

eventration: protrusion of the bowel through the viscera of the abdomen

evisceration: pulling the viscera outside of the body through an incision

excision: it is full-thickness removal of a lesion that may include simple closure

excisional: removal of an entire lesion for biopsy

Exclusive Provider Organization (EPO): similar to a Health Maintenance Organization except that the providers of the services are not prepaid, but rather are paid on a fee-for-service basis

exenteration: removal of an organ all in one piece

exostosis: bony growth

exstrophy: condition in which an organ is turned inside out

false aneurysm: sac of clotted blood that has completely destroyed the vessel and is being contained by the tissue that surrounds the vessel

fasciectomy: excision of fascia

FDA (Food and Drug Administration): responsible for the safety of food and drugs in America; is an agency within the U.S. Public Health Service, which is part of the Department of Health and Human Services

Federal Register: official publication of all "Presidential Documents," "Rules and Regulations," "Proposed Rules," and "Notices"; government-instituted national changes are published in the *Federal Register*

fenestration: creation of a new opening in the inner wall of the middle ear

fimbrioplasty: surgical repair of the fringe of the uterine tube

first-listed diagnosis: outpatient diagnosis

Fiscal Intermediary (FI): handles administration of Medicare claims but will be phased out by 2011 into MACs

fistula: abnormal opening from one area to another area or to the outside of the body

fluoroscopy: procedure for viewing the interior of the body using x-rays and projecting the image onto a television screen

fracture: break in a bone

fulguration: use of electric current to destroy tissue

fundoplasty: repair of the bottom of an organ or muscle

gastro-: prefix meaning stomach

gastrointestinal: pertaining to the stomach and intestine

gastroplasty: operation on the stomach for repair or reconfiguration

gastrostomy: artificial opening between the stomach and the abdominal wall

general anesthesia: a state of unconsciousness produced by the administration of a drug; it can be administered by inhalation or intramuscularly, rectally, or intravenously

gloss(o)-: prefix meaning tongue

gonioscopy: use of a scope to gain a view of the iridocorneal angle, or the anatomical angle formed between the eye's cornea and iris

Group Practice Model: an organization of physicians who contract with a Health Maintenance Organization to provide services to the enrollees of the HMO

grouper: computer used to input the principal diagnosis and other critical information about a patient and then provide the correct MS-DRG code

Guidelines: provide specific instructions about coding for each section of the CPT manual; the Guidelines contain definitions of terms, applicable modifiers, explanation of notes, subsection information, unlisted services, special reports information, and clinical examples

HCFA: Health Care Financing Administration, now known as Centers for Medicare and Medicaid Services (CMS)

Health Maintenance Organization (HMO): a health care delivery system in which an enrollee is assigned a primary care physician who manages all the health care needs of the enrollee

hemodialysis: cleansing of the blood outside of the body

hepat(o)-: prefix meaning liver

hepatography: radiographic recording of the liver

hernia: organ or tissue protruding through the wall or cavity that usually contains it

histology: study of the minute structures, composition, and function of tissues

Hodgkin's disease: malignant lymphoma

hydrocele: sac of fluid

hypertension, uncontrolled: untreated hypertension or hypertension that is not responding to the therapeutic regimen

hypertensive heart disease: secondary effects on the heart of prolonged, sustained systemic hypertension; the heart has to work against greatly increased resistance, causing increased blood pressure

hypogastric: lowest middle abdominal area

hyposensitization: decreased sensitivity

hypospadias: congenital deformity of the urethra in which the urethral opening is on the underside of the penis rather than at the end

hypotension: abnormally low blood pressure; sometimes induced during surgical procedures

hypothermia: low body temperature; sometimes induced during surgical procedures

hysterectomy: surgical removal of the uterus

hysterorrhaphy: suturing of the uterus

hysterosalpingography: radiographic recording of the uterine cavity and fallopian tubes

hysteroscopy: visualization of the canal of the uterine cervix and cavity of the uterus using a scope placed through the vagina

hysterotomy: incision into the uterus

ileostomy: artificial opening between the ileum and the abdominal wall

imbrication: overlapping

immunotherapy: therapy to increase immunity

incarcerated: regarding hernias, a constricted, irreducible hernia that may cause obstruction of an intestine

incision: surgically cutting into

incision and drainage: to cut and withdraw fluid

incisional: *see* incision

Individual Practice Association (IPA): an organization of physicians who provide services

for a set fee; Health Maintenance Organizations often contract with the IPA for services to their enrollees

infectious disease carrier: person who has a communicable disease but is symptom free despite having the disease

infectious disease contact: encounter with a person who has a disease that can be communicated or transmitted

inferior: away from the head or the lower part of the body; also known as caudal

inguinofemoral: referring to the groin and thigh

injection: introduction of fluid into a tissue, vessel, or cavity

inpatient: one who has been formally admitted to a health care facility

in situ: malignancy that is within the original site of development and has not invaded neighboring tissue

internal/external fixation: application of pins, wires, screws, and so on to immobilize a body part; they can be placed externally or internally

intracardiac: inside the heart

intramural: within the organ wall

intramuscular: into a muscle

intraoperative: period of time during which a surgical procedure is being performed

intravenous: into a vein

intravenous pyelography (IVP): radiographic recording of the urinary system

introitus: opening or entrance to the vagina

intubation: insertion of a tube

invasive: entering the body, breaking the skin

iontophoresis: introduction of ions into the body

ischemia: deficient blood supply due to obstruction of the circulatory system

isthmus: connection of two regions or structures

isthmus, thyroid: tissue connection between right and left thyroid lobes

isthmusectomy: surgical removal of the isthmus

italicized code: an ICD-9-CM code that can never be sequenced as the principal or primary diagnosis

jejunostomy: artificial opening between the jejunum and the abdominal wall

joint movement:

    abduction: movement of a limb away from the midline of the body

adduction: movement of a limb toward the midline of the body

circumduction: circular movement of a limb

extension: movement by which two parts are drawn away from each other

flexion: movement by which two parts are drawn toward each other

hyperextension: excessive extension of a limb

pronation: applied to the hand, the act of turning the palm down

supination: applied to the hand, the act of turning the palm up

jugular nodes: lymph nodes located next to the large vein in the neck

kerat/o-: prefix meaning cornea

keratoplasty: surgical repair of the cornea

key components: the history, examination, and medical decision-making complexity of an E/M service

Kock pouch: surgical creation of a urinary bladder from a segment of the ileum

kyphosis: humpback, the abnormal curvature of the spine

labyrinth: inner connecting cavities, such as the internal ear

laminectomy: surgical excision of the lamina

laparoscopy: exploration of the abdomen and pelvic cavities using a scope placed through a small incision in the abdominal wall

laryngeal web: congenital abnormality of connective tissue between the vocal cords

laryngectomy: surgical removal of the larynx

laryngo-: prefix meaning larynx

laryngography: radiographic recording of the larynx

laryngoplasty: surgical repair of the larynx

laryngoscope: an endoscope used to view the inside of the larynx

laryngoscopy: viewing of the larynx using a fiberoptic scope

laryngotomy: incision into the larynx

late effect: residual effect (that a condition produced) after the acute phase of an illness or injury has terminated

lateral: away from the midline of the body (to the side)

lavage: washing out of an organ

lesion: abnormal or altered tissue, e.g., wound, cyst, abscess, or boil

ligament: a band of fibrous tissue that connects cartilage or bone and supports a joint

ligation: binding or tying off, as in constricting the bloodflow of a vessel or binding fallopian tubes for sterilization

litholapaxy: lithotripsy

lithotomy: incision into an organ or a duct for the purpose of removing a stone

lithotripsy: crushing of a gallbladder or urinary bladder stone followed by irrigation to wash the fragment out

lobectomy: surgical excision of a lobe of the lung

lymph node: station along the lymphatic system

lymphadenectomy: excision of a lymph node or nodes

lymphadenitis: inflammation of a lymph node

lymphangiography: radiographic recording of the lymphatic vessels and nodes

lymphangiotomy: incision into a lymphatic vessel

lysis: releasing

M-mode: one-dimensional display of movement of structures

MAAC (Maximum Actual Allowable Charge): limitation on the total amount that can be charged by physicians who are not participants in Medicare

MAC (Medicare Administrative Contractor): an entity that manages the process claims for CMS

magnetic resonance imaging (MRI): procedure that uses nonionizing radiation to view the body in a cross-sectional view

malignancy: used in reference to a cancerous tumor

malignant: used to describe a cancerous tumor that grows worse over time

malignant hypertension: accelerated, severe form of hypertension, manifested by headaches, blurred vision, dyspnea, and uremia; usually causes permanent organ damage

mammography: radiographic recording of the breasts

Managed Care Organization (MCO): a group that is responsible for the health care services offered to an enrolled group of persons

mandated service: a service required by an agency or organization to be performed for a patient; usually the agency or organization pays all or a portion of the patient's medical bills

manifestation: sign of a disease

manipulation or reduction: words used interchangeably to mean the attempted restoration of a fracture or joint dislocation to its normal anatomic position

marsupialization: surgical procedure that creates an exterior pouch from an internal abscess

mast-: prefix meaning breast

mastoid-: prefix meaning posterior temporal bone

MDC (Major Diagnostic Categories): the division of all principal diagnoses into 25 mutually exclusive principal diagnosis areas within the MS-DRG system

meatotomy: surgical enlargement of the opening of the urinary meatus

medial: toward the midline of the body

mediastinoscopy: use of an endoscope inserted through a small incision to view the mediastinum

mediastinotomy: cutting into the mediastinum

mediastinum: area between the lungs that contains the heart, aorta, trachea, lymph nodes, thymus gland, esophagus, and bronchial tubes

Medicare Administrative Contractor (MAC): handles the administration of Medicare claims and will be the only administrators by 2011

Medicare Risk HMO: a Medicare-funded alternative to the standard Medicare supplemental coverage

MEI (Medicare Economic Index): government-mandated index that ties increases in the Medicare prevailing charges to economic indicators

MeV: megaelectron volt

MFS (Medicare Fee Schedule): schedules that list the allowable charges for Medicare services

modality: treatment method

moderate (conscious) sedation: a decreased level of consciousness in which the patient is not completely asleep

modifiers: added to codes to supply more specific information about the services provided

monofocal: eyeglasses with one vision correction

morbidity: condition of being diseased or morbid

morphine: a narcotic analgesic

morphology: the science of the form and structure of organisms

mortality: death

MS-DRG (Medicare Severity Diagnosis Related Groups): a system of classifying patient groups by related diagnoses

MSLT: multiple sleep latency testing

multiple coding: also known as dual coding, use of more than one ICD-9-CM code to identify both etiology and manifestation of a disease, as contrasted with combination coding

muscle: fibrous structures that can contract and facilitate movement of the body. There are three types of muscles: smooth, skeletal, and cardiac

MVPS (Medical Volume Performance Standards): government's estimate of how much growth is appropriate for nationwide physician expenditures paid by the Part B Medicare program

myasthenia gravis: syndrome characterized by muscle weakness

myelography: radiographic recording of the subarachnoid space of the spine

myocardial infarction (MI): necrosis of the myocardium resulting from interrupted blood supply

myring-: prefix meaning eardrum

nasal button: a synthetic circular disk used to cover a hole in the nasal septum

nasopharyngoscopy: use of a scope to visualize the nose and pharynx

NCPAP: nasal continuous positive airway pressure

NEC: not elsewhere classifiable

neoplasm: new tumor growth that can be benign or malignant

nephrectomy, paraperitoneal: surgical removal of a kidney by a cut through the side along the twelfth rib

nephro-: prefix meaning kidney

nephrocutaneous fistula: a channel from the kidney to the skin

nephrolithotomy: removal of a kidney stone through an incision made into the kidney

nephrorrhaphy: suturing of the kidney

nephrostolithotomy: procedure to establish an artificial channel between the skin and the kidney

nephrostomy: creation of a channel into the renal pelvis of the kidney

nephrostomy, percutaneous: creation of a channel from the skin to the renal pelvis

nephrotomy: incision into the kidney

new patient: a patient who has not received any face-to-face professional services from the physician or another physician of the same specialty in the same group within the past 3 years

newborn care: the evaluation and determination of care management of a newly born infant

noninvasive: not entering the body, not breaking the skin

NOS: not otherwise specified

nuclear cardiology: diagnostic specialty that uses radiopharmaceuticals to aid in the diagnosis of cardiologic conditions

nystagmus: rapid involuntary eye movements

OBRA (Omnibus Budget Reconciliation Act of 1989): act that established new rules for Medicare reimbursement

ocul/o-: prefix meaning eye

ocular adnexa: orbit, extraocular muscles, and eyelid

office visit: a face-to-face encounter between a physician and a patient in the physician's private office to allow for primary management of a patient's health care status

Official Guidelines for Coding and Reporting: rules of coding diagnosis codes (ICD-9-CM) published by the Editorial Advisory Board of Coding Clinic

omentum: peritoneal connection between the stomach and other internal organs

oophor-: prefix meaning ovary

oophorectomy: surgical removal of the ovary(ies)

opacification: area that has become opaque (milky)

open treatment: fracture site that is surgically opened and visualized

ophthalmodynamometry: test of the blood pressure of the eye

ophthalmology: body of knowledge regarding the eyes

optokinetic: movement of the eyes to objects moving in the visual field

orchiectomy: castration

orchiopexy: fixation or suturing of an undescended testicle to secure it in the scrotum

orthoptic: corrective; in the correct place

osteotomy: cutting into bone

ostomy: artificial opening

oto-: prefix meaning ear

-otomy: suffix meaning incision into

outpatient: a patient who receives services in an ambulatory health care facility and is currently not an inpatient

overdose: excessive dose

oviduct: fallopian tube

pacemaker: electrical device that controls the beating of the heart by electrical impulses

paraesophageal hiatal hernia: hernia that is near the esophagus

parathyroid: produces a hormone to mobilize calcium from the bones to the blood

paring: removal of thin layers of skin by peeling or scraping

Part A: Medicare's Hospital Insurance; covers hospital/facility care

Part B: Medicare's Supplemental Medical Insurance; covers physician services and durable medical equipment that are not paid for under Part A

Part C: Medicare Advantage is a set of health care options from which beneficiaries choose health care providers

Part D: Medicare's prescription drug program

participating provider program: Medicare providers who have agreed in advance to accept assignment on all Medicare claims; now termed QIO

patient-controlled analgesia (PCA): a system that allows the patient to self-administer an analgesic drug, such as morphine, to control pain. A hand-held device is attached to a pump holding the drug and the patient can depress a button to administer a dose of the drug. In this way, the patient can control the amount of the drug, frequency of administration, and manage postoperative pain. The system is used with patients with chronic pain.

pelviolithotomy: pyeloplasty

penoscrotal: referring to the penis and scrotum

percutaneous: through the skin

percutaneous skeletal fixation: considered neither open nor closed; the fracture is not visualized, but fixation is placed across the fracture site under x-ray imaging

pericardiocentesis: procedure in which a surgeon withdraws fluid from the pericardial space by means of a needle inserted percutaneously into the space

pericarditis: inflammation of the sac surrounding the first few centimeters of great vessels and the heart

pericardium: membranous sac enclosing the heart and the ends of the great vessels

perineal approach: surgical approach in the area between the thighs

perinephric cyst: cyst in the tissue around the kidney

perineum: area between the vulva and anus; also known as the pelvic floor

peripheral nerves: 12 pairs of cranial nerves, 31 pairs of spinal nerves, and autonomic nervous system; connects peripheral receptors to the brain and spinal cord

perirenal: around the kidney

peritoneal: within the lining of the abdominal cavity

peritoneoscopy: visualization of the abdominal cavity using one scope placed through a small incision in the abdominal wall and another scope placed in the vagina

perivesical: around the bladder

perivisceral: around an organ

pharyngolaryngectomy: surgical removal of the pharynx and larynx

phlebotomy: cutting into a vein

phonocardiogram: recording of heart sounds

photochemotherapy: treatment by means of drugs that react to ultraviolet radiation or sunlight

physical status modifiers: modifying units in the Anesthesia section of the CPT manual that describe a patient's condition at the time anesthesia is administered

physics: scientific study of energy

-plasty: suffix meaning technique involving molding or surgically forming

plethysmography: determining the changes in volume of an organ part or body

pleura: covering of the lungs and thoracic cavity that is moistened with serous fluid to reduce friction during respiratory movements of the lungs

pleurectomy: surgical excision of the pleura

pneumo-: prefix meaning lung or air

pneumoncentesis: surgical puncturing of a lung to withdraw fluid

pneumonolysis: surgical separation of the lung from the chest wall to allow the lung to collapse

pneumonostomy: surgical procedure in which the chest cavity is exposed and the lung is incised

pneumonotomy: incision of the lung

pneumoplethysmography: determining the changes in the volume of the lung

polyp: tumor on a pedicle that bleeds easily and may become malignant

posterior (dorsal): in back of

posterior segment: those parts of the eye behind the lens

posteroanterior: from back to front

postoperative: period of time after a surgical procedure

postpartum: after childbirth

Preferred Provider Organization (PPO): a group of providers who form a network and who have agreed to provide services to enrollees at a discounted rate

preoperative: period of time prior to a surgical procedure

priapism: painful condition in which the penis is constantly erect

primary diagnosis: first-listed diagnosis, used in the outpatient setting to identify the reason for the encounter

primary site: site of origin or where the tumor originated

principal diagnosis: defined in the Uniform Hospital Discharge Data Set (UHDDS) as "that condition established after study to be chiefly responsible for occasioning the admission of the patient to the hospital for care"; the principal diagnosis is sequenced first

proctosigmoidoscopy: fiberscopic examination of the sigmoid colon and rectum

professional component: term used in describing physician's services in radiology or pathology

prognosis: probable outcome of an illness

prophylactic: substance or agent that offers some protection from disease

PROs (Peer Review Organizations): groups established to review hospital admission and care; now termed QIO

prostatotomy: incision into the prostate

PSRO (Professional Standards Review Organization): voluntary physicians' organization designed to monitor the necessity of hospital admissions, treatment costs, and medical records of hospitals

punch: use of a small hollow instrument to puncture a lesion

pyelo-: prefix meaning renal pelvis

pyelocutaneous: from the renal pelvis to the skin

pyelography: radiographic recording of the kidneys, renal pelvis, ureters, and bladder

pyelolithotomy: surgical removal of a kidney stone from the renal pelvis

pyeloplasty: surgical reconstruction of the renal pelvis

pyeloscopy: viewing of the renal pelvis using a fluoroscope after injection of contrast material

pyelostolithotomy: removal of a kidney stone and establishment of a stoma

pyelostomy: surgical creation of a temporary diversion around the ureter

pyelotomy: incision into the renal pelvis

pyloroplasty: inision and repair of the pyloric channel

QIO (Quality Improvement Organization): consists of a national network of 53 entities that work with consumers, physicians, hospitals, and caregivers to refine care delivery systems

qualifying circumstances: five-digit CPT codes that describe situations or conditions that affect the administration of anesthesia

qualitative: measuring the presence or absence of

quantitative: measuring the presence or absence of and the amount of

rad: radiation absorption dose, the energy deposited in patients' tissues

radiation oncology: branch of medicine concerned with the application of radiation to a tumor site for treatment (destruction) of cancerous tumors

radiograph: film on which an image is produced through exposure to x-radiation

radiologist: physician who specializes in the use of radioactive materials in the diagnosis and treatment of diseases and illnesses

radiology: branch of medicine concerned with the use of radioactive substances for diagnosis and therapy

RBRVS (Resource-Based Relative Value Scale): scale designed to decrease Medicare expenditures, redistribute physician payment, and ensure quality health care at reasonable rates

real time: two-dimensional display of both the structures and the motion of tissues and organs, with the length of time also recorded as part of the study

reanastomosis: reconnection of a previous connection between two places, organs, or spaces

rectocele: herniation of the rectal wall through the posterior wall of the vagina

reducible: able to be corrected or put back into a normal position

referral: the transfer of the total or a specific portion of care of a patient from one physician to another that does not constitute a consultation

regional anesthesia: the interruption of the sensory nerve conductivity in a region of the body, which is produced by field block (forming a wall of anesthesia around the site by means of local injections) or by nerve block (injection of the area close to the major sensory nerve supplying a field); also known as block anesthesia, block, or conduction anesthesia

Relative Value Guide: comparison of anesthesia services; published by the American Society of Anesthesiologists (ASA)

renal pelvis: funnel-shaped sac in the kidney where urine is received

repair: to remedy, replace, or heal (in the Integumentary subsection pertains to suturing a wound)

residual: that which is left behind or remains

resource intensity: refers to the relative volume and type of diagnostic, therapeutic, and bed services used in the management of a particular illness

retrograde: moving backward or against the usual direction of flow

retroperitoneal: behind the sac holding the abdominal organs and viscera (peritoneum)

rhino-: prefix meaning nose

rhinoplasty: surgical repair of the nose

-rrhaphy: suffix meaning suturing

rubric: heading used as a direction or explanation as to what follows and the way in which the information is to be used. In ICD-9-CM coding, the rubric is the three-digit code that precedes the four- and five-digit codes

rule of nines: rule used to estimate burned body surface area in burn patients

RUQ: right upper quadrant

RVU (Relative Value Unit): unit value that has been assigned for each service

salpingectomy: surgical removal of the uterine tube

salping(o)-: prefix meaning tube

salpingostomy: creation of a fistula into the uterine tube

scan: mapping of emissions of radioactive substances after they have been introduced into the body; the density can determine normal or abnormal conditions

sclera: the white, outer covering of the eye

scoliosis: abnormal lateral curvature of the spine

secondary site: place to which a malignant tumor has spread; metastatic site

section: slice of a frozen block

sections: the six major areas into which all CPT codes and descriptions are categorized

See: a cross-reference term within the index of the CPT manual used to direct the coder to another term or other terms. The *See* indicates that the correct code will be found elsewhere

segmentectomy: surgical removal of a portion of a lung

seminal vesicle: gland that secretes fluid into the vas deferens

separate procedures: minor procedures that when done by themselves are coded as a procedure, but when performed at the same time as a major procedure are considered incidental and not coded separately

septoplasty: surgical repair of the nasal septum

sequela: a condition that follows an illness

severity of illness: refers to the levels of loss of function and mortality that may be experienced by patients with a particular disease

shaving: horizontal or transverse removal of dermal or epidermal lesions, without full-thickness excision

shunt: divert or make an artificial passage

sialography: radiographic recording of the salivary duct and branches

sigmoidoscopy: fiberscopic examination of the rectum and sigmoid colon that may include a portion of the descending colon

single chamber pacemaker: the electrode of the pacemaker is placed only in the atrium or only in the ventricle, but not placed in both

sinography: radiographic recording of the sinus or sinus tract

sinuses: cavities within the facial bones (maxillary, frontal, sphenoid, and ethmoid)

sinusotomy: surgical incision into a sinus

skin graft: transplantation of skin tissue

skull: entire skeletal framework of the head

slanted brackets: indicate that the ICD-9-CM code can never be sequenced as the principal or primary diagnosis

soft tissue: tissues (fascia, connective tissue, muscle, and so forth)

somatic nerve: sensory or motor nerve that supplies a dermatome

special reports: detailed reports that include adequate definitions or descriptions of the nature, extent, and need for the procedure and the time, effort, and equipment necessary to provide the services

specimen: sample of tissue or fluid

spermatocele: cyst filled with spermatozoa

spirometry: measurement of breathing capacity

splenectomy: excision of the spleen

splenography: radiographic recording of the spleen

splenoportography: radiographic procedure to allow visualization of the splenic and portal veins of the spleen

Staff Model: a Health Maintenance Organization that directly employs the physicians who provide services to enrollees

stem cell: immature blood cell

stent: mold that is surgically placed to reinforce or hold open an area

stereotaxis: method of identifying a specific area or point in the brain

strabismus: extraocular muscle deviation resulting in unequal visual axes

subcutaneous: tissue below the dermis, primarily fat cells that insulate the body

subsections: the further division of sections into smaller units, usually by body systems

superior: toward the head or the upper part of the body; also known as cephalic

supine: lying on the back

surgical package: bundling together of time, effort, and services for a specific procedure into one code instead of reporting each component separately

suture: to unite parts by stitching them together

Swan-Ganz catheter: central venous catheter

symbols: special guides that help the coder compare codes and descriptors with the previous edition. A bullet (•) is used to indicate a new procedure or service code added since the previous edition of the CPT manual. A solid triangle (▲) placed in front of a code number indicates that the code has been changed or modified since the last edition. A plus (+) is used to indicate an add-on code. A circle with a line through it (⊘) is used to identify a modifier -51 exempt code. Right and left triangles (►◄) indicate the beginning and end of the text changes. A bullseye (⊙) indicates procedures that include moderate sedation. New in 2006 is a lightning bolt symbol (⚡) that identifies codes that are being tracked by the AMA to monitor FDA status for approval of a drug.

sympathetic nerve: part of the peripheral nervous system that controls automatic body function and sympathetic nerves activated under stress

symphysiotomy: cutting of the pubic cartilage to help in birthing

systemic: affecting the entire body

tarsorrhaphy: suturing together of the eyelids

technical component: term used in describing the services provided by the facility

TEFRA (Tax Equity and Fiscal Responsibility Act): act that contains language to reward costconscious health care providers

tenodesis: suturing the end of a tendon to a bone

tenorrhaphy: suturing together two parts of a tendon

term location methods: service/procedure, anatomic site/body organ, condition/disease, synonym, eponym, and abbreviation

thermogram: written record of temperature variation

thoracentesis: surgical puncture of the thoracic cavity, usually using a needle, to remove fluids

thoracic duct: collection and distribution point for lymph, and the largest lymph vessel located in the chest

thoracoplasty: surgical procedure that removes rib(s) to allow the collapse of a lung

thoracoscopy: use of a lighted endoscope to view the pleural spaces and thoracic cavity or perform surgical procedures

thoracostomy: surgical incision into the chest wall and insertion of a chest tube

thoracotomy: surgical incision into the chest wall

thrombosis: blood clot

thymectomy: surgical removal of the thymus

thymus: gland that produces hormones important to the immune response

thyroglossal duct: a duct in the embryo between the thyroid primordium and the posterior tongue

thyroglossal duct cyst: a cyst of the neck caused by persistence of portions of or by the lack of closure of the primitive thyroglossal duct

thyroid: part of the endocrine system that produces hormones that regulate metabolism

thyroidectomy: surgical removal of the thyroid

thyroiditis: a thyroid gland inflammation

tissue transfer: piece of skin for grafting that is still partially attached to the original blood supply and is used to cover an adjacent wound area

tocolysis: repression of uterine contractions

tomography: procedure that allows viewing of a single plane of the body by blurring out all but that particular level

tonography: recording of changes in intraocular pressure in response to sustained pressure on the eyeball

tonometry: measurement of pressure or tension

total pneumonectomy: surgical removal of an entire lobe of a lung

tracheostomy: creation of an opening into the trachea

tracheotomy: incision into the trachea

traction: application of force to a limb

transabdominal: across the abdomen

transcutaneous: entering by way of the skin

transesophageal echocardiogram (TEE): echocardiogram performed by placing a probe down the esophagus and sending out sound waves to obtain images of the heart and its movement

transfer order: official document that transfers the care of a patient from one physician to another; often required by third-party payers to legally transfer the care of a patient

transglottic tracheoplasty: surgical repair of the vocal apparatus and trachea

transhepatic: across the liver

transmastoid antrostomy: called a simple mastoidectomy, it creates an opening in the mastoid for drainage

transplantation: grafting of tissue from one source to another

transseptal: through the septum

transthoracic: across the thorax

transtracheal: across the trachea

transureteroureterostomy: surgical connection of one ureter to the other ureter

transurethral resection, prostate: procedure performed through the urethra by means of a cystoscopy to remove part or all of the prostate

transvenous: across a vein

transverse: horizontal

transvesical ureterolithotomy: removal of a ureter stone (calculus) through the bladder

trocar needle: a sharp-pointed instrument equipped with a cannula, used to puncture the wall of a body cavity and withdraw fluid

tumescence: state of being swollen

tumor: swelling or enlargement; a spontaneous growth of tissue that forms an abnormal mass

tunica vaginalis: covering of the testes

tympanic neurectomy: excision of the tympanic nerve

tympanometry: procedure for evaluating middle ear disorders

UHDDS: Uniform Hospital Discharge Data Set

ultrasound: technique using sound waves to determine the density of the outline of tissue

unbundling: assigning multiple CPT codes when one CPT code would fully describe the service or procedure

uncertain behavior: refers to the behavior of a neoplasm as being neither malignant nor benign but having characteristics of both kinds of activity

uncertain diagnosis: diagnosis documented at the time of discharge as "probable," "suspected," "likely," "questionable," "possible," or "rule out"

unilateral: occurring on one side

unlisted procedures: procedures that are considered unusual, experimental, or new and do not have a specific code number assigned; unlisted procedure codes are located at the end of the subsections or subheadings and may be used to identify any procedure that lacks a specific code

unspecified hypertension: hypertensive condition that has not been specified as either benign or malignant hypertension

unspecified nature: when the behavior or histology of a neoplasm is not known or is not specified

uptake: absorption of a radioactive substance by body tissues; recorded for diagnostic purposes in conditions such as thyroid disease

ureterectomy: surgical removal of a ureter, either totally or partially

ureterocolon: pertaining to the ureter and colon

ureterocutaneous fistula: the channel from the ureter to the exterior skin

ureteroenterostomy: creation of a connection between the intestine and the ureter

ureterolithotomy: removal of a stone from the ureter

ureterolysis: freeing of adhesions of the ureter

ureteroneocystostomy: surgical connection of the ureter to a new site on the bladder

ureteroplasty: surgical repair of the ureter

ureteropyelography: ureter and bladder radiography

ureteropyelonephrostomy: surgical connection of the ureter to a new site on the kidney

ureteropyelostomy: ureteropyelonephrostomy

ureterosigmoidostomy: surgical connection of the ureter into the sigmoid colon and out through a new opening in the skin

ureterotomy: incision into the ureter

ureterovisceral fistula: surgical formation of a connection between the ureter and the bladder

urethrocutaneous fistula: surgically created channel from the urethra to the skin surface

urethrocystography: radiography of the bladder and urethra

urethromeatoplasty: surgical repair of the urethra and meatus

urethroplasty: surgical repair of the urethra

urethrorrhaphy: suturing of the urethra

urethroscopy: use of a scope to view the urethra

urography: same as pyelography; radiographic recording of the kidneys, renal pelvis, ureters, and bladder

uveal: vascular tissue of the choroid, ciliary body, and iris

V codes: numeric designations in the ICD-9-CM preceded by the letter "V"; used to classify persons who are not currently sick when they encounter health services

vagina: canal from the external female genitalia to the uterus

vagotomy: surgical separation of the vagus nerve

Valium: a sedative

varicocele: swelling of a scrotal vein

vas deferens: tube that carries sperm from the epididymis to the urethra

vasogram: recording of the flow in the vas deferens

vasotomy: creation of an opening in the vas deferens

vasovasorrhaphy: suturing of the vas deferens

vasovasostomy: reversal of a vasectomy

VBAC: vaginal delivery after a previous cesarean delivery

vectorcardiogram (VCG): continuous recording of electrical direction and magnitude of the heart

vein: vessel that carries unoxygenated blood to the heart from body tissues; pulmonary veins carry oxygenated blood back to the heart

vena caval thrombectomy: removal of a blood clot from the blood vessel (inferior vena cava or superior vena cava)

venography: radiographic recording of the veins and tributaries

ventricle: chamber in the lower part of the heart

version: turning of the fetus from a presentation other than cephalic (head down) to cephalic for ease of birth

vesicostomy: surgical creation of a connection of the bladder mucosa to the skin

vesicovaginal fistula: creation of a tube between the vagina and the bladder

vesiculectomy: excision of the seminal vesicle

vesiculography: radiographic recording of the seminal vesicles

vesiculotomy: incision into the seminal vesicle

vitre/o-: prefix meaning pertaining to the vitreous body of the eye

vulva: external female genitalia including the labia majora, labia minora, clitoris, and vaginal opening

World Health Organization (WHO): group that deals with health care issues on a global basis

wound repair, complex: involves complicated wound closure, including revision, debridement, extensive undermining, and more than layered closure

wound repair, intermediate: requires closure of one or more subcutaneous tissues and superficial fascia, in addition to the skin closure

wound repair, simple: superficial wound repair, involving epidermis, dermis, and subcutaneous tissue, requiring only simple, one-layer suturing

xeroradiography: photoelectric process of radiographs

References are to pages. Current Procedural Terminology (CPT) codes begin on page 855; ICD-9-CM and ICD-10 codes begin on page 862; HCPCS codes begin on page 866.

CURRENT PROCEDURAL TERMINOLOGY (CPT) CODES

0000F:	7
00100-01999:	9, 106
00142:	98
0030T:	18
00400:	99
00566:	92
00740:	103
00810:	103
0090T:	136
01916-01936:	92
01922:	92
01925:	92
01951-01953:	92
01958-01969:	92
01990-01999:	92
01999:	102
10021:	290
10021-10022:	140
10021-69990:	9, 116, 132
10022:	215, 290
10040-10180:	141, 142
10080:	138
10081:	138
10160:	141
11000:	5, 142
11000-11044:	142, 156
11001:	5, 142
11004-11006:	142
11040-11044:	142, 424
11055-11057:	145
11100:	113, 146, 169, 204
11101:	113, 146, 169
11200:	146
11201:	146
11300-11313:	148
11400-11471:	148
11402:	111
11423:	111
11450-11471:	144
11600-11646:	149
11719:	150
11719-11765:	150
11720:	150

11730:	150
11732:	150
11740:	150
11750-11752:	150
11755:	150
11770-11772:	150
11900:	151
11900-11983:	151
11901:	151
11920-11922:	152
11950-11954:	152
11960-11971:	152
11975-11977:	152
11980:	152
12001:	156
12001-12021:	153
12004:	140
12014:	139
12020-78:	139
12031-12057:	156
12031-13160:	149
13100-13160:	156
13131-13153:	309
14000-14350:	157
14040-14300:	311
15002-15005:	159
15002-15431:	159
15050:	159
15100:	159
15101:	159
15110-15116:	159
15120:	159, 343, 348
15121:	159, 343, 348
15130-15136:	159
15150-15157:	160
15170-15176:	160
15260:	343
15261:	343
15300-15321:	160
15300-15366:	161
15400-15431:	161
15570-15738:	161, 164
15740-15750:	162
15740-15776:	162
15780-15783:	163
15780-15879:	163

15786:	163
15787:	163
15788-15793:	163
15819:	163
15820-15823:	163
15824-15829:	163
15830-15839:	163
15840-15845:	163
15850-15852:	163
15876-15879:	163
15920-15999:	163, 164
16000-16036:	165
16020-16030:	165
16035:	165
16036:	165
17000-17250:	148
17000-17286:	168
17260-17286:	149
17311-17315:	168, 169, 341
19000-19499:	170
19100:	136, 137, 140
19101:	140
19290:	113, 170
19291:	113
19303:	110, 116
19307:	137
19342:	152
19357:	152
20000:	181, 182
20000-69990:	121
20005:	182
20100-20103:	182
20150-20251:	184
20206:	184, 185
20520:	13
20520-20525:	185
20525:	13
20550:	185
20551:	185
20553:	185
20600-20610:	185
20650:	186
20665:	187
20670:	187
20680:	187
20690:	187

ICD-9-CM AND ICD-10 CODES

HCPCS CODES

INDEX

Index

Liver, 320
  abnormal scan, 566
  biopsy, 320
  transplant, 320–321
Local anesthesia, 90, 91f
Long-term care facility, 69
Lumbar puncture, 338, 339f
Lund-Browder chart/classification of
  burns, 166f, 572f
Lungs and pleura, 213
  excision, 215–216
  incision, 213–214
  pneumonolysis, 216
  pneumothorax injection, 216
  thoracoplasty, 216
Lymphadenectomies, 332
Lymphatic system. *See* Hemic and
  lymphatic systems
Lymph nodes, 332

M

Magnetic resonance angiography,
  367–368, 369f
Magnetic resonance imaging, 357,
  367–368, 369f. *See also*
  Radiology
  cardiac MRIs, 255
Magnifying loupes, 351
Male genital system
  diseases of, 552–553
  epididymis, 284–285
  format of subsection, 280
  ICD-9-CM manual, 552–553
  intersex surgery, 292–293
  penis. *See* Penis
  prostate. *See* Prostate
  scrotum, 285
  seminal vesicles, 286–287
  spermatic cord, 286
  testis, 283–284
  tunica vaginalis, 285
  vas deferens, 285–286
Malignancies. *See* Cancer
Mammography, 368
Managed Care Organizations (MCOs),
  637
Managed health care, 636–638
Manometric studies, 300
Mapping, 250
Mastectomies, 116, 170
Maternity care and delivery
  abortion services. *See* Abortion
    services
  antepartum services, 272, 273
    amniocentesis, 273
    cordocentesis, 273
    excision, 273–274
    introduction codes, 274–275
    repair services, 275
  complications of, 553–559
    ICD-9-CM Official Guidelines for
      Coding and Reporting,
      678–683
  congenital anomalies and
    conditions originating in the
    perinatal period, 562, 564,
    565, 686, 688
  estimated date of delivery, 272
  format of subsection, 272
  HIV-infected persons, 557, 680–681
  ICD-9-CM manual, 553–559
    Official Guidelines of Coding and
      Reporting, 678–683
  normal delivery, 557–558

Maternity care and delivery
  (*Continued*)
  outcome of delivery, 521
  postpartum care, 272
  postpartum complications, 682
  routine obstetric care, 272–273
  V codes, 521, 706–707
MCOs, 637
Meckel's diverticulum, 319
Mediastinum, 323–324
  biopsy, 215
Medical decision making, 42
  complexity levels, 43
  complications or death, risk of,
    44–46
  data to be reviewed, 44
  diagnoses, number of, 43
  Documentation Guidelines,
    776–779, 804–806
  elements of, 46f
  examples, 44–45, 47
Medical examination. *See* Examination
Medically Unlikely Units, 366
Medical necessity, certificates of
  oxygen necessity, 437f
  transcutaneous electrical nerve
    stimulation, 436f
Medical records
  documentation, 30
    general principles of, 771–772,
      782–783
    importance of, 771, 782
    1995 Guidelines, 81–84. *See also*
      E/M services
    payers, rights as to, 771, 782
    what is, 771, 782
  management options, 43
  patient history. *See* History
  risk of complications or death, 44–46
Medical team conferences, 75
Medicare Administrative Contractors
  (MACs), 607, 608f
Medicare Advantage, 610, 637–638
Medicare fraud and abuse
  form of fraud, 633
  "incident to" services, 634
  protecting yourself from, 635
  regulations, 634
  violators, 633
  what constitutes, 632–633
  who determines, 634
Medicare program, 606–607
  abuse. *See* Medicare fraud and abuse
  accepting assignment, 609
  add-on anesthesia codes, 97
  ambulatory payment classifications,
    630, 631f, 632f
  coinsurance payments, 607
  diagnosis-related groups. Inpatient
    diagnosis-related groups, *see
    below*
  DRGs. Inpatient diagnosis-related
    groups, *see below*
  Federal Register, 611–612, 613f
  fee schedule, 624
  fraud. *See* Medicare fraud and abuse
  hospital insurance, 609–610
  inpatient diagnosis-related groups
    adjustments, 615–616
    grouper and ICD-9-CM codes, 617
    major diagnostic categories, 616,
      617f, 618f, 619f, 620f, 621f
    relative weights, 615–616
    setting payment rates, 615

Medicare program (*Continued*)
  inpatient prospective payment
    system, 614–615
  Medicare Advantage, 610, 637–638
  outpatient Medicare reimbursement
    system, 629–630
    ambulatory payment
      classifications, 630, 631f,
      632f
  outpatient resource-based relative
    value scale, 623–624
    adjustments, 626–627
    beneficiary protection, 626
    conversion factor, 624–625
    5-year transitional phase-in, 625
    Geographic Practice Cost Index,
      624
    limiting charge, 626
    Medicare Volume Performance
      Standards, 625
    national fee schedule, 624
    relative value unit, 624
    site-of-service limitations, 627
    surgical modifier circumstances,
      627–629
    uniformity provision, 626–627
  Part A, 609–610
  Part B, 610
  Part C, 610
  Part D, 610
  prescription drugs, 610
  Quality Improvement Organizations
    agreements with, 607, 609
    purpose of, 621–622
  RBRVS. Outpatient resource-based
    relative value scale, *see above*
  skilled nursing facilities, 629
  skin closures, 156
  supplementary insurance, 610
  volume performance standards, 625
Medicine codes, 402
  allergen immunotherapy, 418
  allergy testing, 417
  anesthesia. *See* Anesthesia
  behavior assessment/intervention,
    420
  biofeedback, 410
  cardiovascular system. *See*
    Cardiovascular system
  chemotherapy. *See* Chemotherapy
  chiropractic manipulative
    treatment, 425
  CNS assessments/tests, 420
  dermatological procedures, special,
    423
  dialysis, 411–412
  gastroenterology, 413
  glucose monitoring, 418
  HCPCS. *See* Healthcare Common
    Procedure Coding System
  home health procedures/services,
    427
  hydration services, 407–408
  immune globulins, 404
  immunization agents, 404–406
    influenza immunizations, 406
    pneumococcal immunizations,
      406
  influenza immunizations, 406
  infusion services, 407, 408
    home infusion procedures
      services, 427
  injection services. *See* Injection
    services

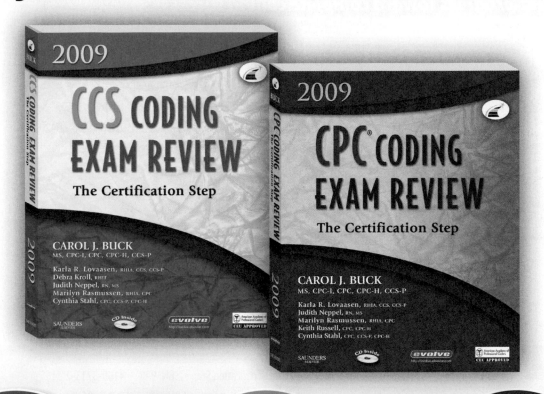
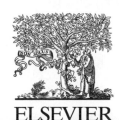

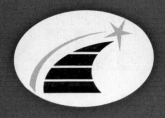

Trust Carol J. Buck and Elsevier for the
resources you need at *each step* of your coding career!

Track your progress toward complete coding success!

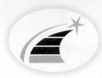

Step 1: Learn

☐ Step-by-Step Medical Coding 2009 Edition • ISBN: 978-1-4160-4566-3
☐ Workbook for Step-by-Step Medical Coding 2009 Edition • ISBN: 978-1-4160-4565-6
☐ Medical Coding Online for Step-by-Step Medical Coding 2009 • ISBN: 978-1-4160-6042-0
☐ Virtual Medical Office for Step-by-Step Medical Coding 2009 Edition

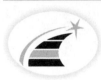

Step 2: Practice

☐ The Next Step: Advanced Medical Coding 2009 Edition• ISBN: 978-1-4160-5679-9
☐ Workbook for The Next Step: Advanced Medical Coding 2009 Edition • ISBN: 978-1-4160-5677-5
☐ Advanced Medical Coding Online for The Next Step:
   Advanced Medical Coding 2009 Edition • ISBN: 978-1-4160-6043-7

Step 3: Certify

☐ CPC®Coding Exam Review 2009: The Certification Step • ISBN: 978-1-4160-3713-2
☐ CCS Coding Exam Review 2009: The Certification Step • ISBN: 978-1-4160-3686-9
☐ The Extra Step: Facility-Based Coding Practice • ISBN: 978-1-4160-3450-6
☐ The Extra Step: Physician-Based Coding Practice 2009 Edition • ISBN: 978-1-4160-6162-5

Step 4: Specialize

☐ Evaluation and Management Step: An Auditing Tool 2009 Edition • ISBN: 978-1-4160-6724-5

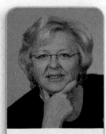

Author and
Educator
Carol J. Buck,
MS, CPC-I, CPC,
CPC-H, CCS-P

Coding References

☐ 2009 ICD-9-CM, Volumes 1 & 2, Professional Edition • ISBN: 978-1-4160-4448-2
☐ 2009 ICD-9-CM, Volumes 1, 2, & 3, Professional Edition • ISBN: 978-1-4160-4450-5
☐ 2009 ICD-9-CM, Volumes 1 & 2, Standard Edition • ISBN: 978-1-4160-4449-9
☐ 2009 ICD-9-CM, Volumes 1, 2, & 3, Standard Edition • ISBN: 978-1-4160-4447-5
☐ 2009 HCPCS Level II Professional Edition • ISBN: 978-1-4160-5203-6
☐ 2009 HCPCS Level II Standard Edition • ISBN: 978-1-4160-5204-3

Get the next resources on your list today!

• Order securely at **www.elsevierhealth.com**
• Call toll-free **1-800-545-2522**
• Visit your local bookstore

SL80281

ELSEVIER